Joint Structure and *Function*

A COMPREHENSIVE ANALYSIS

THIRD EDITION

Pamela K. Levangie, DSc, PT
Associate Professor
Physical Therapy Program
Sacred Heart University
Fairfield, Connecticut

Cynthia C. Norkin, EdD, PT
Former Director and Associate Professor
School of Physical Therapy
Ohio University
Athens, Ohio

F. A. Davis Company ■ Philadelphia

F. A. Davis Company
1915 Arch Street
Philadelphia, PA 19103

Printed in Canada

Last digit indicates print number: 10 9 8 7 6 5 4 3 2 1

Acquisitions Editor: Jean-François Vilain
Developmental Editor: Christa Fratantoro
Production Editor: Elena Coler
Designer: Bill Donnelly
Cover Designer: Louis J. Forgione

As new scientific information becomes available through basic and clinical research, recommended treatments and drug therapies undergo changes. The author(s) and publisher have done everything possible to make this book accurate, up to date, and in accord with accepted standards at the time of publication. The authors, editors, and publisher are not responsible for errors or omissions or for consequences from application of the book, and make no warranty, expressed or implied, in regard to the contents of the book. Any practice described in this book should be applied by the reader in accordance with professional standards of care used in regard to the unique circumstances that may apply in each situation. The reader is advised always to check product information (package inserts) for changes and new information regarding dose and contraindications before administering any drug. Caution is especially urged when using new or infrequently ordered drugs.

Library of Congress Cataloging in Publication Data

Levangie, Pamela K.
    Joint structure and function : a comprehensive analysis / Pamela K. Levangie,
Cynthia C. Norkin.—3rd. ed.
        p. ; cm.
    Norkin's name appears first on the earlier edition.
    Includes bibliographical references and index.
    ISBN 0–8036-0710-5 (alk. paper)
    1. Human mechanics. 2. Joints.
    [DNLM: 1. Joints—anatomy & histology. 2. Joints—physiology. WE 300 L655j 2001] I. Norkin,
Cynthia C. Joint structure & function.   II. Title.
QP303.N59   2001
612.7'5—dc21

                                                                00-060203

Dedication

We wish to dedicate the third edition of **Joint Structure and Function** to Dr. Linda Crane and to the fight against breast cancer. Dr. Crane was the originator of the Thorax and Chest Wall chapter of our text. Her friends and family and the physical therapy community lost her to breast cancer in March 1999. Breast cancer has cast a strong shadow over the authors and contributors to this text. As we think of those already diagnosed and those yet to be diagnosed with breast cancer, we hope that the fourth edition of **Joint Structure and Function** will be published in a world that has fulfilled the promises of today's research.

PREFACE TO THE THIRD EDITION

Twenty years ago, we set out to put together a text that would fill a perceived void in the relatively scant offerings available to those interested in studying and understanding human musculoskeletal function and dysfunction. Today a new generation of readers can choose from a wide variety of print and multimedia offerings with varying degrees of breadth and depth of topic. Our goal in this third edition, however, remains essentially unchanged. We offer a basic but comprehensive preparation in the principles needed to understand human kinesiology and pathokinesiology.

While the human body has not changed in the last 20 years, the technology we use to study it and the information we have gained about the body and its function have changed and grown markedly. We attempt again with this edition to strike the delicate balance between informing the reader of new research and hypotheses that are part of the burgeoning developments in health care, while maintaining the text's role as a tool of basic (albeit changing) professional education. By referencing our sources carefully, we hope to encourage readers to seek additional depth and alternative sources as they pursue their professional education and development. In addition to clarifying text, we reorganized selected chapters and added new summary tables, as well as many new figures. We hope, with this edition, to continue our tradition of offering an informative, readable and concise reference that will lay an appropriate foundation for our readers in their quest to understand human function.

Pamela K. Levangie

Cynthia C. Norkin

PREFACE TO THE SECOND EDITION

Our goals in writing the second edition have been threefold. One, we wished to ensure that this edition included the important aspects of the large volume of research published in recent years. New information and revised theories are more notable in the areas of tissue composition and response, muscle physiology, and in the specific reactions of regional structures to the application of normal and abnormal forces. Two, we tried to respond to the comments and suggestions of both students and instructors. Three, we attempted to maintain the fairly basic level of the text so that it remained an appropriate resource for those who wish to have a simple reference that gives a comprehensive overview of the principles needed to understand human function and dysfunction.

Our pursuit of the first two of our three goals, you will find, has caused the text to grow substantially. We have not only updated content but also have expanded explanations to improve clarity and supplemented the text with more than 250 new figures and summary tables. Responding to the clinical needs of our readers, we have added chapters on the temporomandibular joint and the chest wall. In meeting our third goal of maintaining the basic level of the text, we have had to make difficult decisions about limiting the inclusion of new information. Details that might be useful to experienced evaluators of human function have not been included unless, in our judgment, they enhanced a basic understanding of the content without overwhelming the reader. Occasionally we have chosen to introduce complex material at a superficial level with the intent of at least exposing the reader to advanced concepts. Readers who wish to pursue such topics in greater depth are encouraged to continue their reading using the reference lists at the ends of the chapters.

We would like to thank the readers who have been so responsive to our efforts to develop a readable and comprehensive text on human musculoskeletal function and would like to encourage you to continue your dialogue with us as we prepare for our third edition.

Cynthia C. Norkin

Pamela K. Levangie

PREFACE TO THE FIRST EDITION

The prototype of this text was developed 8 years ago in response to a perceived need for a single source that would provide entry-level knowledge in biomechanics, muscle physiology, joint structure, and coordinated muscular function for physical therapy students. Through the years the content was modified and broadened in response to feedback from students and practitioners, as well as reviews of recent literature. What evolved was a *transdisciplinary* text that not only encompasses basic theory required to understand normal and pathologic function, but also provides the foundation for understanding current trends in musculoskeletal evaluation and treatment.

The text is organized around general principles of structure and function that are then applied to individual joint complexes using a cephalo-caudal, proximal-distal approach. The concepts developed in the earlier chapters are integrated with and applied to total body function by examining the complex tasks of posture and gait. Educational features of the text include learning objectives and review questions for each chapter, models that take the reader through the process of identifying the relationship between normal and abnormal function, and liberal use of diagrams.

The authors would like the process of feedback and modification to continue as the reading audience widens, and we hope that subsequent editions can respond to the changing needs of those involved in human evaluation and treatment.

Cynthia C. Norkin

Pamela K. Levangie

ACKNOWLEDGMENTS

We must first recognize our continuing and new contributors, whose efforts were key elements in our endeavor. Professors Chleboun, Dalton, Perry, and Starr applied their considerable educational expertise to maintaining currency and comprehensiveness of the text while increasing readability. Mr. Tim Malone, our capable and responsive artist, continues to successfully interpret our thoughts into clear visual images that significantly enhance the principles we present. We also wish to express our gratitude to the continued support of our families who, as they've aged and grown, have become more direct contributors to our efforts. In particular, we wish to thank Taylor Field for her efforts on our behalf. We also acknowledge the important support we have received from F. A. Davis and its staff, with Jean-François Vilain earning our special gratitude. Finally, we must thank and acknowledge the thousands of faculty members and students who continue to shape this book and allow us to contribute to, and be part of, their professional education.

CONTRIBUTORS

Gary Chleboun, PhD, PT
Associate Professor
School of Physical Therapy
Ohio University
Athens, Ohio

Diane Dalton, MS, PT, OCS
Clinical Assistant Professor
Department of Physical Therapy
Sargent College of Allied Health
    Professionals
Boston University
Boston, Massachusetts

Jan F. Perry, EdD, PT
Professor and Chair
Department of Physical Therapy
School of Allied Health
Medical College of Georgia
Augusta, Georgia

Julie Ann Starr, MS, PT
Clinical Assistant Professor
Department of Physical Therapy
Sargent College of Allied Health
    Professionals
Boston University
Boston, Massachusetts

CONTENTS

CHAPTER 1

BASIC CONCEPTS IN BIOMECHANICS

. . . .

. . . .

OBJECTIVES

Following the study of this chapter, the reader should be able to:

Define

1. The terminology used in biomechanics.

Describe

1. Four types of motion.
2. The plane in which a given joint motion occurs, and the axis around which the motion occurs.
3. The location of the center of gravity of a rigid object; the location of the center of gravity of a segmented object; the location of the center of gravity of the human body.
4. The action line of a single muscle.
5. The name, point of application, direction, and magnitude of any interaction force, given its reaction force.
6. A linear force system, a concurrent force system, a parallel force system.
7. The relationship among torque, moment arm, and rotatory force component.
8. Two methods of determining torque for the same given set of forces.
9. How an anatomic pulley changes muscle action lines, moment arms, and torque of muscles.
10. In general terms, the point in the range of motion at which a muscle acting over that joint is biomechanically most efficient.
11. How external forces can be manipulated to maximize torque.
12. Friction, and its relationship to contacting surfaces and to the shear forces.

Determine

1. The identity (name) of diagrammed forces on an object.
2. The new center of gravity of an object when segments are rearranged, given the original centers of gravity.
3. The resultant vector in a linear force system, a concurrent force system, and a parallel force system.
4. If a given object is in linear and rotational equilibrium.
5. The magnitude and direction of acceleration of an object not in equilibrium.
6. Which forces are joint distraction forces and which are joint compression forces. What are the equilibrium forces for each?
7. The magnitude and direction of friction in a given problem.
8. The class of lever in a given problem.

Compare

1. Mechanical advantage in a second- and third-class lever.
2. Work done by muscles in a second- and third-class lever.
3. Stability of an object in two given situations in which location of the center of gravity and the base of support of the object vary.

Draw

1. The action line of a muscle.
2. The rotatory force component, the translatory force component, and the moment arm for a given force of a lever.

· ·

Introduction

The human body is a highly sophisticated machine composed of a large but finite number of components. These components can combine to produce an infinite variety of postures and movements. It is the intention of this text to investigate the nature of this machine, with the goal of understanding how joint structure and muscle function meet the concomitant but contradictory needs of the human body for both mobility and stability. A knowledge of the physical principles that govern the body and of the forces that affect the body is prerequisite to examination of the structure and function of individual components. This knowledge is gained through the study of mechanics. The study of mechanics in the human body is referred to as **biomechanics** and consists of the areas of **kinematics** and **kinetics.** Kinematics is the area of biomechanics that includes descriptions of motion without regard for the forces producing the motion. Kinetics is the area of biomechanics concerned with the forces producing motion or maintaining equilibrium.

The focus of this chapter will be on biomechanics that relate to rigid objects; that is, we will for the most part be treating the body as if it

were made up of rigid bony levers. In fact, however, neither the bones nor the structures that attach to them are rigid. Rather, the tissues that make up these structures respond internally to the forces applied to them in ways characteristic of their tissue composition. These internal responses to forces, or material properties, of the body are discussed in Chapter 2.

Kinematics: Description of Motion

The human skeleton is, quite literally, a system of components or levers. A lever can have any shape, and each long bone can be visualized as a rigid bar that can transmit, accept, and modify force and motion. Kinematic variables for a given movement may include (1) the type of motion that is occurring, (2) the location of the movement, (3) the direction of the motion, (4) the magnitude of the motion, and (5) the rate or duration of motion.

Types of Motion

There are four types of movement that can be attributed to any rigid object or four pathways through which a rigid object can travel. In the human body, one can describe the path taken by the body as a whole, or describe the path taken by one or more of its component levers.

Rotatory (angular) motion is movement of an object or segment around a fixed axis in a curved path. Each point on the object or segment moves through the same angle, at the same time, at a constant distance from the axis of rotation. Because all human movement must occur at joints, the goal of most muscles would appear to be to rotate a bony lever around a relatively fixed axis (Fig. 1–1). In actuality, few if any joints in the human body move around truly fixed axes. Nor is it usual for one lever to remain completely fixed while the other moves. Even so, for purposes of simplicity, joint motion is commonly described as if it were a pure rotation of one moving segment on another fixed segment. This oversimplification will suffice for some applications, but not for all.

Translatory (linear) motion is the movement of an object or segment in a straight line. Each point on the object moves through the same distance, at the same time, in parallel paths. Translation of a body segment without some concomitant rotation rarely occurs. Oversimplifying once again, we can illustrate translatory motion of a segment by the movement of the combined forearm/hand segment to grasp an object (Fig. 1–2). In this example, all points on the forearm/hand segment move through the same distance at the same time. It must be noted, however, that translation of the forearm/hand segment is actually produced by rotation of both the shoulder and the elbow joints. This is similar to the "translation" of the head through space when walking on level

ground. The head translates through space as one walks, but it does so through a series of joint motions taking place predominantly in the lower extremities.

Although we tend to think of human joint motion in terms of joint rotations, the shape of surfaces (and the forces that produce the motion) result in translatory motion between joint surfaces that, even when very small in magnitude, are important for understanding joint stress and joint stability. True translatory motion of a bony lever without concomitant joint rotation can occur to a limited extent when a bone is pulled directly away from its joint or pushed directly toward its joint. Another form of translation could occur if the articular surface of one bone moved parallel to the flat articular surface of a contiguous bone. This type of translatory motion of a bone is known as **gliding.** In reality, however, most joint surfaces are at least slightly curved, so most joint glides are not pure translatory motion.

Rotatory and translatory motions in human joints most commonly occur together. Although rotation may predominate at most joints, there is enough concomitant gliding for

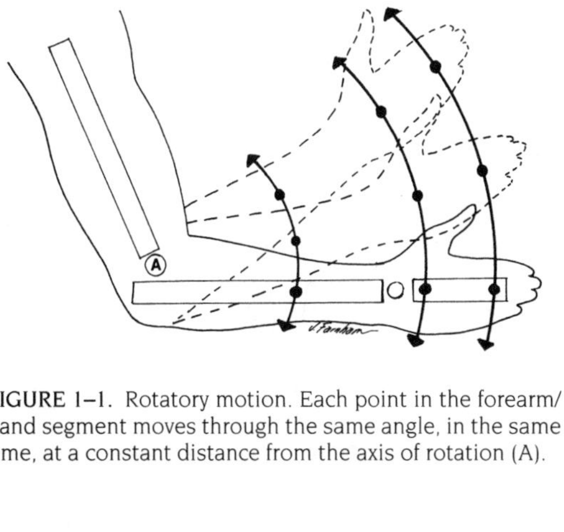

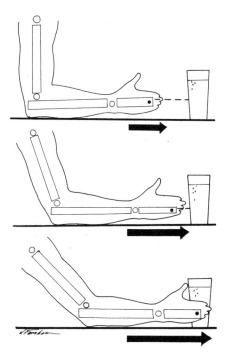

FIGURE 1–1. Rotatory motion. Each point in the forearm/hand segment moves through the same angle, in the same time, at a constant distance from the axis of rotation (A).

FIGURE 1–2. Translatory motion. Each point on the forearm/hand segment moves through the same distance, at the same time, in parallel paths.

the axis of rotation to move in space. When an object rotates about an axis and moves through space at the same time, the object describes a third pathway known as **curvilinear motion.** The classic example of curvilinear motion outside the body is that of a thrown ball, where the ball both moves through space and rotates on its own axis concomitantly. In this context, curvilinear motion is rotation of a rigid object through space. Curvilinear motion in the human body is the most common path that a rigid bony segment takes at a joint. However, the translatory component of the motion may be quite subtle and is frequently ignored when we discuss joint rotations. A more obvious example of combined rotation and translation is shown in Figure 1–3. Here, the forearm/hand segment holding the glass is rotating around the elbow joint axis while the elbow joint is being moved forward in space by shoulder flexion. Because the elbow joint axis is translating at the same time that the forearm/hand segment is rotating around it, the forearm/hand segment holding the glass describes a parabolic pathway.

Location of Motion

A kinematic description of motion must include the segments and joints being moved, as well as the place, or plane, of the movement.

Borrowing from the universal three-dimensional coordinate system used in mathematics, motion at a joint may be described as occurring in the **transverse (horizontal), frontal (coronal),** or **sagittal (anterior-posterior** or **A-P) planes.** Motion in any one of these planes means that a body segment is being rotated about its axis or translated in such a way that the segment is moving through a path that is parallel to one of the three cardinal planes. Human motion is not constrained to cardinal planes and, in fact, infrequently occurs or remains in specific planes. The system of planes and axes, however, provides a simple way of describing the motions that are available at a given joint. Because the plane of a movement could theoretically change if the position of the body changed (e.g., standing versus lying down), it is traditional to refer to motions as if they were occurring with the person standing in what is known as **anatomic position.** In anatomic position, a person stands, looking forward, with the palms of the hands facing forward.

The universal x-coordinate corresponds to the cardinal transverse plane. This plane divides the body into upper and lower halves (Fig. 1–4). Movements in the transverse plane occur parallel to the ground. For example, in rotation of the head, the nose moves parallel to

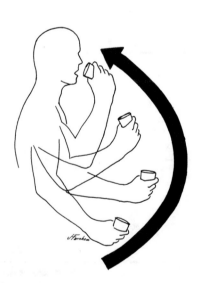

FIGURE 1–3. Curvilinear motion. The forearm/hand segment moves in a parabolic path as it rotates around the elbow joint. The elbow joint is moved through space by shoulder joint rotation.

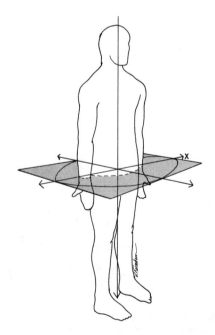

FIGURE 1–4. Transverse plane.

the ground. Rotatory motions in the transverse plane occur around a **vertical** or **longitudinal axis** of motion. The term longitudinal axis is used when the axis of motion passes through the length of a long bone. The axis of any cardinal plane movement is always found perpendicular to its corresponding plane.

The y-coordinate corresponds to the frontal (coronal) plane. The frontal plane divides the body into front and back halves (Fig. 1–5). Movements in the frontal plane occur as side-to-side movements such as bringing the head to each of the shoulders. Rotatory motion in the frontal plane occurs around an **anterior-posterior (A-P) axis.**

The z-coordinate corresponds to the sagittal plane and divides the body into right and left halves (Fig. 1–6). Movements in this plane include forward and backward motions such as nodding of the head. Rotatory motion in the sagittal plane occurs around a **coronal axis.**

Direction of Motion

Narrowing movement down to a single plane does not indicate the direction of movement in that plane. We need further descriptors. For rotatory motions, the direction of movement of a

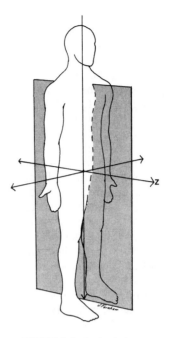

FIGURE 1–6. Sagittal plane.

lever around an axis can be described as occurring in a clockwise or counterclockwise direction. However, these terms are dependent on the perspective of the viewer (as viewed from the left side, bending the elbow is a clockwise movement; if the subject turns around and faces the opposite direction, the same movement is now seen by the viewer as a counterclockwise movement). Positive and negative signs are traditionally assigned to counterclockwise and clockwise movements, respectively. Anatomic terms describing human movement are independent of viewer perspective and, therefore, more useful to us. **Flexion** refers to rotation of one or both bony levers around a joint axis so that ventral surfaces are being approximated. Rotation in the same plane in the opposite direction (approximation of dorsal surfaces) is termed **extension.** Flexion and extension generally occur in the sagittal plane around a coronal axis, although exceptions exist (carpometacarpal flexion and extension of the thumb).

Abduction is rotation of one or both segments of a joint around an axis so that the distal segment moves away from the midline of the body. **Adduction** occurs in the same plane, but in the opposite direction (movement of the distal lever of the joint occurs toward the midline of the body). When the segment that is

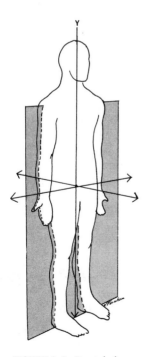

FIGURE 1–5. Frontal plane.

moving is part of the midline of the body (e.g., the trunk and the head), the movement is commonly termed **lateral flexion.** Abduction/adduction and lateral flexion generally occur in the frontal plane around an A-P axis, although, again, some exceptions exist (carpometacarpal abduction and adduction of the thumb).

Motion of a body segment in the transverse plane around a vertical or longitudinal axis is generally termed medial or lateral rotation. **Medial** (or internal) **rotation** refers to rotation toward the body's midline; **lateral** (or **external) rotation** refers to the opposite motion. When the segment is part of the midline, the movement in the transverse plane is simply called rotation to the right or rotation to the left. The exceptions to the general rules for naming motions must be learned on a joint-by-joint basis.

Descriptions of direction of translatory movements are conventionally given signs. Motions that are up or to the right are given positive values; motions down or to the left are given negative values. As will be described in further detail later, we can also refer to translatory movement of a segment toward its joint as **compression,** whereas translatory motion of a segment away from the joint can be termed **distraction.**

Magnitude of Motion

The magnitude or quantity of a rotatory motion (range of motion) can be given either in degrees or in radians. If a segment describes a complete circle, it has moved through 360° or 6.28 radians. A radian is the ratio of an arc to the radius of its circle (Fig. 1–7). One radian is equal to

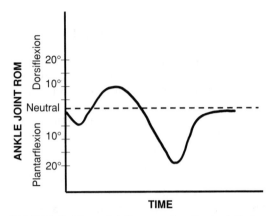

FIGURE I–8. When a joint's range of motion is plotted on the vertical (y) axis and time is plotted on the horizontal (x) axis, the resulting time-series plot portrays the change in joint position over time. The slope of the plotted line reflects the velocity of the joint change.

57.3°; 1° is equal to 0.01745 radians. The most widely used standardized method of clinical joint range measurement is goniometry, with units in degrees. Magnitude of motion may also be given as the number of degrees through which an object rotates per second (**angular speed** or **rate**). When angular speed (a magnitude of motion only) is given a designated direction, it becomes the vector quantity **velocity.**

A number of instruments are now available that will allow documentation of the change in joint angles and angular velocity over time. A computer-generated time-series plot such as that in Figure 1–8 graphically portrays not only the joint angle between two bony segments at each point in time but also the direction of motion. The steepness of the slope of the graphed line represents the angular velocity.

Translatory motions are quantified by the linear distance (displacement) through which the object or segment has moved. Units may vary but will be given in this text as pounds/inches/seconds, using the English system of measurement. Displacement per unit time with direction (velocity) or without direction (speed) may also be considered as a description of magnitude of motion.

Kinetics: Analysis of Forces

Definition of Forces

Kinematic descriptions of human movement permit us to visualize motion but do not give us an understanding of why the motion is oc-

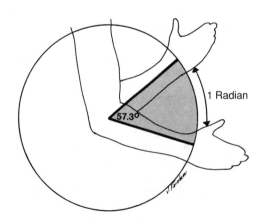

FIGURE I–7. An angle of 57.3° describes an arc of one radian.

curring. This requires a study of forces. Whether a body or body segment is in motion or at rest depends on the forces exerted on that body. A **force,** simplistically speaking, is a push or a pull exerted by one material object or substance on another. All forces can, in fact, be described as the push or pull of object A on object B. The concept of a force as a push or pull also can be used to describe the forces encountered in evaluating human motion.

External forces are pushes or pulls on the body that arise from sources outside the body. **Gravity** is an external force that under normal conditions constantly affects all objects. For that reason, the force of gravity should always be the first external force on the human body to be considered. Gravity is the pull of the earth on objects within its sphere of influence, or more specific to our purposes, it is the *pull of the earth on a body* (or its segments). Gravity is only one of an infinite number of external forces that can affect the human body. Other objects or substances that may exert a push or pull on the human body or its segments are (to name only a few) wind (push of air on the body), water (push of water on the body), other people (push of Mr. Jones's shoulder, pull of Mr. Jones's hand on Mr. Smith's hand), and other objects (the push of floor on the feet, the pull of a briefcase on the arm).

Internal forces are forces that act on the body but arise from sources within the human body. Examples are muscles (pull of the biceps brachii on the radius), ligaments (pull of a ligament on bone), and bones (the push of one bone on another bone). Internal forces are essential to human function because external forces are difficult to depend on to create purposeful movement of a body segment. More importantly, internal forces serve to counteract those external forces that jeopardize the integrity of human joint structure. Some forces, such as friction and atmospheric pressure, also can act both external to and within the body.

Force Vectors

All forces, despite the source or the object acted on, are **vector** quantities and can be defined by:

- A point of application on the object being acted on
- An action line and direction indicating a pull toward the source or a push away from the source

- A magnitude, that is, the quantity of force being exerted

A vector is traditionally represented by an arrow, so a force is represented by an arrow that (1) has a base on the object being acted on (point of application), (2) has a shaft and arrowhead in the direction of the force being exerted (action line, direction), and (3) has a length drawn to represent the amount of force being exerted (magnitude). In the English system, the unit of measure for the magnitude of a force is the **pound.** The corollary unit of measure in the metric system is the **newton.** Figure 1–9 shows a hand pushing on a book. The force called hand-on-book is represented by vector HB. The point of application is on the book; the action line and direction indicate the direction of the push; and the length is drawn to represent the magnitude of the push. The length of a vector is usually drawn proportional to the magnitude of the force using a given scale. For example, if the scale is specified as 0.25 = 10 lb of force, an arrow of 0.375 inches would represent 15 lb of force. The length of a vector, however, need not be drawn to scale. The action line of any vector can be considered infinitely long; that is, any vector can be extended infinitely in either direction if this is useful in determining relationships of the vector to other vectors or objects. The length of a vector should not be arbitrarily drawn, however, if a scale has been specified.

An example of a vector that depicts the force of a muscle acting on a bony lever in the body is shown in Figure 1–10. The force can be named muscle-on-bone (MB). The point of application of the force is *on the bone*, which is the object being acted on; the action line and di-

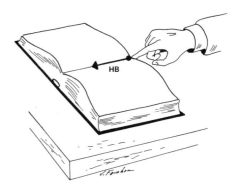

FIGURE 1–9. Vector HB represents the push of the hand on the book with a magnitude of 15 lb (0.25 in = lb).

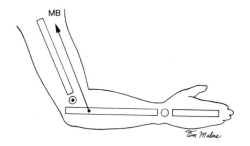

FIGURE 1–10. Vector MB represents the pull of a muscle on a bone, with a magnitude of 20 lb.

rection are in the direction of pull of the muscle; and the magnitude of the muscle force (using a scale of 0.5 inches = 10 lb) is 20 lb.

Naming Forces

When the naming convention of *object-on-object* is used to identify forces, the first part of the force name will always identify the object that is the *source* of the force; the second part of the force name will always identify the object that is *being acted on*. This means that the point of application will always be found on the second object named (the object to which the force is applied will always be the "last name" of the force). The action line and direction of a force will be toward the source in the case of a pull, or away from the source in the case of a push. The source of the push or pull will always be the "first name" of the force.

Figure 1–11 shows a man holding a 30-lb box in both hands. The two vectors in the figure can be identified and named using the naming convention just described. The point of applica-

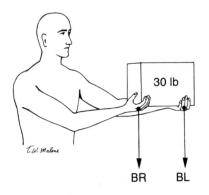

FIGURE 1–11. Vectors BR and BL represent the contact (or push) of the 30-lb box on each hand. BR = **box-on-right-hand**; BL = **box-on-left-hand**.

tion of vector BR is on the right hand and vector BL on the left hand. Preliminarily, therefore, BR can be named "object-on-right-hand" and BL can be named "object-on-left-hand."

The second step in the process of identification and naming is to determine the source of the force. This is considerably easier when it is recognized that the source of most forces that may act on an object must *touch* or *contact* the object. The major exception to this rule when considering forces on the human body is the force of gravity. If permitted the conceit that gravity "contacts" all objects on earth, we can circumvent this exception and maintain the rule that *any* force acting on a segment of the human body must come from something touching the segment.

- Forces on an object are exerted by things that touch that object.
- Gravity exerts a force on all objects on the earth (is always touching an object).

In Figure 1–11, the hands are clearly being contacted by the box. Each hand segment is also being contacted by the adjacent segment of the forearm. In addition to the contact of the box on the hand and the contact of the forearm on the hand, each hand is also being "contacted" by gravity. We now have three possible first names for the unidentified vectors. We can further narrow down the first name (the source) by recognizing that the source can only exert a push (that will be directed away from the source) or pull (that will be directed toward the source). A push or pull by the forearm segments would have to be in line with the forearms. Because BR and BL are not in line with the forearms, we can eliminate the forearms as the source of the vectors. The box would push on the hands and, therefore, is a possible source of vectors BR and BL. Gravity is also a possibility because it is the pull of the earth on the hands. Without further information, we could not determine whether the source of vectors BR and BL was gravity on the left and right hands or the box on the left and right hands.

If the scale and length of vectors BR and BL were known, it would be possible to make the final determination about the identity of the vectors. If we specify the scale as 1 inch = 20 lb, and vectors BR and BL are each 0.75 inches long, the magnitude of each force would be 15 lb. Because the box would exert a force of 15 lb on each hand (30 lb with half distributed to each hand), the box is the likely source of vectors BR and BL. It is unlikely that the hands would each weigh 15 lb (gravity is the pull of the earth on the hand segments and is better known as the weight of the hand segments). Vectors BR and BL can now be named as box-on-right-hand and box-on-left-hand.

Force of Gravity

Gravity is the attraction of the mass of the earth for the mass of other objects and, on earth, has a magnitude of 32 ft/s². The force of gravity gives an object **weight,** which is actually the mass of the object times the acceleration of gravity.

$$\text{Weight} = \text{mass} \times 32 \text{ ft/s}^2$$

The magnitude of weight, being a force, is expressed in pounds (or in newtons using the metric system). It should be noted that the proper unit for mass in the English system is the slug (lb × s²/ft). In the metric system, the unit of mass is the kilogram. The units of mass are scalar units (without action line or direction), whereas the pound and newton are force units having vector characteristics.

Gravity is the most consistent force encountered by the human body and behaves in a predictable manner. As a vector quantity, it can be fully described by point of application, action line/direction, and magnitude. Although gravity acts at all points on an object or segment of an object, its point of application is given as the **center of gravity (COG)** or **center of mass** of that object or segment. The COG is a hypothetical point at which all mass would appear to be concentrated and is the point at which the force of gravity would appear to act.

In a symmetrical object, the COG is located in the geometric center of the object (Fig. 1–12a). In an asymmetrical object, the COG will be located toward the heavier end where the mass will be evenly distributed around the point (Fig. 1–12b). The crutch in Figure 1–12c demonstrates that the COG is only a hypothetical point; it need not lie within the object being acted on. Even when the COG lies outside the object, it is still the point at which gravity *appears* to act. The location of the COG of any object actually can be determined by a number of methods not within the scope of this text. However, the COG of an object can be approximated if one considers it as the balance point of the object (assuming you could balance object on one finger).

The action line and direction of the force of gravity on an object are always vertically downward toward the center of the earth regardless of the orientation in space of the object. The gravity vector is commonly referred to as the **line of gravity (LOG).** The length of the LOG can be drawn to scale, or it may be extended somewhat arbitrarily when other relationships are being explored. The LOG can best be visualized as a string with a weight on the end (a plumb line), with the string attached to the COG of an object. A plumb line applied to the COG of an object gives an accurate representation of the point of application, direction, and action line of gravity, although not the magnitude.

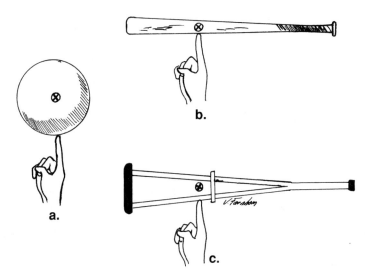

FIGURE 1–12. (a) Center of gravity of a symmetrical object. (b) Center of gravity of an asymmetrical object. (c) The center of gravity may lie outside the object.

Segmental Centers of Gravity

Each segment in the body is acted on by the force of gravity and has its own COG. One can group together two or more adjacent segments if they are going to move together as a single rigid segment. When segments are combined, gravity acting on the combined segments can be represented by a single COG. Figure 1–13a shows the location of the gravity vectors at the centers of the arm (GA), the forearm (GF), and the hand (GH) segments, considering the hand as a single rigid segment. The COGs approximate those identified in studies done on cadavers and on *in vitro* body segments that have yielded standardized data on centers of mass and segmental body weights of individual and combined body segments.[1]

When two adjacent segments are combined and considered as one rigid segment, the new larger segment will have a COG that is located between and in line with the original two COGs. When the segments are not equal in mass, the new COG will lie closer to the heavier segment. Figure 1–13b shows vector GA on the arm and new vector GFH on the forearm/hand segment. The forearm and hand have been combined into a single segment. The new COG for the combined forearm/hand segment is located between the original two COGs with a magnitude equal to the sum of GF and GH. Figure 1–13c has combined all three segments into a single rigid object, with the force of gravity (GAFH) acting at the new COG located between GA and GHF. The magnitude of GAFH is equal to the sum of the magnitudes of its component segments.

The COG for any rigid object or fixed series of segments will remain unchanged regardless of

the position of that object in space. However, when an object is composed of two or more linked and movable segments, the location of the COG of the combined unit will change if the segments are rearranged relative to each other. In Figure 1–13d the arm segment and the forearm/hand segment have been rearranged. The magnitude of the force of gravity will not change because the segments have not changed their mass, but the location of vector GAFH is now different from that in Figure 1–13c. The new location of the COG is still found on a line between the original two. Here, we have another example in which the COG lies outside the rigid arm/forearm/hand segment.

Center of Gravity of the Human Body

When all the segments of the body are combined and the body is taken as a single rigid object in anatomic position, the COG of the body lies approximately anterior to the second sacral vertebra (Fig.1–14). The precise location of the COG for a person in anatomic position depends on the proportions of that person, with the magnitude equal to the weight of the individual. If the person were a rigid object, the COG would not change its position regardless of whether the body were standing up, lying down, or leaning forward. Although the COG does not change its location in the rigid body regardless of position in space, the LOG does change its *relative* position in the body. In Figure 1–14, the LOG falls between the person's feet and is parallel to the body. Because the LOG remains vertically downward regardless of the position of the body in space, the LOG projecting from the COG of a body that is lying down

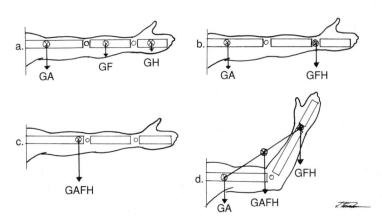

FIGURE 1–13. (a) Gravity acting on the arm (GA), the forearm (GF), and the hand (GH). (b) Gravity acting on the arm and forearm/hand (GFH). (c) Gravity acting on the arm/forearm/hand segment (GAFH). (d) GAFH relocates when segments are rearranged.

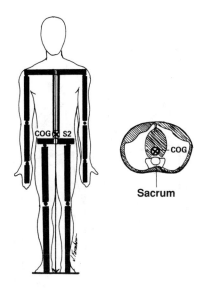

FIGURE 1–14. The center of gravity (COG) of the human body lies approximately at S2, anterior to the sacrum (inset).

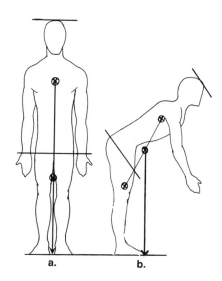

FIGURE 1–15. (a) Location of the COGs of the upper trunk and lower limb segments. (b) Rearrangement of segments produces a new combined COG.

would lie perpendicular to the body rather than parallel to the body as it does in the standing position. In reality, of course, people are not rigid, do not remain in anatomic position, and are constantly rearranging the position of segments relative to each other as they function. With each rearrangement of body segments, the location of the individual's COG will potentially change. The amount of change in the location of the COG depends on how disproportionately the segments are rearranged.

If the body is considered to be composed of a rigid upper-body and a rigid lower-limb segment, the COGs for each of the two segments will be located approximately as given in Figure 1–15a. The combined COG for these two segments in anatomic position as shown will still lie at S-2. When the trunk is inclined forward, however, the location of the new COG lies outside the body (Fig. 1–15b). Figure 1–16 shows a more disproportionate rearrangement of segments. The two lower-limb and single upper-body segments have produced a new COG located at point ABC.

Stability and the Center of Gravity

In Figure 1–16, the LOG (GABC) falls outside the football player's left toes that serve as his **base of support** (**BOS**). The LOG has been extended to indicate its relationship to the BOS. By extending the LOG, it no longer represents the *magnitude* of the football player's weight, al-

though the point of application, action line, and direction remain accurate. For an object to be stable, the LOG *must fall within the* BOS. When the LOG falls outside the BOS, the object will fall. In the case of the football player in Figure 1–16, the LOG falls anterior to his BOS and it

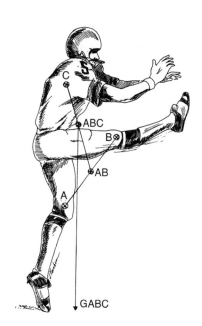

FIGURE 1–16. COG of the left leg (A) and the right leg (B) combine to form the COG for the lower limbs (AB). AB combines with the upper trunk center of gravity (C) to produce the COG for the entire body (ABC).

would be impossible for the player to hold this pose. As the football player has moved from a starting position of standing on both feet with his arms at his side, two factors changed as he assumed the position in Figure 1–16. He reduced his BOS from the area between and including his two feet to the much smaller area of the toes of one foot. His COG, with his rearrangement of segments, has risen above S-2. These two factors, combined with a slight forward lean, influenced the shift in his LOG and contributed to his instability.

When the BOS of an object is large, the LOG has more freedom to move without passing beyond the limits of the base. When a person stands with his or her legs spread apart, the base is larger side to side and the trunk can move a good deal in that plane without displacing the LOG from the BOS (Fig. 1–17). When a person grasps or leans on another object, that object can become part of the BOS. In Figure 1–18, the dancer is in a similar position to the football player. She can maintain the position, however, because her BOS includes not only her left toes, but all the space between it and the bar she is holding. She remains stable as long as her LOG remains somewhere within the extended BOS.

When the COG is low, movement of the object in space is less likely to cause the COG (and LOG) to fall outside the BOS. If one holds a 3-ft long plumb line in one's hand and dangles it just above the ground, the plumb line will swing through a wide arc on the floor

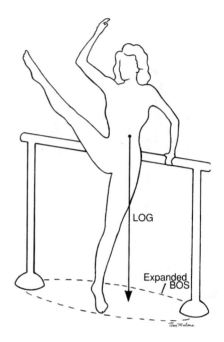

FIGURE 1–18. Although the rearrangement of body segments in this figure raises the COG and displaces the LOG outside her foot, she remains stable because her LOG falls well within the expanded base of support provided by the exercise bar.

with relatively little movement of the hand. Conversely, a plumb line that is 6 inches long and held just above the ground will move through a much smaller arc. The longer the LOG (the higher the COG), the less stable the object. The shorter the LOG (the lower the COG), the more stable the object. Figure 1–19 shows a punching bag as it moves from side to

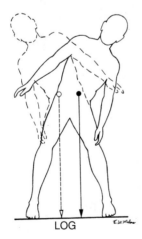

FIGURE 1–17. A wide base of support permits a wide excursion of the line of gravity (LOG) without the LOG falling outside the base of support.

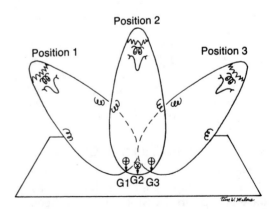

FIGURE 1–19. Given the very low COG of the punching bag, the LOG remains within the base of support regardless of the tipping of the bag from one position to another.

side. The base of the punching bag is filled with sand and the remainder is air. This creates a COG that nearly lies on the ground. The position of the COG of the punching bag remains the same within the punching bag regardless of how tipped the bag might be. The punching bag leans from side to side as much as or more than the man in Figure 1–17 even though the BOS for the punching bag is smaller. The punching bag is extremely stable because it is nearly impossible to get the very short LOG to fall outside the BOS.

When stability of an object or the human body is considered:

- The larger the BOS of an object, the greater the stability of that object.
- The closer the COG of the object is to the BOS, the more stable is the object.
- An object cannot be stable unless its LOG falls within its BOS.

Relocation of the Center of Gravity

The location of the COG of an object or the body depends not only on the arrangement of segments in space but also on the distribution of mass of the object. People certainly gain weight and may gain it disproportionately in the body (thus shifting the COG). However, the most common way to functionally (as opposed to literally) redistribute mass in the body is to add external mass. Every time we add an object to the body by wearing it (a backpack), carrying it (a box), or using it (a power drill), the new COG for the combined body and external mass will shift toward the additional weight; the shift will be proportional to the weight added.

The man in Figure 1–20 has a cast applied to the right lower limb. This resulted in the shift of the COG down and to the right. Because his COG is now lower, he is theoretically more stable. However, his BOS has also been reduced to consist only of the left foot, because his right leg is now nonweight bearing. Rather than require the patient to shift his LOG considerably to the left, crutches have been added. The crutches and the left foot combine to form a much larger BOS, adding to the patient's stability and avoiding a large compensatory weight shift to the left.

In Figure 1–21, the man is holding a heavy suitcase in his right hand (suspending the suitcase from his shoulder girdle). This results in a shift of the COG up and to the right. Because the LOG would move toward the right foot (and potentially to the lateral aspect of the right foot

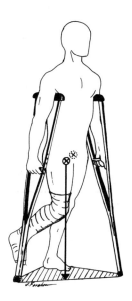

FIGURE 1–20. The addition of the weight of the cast has shifted the COG. Addition of crutches enlarges the base of support to improve stability.

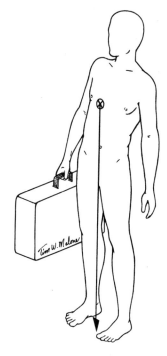

FIGURE 1–21. The weight of the suitcase added to the shoulder girdle causes the COG to shift up and to the right. The man laterally leans to the left to bring the LOG back to the middle of his base of support.

if the suitcase is of sufficient weight), the man leans to the left to "compensate." The small rearrangement of segments caused by leaning the trunk does relatively little to relocate the COG. Rather, the main effect of leaning the trunk is to bring the LOG from the right foot back to the middle of the base of support. The body segments are reoriented in space, not to relocate the COG, but to swing the LOG back toward the center of the base of support.

Reaction Forces

Newton's Law of Reaction

When studying the source and application of forces, one must consider a critical property of forces; that is, that *forces always come in pairs.* Newton's third law, the **law of reaction,** reflects this concept. Newton's third law is commonly stated as: For every action there is an equal and opposite reaction. This statement is misleading because it seems to result in the *incorrect* interpretation shown in Figure 1–22. Newton's third law can be restated more clearly: When one object applies a force to the second object, the second object *must* simultaneously apply a force equal in magnitude and opposite in direction to the first object. These two forces on the two contacting objects constitute an **interaction pair,** or **action-reaction forces.** The simplicity of Newton's third law can better be appreciated when we recall the concept that a force on an object always arises from something that contacts that object. For example, a force applied to object A arises from something touching object A—perhaps a hand. Of course, if the hand is touching object A, then object A *must* also be touching the hand with exactly the same magnitude of force. We have already established that forces applied to

an object come from things touching that object. Now we will expand that concept to say that *anything that touches an object will exert a force on the object.* If object A is touching the hand, object A must also be exerting a force on the hand. If all forces come from things that touch and if all things that touch exert forces, then any two contacting objects must exert forces on each other. Newton noted this phenomenon and concluded the all forces come in pairs that are equal in magnitude, opposite in direction, and applied to adjacent contacting objects. The relation of action-reaction pairs to the concept of contacting objects allows us to also refer to reaction forces as **contact forces.**

EXAMPLE 1: In Figure 1–23 a book is resting on the table. Whenever two objects are in contact, each exerts a force on the other. The book must exert a force on the table, and the table must exert a force on the book. The magnitudes will be equal and the vectors opposite in direction. The forces exerted would be named book-on-table (BT) and table-on-book (TB). Vector BT is applied to the table; its source is a push from the book directed downward with a magnitude equal, in this instance, to the weight of the book. Vector TB is applied to the book; it results from a push of the table upward with a magnitude equal to that of BT. Forces BT and TB can be referred to as action-reaction pairs, as reaction forces, or as contact forces.

It is important to note that in any interaction pair the points of application are on *different objects,* not on the same object as shown incorrectly in Figure 1–22. In Figure 1–23, the book

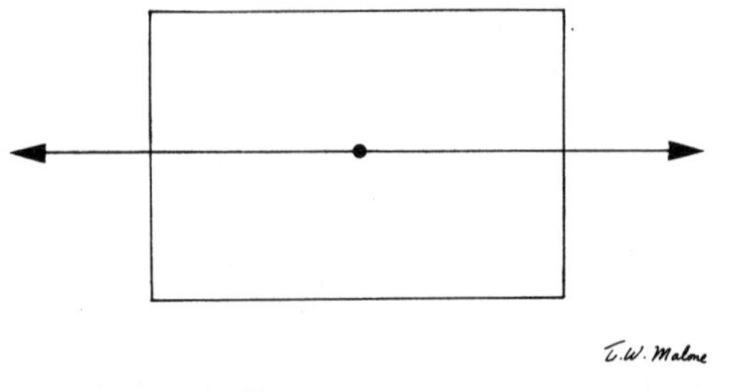

FIGURE 1–22. Newton's third law ("for every action there is an equal and opposite reaction") is commonly *but incorrectly* represented by two vectors acting on the same object.

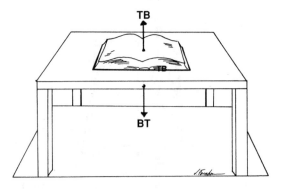

FIGURE 1–23. Reaction forces **book-on-table** (BT) and **table-on-book** (TB).

acted on the *table* while the table simultaneously acted on the *book*. The interaction pair or reaction forces thus always bear names that are the inverse of each other. In Figure 1–11, the vectors were named box-on-left-hand and box-on-right-hand. Because forces come in pairs and objects that are in contact exert forces on each other, we must also have two additional forces called right-hand-on-box and left-hand-on-box. These vectors would each be applied to the *box* in an upward direction with a magnitude of 15 lb.

Because the force of gravity does not actually touch an object, one might think that gravity, or the force of earth-on-object, does not have a mate. Gravity, too, must have a reaction. The earth exerts an attraction for all objects with mass; likewise these objects exert an attraction for the earth equal in magnitude and opposite in direction. Because the attraction of a small object for the large earth seems inconsequential compared to the attraction of the earth for the small object, object-on-earth tends to be ignored (but does exist!). We can continue to consider that anything touching the body or its segments has a reaction or interaction pair.

Whenever one is trying to account for forces on an object or set of objects, one must remember that:

- Forces on an object are exerted by things that touch that object.
- Gravity exerts a force on all objects (is always touching an object).
- Whenever two objects contact, they exert a force on each other (all forces come in pairs).

Equilibrium

The primary concern, when looking at forces that act on an object (or the body in particular), is the effect that the forces will have on the object or body. Whether an object is in translatory, rotatory, or curvilinear motion depends on the forces acting on that object. It is also possible to have forces applied to an object without causing movement of the object. Statics is the study of the conditions under which objects remain in **equilibrium** (at rest or in uniform motion) as a result of the forces acting on them.

Newton's Law of Inertia

Newton's first law, the **law of inertia,** deals with objects in equilibrium. The law states that

an object will remain at rest or in uniform motion unless acted on by an unbalanced force. Uniform motion occurs when an object is moving with a constant velocity; when that constant velocity is zero, the object is at rest. **Inertia** is the property of an object that resists both the initiation of motion and a change in motion. **Velocity** is a vector quantity with both magnitude (speed) and direction. Constant velocity implies, therefore, both constant speed of an object and movement in a constant direction. Velocity can be linear (as for translatory motion) or angular (as for rotatory motion). When dealing with the human body and its segments, moving equilibrium (or uniform motion) occurs infrequently. Therefore, within the scope of this text, equilibrium can be simplified to mean an object at rest unless otherwise specified.

Newton's law of inertia (or law of equilibrium) can be restated: For an object to be in equilibrium, the sum of all the forces *applied to that object* must equal zero, $\Sigma F = 0$. An object cannot be in equilibrium if only one force is acting on that object, because there would be nothing to counteract that force. If a force exists, it must have magnitude; the magnitude of one force cannot be zero.

Determining Equilibrium of an Object

Using what has been reviewed so far, all the forces acting on a body at rest can be accounted for. Figure 1–24 shows a book resting on a table. Assuming the book is in equilibrium (i.e., it remains at rest on the table), the identity and the magnitude of all the forces acting on the book can be accounted for (note that we

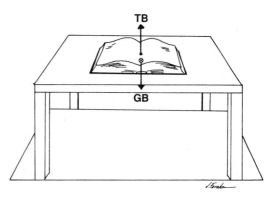

FIGURE 1–24. Equilibrium vectors **gravity-on-book** (GB) and **table-on-book** (TB).

are focusing on the book and *not* the table at this point).

• Gravity acts on all objects. Therefore, gravity must be acting on the book at the book's COG, with a magnitude proportional to the mass of the book: vector GB = gravity-on-book.

Because an object with only one force cannot be in equilibrium, at least one other force must exist on the book.

• Whenever objects touch, each object exerts a force on the other. The book is being contacted by the table; therefore, the table must be exerting a force on the book (TB = table-on-book).

As diagrammed in Figure 1–24, nothing else is touching the book, so there are no other forces to consider. Because vectors GB and TB are applied to the same object and have action lines that lie in the same line, GB and TB are part of a linear force system. To prevent confusion in the figures, vectors with coinciding points of application and action lines will be diagrammed as if they were next to each other. A **linear force system** exists whenever two or more forces act *on the same object* and in the same line. Vectors in the same linear force system will overlap if the vector lengths are extended. Vectors that overlap but are applied to *different* objects cannot be part of the same linear force system. Because linear forces cause translatory motion, the magnitudes of linear forces are given signs using the convention previously described for translatory forces. Forces applied up or to the right are considered positive, whereas forces applied down or to the left are considered negative. Vectors in opposite directions should always have magnitudes of opposite sign. The net effect, or resultant, of all forces that are part of the same linear force system can be determined by finding the arithmetic sum of the magnitudes of each of the forces in the same force system, taking into account its positive or negative value. For the sum of gravity-on-book and table-on-book to be zero, the magnitudes must be equal but opposite in sign and direction. If the book weighed 2.5 lb, GB would be −2.5 lb. Vector TB would then have to have a magnitude of +2.5 lb.

Shifting our attention now from the book to the *table* in Figure 1–25, we can establish the equilibrium of the table in a similar manner. The table is being "touched" or contacted by gravity and by the book. Gravity will exert a downward force (GT) on the table that is the

table's weight and is applied at the COG of the table. Presuming the table weighs 20 lb, GT has a magnitude of −20 lb. Because the table touched the book, so too must the book touch the table. The two "touches" will be equal in magnitude and opposite in direction, but applied to the different and touching objects (law of reaction). Therefore, book-on-table (BT) is equal in magnitude and opposite in direction to vector TB. Consequently, BT must be −2.5 lb.

In Figure 1–25, presuming that the book is placed symmetrically in the middle of the table, two forces are now acting on the table at the same point and in the same line (vectors GT and BT are diagrammed separately to avoid overlap). Gravity-on-table and book-on-table are part of the same linear force system. The net effect on the table of GT and BT can be represented by a new vector applied to the COG of the table, with a magnitude of −22.5 lb. The table cannot be in equilibrium with such a net force acting on it. At least one other force must exist on the table.

The source of any additional force acting on the table must be something contacting the table. The only other contact on the table in Figure 1–25 is made by the floor. Because any contact between two objects creates a force, there must be a vector applied to the table called floor-on-table (FT). If the table is at rest, the sum of the forces acting on the table must be zero. Consequently, FT must be equal in magnitude and opposite in direction to the net

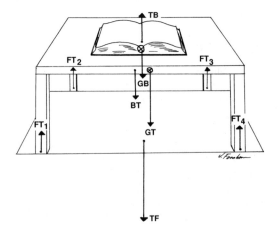

FIGURE 1–25. Equilibrium of the table is established with the forces of **gravity-on-table** (GT), **book-on-table** (BT), and **floor-on-table** (FT$_1$ + FT$_2$ + FT$_3$ + FT$_4$). **Table-on-floor** (TF) is the reaction to FT and does not have a direct effect on the equilibrium of the table.

EXAMPLE 2: In Figure 1–26, three forces were identified as being applied to the hand. Each of these *must* have a reaction force, although the reaction is not significant to the establishment of equilibrium of the hand. The reaction forces (interaction pairs) to each of these forces are:

Original Force Vector	Reaction Vector	Affected Object
Gravity (earth-on-hand)	Hand-on-earth (HE)	Earth
Briefcase-on-hand (BH)	Hand-on-briefcase (HB)	Briefcase
Forearm-on-hand (FH)	Hand-on-forearm (HF)	Forearm

---

effect of GT and BT. FT has a magnitude of +22.5 lb. The point of application of FT can be placed at the COG on the table, because that is the hypothetical point at which the mass of the table is concentrated. FT can also be applied at the actual points of contact; that is, at each leg of the table. Figure 1–25 shows FT distributed over the four legs to avoid redundant lines in the diagram, but it should be understood that FT can be considered to act at the COG of the table and is therefore part of the same linear force system as GT and BT. ($FT = FT_1 + FT_2 + FT_3 + FT_4$).

Figure 1–25 includes one other force vector. Table-on-floor (TF) is the reaction to floor-on-table (FT). TF must exist because the contact of the table and floor requires that the floor and table exert forces on each other. TF is equal in magnitude and opposite in direction to FT. It does *not*, however, have a direct influence on the equilibrium of the table, because only those forces that have a *point of application on an object* can contribute to the equilibrium of that object. Similarly, table-on-book and gravity-on-book, if diagrammed in their precise locations, would overlap with gravity-on-table and book-on-table. Although coinciding, these four vectors are *not* part of the same linear force system because they are applied to two different objects.

In Figure 1–26, the hand segment of the man holding a briefcase is in equilibrium. The hand segment is touched by gravity, by the briefcase, and by the distal forearm segment. Hand vectors GH (gravity-on-hand), BH (briefcase-on-hand), and FH (forearm-on-hand) each act on and have coinciding points of application and action lines on the hand. They are, therefore, parts of the same linear force system. Gravity (GH) and the pull of the briefcase on the hand (BH) both act in a negative (downward) direction. The magnitude of GH is equal to the

weight of the hand (2 lb). The magnitude of BH can also be identified if we first look at the briefcase. If the briefcase weighs 8 lb (gravity-on-briefcase), then hand-on-briefcase (HB) must be +8 lb if nothing else is touching the briefcase and the briefcase is in equilibrium. If the hand is pulling on the briefcase with a force of +8 lb, then the briefcase is also pulling on the hand with a force of −8 lb. Therefore, BH has a magnitude of −8 lb. Given the two downward forces (BH and GH), if the hand is in equilibrium, the pull of the forearm on the hand (FH) must be positive in direction and must be equivalent to the sum of GH and BH (or +10 lb).

Although it is true that forces that result from the contact of objects always come in pairs and are always applied to different and touching objects, the reaction to a force on one object can be ignored if it does not affect the problem at hand (see Example 2). Although the

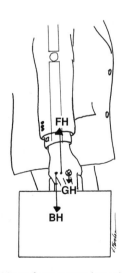

FIGURE 1–26. Linear force system formed by the forces of **gravity-on-hand** (GH), **briefcase-on-hand** (BH), and **forearm-on-hand** (FH).

reaction forces HE, HB, and HF in Figure 1–26 can, for the most part, be ignored for our purposes, the reaction force or forces can sometimes be very important.

In Figure 1–27, a person is standing on a scale with the intent of recording his weight, gravity-on-person (GP). The scale cannot, however, measure or record a force applied to the person but can only record a force applied to the scale. What is actually being recorded on the scale is the *contact* of the person-on-scale (PS) and not the weight of the person. Under usual conditions of weighing oneself, this distinction is not a particularly important one. Vector PS will always be equal in magnitude and opposite in direction to its reaction, scale-on-person (SP). As long as the person is in equilibrium *and* nothing else is touching the person, scale-on-person and gravity-on-person will have equal magnitudes. Consequently, the magnitude of PS and GP will be equivalent to each other.

The distinction between GP and the reaction force PS can be very important if something else is touching the person or the scale. If the person being weighed is holding something, the person's weight (GP) does not change, but the contact forces (PS and SP) will increase. Similarly, we are all familiar with the phenomenon where a gentle pressure down on the bathroom countertop as we weigh ourselves will result in a weight reduction. The pressure of the fingers down on the countertop creates an upward reaction of countertop-on-person (CP). Now scale-on-person equals (−GP) + (+CP), a sum less than the magnitude of GP alone. The contact between the person and the countertop has created an additional reaction force acting on the person, resulting in what appears to be a weight reduction. It is not a decrease in GP, of course, but a decrease in PS.

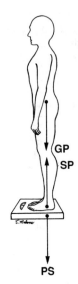

FIGURE 1–27. Although a scale is commonly thought to measure the weight of the person (**gravity-on-person** [GP]), it is actually recording the contact of the **person-on-scale** (PS). Vectors GP and PS are equal in magnitude as long as nothing else is touching the person.

Because the scale is *not* actually measuring the person's weight but the reaction force of person-on-scale, PS will be equal to GP only if no other forces are applied to the person. In this example, the reaction force (PS) *cannot* be ignored because it is the variable of interest.

Objects in Motion

When a state of equilibrium exists, all forces applied to the object are balanced (the sum of all the forces applied to the object is zero). When unbalanced forces are applied to an object, **acceleration** of the object will necessarily result. Figure 1–28 shows three people pulling

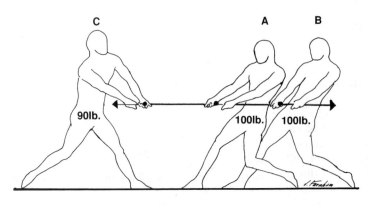

FIGURE 1–28. Unbalanced forces on the rope produce acceleration of the rope toward men (A) and (B).

on a rope. Person A and person B are exerting a force of 100 lb each on the rope. Person C is exerting a force of 90 lb in an opposite or negative direction. Each force is acting on the same object (the rope) along the same line and so are part of one linear force system. Because the people are the only objects touching the rope (the negligible effect of gravity is ignored in this very light rope), the resultant force R acting on the rope is (+100 lb) + (+100 lb) + (−90 lb); that is, R = +110 lb. The net effect on the rope is a linear force of 110 lb acting to the right, causing the rope to move and accelerate in that direction. Once an object begins to accelerate, new forces are introduced and kinetic analysis becomes far more complex. We will maintain a fairly simple (and simplified) approach that will not include more advanced concepts in dynamics.

Newton's Law of Acceleration

The magnitude of acceleration of a moving object is defined by Newton's second law, the **law of acceleration.** Newton's second law states that the acceleration of an object is proportional to the unbalanced forces acting on it and inversely proportional to the mass of that object:

$$a = F/m$$

That is, a large push (F) applied to an object of constant mass (m) will produce more acceleration (a) than a small push. A push on an object of large mass will produce less acceleration than an equal push on an object of smaller mass. Acceleration may occur as a change in speed of an object or as a change in direction of movement or both. From the law of acceleration it can be seen that inertia, a body's or object's resistance to change in movement (or change in acceleration), is proportional to the mass of the body or object. The greater the mass of an object, the greater the magnitude of net force needed either to get the object moving or to change its motion. A very large woman in a wheelchair has more inertia than a small woman; an aide must exert a greater push on a wheelchair with a large woman in it than on the wheelchair with a small woman in it to obtain the same acceleration.

Examples of Dynamics

In Figure 1–29a, a 200-lb man is taking a step forward on the floor. At the particular moment

in time captured in the figure, approximately half of the man's 200-lb body weight, gravity-on-man (G_1), is acting down the right leg. The right leg at that moment is in equilibrium only if there is another force equal in magnitude and opposite in direction applied to the right leg by the contacting floor. Floor-on-right-leg (FL) is applied to the leg and is a result of the floor's ability to react to the force of right-leg-on-floor (LF). Because nothing else is touching the leg and body other than the floor, FL must be equal in magnitude to G_1 or also 100 lb. Ordinarily, no matter how large in magnitude G_1 might be, the floor can exert an equal force back on the leg (we count on this whenever we cross the floor!). However, in Figure 1–29b, the force of FL (and, therefore, its reaction LF) is smaller in magnitude (75 lb) than G_1. The floor has been weakened and is not capable of pushing back adequately. Because the sum of G_1 and FL is not zero, the person's leg cannot be in equilibrium. The leg will accelerate downward through the floor with an unbalanced force of 25 lb.

The magnitude of acceleration of the leg through the floor can be easily determined by using Newton's second law if the problem is treated as one in statics rather than dynamics. Once the floor actually begins to break, the force the floor exerts on the leg (FL) will diminish until it reaches zero, changing the unbalanced force acting on the leg continuously until that point. The problem can be simplified

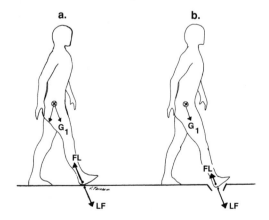

FIGURE 1–29. (a) A man in equilibrium. Gravity (G_1) acting down the right leg is opposed by the equal and opposite force of **floor-on-leg** (FL). (b) A man not in equilibrium. The push of FL is not equal to gravity; therefore the leg accelerates down through the floor.

by considering only the point in time at which FL and LF equals 75 lb.

The acceleration of the leg through the floor can be found using the equation a = F/m. One must know both the magnitude of the unbalanced force (25 lb) and the mass of the accelerating segment (half the mass of the body acting through the right leg). The direction (downward through the floor) will remain relatively unchanged and can be ignored for the purposes of this calculation. The body weight (or the force acting through the right leg) was given as 100 lb. The force unit of the pound will have to be converted to a mass unit (slugs); 100 lb of force is equal to 3.125 sl (1 lb = 1/32 sl). The slug can also be written using the units lb*s^2/ft. Therefore,

$$a = 25 \text{ lb} \div 3.125 \text{ lb} \times s^2/\text{ft}$$
$$a = 8 \text{ ft/s}^2$$

The calculated acceleration of 8 ft/s^2 will occur only at the point in time that the floor breaks. As the floor gives less support, FL diminishes in magnitude. As FL diminishes in magnitude, the net unbalanced force downward increases, as does the acceleration. The acceleration will continue to increase until the floor no longer exerts any force on the leg at all or, more likely, until a new force is encountered (e.g., contact of the leg with the subflooring) that will restore equilibrium to the leg.

Creating a static situation by capturing a single point in time simplifies an analysis. However, oversimplification can lead to incorrect conclusions. Figure 1–30 shows the pelvis of a person lying on a table with the skin of the buttocks in between. The pelvis is contacted by gravity (gravity-on-pelvis or GP) and by the skin

(skin-on-pelvis or SP). The skin is contacted by gravity (gravity-on-skin or GS), by the table (table-on-skin or TS), and by the pelvis (pelvis-on-skin or PS). If everything is in equilibrium, then: GP = SP and GS + PS = TS. It is possible, however, for the ability of the skin to "push" back on the pelvis to be compromised by, for example, poor nutrition. If the skin is limited in its ability to push back, then SP may be *slightly* smaller in magnitude than GP. In this instance, then, there is a net unbalanced force acting on the pelvis, causing it to accelerate downward *very slowly* because the net unbalanced force is very small. The skin will not move downward with the pelvis, however. If the magnitude of PS is slightly diminished (as it will be if SP is slightly diminished), then the magnitude of TS will also diminish. That is, if there is less net downward force on the skin, there will be less contact between the skin and the table. The result of the scenario here is that the pelvis will *slowly* accelerate downward through the skin while the skin remains in place. The result is a bed sore, or decubitus ulcer. The static analysis masked what was actually a progressive dynamic situation.

We have just seen that analyzing linear forces as if equilibrium always existed (statics) can lead to inaccuracies. As soon as there is acceleration, new forces come into place that we have ignored. Similarly, angular acceleration of a bony lever rotated about a joint axis also produces new forces that will complicate an analysis beyond what can be covered in this basic biomechanics unit. A segment can be rotating around an axis with a constant speed (degrees of movement per unit time). Although the magnitude of the angular velocity of the segment

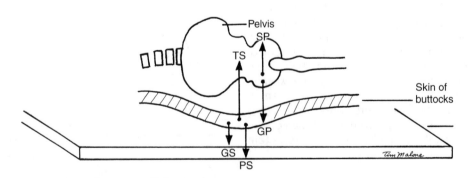

FIGURE 1–30. The pelvis is not in equilibrium because **gravity-on-pelvis** (GP) is greater in magnitude than **skin-on-pelvis** (SP). The skin remains in equilibrium as long as the sum of vectors **gravity-on-skin** (GS), **pelvis-on-skin** (PS) and **table-on-skin** (TS) is zero. In this instance, the pelvis will "accelerate" downward through the skin, creating a pressure sore.

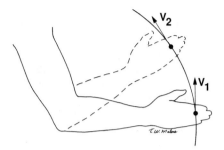

FIGURE 1–31. Although the magnitude of angular velocity (V_1, V_2) may be constant, the direction of angular velocity of a rotating limb segment changes as the limb segment moves around its axis. The angular velocity is always tangential to the arc of motion.

may be constant, the *direction* will not be. The direction of the angular velocity vectors (v_1 and v_2) is always tangential to the arc (or perpendicular to the moving segment) as shown in Figure 1–31. The constantly changing vector of angular velocity can make an analysis inaccurate if not taken into consideration. When torque (the magnitude of rotation of an object) is discussed later in this chapter, we will remind the reader again that a simple static analysis will underestimate the forces actually acting on the lever under consideration.

Joint Distraction in a Linear Force System

Knowledge of the principles of Newton's laws and of linear force systems can be used to understand how skeletal traction produces joint distraction. Figure 1–32 shows skeletal traction applied to the leg. We will show how hanging a 10-lb weight on this pulley system produces separation between the tibia and the femur at the knee joint. Follow each force carefully as it is described.

We will begin by assuming that the objects in Figure 1–32 are all in equilibrium. Because

we chose a 10-lb weight to hang on the rope, we know that the force of gravity-on-weight (GW) has a magnitude of −10 lb acting vertically downward. For the weight to be in equilibrium, a +10-lb force must also exist on the weight, coming from something touching the weight. Because the rope is the only other object contacting the weight, the +10-lb force must be rope-on-weight (RW). RW must have a reaction force weight-on-rope (WR), which is equal in magnitude and opposite in direction (−10 lb) to RW.

Assuming we have a frictionless pulley system, tension in the rope must be the same throughout the rope; that is, the magnitude of force applied to each end of the rope must be the same. Because WR represents the pull of the weight or tension (T_1) in the vertical rope segment, an equal tension vector (T_2) must exist at the other end of the rope. To create tension at both ends of the rope, T_2 must be applied in the opposite direction from T_1. Given that the pulley changes the direction of the force, T_2 in this instance is horizontal and to the left (with a magnitude of 10 lb). If the rope was not "bent" around the pulley, T_1 and T_2 would be directly opposite each other.

Given that we know that T_2 exists, we must identify it by name. The force T_2 must originate from something that contacts the horizontal rope segment and is capable of exerting a force of 10 lb to the left. Both the pulley and the leg sling touch the horizontal rope segment. Both the sling and the pulley can only "pull" on the rope (a "push" on the rope would tend to make it slack. Also, if a pulley could push, it would not be called a pulley!). Because a pull is always toward its source, only the sling could exert a pull to the left. To simplify things, we will treat the sling and leg as one rigid object known as **leg.** Consequently, T_2 must be leg-on-rope (LR) and, as tension vector T_2, must have a magnitude of −10 lb. Leg-on-rope has a reaction, rope-on-leg (RL), applied to the leg with a magnitude of +10 lb.

The leg (a term referring to the body segment below the knee) is contacted by gravity (GL), the knee ligaments, and the rope. The force exerted by the rope has already been identified. Vector GL is vertically downward and not in line with RL. GL is not part of a linear force system with RL and will be ignored for now. We will only consider the horizontal forces acting on the leg or femur segments that we are trying to separate (distract). The force of knee-

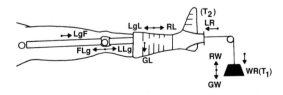

FIGURE 1–32. Traction applied to the foot sets up numerous forces that result in joint distraction at the knee.

ligaments-on-leg (LgL) would potentially pull on the leg, creating a force to the left that would be part of the same linear force system as RL. (Although the joint capsule is also part of the ligamentous force acting on the leg, only the ligaments will be referenced for purposes of simplicity.) If the net effect of the two forces LgL and RL is no movement (equilibrium), the forces must be balanced and their sum must be zero. Therefore, LgL must have a magnitude of −10 lb.

Vector LgL must have a reaction force; the leg must exert an equal and opposite force of +10 lb on the ligaments, leg-on-ligaments (LLg). For the ligaments to be in equilibrium, an equal force of −10 lb must be exerted on the ligaments by the femur, femur-on-ligaments (FLg) because the femur is the only other object contacting the ligaments (again ignoring the vertical effect of gravity on the ligaments). FLg will have a reaction force, ligaments-on-femur (LgF), of +10 lb. Assuming the femur is in equilibrium without examining all forces acting on it, all forces relevant to joint distraction have now been identified.

Equilibrium of each object identified in Figure 1–32 depends on the ability of the object to generate the required force (the ability to push back or pull back sufficiently to balance forces). In the case of the suspended weight, the rope, and the leg, each is quite capable of exerting the required 10-lb force as long as no defects exist. The ligaments, however, cannot exert any significant force on the leg when the ligaments are slack. The ligaments will, in fact, be slack when the weight is first put on the traction system because the femur and leg are close to each other (the goal of the traction is to separate them). Initially, the force of LgL (and LLg) might be as little as 1 lb, and a net force of 9 lb to the right will exist on the leg (the pull of the rope on the leg will not be completely offset by the pull of the ligaments on the leg).

Given the unbalanced force acting on the leg, the leg will accelerate to the right. As the leg moves to the right, the tension in the ligaments will increase as the bones separate. The tighter the ligaments become, the less unbalanced force exists and the less acceleration there is. Once the ligaments are pulled taut by the movement of the leg, the ligaments are capable of exerting the 10-lb force needed to establish equilibrium of the leg. Ligaments have a tremendous tensile strength and are capable

of withstanding far greater forces than the force applied in this example for at least short periods of time. As shall be seen in subsequent chapters, prolonged loading may result in gradual elongation of the ligaments. The example of joint distraction created by acceleration of the leg to the right, directly away from the joint, is an example of pure translatory motion without concomitant joint rotation. It is also an example of how important even small unbalanced forces can be.

Equilibrium of the leg has now been established in a position in which the ligaments are taut and the joint surfaces are separated by a distance permitted by the length of the ligaments. Note that in this example the muscles that cross the knee joint were assumed to be inactive because no muscle forces were included. In the case of a bone fracture, the process of distraction of bone fragments required for proper alignment and healing is similar to that described in joint distraction. The fracture acts as a false joint and distraction is resisted by the muscles crossing the fracture site. Overactivity of the muscles initially accelerates the distal fragment toward the proximal one. Traction is applied to realign the bones. As the muscle spasm subsides and the muscle fatigues, the muscle exerts less and less force, until the force of the traction rope on the distal fragment exceeds the force of the muscles on that fragment; the direction of movement will then cause the fragments to separate and realign. Equilibrium is reestablished when the structures crossing the fracture site become taut once again.

In the example of leg traction, we ignored the force of gravity on the leg and on the ligaments, stating that the vertical forces of gravity were not part of the same linear force system as the distraction forces and, therefore, could be ignored when calculating the magnitude of these forces. In fact, this can lead to a further refinement of Newton's first law or law of equilibrium:

- For an object to be in equilibrium, the sum of all the vertical forces on the object must be zero and, independently, the sum of all the horizontal forces must be zero.

$$\Sigma F_V = 0$$
$$\Sigma F_H = 0$$

We accounted for the sum of the horizontal forces, but ignored the sum of the vertical forces. Having identified only gravitational vertical forces (applied vertically downward), we did *not* take into consideration the vertical equilibrium of the leg in the traction example. Even if we conveniently ignored the negligible magnitude of gravity on rope, we would still have to consider the effect of gravity on leg. We could offset GL by resting the leg on a bed (creating an upward contact force, bed-on-leg) but would then potentially introduce a new force, the force of friction.

Force of Friction

The **force of friction (Fx)** potentially exists whenever two objects contact. The contact results in reaction forces on each of the two touching objects. For friction to have magnitude, however, some other force must be moving or attempting to move one of the touching objects on the other. The force that moves or attempts to move one object on another is known as a **shear force.** By definition the shear force is that force (or the component of the force) that is applied parallel to contacting surfaces in the direction of attempted movement. The magnitude of a friction force on an object is a function of the magnitude of contact between the objects, the slipperiness or roughness of the contacting surfaces and, for objects that are not moving, the magnitude of the shear force.

When two contacting objects are *not* moving on each other, but there is a shear force applied to the object that attempts to move that object on the one below it, then *maximum* magnitude of the force of friction on that object is the product of a constant known as the coefficient of static friction (μ_s) and the reaction or contact force (F_c) exerted by the contacting object. That is,

$$Fx \leq \mu_s F_c$$

The coefficient of static friction is a constant value for given materials. For example, μ_s for ice on ice is approximately 0.05; the value of μ_s for wood on wood is approximately 0.25. As the contacting surfaces become softer or rougher, μ_s increases. The contact force, F_c, increases with the magnitude of contact of the adjacent objects. A heavier object generally has a greater magnitude of contact with an object beneath it than a lighter object (assuming no other supporting forces). The greater the contact force on an object and the rougher the contacting surfaces, the greater the maximum potential force of friction. When using friction to warm your hands, the contact of the hands warms both of them (friction forces exist on both the right and the left hands). If you wish to increase the friction, you press your hands together harder (increase the contact force) as you rub. Increasing the pressure increases the contact force between the hands and increases the maximum value of friction (the coefficient of friction remains unchanged because the surface remains skin on skin).

Friction is given as a *maximum potential* force because it has magnitude (or is "activated") only if an attempt is made to move one object on another. In Figure 1–33, a large box weighing 100 lb is resting on the floor. Assessing the equilibrium of the box, the maximum *potential* friction force on the box (FX) is a product of the coefficient of static friction of wood box on

FIGURE 1–33. In (a), the box is acted on by the forces of gravity (G) and the contact of the floor (FB). The force of friction does not exist because it does not have magnitude. In (b), the force of the man pushing on the box (MB) causes an opposing friction force (FX).

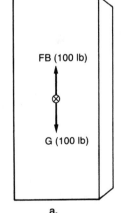

a.

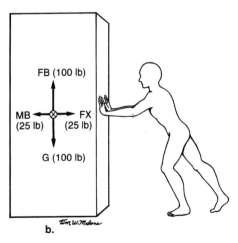

b.

wood floor (0.25) and the contact or reaction force of floor-on-box (FB) is 100 lb.

$$FX \le (0.25)(100)$$
$$FX \le 25 \text{ lb}$$

As long as no other forces are applied to the box, friction will not have magnitude. However, as an external shear force (the man pushing on the box) is applied to the left, friction will increase its magnitude to balance or offset the magnitude of the shear force. Friction in this instance can only increase up to a magnitude of 25 lb of force to the right; a shear force of more than 25 lb to the left will cause the box to accelerate to the left because there will be a net unbalanced force to the left. Note that only the forces applied horizontally to the box (friction and shear) affect its horizontal equilibrium.

Once an object is moving, friction between any two objects is a constant value, equal to the product of the reaction force and the coefficient of *kinetic friction* (μ_k). The coefficient of kinetic friction (μ_k) is less than the maximum value of static friction for any set of contacting surfaces. The shear force attempting to move the object must be larger than the maximum value of static friction before movement will begin (at least a small net unbalanced force must exist in the direction of movement). However, once movement is initiated, the value of friction drops from its maximum value to its smaller kinetic value, suddenly increasing the net unbalanced force if the external shear force remains unchanged. The sudden drop in magnitude of friction results in the classic situation in which the man pushes harder and harder to get the box moving along the floor and then suddenly finds himself and the box accelerating too rapidly. Again calling attention to the more detailed restatement of Newton's law of equilibrium, note that a box pushed along the floor by an external force is not in horizontal equilibrium, but is in *vertical* equilibrium (G and FB are balanced). It should not be assumed that vertical equilibrium and horizontal equilibrium will occur concomitantly.

- Friction may exist on an object whenever two objects touch.
- Friction has magnitude only when there is a shear force applied to an object; that is, friction has magnitude only when two contacting objects move or attempt to move on each other.
- Friction forces (like all forces) come in pairs, are applied to each of the contacting objects, are equal in magnitude and are opposite in direction on the two contacting objects.
- The action line of friction forces always lies parallel to the contacting surfaces.
- The direction of the force of friction on an object is always opposite to the direction of potential or relative movement of the objects (opposite in direction to the shear force).
- The friction force and its relevant shear force on an object are part of the same linear force system.

In the example of the leg in traction (Fig. 1–32), if the leg were to rest on the bed we would add a vertical contact force (bed-on-leg) that would oppose gravity (GL), but would also add a potential friction force. The potential friction force would be parallel to the contacting surfaces (the leg and the bed) and so would be a horizontal force applied in the direction opposite to potential movement of the leg away from the femur; that is, friction-on-leg would be opposite to the shear force attempting to move the leg along the bed (RL).

The maximum magnitude of the friction force on the leg (Fx_L) would be the product of bed-on-leg (the contact force) and an unknown coefficient of static friction. In this example, μ_s would be fairly large, because the skin and the sheet do not slide easily on each other. We can assume the Fx_L is fairly large and could potentially completely offset the shear force of rope-on-leg. The leg would not move because there would be no net unbalanced force acting on the leg. No distraction between the femur and the leg would occur and the ligaments would remain slack. To maintain the effectiveness of the traction the leg would either have to be supported off the surface of the bed or friction minimized in some other way.

Concurrent Forces

When identifying equilibrium forces and reaction pairs, the forces presented so far in this chapter were part of linear force systems applied to the object. More commonly, however, forces applied to an object are not in a line but have action lines that lie at angles to each other. Two or more forces acting at a common point of application on an object but in divergent directions are part of a **concurrent force system.** Two or more forces applied to the same object can also be part of the same concurrent force system when the vectors have different points of application on the object as long as the vectors intersect when extended in length. The net effect, or resultant, of concurrent forces appears to occur at the common point of application or at the point of intersection and can be represented by a single new vector through the process known as composition of forces.

Composition of Forces

In Figure 1–34 man A and man B are each pulling on the block at a right angle to each other with a force of 75 lb each. The action lines of man-A-on-block (AB) and man-B-on-block (BB) are in different directions but are commonly applied through the COG of the block (because vectors can be extended, the ropes do not need to be attached at the COG of the block). The net effect, or resultant action, of the two pulls will be in a line that lies between the men. Figure 1–34 (inset) shows a graphic solution of the problem by the polygon method. Vectors AB and BB are drawn to scale with a common point of application, maintaining the 90° angle between them. Line (AB)$_1$ is then drawn parallel to AB from the end of BB; line (BB)$_1$ is drawn parallel to BB from the end of AB, forming a polygon. The resultant force R is diagrammed with its point of application at the intersection of AB and BB; its action line and magnitude are drawn so that the arrowhead lies at the intersection of lines (AB)$_1$ and (BB)$_1$. The resultant vector is always the diagonal of the polygon formed by the original two vectors.

The net effect of forces AB and BB (75 lb each) would be a force of 106.25 lb in the direction of R (given the proportional size of R to AB and BB). It is important to note that the magnitude of R is not equal to the sum of the magnitudes of AB and BB. The block can be pulled more efficiently if a single force of 106.25 lb is applied in the direction of R, rather than with two divergent forces of 75 lb each.

Muscle Action Lines

TOTAL MUSCLE FORCE VECTOR

The force applied by a muscle to a bony segment is actually the resultant of the pull on a common point of attachment of all the fibers that compose the muscle. Because each muscle fiber can be represented by a vector (Fig. 1–35), the fibers taken together form a concurrent force system with a resultant that is the total muscle force vector (Fms). Fms has a point of application at the attachment of the muscle and an action line that is the direction of the resultant pull of all the muscle's fibers. An actual graphic solution could be attempted by taking the pull of two fibers initially, composing them into a single pull, and adding another fiber. This would have to be repeated until all the fibers have been taken into account. The resultant pull can also be approximated by putting the point of application at the muscle's attachment on the bone and drawing a resultant action line symmetrically toward the middle of the muscle's fibers. The direction of pull for all muscles is toward the center of the muscle. The magnitude or length of Fms may be drawn arbitrarily

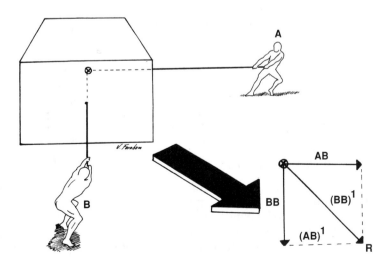

FIGURE 1–34. Man A and man B pulling at angles to each other through the COG of the block represent a concurrent force system. Inset shows the composition of forces from man A (AB) and man B (BB) to give resultant R.

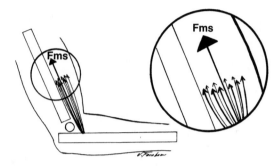

FIGURE 1–35. The total muscle force (Fms) is the resultant of all fiber pulls taken together.

unless a hypothetical magnitude is specified. The actual force of active pull of either individual muscle fibers or the total force muscle cannot be determined in the living person.

Every muscle pulls on each of its ends every time the muscle exerts a force. Therefore, every muscle creates a minimum of two force vectors, one on each of the bones to which the muscle is attached. Movement created by a muscle depends on the net forces acting on each of its levers, and *not* on the designation of the attachment as "origin" or "insertion." As we analyze motion, we commonly choose to confine our analysis to only one of the segments on which the muscle is acting. Although we may do this, we must also recognize that we are purposefully ignoring forces on one or more other segments. For instance, if consideration is being given to flexion of the forearm at the elbow joint, all the forces (external and internal) acting on the *forearm* must be considered. Although muscles acting on the forearm will act on at least one other segment, the action on the other segment (e.g., humerus or scapula) can be ignored until that segment is analyzed.

- Muscles pull on all segments to which they are attached whenever a muscle force is exerted.
- Muscles create movement based on the net forces applied to each of their segments, *not* based on which is the so-called origin or insertion.

DIVERGENT MUSCLE PULLS

The concepts of a concurrent force system can be used to determine the resultant of two or more segments of one muscle, or two muscles when the muscles have a common attachment. Figure 1–36 shows the resultant force of the an-

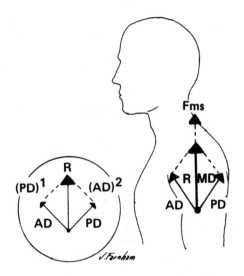

FIGURE 1–36. The pulls of the anterior deltoid (AD), the middle deltoid (MD), and the posterior deltoid (PD) form a concurrent force system with resultant pull Fms found by composition of forces. AD + PD = R; R + MD = Fms.

terior portion of the deltoid muscle (AD) and the resultant force of the posterior portion of the deltoid muscle (PD) acting on the humerus. Using the polygon method of composition of forces, the resultant force vector for the constructed polygon (see Fig. 1–36, inset) is vector R. Vector R, therefore, represents the vector sum of AD and PD. The deltoid muscle is also composed of a middle segment (MD) that is located between AD and PD. Because R and MD coincide and have a common point of application, they are part of a linear force system. The resultant in a linear force system is found by finding the arithmetic sum of vectors R and MD; that is, the new resultant vector Fms will be equal in magnitude to R + MD and in the same direction. Vector Fms represents the total pull of the three segments of the deltoid, producing abduction of the arm as the muscle exerts a force on the humerus.

Figure 1–37 shows another example of composing forces to find the total muscle pull. In this instance the resultant force of the clavicular portion of the pectoralis major muscle (CPM) and the resultant force of the sternal portion of the pectoralis major muscle (SPM) are shown with a common attachment on the humerus. When both portions of the pectoralis major contract simultaneously, the resultant force on the humerus Fms is produced. Fms is in a new direction and would produce adduction and medial rotation of the humerus.

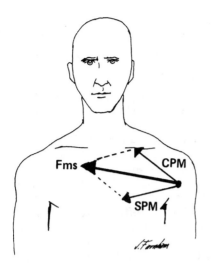

FIGURE 1–37. The clavicular portion of the pectoralis major (CPM) and the sternal portion of the pectoralis major (SPM) can be composed to find Fms.

ANATOMIC PULLEYS

Frequently the fibers of a muscle or a muscle tendon wrap around a bone or are deflected by a bony prominence. When the direction of pull of a muscle is altered, the bone or bony prominence causing the deflection forms an anatomic pulley. Pulleys change the direction without changing the magnitude of the applied force.

In Figure 1–38, a schematic representation of the shoulder is shown on the left, treating the shoulder as a link between two straight levers. The deltoid muscle force vector (Fms) for abduction of the arm has been drawn as it would exist in this hypothetical situation. The right figure shows a more anatomic representation of the shoulder, including the rounded head of the humerus, and the overhanging acromion with the clavicle. These anatomic features

change the direction of the fibers of the deltoid muscle. When Fms is drawn, the point of application will still be on the humerus. The action line of the muscle is in the direction of pull of the muscle fibers *at the point of attachment*. In this example, the action line follows the pull of the fibers of the middle deltoid (recalling that the total pull of the deltoid in abduction of the humerus was determined to be in line with the middle deltoid). The action line of the deltoid continues in a straight line even though the muscle is wrapping around the humeral head because vectors are always straight lines; that is, the effect of a muscle on a bone is governed by the direction of pull of the muscle at the point of bony attachment and *not* by subsequent shifts in fiber direction. The action line and direction of Fms are significantly different between the left portion of Figure 1–38 and the right portion, although the point of application and magnitude of the force are the same in each figure.

Because anatomic pulleys are commonly encountered by muscles in the body, the pull of a muscle (Fms) should be visualized for any given muscle or muscle segment in such a way that:

- The point of application is located on the segment under consideration, at the point of attachment of the muscle on that segment.
- The muscle action line is in the direction of pull that the fibers or tendons of the muscle create *at the point of application*.
- Vectors are straight lines and do not change directions, regardless of any change in direction of muscle fiber or tendon.
- Magnitude (length) of muscle vectors, unless given a specific hypothetical value,

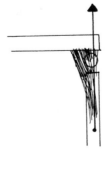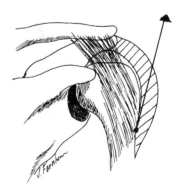

FIGURE 1–38. Action line of the deltoid muscle on a schematic representation of the clavicle and humerus (left). Action line of the deltoid is deflected by the bony contours that form anatomic pulleys (right).

are usually arbitrary because we cannot measure the absolute force of a muscle's pull on bone in most living subjects.

Parallel Force Systems

The forces we have examined thus far have had action lines that either coincided or intersected. One may also find forces on the levers of the human body that have action lines that do not coincide and will not intersect. One commonly finds in the human body forces that act on the same object and are parallel to each other. A **parallel force system** exists whenever two or more parallel forces act on the same lever but at some distance from each other *and* at some distance from the axis about which the lever will rotate. Each of the forces in a parallel force system will create or tend to create rotation of the lever about its axis. To further understand the effect that parallel force systems have on the rigid levers of the skeleton, we need to examine the principles of levers.

First-Class Levers

A **first-class lever system** exists whenever two parallel forces (or parallel resultant forces) are applied on either side of an axis at some distance from that axis, creating (or tending to create) rotation of the lever in opposite directions. A first-class lever is commonly exemplified by a seesaw (Fig. 1–39a). The lever, or seesaw, is being subjected to four forces (because four things touch the lever). These are the contact of man A, the contact of man B, the contact of the wedge, and the contact of gravity. Figure

1–39b shows a schematic representation of the lever and the forces acting on it. Wedge-on-seesaw (WS) and gravity-on-seesaw (GS) are applied to the COG of the seesaw and are part of a linear force system. Because these two forces do not lie at a distance from each other (they are part of a linear force system) or do not lie at some distance from the axis (the wedge), we will ignore them for the moment and focus on the effects of vectors A and B. Figure 1–40 shows the seesaw and its forces diagrammed once again, but labeled differently than in Figure 1–39b. Force B has been renamed the effort force (EF). The **effort force** is defined as the force that is *causing the rotation of the lever.* Force A has been labeled the resistance force (R). The **resistance force** is the force that is *opposing the rotation of the lever* (pulling in a direction opposite to the rotation that is occurring). This assumes, of course, that man B is causing the rotation of the seesaw; that is, that the seesaw is going down on the side of man B. If the seesaw were balanced (in equilibrium), neither force would be *causing* motion because none is occurring. When there is equilibrium, it is arbitrary as to which force is identified as the effort and which as the resistance. Whenever equilibrium does not exist (whenever the lever is rotating), rotation of the lever will *always* occur in the direction exerted by the effort force or, more correctly stated, the effort force is the force pulling in the direction of movement.

The **lever arm (LA)** in a parallel force system is the distance from the axis to the point at which a force is applied to the lever. The term *lever arm* is used in this text to specifically describe how far away from the axis the force is applied; it does *not* refer to the length of the lever. The **effort arm (EA)** refers specifically to the lever arm of the effort force or how far the effort force lies from the axis. Similarly, the **resistance arm (RA)** refers to the lever arm of the resistance force or how far the resistance force lies from the axis (see Fig. 1–40). In a first-class

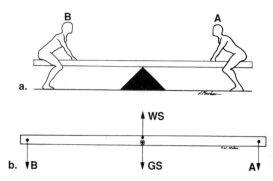

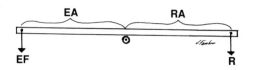

FIGURE 1–39. (a) A seesaw is commonly used to represent a lever to which forces are applied. (b) The lever is contacted by man A, man B, gravity on the seesaw (GS), and the wedge (WS) that serves as its axis.

FIGURE 1–40. First-class lever system. EF is the effort force that lies at a distance EA (effort arm) from the axis. R is the resistance that lies at a distance RA (resistance arm) from the axis.

Basic Concepts in Biomechanics

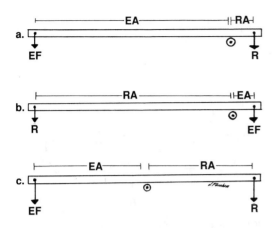

FIGURE 1–41. In a first-class lever system, EA may be (a) greater than RA, (b) smaller than RA, or (c) equal to RA.

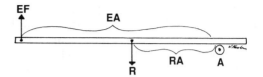

FIGURE 1–43. Second-class lever system. The effort arm (EA) is always larger than the resistance arm (RA).

Second-Class Levers

A **second-class lever** exists whenever two parallel forces (or parallel resultant forces) are applied at some distance from the axis, with the resistance force applied closer to the axis than the effort force (Fig. 1–43). In a second-class lever EA is *always* greater than RA. Second-class levers in the human body commonly occur when gravity is the effort force and muscles are the resistance. There are also examples of second-class levers in which the muscle is the effort force, but the distal segment to which the muscle is attached is weight bearing. The result is movement of the proximal rather than distal lever. Figure 1–44 shows the action of the triceps surae (gastrocnemius, soleus, and plantaris) lifting the body around the axis of the toes (metatarsophalangeal joints). The superimposed body weight acting on the foot through the LOG is the resistance (R). Because the muscles are the effort and the body weight is the resistance, a second-class lever system is formed.

There are no apparent examples in the human body of second-class levers in which the muscle is the effort force, causing movement of its distal lever against the resistance of gravity.

lever, EA may be greater than, smaller than, or equal to RA (Fig. 1–41) because the axis may be located anywhere between the effort force and the resistance force without changing the classification of the lever.

The human body has relatively few first-class levers. Figure 1–42 shows two parallel forces acting on the forearm lever; one is the force of the triceps at the olecranon, creating a clockwise rotation, and the other is a resultant external force pushing up on the forearm in a counterclockwise direction. This constitutes a first-class lever regardless of which force is labeled the effort and which is labeled the resistance because the axis lies between the two forces. If the forearm were to extend, the triceps brachii would be the effort force. If the external force overcame the triceps force and the forearm flexed, the external force would be the effort.

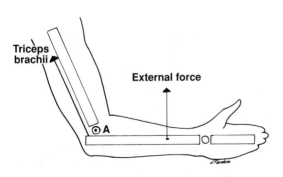

FIGURE 1–42. First-class lever in the human body. The force of the triceps muscle on the olecranon of the ulna and an external force on the ulna are separated by the axis (A).

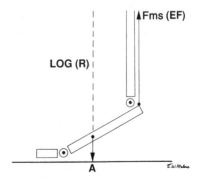

FIGURE 1–44. As the triceps surae (Fms) actively contract, the weight of the body (LOG) is lifted around the metatarsophalangeal (MTP) axis of the toes. The force of Fms (EF) and the force of gravity (R) act on a second-class lever with the axis at the MTP joints.

In such an instance the point of application of the muscle would have to lie farther from the axis than the COG of the limb being moved. No muscles have attachments that meet this requirement. Consequently, all second-class levers in the body occur either with a muscle eccentrically contracting against an external moving force or in some circumstances when a muscle is acting on its proximal segment while the distal segment is fixed.

Third-Class Levers

A **third-class lever** exists whenever two parallel forces (or parallel force components) on a lever are applied so that the effort force lies closer to the axis of the lever than does the resistance (Fig. 1–45). In a third-class lever, EA will *always* be smaller than RA. In the human body, most muscles creating rotation of their distal segments are part of third-class lever systems. The point of attachment of the muscle causing the motion is almost always closer to the joint axis than the external force that is usually resisting the motion. Figure 1–46 shows an example of a third-class lever system with the biceps brachii performing flexion of the forearm/hand segment against the resistance of gravity. Because the biceps force is labeled as EF, the rotation must be occurring in the direction of the biceps force. Gravity is opposing the motion and is labeled R.

Torque

Regardless of the class of the lever, the rotation of the segment depends both on the magnitude of force exerted by the effort and resistance forces and on the *distance the forces lie from the axis*. The ability of any force to cause rotation of the lever is known as **torque** or **moment of force.** Torque (T) is a product of the magnitude of the applied force (f) and the distance (d) that force lies from the axis of rotation. The distance (d) is the *shortest* distance between the action

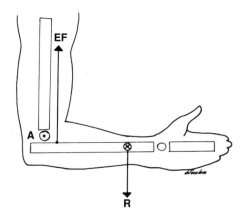

FIGURE 1–46. Third-class lever in the human body. The biceps brachii, as the effort force (EF), lies closer to the axis (A) than gravity (R).

line of the applied force and the axis of the lever; it is the length of a line drawn perpendicular to the action line of the force and intersecting the axis. Therefore,

$$T = (F)(\perp d)$$

In the schematic example of a second-class lever in Figure 1–43, $\perp d$ for the effort force and the resistance force would correspond to the lever arms EA and RA, respectively. In this example EA and RA are already perpendicular to their respective forces and, therefore, represent the shortest distance between the forces and the axis.

If hypothetical magnitudes and distances were given in Figure 1–46, the net torque acting on the lever could be determined. Assume that the biceps brachii (EF) is contracting with a force of 120 lb applied at a distance (EA) of 1 inch from the axis. The weight of the forearm/hand segment (R) is 10 lb and the COG of the segment lies 10 inches (RA) from the axis. Then:

$T_{EF} = (F)(EA)$	$T_R = (F)(RA)$
$T_{EF} = (120\text{ lb})(1\text{ in})$	$T_R = (10\text{ lb})(10\text{ in})$
$T_{EF} = 120\text{ in-lb}$	$T_R = 100\text{ in-lb}$

The biceps brachii exerts a torque of 120 in-lb on the forearm in a counterclockwise or positive direction ($T_{EF} = +120$ in-lb). The torque exerted by gravity is in a clockwise or negative direction ($T_R = -100$ in-lb).

- The **net rotation** (or **resultant torque**) of a lever can be determined by finding the sum of all the torques acting on the lever (maintaining appropriate positive and negative signs).

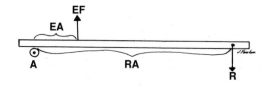

FIGURE 1–45. Third-class lever system. The effort arm (EA) is always smaller than the resistance arm (RA).

• Forces that act through an axis (at no distance from it) cannot produce torque on that lever.

The second bulleted point addresses why we were able to ignore the effect of the gravity and the contact of the wedge on the seesaw in Figure 1–39. Because both of these forces acted through the axis of rotation of the seesaw (the wedge), neither created a torque on the seesaw and was not relevant to determining the resultant torque of the seesaw.

When the sum of all the torques is zero, the torques are balanced and the lever will not rotate. The lever is in rotational equilibrium when

$$\Sigma_T = 0$$

In the example above where the torque of the biceps (EF) was +120 in-lb and the torque of gravity was −100 in-lb, the resultant torque is +20 in-lb or 20 in-lb of torque in a counterclockwise direction (flexion of the forearm/hand segment).

COMPOSITION OF FORCES IN A PARALLEL FORCE SYSTEM

Figure 1–47 shows the forearm/hand segment being acted on by three forces: the muscle force of the biceps brachii on the forearm at its attachment (Fms = 120 lb), the force of gravity on the forearm/hand at the COG (G = 10 lb), and the contact of the weight ball on the forearm/hand at its point of contact (WH = 5 lb). The lever arms of these forces are 1, 10, and 15 inches, respectively. We can find the net torque acting on the lever by finding the sum of the torques created by each force. If we also wish to determine the class of the lever, the task is simplified if we compose forces until there is a single effort force and a single resistance.

In a parallel force system, all forces causing rotation in one direction can be represented by a single vector that acts in the same direction and has a magnitude equal to the sum of the magnitudes of the composing forces. Vectors G and WH can be combined and represented by vector GWH. The point of application of the resultant vector GWH will lie on a line between the original two vectors. This is how the new COG was located when the COGs of two composing segments were known. Now the precise point of application of the new resultant force can be determined:

• When two or more parallel forces applied to a lever are composed into a single resultant force, the magnitude of the resultant force will be equal to the sum of the magnitudes of the original forces and will be applied in the same direction.

• When two or more parallel forces applied to a lever are composed into a single resultant force, the torque produced by the resultant will be the same as the net torque produced by the original forces.

• The point of application of the resultant force can be found once its magnitude and the torque it produces are known by solving the torque equation for the perpendicular distance:

$$\bot d = T \div F$$

GWH will be equal in magnitude to the magnitudes of the composing forces G and WH:

$$GWH = (10 \text{ lb}) + (5 \text{ lb})$$
$$GWH = 15 \text{ lb}$$

The torque of GWH will be the same as the net torques produced by vectors G and WH:

$$T_G = (-10 \text{ lb}) (10 \text{ in}) \qquad T_{WH} = (-5 \text{ lb}) (15 \text{ in})$$
$$T_G = -100 \text{ in-lb} \qquad T_{WH} = -75 \text{ in-lb}$$

Therefore, T_{GWH} must be:

$$T_{GWH} = (-100 \text{ in-lb}) + (-75 \text{ in-lb})$$
$$T_{GWH} = -175 \text{ in-lb}$$

Because both the torque and magnitude of GWH are known, the distance ($\bot d$) from the axis can be determined.

$$\bot d = T \div F$$
$$\bot d = -175 \text{ in-lb} \div 15 \text{ lb}$$
$$\bot d = 11.67 \text{ in}$$

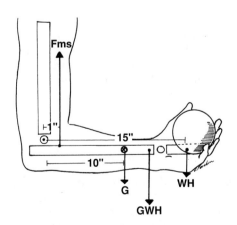

FIGURE 1–47. The class of the lever can be identified by determining the net torque acting on the lever. The net rotation will be in the direction of force EF.

The resultant force GWH in Figure 1–47 has a magnitude of 15 lb, lies 11.67 inches from the joint axis, and applies a torque of 175 in-lb in a clockwise direction.

Although the number of forces acting on the forearm/hand segment has been reduced to two (Fms and GWH), the class of the lever cannot be determined until it has been determined which is the effort force and which is the resistance force. To determine this, the direction of movement must be ascertained. The effort force is the force *producing* the motion in the direction of the net torque. To determine the net torque acting on the forearm/hand segment in Figure 1–47, the torque exerted by the muscle (Fms) must be found. The torque produced by Fms would be:

$$T_{Fms} = (+120 \text{ lb}) (1 \text{ in})$$
$$T_{Fms} = +120 \text{ in-lb}$$

The resultant torque on the lever will be the sum of the torques produced by GWH and Fms:

$$T = T_{Fms} + T_{GWH}$$
$$T = (+120 \text{ in-lb}) + (-175 \text{ in-lb})$$
$$T = -55 \text{ in-lb}$$

The forearm/hand segment is rotating in a clockwise direction (elbow extension) with a magnitude of 55 in-lb of torque. Because rotation is occurring in the direction of GWH, GWH must be the effort force and Fms the resistance. The resistance lies between the axis and the effort, so these two forces are operating in a second-class lever.

The example just analyzed points out that simply describing that the elbow is extending (a kinematic description) can lead to erroneous conclusions about what muscles might be active (kinetics). In this instance, the elbow is extending despite the fact that there are no active *elbow extensors*. In fact, the only active muscle is an elbow flexor! An understanding of the muscles and other forces involved in any movement can only occur through a kinetic analysis of the motion (a dynamic analysis) and not simply by describing the location, direction, or magnitude of motion.

In the examples given for both Figures 1–46 and 1–47, the biceps brachii, an elbow flexor, is exerting a 120-lb force. In one instance, however, the elbow is flexing (Fig.1–46) and in one instance the elbow is extending (Fig. 1–47). The force of the muscle, while consistently applied toward flexion, is losing to the combined forces of gravity and the weight in the latter ex-ample. The elbow flexor in effect is acting as a brake or *control* to the two external forces. Because the muscle is pulling the lever in one direction, yet the lever is moving in the opposite direction, the muscle must be getting longer (its two attachments are moving away from each other). When an *active* muscle is lengthening, it is contracting **eccentrically.** An eccentric contraction can only occur when the muscle is acting as the resistance force; that is, an eccentric contraction is resisting the force causing the motion. When an *active* muscle is shortening (as it will any time the muscle is the effort force), it is contracting **concentrically.** When the biceps brachii was the effort force and was *producing* elbow flexion, the forearm/ hand segment was a third-class lever. When the muscle became the *resisting* force, the forearm/hand segment became second class. Because most muscles in the body act on third-class levers when the muscle is contracting concentrically *and* distal lever free, the most common second-class lever in the human body is when the same muscles work eccentrically as brakes (the controlling resistance) to external forces.

- When an active muscle shortens (performs a concentric contraction), it must be moving the segment under consideration in the direction of its pull so that the muscle will be the effort force.
- When an active muscle lengthens, it is contracting eccentrically and must be pulling in a direction opposite to motion of the segment under consideration; that is, it is the resistance force and serves to control (slow down) the force producing the motion.
- When a lever is in rotational equilibrium, muscles acting on the segment under consideration are neither shortening nor lengthening. Such muscles would be performing an **isometric** contraction (iso = same; metric = length). In such a case, labeling of the muscles as effort or resistance forces is arbitrary.

Mechanical Advantage

Mechanical advantage (M Ad) is a measure of the efficiency of the lever (the relative effectiveness of the effort force compared to the resistance). M Ad is related to the classification of a lever and can be used to develop an understanding of the relevance of the concept of classes of levers. M Ad is the ratio of the *effort arm* to the *resistance arm*, or

$$M\ Ad = EA \div RA$$

When the effort arm (EA) is larger than the resistance arm (RA), the M Ad will be greater than 1. When the M Ad is greater than 1, the magnitude of the effort force can be smaller than the magnitude of the resistance and still "win" (cause movement in the direction of its pull). Recall that the torque of the effort force by definition will always be greater than the torque of the resistance force, or

$$(EF)\ (EA) > (R)\ (RA)$$

When EA is larger than RA (as it is when the M Ad > 1), then EF can be smaller than R and still create more torque. The greater the ratio of EA to RA, the smaller EF can be compared to R and still "win." The advantage to a lever with a M Ad greater than 1 is simply that the effort can overcome the resistance without expending as much force as the resistance.

In the example shown in Figure 1–47, EF was vector GWH applied 11.67 inches from the axis. R was the force of the biceps brachii applied 1 inch from the axis. Therefore,

$$M\ Ad = 11.67\ in \div 1\ in = 11.67$$

The forearm/hand segment, a second-class lever, was efficient because it took only 15 lb of force GWH to overcome 120 lb of force exerted by the biceps brachii. A second-class lever (EA > RA) is always efficient or has a M Ad greater than 1, although the magnitude of the M Ad will vary with the lever and the forces applied to it. It should be noted here that M Ad is determined by the lengths of the lever arms and *not* by the magnitudes of the effort and resistance forces. Although the effort force *may* be smaller than the resistance force in a second-class lever, it does not have to be. That is, if GWH in Figure 1–47 had a magnitude of 150 lb and Fms still had a magnitude of 120 lb, GWH would still create a larger torque (a much larger torque!) and would still be the effort force. The lever would still have a mechanical advantage of 11.67.

In third-class levers, EA is always smaller than RA because the effort force lies closer to the axis than the resistance. The M Ad of a third-class lever, therefore, will always be less than 1. A third-class lever is inefficient in that the magnitude of the effort required to move the lever *must* be *greater* than the magnitude of the resistance. To generate more torque than the resistance force, the effort force must be greater in magnitude because it works through a smaller distance.

- In all second-class levers, the M Ad of the lever will always be greater than 1. The magnitude of the effort force can be (but is not necessarily) less than the magnitude of the resistance.
- In all third-class levers, the M Ad of the lever will always be less than 1. The magnitude of the effort force *must* be *greater* than the magnitude of the resistance for the effort to produce greater torque.
- First-class levers follow no rules relative to M Ad. EA can be greater than, less than, or equal to RA. It is level dependent.

TRADE-OFFS OF MECHANICAL ADVANTAGE

It has already been observed that the majority of the muscles in the human body act as part of third-class lever systems when contracting both concentrically and distal lever free. It would appear, then, that the human body is structured inefficiently. In fact, the muscles of the body are structured to take on the burden of "mechanical disadvantage" to achieve the goal of moving the lever through space.

Figure 1–48a shows the forearm/hand segment being flexed (rotated counterclockwise) through space by a concentrically contracting muscle (Fms) against the resistance of gravity (G). This is a third-class lever, because the effort force lies closer to the axis than the resistance. It has already been shown that the magnitude of Fms must be much larger than the magnitude of G for flexion of the forearm/hand segment to occur. The system is, indeed, inefficient. However, as Fms pulls its point of application (on the proximal forearm/hand lever) through a very small arc, the distal portion of the lever is displaced through a much greater arc. Although the muscle force needed to create the movement was large compared to the resistance, the result was a large angular displacement and angular velocity for the distal portion of the segment. Where the goal in human function is to maximize angular displacement of a distal segment through space (at the expense of energy cost), the use of third-class lever systems achieves the desired goal. In fact, the shorter the lever arm of the effort force (resulting in a diminishing mechanical advantage), the greater is the angular displacement and angular velocity of the distal end of the lever for a given arc of displacement of the effort force.

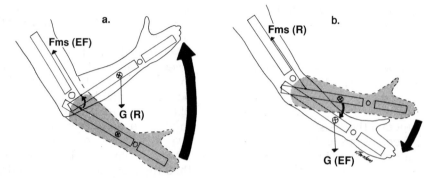

FIGURE 1–48. (a) In a mechanically inefficient third-class lever, movement of the point of application of EF (Fms) through a small arc produces a large arc of movement of the lever distally. (b) In a mechanically efficient second-class lever, movement of the point of application of EF (G) through a small arc produces little increase in the arc distally.

In second-class levers in the human body, the effort force is usually (but not always) the external force. Although the effort force in a second-class lever can be smaller in magnitude than the resistance, less is gained in angular displacement and velocity at the distal end of the segment. A small arc of movement at the point of application of the effort force (G) results in only a small increase in angular displacement of the more distal segment (see Fig. 1–48b). In any second-class lever (and in a first-class lever where EA > RA), the lever is efficient in terms of force output to torque production, but relatively less is gained in terms of angular displacement of the distal end of the segment through space. In fact, the larger EA becomes (resulting in a greater mechanical advantage), the less angular displacement there is distally for a given displacement of the effort force.

- When the muscle is the effort force and the EA is smaller than the RA, the magnitude of the effort force must be large, but the necessary expenditure of muscle force is offset by gains in angular displacement and angular velocity of the distal portions of the segment. This is true (to varying degrees) for all third-class levers and for first-class levers in which RA is greater than EA.
- When the external force is the effort force and the EA is larger than the RA, the magnitude of the effort can be small as compared to the resistance, but less is gained in angular displacement and velocity. This is true (to varying degrees) for all second-class levers and for first-class levers in which EA is greater than RA.

When one is looking at the advantages and disadvantages of each lever class, it is impor-

tant to keep in mind the role of the muscle. In the typical second-class lever in the body (distal lever free), the external effort force is the efficient force on the lever. The muscle is still expending a large amount of eccentric resistance force to control motion of the lever. In a third-class lever, the muscle effort force overcomes the resistance, but at the cost of large force requirements. Consequently, the muscle must be able to create large forces regardless of the class of the lever. As shall be shown in Chapter 3, the muscle is structured to optimize production of the large forces required both to produce large angular displacements of the distal segments of the body in mechanically inefficient lever systems and to resist the external forces in mechanically efficient lever systems.

Work

A more thorough understanding of the functional significance of classification of levers and of the role of muscles in human lever systems can be achieved by looking at the mechanical concept of work and the related concept of energy. In mechanical terms, **work** is done by a force applied to an object whenever the force is applied parallel to motion of the object. The magnitude of work is directly proportional to the applied force (F) and to the magnitude of displacement (d) of the object to which the force is applied. Most simply, this relationship can be expressed by

$$W = (F)(d)$$

where the direction of the applied force is parallel to the movement produced. When this is not the case, only the portion of the force that *is* parallel to the direction of movement ($f_\parallel$) will contribute to work. That is,

$$W = (f_\parallel)(d)$$
$$\text{or}$$
$$W = F\,d\cos\theta$$

where θ is the angle between F and d.

Work is given in units of foot-pounds (ft-lb). The sign given to work will be positive if the force is exerted in the same direction as the motion and negative if the force is exerted in a direction opposite to the motion. When the movement being produced is rotatory, as it is when a lever is moving around a joint axis, then

$$W = (T)\theta$$

where T is the torque of the applied force (EF × EA) and θ is the angular displacement of the point of application of the force.

The net work done on an object is always the sum of the work produced by each of the forces applied to the object.

In Figure 1–48a and b, the muscle (Fms) displaces its point of application through a smaller distance than does the force of gravity because Fms is located closer to the axis than G. In Figure 1–48b, the muscle is doing negative work, because it exerts its force in a direction opposite to the motion that is occurring (it is performing an eccentric contraction). The fact that muscles can do negative work shows that the term *work* is a mechanical, rather than biomechanical, concept. A muscle doing an eccentric contraction is still expending energy. We humans tend to consider any expenditure of energy on our part as work, but this is not true mechanically during an eccentric contraction. If the resistance in a second-class lever were a spring rather than a muscle, virtually no energy would be expended by the spring; in fact, it would store energy (potential energy) because it is having work done on it. As we shall see in Chapter 3, the active contractile components of a muscle are not analogous to a mechanical spring. However, some parts of the muscle (the passive parallel and series connective tissue components) do behave somewhat as the spring does; these portions of the muscle store energy as they are elongated. The effect of negative work done by a muscle is that it takes *less* energy to exert 120 lb of eccentric muscle force through a given displacement than it does to exert 120 lb of concentric force through the same displacement. The reasons for this phenomenon are more complex than

the springlike qualities of the muscle and will be explored further in Chapter 3. To summarize:

- When a muscle is the effort force in a third-class lever, it does a concentric contraction and positive work. It expends additional force and energy to gain angular displacement and velocity.
- When a muscle is the resistance force in a second-class lever, it does an eccentric contraction and negative work, using less energy than a muscle producing the same force concentrically.

Moment Arm of Force

In the examples in which torque ($T = |F||\perp d|$) has been computed thus far, $\perp d$ has been equivalent to the lever arm of the force. Whenever the action line of the force is applied at 90° to the segment, $\perp d$ will lie along the lever and coincide with the lever arm for that force. Most often in the human body, however, forces are applied at some angle other than 90°. This is certainly true of the forces produced by muscles. The action lines of muscles rarely approach an angle of 90° because this would mean that the muscle would lie perpendicular to the bone. Humans would have an unusual shape if this were the rule, rather than the exception. Most muscles have action lines that are closer to being parallel to the bones to which they attach. When the force is not applied at 90° to the lever, the lever arm is no longer the shortest distance between the action line of the force and the joint axis. The **moment arm (MA)** is always the shortest distance between the action line and the joint axis and is found by measuring the length of a line drawn perpendicular to the force vector, intersecting the joint axis. Consequently,

$$MA = \perp d$$
$$\text{and}$$
$$T = (F)(MA)$$

When a force is applied at 90° to a segment, the MA and the lever arm (LA) are equivalent. At all other angles, as shall be seen, the MA will be smaller than the LA.

Moment Arm of a Muscle Force

In Figures 1–49a to c, the force applied to the lever has a constant magnitude, but is changing its angle of application to the lever and,

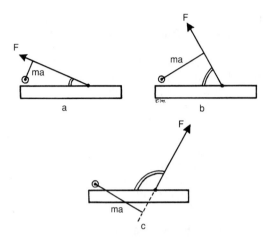

FIGURE 1–49. The angle of pull of the force is the angle between the lever and the vector on the side of the joint axis. As the angle of pull changes, so does the size of the moment arm of the force.

consequently, the length of its moment arm. The **angle of application of a force** is the angle between the action line and the lever *on the side of the joint axis*. The lever arm, as previously defined, is the distance from the point of application of the force to the joint axis. The LAs in Figures 1–49a to c do not change. However, the MA changes with a change in the angle of application of the force. The torque exerted by the force is the product of the magnitude of F in pounds and the size of the MA in inches for each of the three positions. Consequently, both the moment arm *and* the torque produced by the force differs for each of the three angles of application.

In Figure 1–50 the muscle vector of the biceps brachii is shown schematically as it applies a force to the forearm with the elbow joint at 35°, 70°, 90°, and 145° of elbow flexion. Please

be careful to note that these angles refer to the *elbow joint angle*, and *not* the angle of application of the muscle force. However, it is the angle of application of the muscle force in which we are interested. We refer to the elbow joint angle because this angle can be measured readily in humans, whereas the angle of application of the muscle force is very difficult or impossible to measure in humans.

The angle of pull of the action line of Fms on the forearm lever (see Fig. 1–50) can be seen to change as the elbow flexion angle changes. As the angle of *application of the force* changes, so does the length of the MA. The MA would appear to be smallest in Figure 1–50a and largest in Figure 1–50c. If the force of the biceps contraction is a constant 50 lb throughout the elbow range of motion, the torque will change in direct proportion to the change in the MA of the force. The torque would be least at 35° of elbow flexion (where the MA is smallest) and greatest at 90° of elbow flexion (where the MA is largest). The ability of the muscle to rotate the joint would vary during the movement, even though the muscle is contracting with a constant force.

The MA is the shortest distance between a vector and a joint axis. This distance can be infinitely small (it is zero whenever the action line passes *through* the joint axis), but it can never be larger than the distance between the point of application of the force and the joint axis (that is, the LA). Because the LA and the MA coincide whenever the force is applied at 90° to its lever, as in Figure 1–50c, the MA of any force will be largest when the force is applied at 90° to the lever. When the MA is greatest the potential for torque production by a force will be at its maximum.

When a force is applied to its lever at an angle *greater than* 90° as in Figures 1–49c and 1–50d

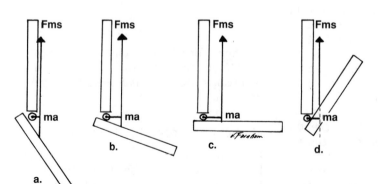

FIGURE 1–50. Schematic representation of the biceps brachii (Fms) exerting a force on the forearm at (a) 35°, (b) 70°, (c) 90°, and (d) 145° of elbow flexion.

(regardless of joint position!), the MA is found by extending the vector (this is the only way a line can be drawn perpendicular to the vector and intersecting the joint axis). Remember that vectors can be extended to assess their effect. The "tail" of the extended vector will get closer to the axis as the vector increases its angle of application. As the vector increases its angle of application past 90°, the MA will continue to get smaller.

- Given a constant force of contraction, the torque generated by a muscle is greatest at the point in the joint range of motion at which the muscle's action line lies farthest from the joint axis.
- The MA of any force is greatest when the action line is applied at 90° to its lever, or when the action line is as close to 90° as possible.

When the goal of a muscle is either to rotate a segment or to resist its rotation, the muscle is biomechanically most effective at the point in the range at which the muscle is capable of generating the greatest torque; that is, the point at which the MA of the muscle is greatest.

The critical factor in optimizing torque is in obtaining an angle of application of a force to a lever that is as close to 90° as possible. The *angle of application of the force* ordinarily is *not* directly related to the *joint angle*. The example of the biceps brachii in Figure 1–50 is unusual in that the angle of elbow flexion is similar to the angle of application of the force. This is true because the action line of the biceps lies con-sistently parallel to the humerus. For most muscles, the angle of application of the muscle force to the bone is quite different from the angle between the two bones forming the joint. Figure 1–51 shows the MA of the deltoid in two different positions of the glenohumeral joint. In Figure 1–51a, the glenohumeral joint is at 0° of abduction, but the angle of pull of the deltoid is about 5° to the humerus. In Figure 1–51b, the glenohumeral joint is at 60° of shoulder abduction, but the action line of the deltoid has only increased to about 15° to the humerus. However, at 60° of abduction of the glenohumeral joint, the deltoid muscle lies as far from the glenohumeral joint axis as it will get; the MA is maximal for this muscle even though the angle of application of the muscle force is still relatively small (although larger than when the joint was at 0°). The MA of any force is greatest when the angle of application of the force is greatest (or closest to 90° to the lever), regardless of joint position.

Moment Arm of Gravity

Any force applied to a lever may change its angle of application as the lever moves through space. The change in angle of application will result in an increase or decrease in the MA of that force. Figure 1–52 shows the forearm at the same ranges of elbow flexion shown in Figure 1–50, with the force of gravity applied to the forearm lever at its COG. As the angle of application of the LOG (the gravitational vector)

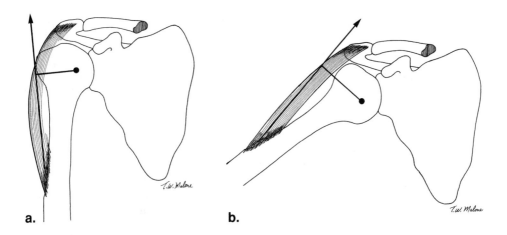

a.   **b.**

FIGURE 1–51. The action line of the deltoid muscle (Fms) at 0° of shoulder abduction (a) and at 60° of shoulder abduction (b). The moment arm (MA) of the deltoid is larger at 60° than at any point in the gleno-humeral range.

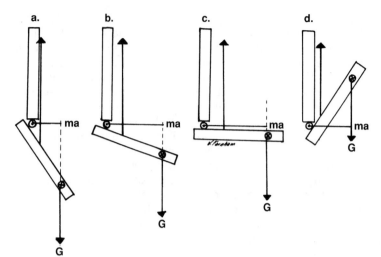

FIGURE 1–52. Gravity (G) acting on the forearm at (a) 35°, (b) 70°, (c) 90°, and (d) 145° of elbow flexion. The MA of gravity changes with the position of the forearm.

changes, so does the length of the MA. As is true for all forces, the MA of the force of gravity is greatest when the force is applied at 90° to the lever. Unlike muscle forces, however, the LOG is always vertical and is completely independent of joint position. For example, Figure 1–53 shows

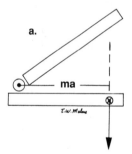

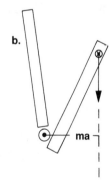

FIGURE 1–53. The LOG remains vertical regardless of the position of the forearm in space. As the angle of application of LOG changes with respect to the forearm, the MA also changes.

two different positions of the forearm and humerus levers in space. In both instances, the elbow is flexed to 135°. Figure 1–53a has a very large MA because the LOG is applied at 90° to the lever (MA is at its maximum value). Figure 1–53b has a much smaller MA because the LOG is only about 30°.

- Because gravity always acts vertically downward, the angle of application of gravity changes as the segment moves in space.
- The force of gravity will be applied perpendicular to a segment whenever the segment is parallel to the ground.
- When a body lever is parallel to the ground, gravity acting on that segment exerts its maximum torque.

Figure 1–54 shows three graded exercises for trunk flexion. The vertebral interspace of L5 to S1 is considered here to be the hypothetical axis about which the segmented head/arms/trunk segment (HAT) rotates. In Figure 1–54a, the arms are raised above the head (the segments are rearranged) causing the COG of HAT to move toward the head (cephalad). The LOG lies at a great distance (MA) from the L5 to S1 axis. The torque generated by gravity is counterclockwise and has a magnitude equivalent to the product of the weight of HAT (two-thirds of body weight) and the MA. For the posture to be maintained (rotational equilibrium), the abdominal muscles must generate an equal torque in the opposite direction.

In Figure 1–54b and c, the COGs move caudally as the arms are lowered. The relocation of the COG of HAT (through rearrangement of the segments) brings the LOG closer to the L5 to

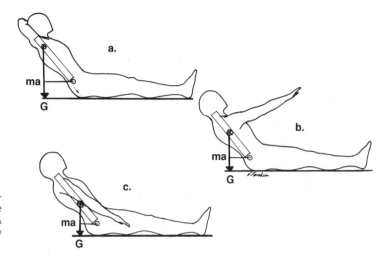

FIGURE 1–54. Changes in arm position in a sit-up cause the COG of the upper body segment to move, the MA to change, and the torque of gravity (G) to decrease from a to c.

S1 axis and reduces the length of the MA. Because the weight of the upper body does not change when the arms are lowered, the magnitude of torque applied by gravity to the upper body diminishes in proportion to the reduction in the MA. The decreased gravitational torque requires less opposing torque by the abdominal muscles to maintain equilibrium. Consequently, it is easiest to maintain the position in Figure 1–54c and hardest to maintain the position in Figure 1–54a.

The angle of pull of the abdominal muscles changes relatively little as the trunk lever moves through space. When increased torque production is needed by the abdominal muscles, the increase will occur predominantly through an increase in the force of contraction of the muscles (Fms). When the abdominal muscles are weak, the muscles may not be capable of exerting the force needed to balance the magnitude of gravitational torque in Figure 1–54a. It may be possible, however, for the muscles to counteract the lesser gravitational torque produced in Figure 1–54b or smallest gravitational torque in Figure 1–54c.

Anatomic Pulleys

It has already been noted that anatomic pulleys change the direction but not the magnitude of a muscle force. The change in direction of the muscle force results, however, in improved ability of the muscle to generate torque. The change in direction or deflection of the action line of a muscle in an anatomic pulley is *away* from the axis of the joint being crossed. By deflecting the action line away

from the joint axis, the MA of the muscle force is increased. Figure 1–55 shows the quadriceps femoris muscle acting on the tibia. Figure 1–55a shows a schematic representation of the action line of the quadriceps without the patella. The action line lies parallel to the femur and close to the knee joint axis; the MA is small. Figure 1–55b shows the deflection of the action line away from the joint axis when the patella is interposed; the MA is significantly larger. If the quadriceps femoris muscle contracted with equal magnitude both with and without the patella, the torque applied to the tibia by the muscle would be much greater with the patella because the force is applied at a greater distance from the joint axis.

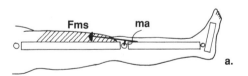

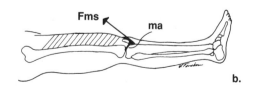

FIGURE 1–55. (a) Schematic representation of the action line of the quadriceps femoris without the patella. (b) The action line of the quadriceps femoris deflected by the patella, increasing the MA.

- Anatomic pulleys change the direction of pull of a muscle.
- Anatomic pulleys deflect the line of pull of a muscle away from the joint axis, thus increasing the MA of the muscle and, consequently, the muscle's ability to produce torque.

Force Components

We have shown that a given magnitude of force applied to a lever at some angle other than 90° will result in less torque than the same force applied at 90°. If the same magnitude of force can produce less torque in one place in the range than in another, some of the applied force must be "wasted" (not producing rotation) when applied at angles other than 90°. Torque, in fact, is produced only by that *portion* of the force that is directed toward rotation.

Although torque is the product of total force and its shortest (perpendicular) distance from the joint axis, it is equivalently a product of the *portion of the force that is directed toward rotation* and its shortest (perpendicular) distance from the joint axis. The portion of the force applied perpendicular to the lever is known as the **rotatory component of the force (f_r)**.

Torque can now be expressed in three equivalent ways. Generically,

$$T = (F)\,(\perp d)$$

When using the magnitude of the total force,

$$T = (F)\,(MA)$$

When using just the magnitude of the proportion of force expended toward rotating the lever:

$$T = (f_r)\,(LA)$$

To find the torque using the magnitude of the rotatory component, its shortest distance from the joint axis will be LA. The LA is the distance between the point of application of the force and the joint axis *along the lever*. Because f_r is drawn perpendicular to the lever, then LA is by definition going to be perpendicular to f_r.

Figure 1–56a shows the biceps brachii force applied at an angle of approximately 80° to the forearm lever. The torque produced by Fms can be determined by calculating $f_r \times$ LA if the f_r and the LA can be ascertained. The magnitude of f_r can be found graphically or mathematically by **resolution** of the vector force Fms into two components. Just as two concurrent forces can be composed into a single resultant vector, a single vector can be resolved into two concurrent components. In this case, the components will be specifically constructed so that one component (f_r) lies perpendicular to the lever. The second component will be the **translatory component (f_t)** and is drawn parallel to the lever. Effectively, the translatory component will pass through the joint axis (although this is not always the case as we shall see). A force that passes through an axis does not create a torque around that axis, but will impose a linear force on the segment. Thus, resolving Fms into perpendicular and parallel components will give both the proportion of Fms applied toward rotation (the portion applied perpendicular to the lever) *and* the portion of Fms affecting the translation of the segment (the portion applied parallel to the lever).

To resolve the resultant vector Fms in Figure 1–56a into its perpendicular and parallel concurrent components, we reverse the process used for composition of forces. A parallelogram will be constructed with the resultant force as the diagonal. For our purposes here, the parallelogram will always be a rectangle because the sides are purposefully drawn perpendicular and parallel to the lever and, therefore, at right angles to each other. To construct the rectangle:

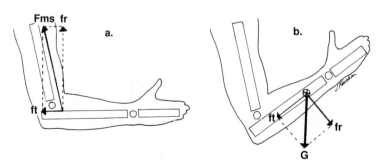

FIGURE 1–56. (a) Resolution of a muscle action line (Fms) into rotatory (f_r) and translatory (f_t) components. (b) Resolution of gravity (G) into rotatory and translatory components.

1. Starting at the point of application of the resultant (total) force, the component f_r is drawn perpendicular to the *long axis of the moving lever.*
2. Starting again at the point of application of the resultant force, component f_t is drawn parallel to the *long axis of the moving lever.*
3. From the head of the resultant vector, a line is drawn that is parallel to f_r.
4. From the head of the resultant vector, a line is drawn parallel to f_t. In this way a rectangle is constructed for which the total force is the diagonal.

Component vectors f_r and f_t are the sides of the constructed rectangle. If the scale of a diagram is known, graphic resolution permits measurement of the components and calculation of magnitudes. For example, if the scale in Figure 1–56a were 1/16 inch = 10 lb, then vector Fms would have a magnitude of 320 lb. The translatory component of Fms would have a magnitude of 50 lb and the rotatory component would have a magnitude of 190 lb. Note that the magnitude of the resultant force is not equal to the sum of its components f_r and f_t. In any concurrent force system, the sum of the component forces will always be greater than the magnitude of the resultant force. Determination of the magnitude of the component vectors could also be obtained trigonometrically. If both the magnitude of the total force and the angle of application of the total force are known:

$$f_r = F \sin \theta$$
$$f_t = F \cos \theta$$

For any given angle of application of a force, the components f_r and f_t will always have the same proportional relationship to the total force and to each other. For example, f_r is almost four times larger than f_t in Figure 1–56. This will be true regardless of the magnitude of the resultant force (Fms in this example). If the magnitude of Fms were to increase or decrease, the magnitudes of both f_r and f_t would increase or decrease proportionally. The magnitue of f_r would remain approximately four times longer than that of f_t.

The translatory component of any force represents that portion of the total force that is applied toward linear movement of the lever. The translatory component of a force is not "wasted" but is simply applied in a direction that contributes to something other than rota-

tion. In the human body, the translatory component of a force can be thought of as either being toward the joint being analyzed or away from the joint being analyzed. A translatory force that is applied *toward a joint* would move or attempt to move the segment to which the force is applied toward its adjacent joint segment. Because this would bring the two joint segments together, a translatory force applied in the direction of the joint is referred to as a **compression component.** A compression component generally contributes to the stability of a joint by maintaining contact between contiguous joint surfaces. Conversely, a translatory force *away from a joint* would tend to separate the adjacent joint segments and is known as a **distraction component.** Distraction forces across the knee joint caused by the application of an external load were shown in the example of traction applied to the leg (see Fig. 1–32).

Figure 1–56b shows the graphic resolution of gravity acting on the forearm into its rotatory and translatory components. In this instance, the resultant force G is applying equal portions of its force toward rotation and translation because the magnitudes of the two components appear to be equal. The translatory force of gravity is applied toward the elbow joint (the axis for forearm motion) and is, therefore, a compression force.

It has been shown that applying a force of constant magnitude to a lever as it rotates around its joint axis is likely to result in a varying angle of application of the force and, consequently, a varying torque. Because the rotatory component of a force is the portion of the total force that produces torque, a change in torque applied by a constant force must mean that there has been a change in the magnitude of the rotatory component. Similarly, a change in the rotatory component must indicate a change in the proportion of the total force applied toward translation, because the magnitudes of the rotatory component and the translatory component are indirectly proportional to each other. That is, when there is an increase in the portion of the total force applied perpendicular to the lever, concomitantly there will be a decrease in the proportion of the total force applied parallel to the lever (and vice versa).

- If the torque of a force of constant magnitude changes as the lever moves through space, the angle of application of the force must be changing.

- If the angle of application of a force changes, the relative magnitudes of the rotatory and translatory components must also change.

The changing torque produced by a constant force as a lever moves around its joint axis can be seen either as a function of the change in MA (distance of the force from the joint axis) or the change in the rotatory component (portion of the force applied perpendicular to the lever). Consequently, it should be seen that these two quantities are directly proportional to each other. Figure 1–50 showed the change in MA of the biceps force with the elbow in four different positions. Figure 1–57 shows the same biceps force at the same elbow positions (35°, 70°, 90°, and 145° of elbow flexion), this time indicating the changing magnitude of the rotatory component. At 90° of elbow flexion, Fms is already applied at 90° to the lever; that is, Fms and f_r coincide and all the force is applied to rotation without any translation. When any force is applied at 90° to a lever, f_r will be maximal because it will be equivalent to the total force. Similarly, the MA has already been shown to be greatest when a force is applied at 90°. When a force is applied at 90°, the two torque formulas (F × MA and f_r × LA) are virtually identical. When a force is applied at 90° to a lever, F and f_r are equivalent and MA and LA are equivalent.

Figure 1–57 shows not only the changing rotatory component but also the change in the translatory component in each position. The translatory component is larger than the rotatory component both at 35° of elbow flexion and at 145° of elbow flexion. As the action line of Fms moves closer to the lever (closer to lying parallel to the lever), f_t increases in size. As the action lines of Fms move farther from the axis as at 70° of elbow flexion), the translatory

component gets smaller. At 90° of elbow flexion, the entire force (Fms) is rotatory and there is no translatory component. The translatory component changes not only in magnitude during the range of elbow flexion, but also in direction. At 35° of elbow flexion the translatory force is toward the joint (compression), whereas at 145° of elbow flexion the translatory component is away from the joint (distraction).

The change of the translatory component from compression to distraction as seen in Figure 1–57 is unusual for a muscle force. In fact, most muscles lie close to their joint axes and nearly parallel to the lever, with action lines almost always directed toward the joint axis regardless of the position of the lever in space. The effect of this arrangement is that muscle forces generally have relatively small rotatory components, with large translatory components that are nearly always compressive. Most of the force generated by a muscle contributes to joint compression, rather than joint rotation! This enhances joint stability, but means that a muscle must generate a large total force to generate the rotatory force necessary to move the lever through space.

Figure 1–58 shows the resultant force of the brachioradialis muscle as it is applied to the forearm with the forearm in increasing flexion. This muscle is more typical of other muscles in the human body than is the biceps brachii. The angle of application of the brachioradialis changes relatively little, with the rotatory component never exceeding the translatory component (although f_r is still maximal at 90° of elbow flexion as is true of f_r for the biceps). The translatory force remains compression regardless of the position of the limb.

- The action line of most muscles is more parallel to the lever than perpendicular to the lever.

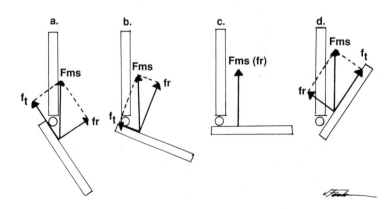

FIGURE 1–57. Resolution of the force of the biceps brachii (Fms) into rotatory (f_r) and translatory (f_t) components at (a) 35°, (b) 70°, (c) 90°, and (d) 145° of elbow flexion.

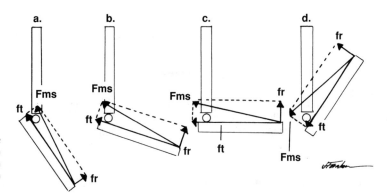

FIGURE 1–58. Resolution of the force of the brachioradialis (Fms) into rotatory (f_r) and translatory (f_t) components at (a) 35°, (b) 70°, (c) 90°, and (d) 145° of elbow flexion.

- The rotatory component of a muscle force is rarely larger than the translatory component.
- The translatory component of most muscle forces contributes to joint compression.

The constraints found to exist on muscle forces in the body do not apply to external forces. Figure 1–59 shows the force of gravity (G) applied to the leg with the leg at different

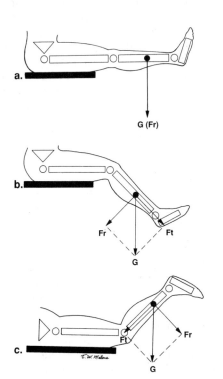

FIGURE 1–59. Resolution of the force of gravity (G) into rotatory (f_r) and translatory (f_t) components with the leg at different locations in space. (a) Gravity is all rotatory. (b) Gravity has rotatory and distraction components. (c) Gravity has rotatory and compression components.

points in space. In Figure 1–59a, the leg is parallel to the ground and force G is applied at 90° to the lever. The entire magnitude of G (G = f_r) is applied toward rotation of the knee joint in a clockwise direction (knee flexion).

In Figure 1–59b and c, force G is applied to the leg such that its rotatory and translatory components are approximately equal in magnitude. The torque applied by f_r to the knee joint is clockwise in both instances. However, the translatory component of vector G is distracting the knee joint in one instance and compressing the knee joint in the other. The change in direction of the translatory component is related to the change in position of the limb and, consequently, the change in angle of application of gravity. Vector G in Figure 1–59b is applied at 135° to the lever, whereas it is applied at 45° to the lever in Figure 1–59c.

In Figure 1–60 a manual external force (R_m) is applied to the leg in an attempt to flex the leg at the knee joint against the resistance of the quadriceps femoris muscle. By creating a clockwise torque with the forearm/hand, the quadriceps femoris muscle must apply a countertorque of equivalent magnitude to maintain the leg in the same position. Figure 1–60a resolves the manual force (R_m) into rotatory and translatory components. Although the majority of the manual force is applied toward rotation (f_r is substantially larger than f_t), some of the manual force is also "wasted" as a distraction force. In this instance, the distraction force serves no useful purpose and actually represents wasted effort for the person applying the manual resistance. The angle of application of the force applied by the forearm/hand, however, can be manipulated so that it lies perpendicular to the lever (see Fig.1–60b). With this shift in forearm-hand orientation, the person applying the manual resistance may con-

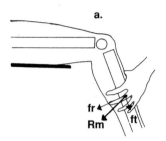 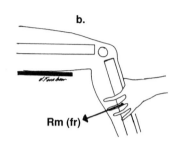

FIGURE 1–60. (a) A manual force (R_m) applied at an angle to the leg wastes force in the direction of distraction. (b) A manual force applied perpendicular to the leg results in a force that is all rotation.

tribute the same force but is able to exert more torque because none of the force is "wasted" as an undesirable translatory force.

Further manipulation of the manual resistance being applied in Figure 1–60 can further increase the biomechanical effectiveness of the applied force. A force will produce the greatest torque when the LA or MA is as large as possible. If the hand were placed at the ankle (instead of upper shin) and if the angle of application of the manual force were maintained at 90°, both the lever arm and rotatory component would be maximal. By maximizing f_r and LA, the greatest torque for a given magnitude of applied force (R_m) can be generated.

- The torque of an external force can be increased by increasing the magnitude of the applied force.
- The torque of an external force can be increased by applying the force perpendicular (or closer to perpendicular) to the lever.
- The torque of an external force can be increased by increasing how far the force is applied from the joint axis.

Equilibrium Levers

Rotational and Linear Equilibrium

When a limb segment in the body does not move, it must be in both rotational and translatory (linear) equilibrium. For a lever to be in **rotational equilibrium,** the sum of all the *torques* applied to that lever must be zero. When the lever is *not* in rotational equilibrium, it will undergo **angular acceleration.** The magnitude of angular acceleration is proportional to the unbalanced torque applied to the lever and inversely proportional to the mass of the lever being moved.

$$a_{angular} = T / m$$

Angular acceleration, as noted earlier, introduces to the lever a new set of forces that are beyond the scope of analysis in this text; it is sufficient to acknowledge that the magnitude of unbalanced torque applied to a lever is an *underestimation* of the forces applied to that lever while it is undergoing angular acceleration.

Forces or force components applied parallel to a lever (presuming they are in line with the joint axis) do not affect the rotation of a lever but will cause the lever to translate. For the lever to be in **linear equilibrium,** the arithmetic sum of all the parallel forces acting on the lever must be zero.

Figure 1–61a shows the force of gravity (G) on the dependent (hanging) leg. The total force of G is parallel to the lever, causing a pure distraction force. Because there are no perpendicular forces or force components applied to the leg, there can be no torques and the leg must be in rotational equilibrium. However, a single translatory force downward (distraction) cannot exist independently on the leg without pulling the knee joint apart. Consequently, there must be a balancing upward (compressive) force of equal magnitude applied to the lever by some other force or set of forces. Muscles predominantly produce compressive forces and a muscle might provide the compressive force in this example. However, if the person is completely relaxed the muscle should be contributing little or no force. The force required to produce linear equilibrium must come from something else that is touching the leg. The force can be provided by the upward pull of the knee joint ligaments that touch the leg and are capable of "pulling" on the leg with the needed amount of force. Because the ligaments surround the knee joint axis, the resultant ligamentous force can be considered in this situation to effectively act *through* the knee joint axis, creating a pure translatory force through the joint.

Figure 1–61b shows the leg being extended at the knee joint by the quadriceps muscle against the resistance of gravity (note: vectors are not drawn to scale). Because the leg is ex-

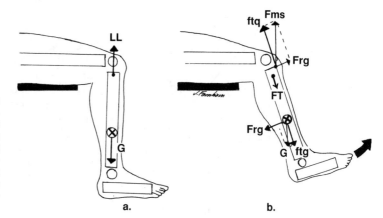

FIGURE 1–61. (a) The dependent leg is in rotatory and linear equilibrium. Gravity is offset by the pull of the knee ligaments on the leg (LL). (b) The quadriceps femoris is causing the leg to extend. Linear equilibrium is produced by the translatory force of the quadriceps (f_{tq}), the translatory force of gravity (f_{tg}), and the push of the femur on the tibia (FT).

tending, there must be a resultant counter-clockwise torque. In this example, the quadriceps force will be the effort force (causing the motion) and gravity will be the resistance force. The force of the quadriceps (Fms) and gravity (G) have been resolved into components. Let's assign the following values to the example:

$$f_{rq} = 100 \text{ lb} \qquad f_{rg} = 10 \text{ lb}$$
$$f_{tq} = 50 \text{ lb } f_{tg} \qquad f_{tg} = 5 \text{ lb}$$
$$\text{LA} = 1 \text{ inches} \qquad \text{LA} = 6 \text{ inches}$$

Although the leg can be rotating into extension and thus undergoing angular acceleration (net T > 0), the leg must be in *linear equilibrium* or the joint would be disrupted and the tibia would accelerate upward past the femur. The sum of the parallel (translatory) components acting on the lever, therefore, *has to be* zero. The translatory component of gravity (f_{tg}) is a 5 lb distraction force. The translatory component of the quadriceps force (f_{tq}) is a compression force of 50 lb. There would appear to be, therefore, a net compression force of 45 lb that would cause the tibia to accelerate toward the femur until the two bones make contact. Once the tibia and femur contact, the two forces of tibia-on-femur (TF) and femur-on-tibia (FT) are introduced. Because we are interested in setting the tibia in linear equilibrium, we can see that FT will be equal in magnitude and opposite in direction to the net compression force on the tibia *if* there are no other forces to account for. The force applied by one segment on its adjacent segment during joint compression is known as a **joint reaction force.** A joint reaction force is simply a special action-reaction pair or set of contact forces that occur between two adjacent bony segments.

Other Effects of Rotatory and Translatory Forces

We now know that forces applied to a lever can be resolved into components that are perpendicular to and parallel to the lever and that rotate and translate, respectively. In reality in the human body, the effects of rotatory and translatory components are a bit more complex. One segment not only rotates around another but, because our bones are *not* truly hinged, one segment can move as if it were simply contiguous to (touching) the segment adjacent to it. The result is that rotatory forces can also translate and translatory forces can also rotate! This can best be explained by example.

Figure 1–62 shows the force of the quadriceps on the tibia. The force Fms is resolved into its rotatory (f_1) and translatory (f_2) components that cause joint rotation and joint compression, respectively, *if* we consider the knee joint to have a fixed axis. However, now note that f_1 not only lies perpendicular to the tibia but also parallel to the tibial plateau. The component f_2 lies not only parallel to the tibia but also perpendicular to the tibial plateau. A force that lies perpendicular to contacting surfaces is a contact force. The fact that f_2 creates contact between the tibia and the femur was already acknowledged when we identified it as a compression force. However, up until this point, we have not seen (or at least acknowledged) that many of the translatory forces such as we see here for f_2 do not truly pass through the joint axis, but lie at some distance from it. Whenever a force is applied at some distance from a joint axis, a torque is created. Given the shape of the articular surfaces and at the point of attach-

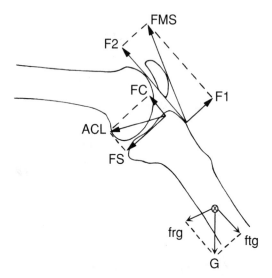

FIGURE 1–62. The rotary force (F_1) of the quadriceps (Fms) not only rotates the tibia at the knee joint, but also creates a shear force between the tibia and the femur. The shear of the quadriceps may be offset in part by the opposing shear force (FS) of the tensed anterior cruciate ligament (ACL) of the knee. Both (F_2) of the quadriceps and FC of the ACL increase the contact between the tibia and the femur.

ment of the quadriceps, the translatory component of the quadriceps force not only compresses joint surfaces, but also creates a small amount of torque!

Just as component f_2 created both translation and a small amount of rotation of the tibia, component f_1 will similarly have a dual effect. A force such as f_1 that lies parallel to contacting surfaces that are free to move on each other (*not* truly hinged) will create or attempt to create *linear* movement between the two contacting surfaces. This is the definition of a shear force. The component f_1 will only rotate the tibia *if* the tibia is prevented from moving linearly (shearing) from beneath the femur. We need to identify another linear force on the tibia that will oppose the shear of f_1. One possibility is the force of gravity (G) acting on the tibia in Figure 1–62. Gravity, like the force of the quadriceps, has components with dual roles. The rotatory force of gravity (f_{rg}) is perpendicular to the tibia, but also parallel to the tibial plateau and in a direction that would move the tibia posteriorly. Consequently, it can oppose the shear of the quadriceps. However, the magnitude of f_1 will be considerably larger than the magnitude of f_{rg}. For the quadriceps to hold the tibia in place or actually extend the tibia at the knee, the torque of the quadriceps force must

be equal to or greater than the torque of gravity. Because gravity is applied at a considerably larger distance than is the quadriceps force, the magnitude of f_1 *must* be substantially larger than the magnitude of f_{rg}. Because shear forces are linear forces, the net shear is found by simply adding up the magnitudes of the shear forces. Given that f_1 is larger than f_{rg}, there still must be a net shear force attempting to move the tibia anteriorly beneath the femur.

Whenever there is a net shear force between two contacting surfaces, there will be an opposing friction force; that is, we potentially have the force of friction-on-tibia created by the compression (contact) between the tibia and the femur. The maximal magnitude of this friction force, however, is likely to be quite small (regardless of the magnitude of contact) because the coefficient of friction (μ_s) for articular cartilage is extremely small ($Fx \leq F_c \times \mu_s$). We are likely to have a net shear on the tibia even after considering both gravity and friction-on-tibia. In reality, the tibia *will* move beneath the femur until ligamentous or capsular tension checks the movement.

In Figure 1–62, we added the pull of the anterior cruciate ligament (ACL) of the knee to the forces on the tibia. The pull of vector ACL has been resolved into components that are perpendicular and parallel *to the tibial plateau.* The contact component (FC) of ACL will simply increase compression between the tibia and femur. The shear component (FS) of ACL will create a countershear to that produced by the quadriceps force (and add to the shear produced by gravity). Presuming the ligament is sufficiently strong, the component FS of the ACL should offset the net shear effect of f_1 of the quadriceps, allowing f_1 to rotate the segment with minimal excursion of the tibia beneath the femur. Most joint capsules and ligaments are arranged not only to tense on pure joint distraction but also to resist net shear forces across the joint surfaces.

- A force or force component that is applied perpendicular to a bony lever *and* is parallel to contacting joint surfaces will create both a torque around the joint axis and a shear between joint surfaces.
- A force or force component that is applied parallel to a bony lever but does not intersect the joint axis will create not only compression or distraction but also a small amount of rotation.
- The sum of the torques around a joint are

commonly greater than zero; that is, it is common to have angular acceleration (a net torque) at a joint.

- The sum of the linear forces (those parallel to the lever *and* those parallel to contact surfaces) *must* eventually result in linear equilibrium or the joint cannot remain intact.

Equilibrium of a lever must ultimately be assessed in terms of:

1. The rotational forces applied around the joint axis (net torque).
2. The translatory forces applied across the joint and perpendicular to joint surfaces (resultant of the joint reaction forces, compressive forces, distractive forces).
3. The translatory forces applied across the joint and parallel to the joint surfaces (resultant of the shear forces, friction forces).

Summary

The physical principles that govern equilibrium or movement of the levers of the human body have been examined at a basic level. This is only a first step, however, in understanding human function. The next step includes a study of joint structures to determine the variable nature of the contacting surfaces and the range of movements permitted at the joints and the ligamentous structure supporting those joints. Also necessary is a study of the structure of muscles, focusing on the properties of a muscle that affect the force (Fms) that either a single muscle or many muscles acting in concert may apply to a lever.

REFERENCES

1. LeVeau, BF: Williams & Lissner's Biomechanics of Human Motion, ed. 3. WB Saunders, Philadelphia, 1992.

SUGGESTED READINGS

Urone, PP: Physics with Health Science Applications. John Wiley & Sons, New York, 1986.
Hall, SJ: Basic Biomechanics, ed. 3. McGraw-Hill, Boston, 1999.
Whiting, WC, and Zernicke RF: Biomechanics of Musculoskeletal Injury. Human Kinetics, Champaign, IL, 1998.

Study Questions

1. In what plane and around what axis does rotation of the head occur?

2. Is naming the plane of motion considered part of kinetics or kinematics? Why?

3. As the foot is brought forward to contact the ground as one walks, what kind of motion of the foot is occurring?

4. To what is the force pencil-on-hand applied? What is its source?

5. What do the forces pencil-on-desk, book-on-desk, glass-on-desk, and blotter-on-desk all have in common?

6. What characteristic(s) does/do all gravity vectors have in common?

7. What generalizations can be made about the LOG (gravity vector) of all stable objects?

8. What happens to the COG of a rigid object when the object is moved around in space?

9. What happens to the COG of the body when the body segments are rearranged? What happens to the COG if the right upper extremity is amputated?

10. Explain how to generally find the resultant (combined) COG for two adjacent objects.

11. A student is carrying all of her books for the fall semester courses in her right arm. What does the additional weight do to her COG? How will her body most likely respond to this change?

12. Why did your Superman punching bag always pop up again?

13. Describe the typical gait of a child just learning to walk. Why does the child walk this way?

14. Give the name, point of application, magnitude and direction of the reaction to body-on-bed when the body is a man weighing 200 lb.

15. What are the reaction forces to each of those forces named in question 5? To what is each of the reactions applied?

16. You see a woman in a waiting room sitting in a chair with a child on her lap. The woman's feet are not touching the floor. Disregarding her clothing, name all the forces responsible for maintaining her equilibrium.

17. Using the example in question 16, what would happen if the magnitude of the force floor-on-chair was equivalent to the sum of the woman's weight and the weight of the child?

18. Are the two forces of an action-reaction pair part of the same linear force system? Defend your answer.

19. What conditions must exist for friction to have magnitude on an object?

20. When is the magnitude of the force of friction always greatest?

21. You have a patient in leg traction similar to that described in the text (Buck's extension traction). There is a 10-lb weight suspended on the rope. The leg weighs 20 lb. Assume the leg is not contacting the bed. Given these forces, is the knee joint being distracted?

22. Repeat question 21. Now, assuming the leg is resting on the bed, and that the coefficient of friction for skin on bed is 0.25, is the knee joint undergoing distraction?

23. A patient is lying in bed with traction applied to her leg. The patient is acted on by the forces of gravity, bed-on-patient, and traction-on-patient. The patient will not be in equilibrium. What additional force(s) is/are necessary to keep the patient in equilibrium?

24. What kind of force system is found in a single muscle? Explain.

25. At which end of a muscle do you place the point of application of Fms?

26. How do you determine the net effect of two muscle pulls applied to the same spot? What is this process called?

27. How do anatomic pulleys affect the magnitude and direction of a muscle force (Fms)?

28. What are the three classes of levers? Give an example of each in the human body.

29. What is torque? Describe how it is determined using an example in the human body of two parallel forces acting on the same lever.

30. How does one determine which is the effort force and which is the resistance force?

31. What factors cause torque to change?

32. A 2-year-old has difficulty pushing open the door into MacDonald's. What advice will you give him as to how to perform the task independently?

33. What is always true of the mechanical advantage of a third-class lever? Of a second? Of a first?

34. What is the "advantage" of a lever with a mechanical advantage greater than one?

35. What kind of work (positive or negative) does a muscle do whenever it is acting as a second-class lever? Why?

36. Using the values below, identify the class of the lever, its mechanical advantage, what kind of contraction the muscle is doing, and the point of application of the resultant force of gravity-on-forearm and ball-on-forearm (the hand will be considered part of the forearm). Here Fms = muscle force, G = gravity-on-forearm, and B = ball-on-forearm (assume that all forces are applied perpendicular to the forearm lever).

> Fms = 50 lb (counterclockwise),
> LA = 1 inch
> G = 7 lb (clockwise), LA = 10 inches
> B = 5 lb (clockwise), LA = 12 inches

37. How do you determine torque if the forces applied to the lever are not perpendicular to the lever or parallel to each other?

38. Describe how the angle of application of a force and the MA of that force are related. When is the MA potentially greatest?

39. Describe how you would position a limb in space so that gravity exerts the least torque on the limb. How would you position the limb to have gravity exert the greatest torque?

40. How do anatomic pulleys affect torque generated by the muscle that passes over the pulley?

41. If not all a muscle's force is contributing to rotation, what happens to the "wasted" force?

42. Describe how a rotatory force or force component applied across a joint can create a shear force at that joint. What are some possible sources of forces to offset that shear force?

CHAPTER 2

JOINT STRUCTURE AND FUNCTION

. . . .

. . . .

OBJECTIVES
Following the study of this chapter, the reader should be able to:

Recall
1. The elementary principles of joint design.
2. The five features common to all diarthrodial joints.
3. The two main types of joints.
4. General composition of connective tissue.
5. Properties and functions of materials used in human joints.
6. Definitions of arthrokinematics and osteokinematics.

Identify
1. The axis of motion for any given motion at a specific joint (knee, hip, metacarpophalangeal).
2. The plane of motion for any given motion at a specific joint (shoulder, interphalangeal, wrist).
3. The degrees of freedom at a given joint.
4. The distinguishing features of a diarthrodial joint.
5. The structures that contribute to joint stability.

Compare the following using examples

1. A synarthrosis with a diarthrosis on the basis of method of construction, materials, and function.
2. A closed kinematic chain with open kinematic chain.
3. The close-packed position of a joint with the loose-packed position.
4. Stress and strain to load and deformation.
5. Motion of a convex surface moving on a concave surface versus a concave surface moving on a convex surface.
6. Theories of joint lubrication.
7. Creep and hysteresis.
8. Composition of the following structures: tendons and ligaments, bone and cartilage.

Diagram

1. A typical load-deformation curve for a ligament and identification of the various regions on the curve.
2. A typical stress-strain curve for a ligament or tendon.

. . . .

Introduction

Joint Design

The joints that are found in the human skeleton are similar to joints used in the construction of buildings, furniture, and machines. Both human and nonhuman joints adhere to the same basic design principles, and both types of joints illustrate the strong interrelationship that exists between structure and function. Function may be said to determine structure, and structure in turn determines function. For example, if one were to design a joint for a piece of furniture or a machine, one would have to know the function of the joint in question to produce an appropriate design. Therefore, in this instance, function determines structure. However, once the joint was designed and constructed, the structure of the joint would determine its function. The joints of the human body already have been designed and constructed, and therefore, human joint structure determines function. However, the reader should keep in mind that human tissue can adapt to the stresses placed on it and thus function may determine structure to some extent. For example, when function of an injured joint is affected, a contiguous joint may change its structure and function in response. Although human joints are the main focus of this chapter, the task of designing a table joint has been selected as a way of introducing the reader to the basic principles of joint design. A table leg joint is easy to conceptualize and illustrates the basic principles of joint design.

Basic Principles

A joint (articulation) is used to connect one component of a structure with one or more other components. The design of a joint and the materials used in its construction depend partly on the function of the joint and partly on the nature of the components. If the function of a joint is to provide stability or static support, the design of the joint will be different from the design used when the desired function is mobility. Therefore, function, at least in part, will determine structure. If one wished to design a joint such as that found between the legs of a table and the tabletop, one would have to consider the function of the joint and the nature of the components. The function of the table joint is stability, and therefore the design must be such that the components are united to form a stable union. If one wished the legs of the table to fold, the joint would have to be designed to provide mobility in one situation and stability in another situation. The design of the folding table joint and the materials used would have to be different from and more complex than that of a purely stable joint. One possible method of designing a folding table joint would be by using a metal brace fitted with a locking device. When the brace is unlocked the leg would be free to move: when the brace is locked, the joint would be stable (Fig. 2–1). The use of such a design would require the application of an external force to produce the locking and unlocking. However, the table joint would not be

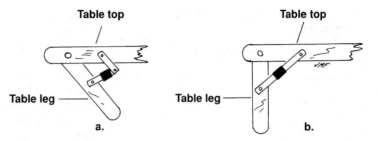

FIGURE 2–1. Folding table joint. (a) The table leg is free to move, and the joint provides mobility when the brace is unlocked. (b) The table leg is prevented from moving, and the joint provides stability when the brace is locked.

able to provide the stability during motion that human joints often must provide.

The table joints have been used as a way of introducing the reader to the elementary principles of joint design that follow, but one should remember that human joints are more complex.

- Joints that serve a single function are less complex than joints that serve multiple functions.
- The design of a joint is determined by its function and the nature of its components.
- Once a joint is constructed, the structure of the joint and the nature of its components will determine its function. However, the function that the joint serves may result in changes in structure.

Materials Used in Human Joints

The fact that the materials used in human joints are composed of living tissue makes human joints unique and difficult to replicate. Living tissue is capable of changing its structure in response to changing environmental or functional demands. It requires nourishment to survive and is subject to disease processes, injury, and the effects of aging. Therefore, to understand the structure and function of the human joints it is necessary to have some knowledge of the nature of the materials that are used in joint construction and the forces that are acting at the joints.

Structure of Connective Tissue

The living material used in the construction of human joints is connective tissue in the form of bones, bursae, capsules, cartilage, disks, fat pads, labra, meniscii, plates, and tendons (Fig. 2–2). The gross anatomic structure and microarchitecture of these connective tissue

structures are extremely varied, and the biomechanical behaviors and composition of capsules, cartilage, specific ligaments, menisci, and tendons are still being investigated.[1–26] Generally, the structure of the connective tissue is characterized by a wide dispersion of cells (cellular component) and the presence of a large **extracellular matrix.** At the microscopic level, the extracellular matrix has both **interfibrillar** (previously referred to as the ground substance) and **fibrillar (fibrous)** components. Table 2–1 summarizes the general composition of connective tissue.

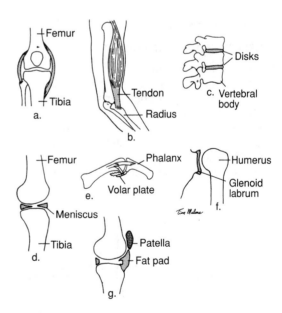

FIGURE 2–2. The shaded areas identify connective tissue structures. (a) Collateral ligaments at the knee support the medial and lateral aspects of the joint. (b) Tendon connects muscle to the bone. (c) Intervertebral disks. (d) Menisci located in the knee joint. (e) Fibrocartilaginous plates at the metacarpophalangeal joints of the fingers. (f) The glenoid labrum extends the area of the glenoid fossa. (g) The patella (largest sesamoid bone in the body) and a fat pad.

Table 2-1. **General Composition of Connective Tissue**

CELLUAR COMPONENT	
Resident Cells	**Circulating Cells**
Chondroblasts	Lymphocytes
Fibroblasts	Macrophages
Osteoblasts	
Tenocytes	

EXTRACELLULAR MATRIX	
Interfibrillar Component	
Proteoglycans	**Glycoproteins**
Aggrecan	Fibronectin
Biglycan	Fibromodulin
Dicorin	Lamimin
Perlecan	Link protein
Versican	Osteopontin
	Tenascin
	Thrombosporin
Fibrillar Component	
Collagen and elastin	

Extracellular Matrix

INTERFIBRILLAR COMPONENT

The interfibrillar component of connective tissue is composed of hydrated networks of proteins: primarily **proteoglycans** and **glycoproteins.** Proteoglycans (PGs) consist of a protein core to which are attached one or more polysaccharide chains called **glycosaminoglycans (GAGs).** The major types of sulfated GAG chains include **chondroitin 4** and **chondroitin 6 sul-**

fate, **karatan sulfate, heparan sulfate,** and **dermatan sulfate. Hyaluronon (HA),** which consists of a very long chain of nonsulfated disaccharides, is an atypical GAG because it is not sulfated and not attached directly to a protein core. A globular region at the end of the protein core binds to HA by way of a glycoprotein called a **link protein.** Twenty-seven **aggregating types** of PGs such as aggrecan and versican bond to HA by link proteins. Aggrecan is composed of a large number of chondroitin sulfate chains (about 100) and a smaller number of keratan sulfate chains (about 30) attached to a protein core (Fig. 2–3). **Nonaggregating** types of PGs such as decorin and biglycan do not bind to HA and possess a relatively small number of GAG chains (Table 2–2).

The proportion of PGs in the extracellular matrix of a particular structure (bone, cartilage, tendon, or ligament) affects its hydration. The GAG chains are negatively charged and the concentration of negatively charged PGs creates a swelling pressure, which causes water to flow into the extracellular matrix. The water flow creates a tensile stress on the surrounding collagen network. The collagen fibers resist and contain the swelling, thus creating the rigidity of the extracellular matrix and its ability to resist compressive forces. In addition to their water-binding function, the PGs and glycoproteins form a supporting substance for the fibrillar and cellular components. The PGs form attachments to collagen fibers and contribute to the strength of the collagen. Tissues that are subjected to high compressive forces have a large PG content, whereas tissues that resist tensile forces have a low PG concentration.[2] Glycoproteins such as **fibronectin** and **laminin**

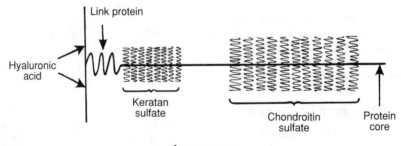

Aggrecan

FIGURE 2–3. A diagrammatic representation of the proteoglycan (PG) aggrecan. The glycosaminoglycan (GAG) chains of chondroitin sulfate and keratan sulfate are shown attached directly to a protein core (represented in the diagram by the horizontal line). The protein core is shown attached indirectly to hyaluronanon (represented in the diagram by a vertical line) by a link protein.

Table 2–2. **Proteoglycans and Glycoproteins**

Proteoglycans	Composition and Function
Aggregating Types	Bond to hyaluronanon. The linkage is stabilized by a glycoprotein link protein.
Aggrecan	Composed of a large number (approx. 100) of chrondroitin sulfate chains and a smaller number (approx. 30) of keratan sulfate chains attached to a protein core.
Versican	Composed of smaller number of chondroitin sulfate chains.
Nonaggregating Types	Do not bind to hyaluronan and possess only a relatively small number of GAG side chains compared to chondroitin sulfate and dermatan sulfate.
Decorin	Composed of only one GAG chain attached to a protein core. Links collagen fibrils.
Biglycan Syndecan	Composed of two GAG chains. Plays a role in regulating cell activity.
Glycoproteins Fibronectin	This large glycoprotein molcule has binding sites for collagen and heparin. It promotes adhesion of collagen in embryonic tissues and facilitates tissue proliferation in wound repair.
Lamimin	This large glycoprotein molecule has binding sites for heparan sulfate and type IV collagen. It forms part of the basal lamina.
Tenascin	Tenascin is associated with the development of hyaline articular cartilage as well as other permanent cartilages.

play an important role in the interaction between adjacent connective tissue cells and in the adhesion of these cells to collagen.

FIBRILLAR COMPONENT

The fibrillar or fibrous component of the extracellular matrix contains two major classes of structural proteins, collagen and elastin.[1] **Collagen** is the most abundant protein in the human body[19] and accounts for 30% of all protein in mammals.[28] Collagen has a tensile strength that approaches that of steel[29] and is responsible for the functional integrity of connective tissue structures.[28,30] Fifteen[31] to 19 (XV–XIX)[2] types of collagen have been identified, but the functions of all of these types have not been determined.[31] The types of collagen and their distribution in joint structures are presented in Table 2–3.

The roman numerals that designate each type of collagen, for example, type I, type II, reflect the order in which each type of collagen was discovered.[1] The fibril-forming collagens (types I, II, III, V, and XI) are the most common. Type I collagen is found in almost all connective tissue including tendon, synovium, bones, labra, and skin.[29] Type I collagen is the predominant type of collagen found in ligaments, tendons, menisci, and the fibrous portion of joint capsules. Type II collagen is the predom-

inant type of collagen found in hyaline articular cartilage. Also, type II collagen is found in the nucleus pulposus in the center of the intervertebral disks.[1,32-34] Types I, II, and IX collagen are found in the annulus fibrosus of the intervertebral disks.[34] Type III collagen is found in the skin and in the stratum synovium of joint capsules.[29]

The basic building block of collagen is a triple helix of three polypeptide chains that is called the **tropocollagen molecule.** It is synthesized in the rough endoplasmic reticulum of the fibroblasts. The tropocollagen molecules are attracted to one another and aggregate to form microfibrils. The microfibrils form subfibrils that in turn combine to form fibrils. The fibrils form a fascicle and the fascicles combine to form fibers. Collagen fibers may be arranged in many different ways and may also vary in size and shape. Collagen fibers are nonelastic, but the arrangement of the fibers in some structures allows a certain amount of elastic-type deformation.[35] In the relaxed state, collagen fibers assume a wavy configuration called **crimp.** When collagen fibers are stretched the crimp disappears.

Elastin (yellow fibrous tissue), as the name implies, has elastic properties that allow elastin fibers to deform under an applied force and to return to their original state following

Table 2–3. **Collagen Types and Distribution in Joint Structures**

Collagen Type	Distribution in Joint Structures
I Fibril-forming collagen—most widely distributed throughout the body	Annulus fibrosus of intervertebral disk,[2,34] bone,[1,2] labra, ligaments,[2,6,37] menisci,[6] tendon,[2,6,32] and synovium
II Fibril-forming collagen	Annulus fibrosus and nucleus pulposus of intervertebral disks,[34] hyaline articular cartilage,[6,39] and menisci[2]
III Fibril-forming collagen usually present with type I	Fibrous joint capsule,[6] ligament,[37] menisci,[2] and tendon[32]
IV Meshwork forming collagen that holds cells together	Nucleus pulposus in young adults[34] and tendon[32]
V Fibril-forming collagen	Hyaline articular cartilage[6,28] and tendon[31]
VI	Hyaline articular cartilage[6,28,39] and intervertebral disks[1]
VII A linking or bridging collagen[1]	Skin[1]
VIII A meshwork-forming collagen	Unknown
IX A collagen associated with fibril forming collagens.[1] It facilitates fibril interaction with proteoglycans[39] and is covalently linked to type II in cartilage.	Hyaline articular cartilage[28,33,40] and intervertebral disks.[33,34]
X A meshwork-forming collagen	Growth plate cartilage,[33] and intervertebral disks with degenerative changes[34]
XI A fibril-forming collagen that regulates fibril size	Hyaline articular cartilage[6,28,39]
XII A fibril associated collagen	Cartilage,[40] ligament, and tendon[6]
XIII Unclassified	
XIV A fibril-associated collagen	Tendon[1,6]
XV Unknown	

removal of that force. Elastin fibers are usually yellowish in color and branch freely. The relative proportion of elastin to collagen fibers in different connective tissue structures varies considerably, but generally elastin fibers make up a much smaller portion of the fibrous component in the extracellular matrix than collagen fibers. Elastin fibers in varying amounts are found in all of the joint structures that follow as well in the skin, tracheobronchial tree, and the walls of arteries.

Specific Connective Tissue Structures

Ligaments

Ligaments are connective tissue structures that connect or bind one bone to another either at or near a joint. Some ligaments are part of, and blend with, the joint capsules. They maybe difficult to identify because they are so closely integrated into the capsule. Other ligaments are distinct, easily recognizable structures often appearing as dense white bands or cords of connective tissue. One notable exception is the **ligamentum flavum,** which has a distinctly yellowish color. Ligaments are usually named descriptively according to their location, shape, bony attachments, and relationship to one another. Occasionally, ligaments are given the name of the individual who first identified the ligament. The anterior longitudinal ligament, which covers most of the anterior surface of the vertebral column, is an example of a ligament that appears to be named both for location (anterior) and shape (longitudinal). The medial and lateral collateral ligaments of the elbow and knee joints that are located on the medial and lateral aspects of these joints are examples of ligaments named for location. Ligaments such as the coracohumeral, which connects the coracoid process of the scapula with the humerus at the shoulder, and the radioulnar ligaments, which connect the radius to the ulna at the distal radioulnar joint, are examples of naming by bony attachment. A ligament named according to shape is the deltoid ligament at the ankle joint. The Y ligament of Bigelow at the hip joint is named both for its inverted Y shape and for an individual. The cruciate ligaments at the knee are so named because they cross each other.

Ligaments, like other connective tissue structures, are heterogenous structures that are composed of a small amount of cells (about 20%) and a large extracellular matrix (about 80% to 90%). The cellular component consists mainly of fibroblasts. The interfibrillar component is composed of PGs and glycoproteins with the most common PG being dermatan sulfate. In comparison to articular cartilage the PG content in ligaments is relatively small, 0.2% dry weight. The fibrillar component of the extracellular matrix in both ligaments and tendons contains a larger collagen than elastin content. However, the relative proportion of collagen to elastin fibers varies considerably among different ligaments. Some ligaments like the **ligamenta nuchae** and the **ligamentum flavum** (see Chap. 4) have more elastin fibers than collagen fibers. Type I collagen predominates in ligaments, whereas types III and VI are present in small amounts.

Ligaments are composed of densely packed type I collagen fibers with a few interspersed cells. The midsubstance of the ligament is composed of bundles of fibrous material that are separated by bundles of loose connective tissue. The two types of bundles and their placement allows interbundle shearing to occur, which allows parts of the ligament to tighten at different joint positions.[36] The cellular appearance and matrix architecture change as the ligament approaches bone. Collagen fibers appear to be cemented into bone during growth and development, forming Sharpey fibers at the ligamentous bony insertion sites (the **enthesis**). The stiffening of the ligament-bone interface decreases the likelihood that the ligament will give way at the enthesis; however, it is a common site for degenerative change.[37]

The arrangement of the collagen fibers and the collagen/elastin fiber ratio in various ligaments determines the relative abilities of these structures to provide stability and mobility for a particular joint. Generally, the collagen fibers in ligaments have a varied arrangement that enables the ligament to resist forces from more than one direction.

Tendons

Tendons connect muscle to bone and are usually named for the muscle to which they are attached, for example, biceps tendon for the biceps brachii or the triceps tendon for the triceps. The Achilles tendon at the ankle is named after a Greek warrior in the Trojan War who was killed by an arrow that struck his heel, the only vulnerable spot on his body.

Tendons, like other connective tissue structures, are composed of a small cellular component (primarily fibroblasts) and a large extracellular matrix.[38] The fibrillar component is composed of varying proportions of collagen and elastin. The interfibrillar component of the extracellular matrix in tendons contains water, PGs, and GAG compounds (primarily dermatan sulfate). Like ligaments, the predominant type of collagen in tendons is type I collagen with lesser amounts of types II, III, IV, and V. Collagen fibrils are composed of microfibrils grouped together to form primary bundles known as fibers. Groups of fiber bundles enclosed by a loose connective tissue sheath are called the **endotendon.** The endotendon, containing types I and II collagen, also encloses nerves, lymphatics, and blood vessels supplying the tendon to form a secondary bundle called a **fascicle.** Individual fascicles are associated with discrete groups of muscle fibers or motor units at the muscle-tendon insertion. Several fascicles may form a larger group (tertiary bundle) that is also enclosed in endotendon. The sheath that covers all secondary bundles is called the **epitenon.** The **peritenon,** or **paratenon,** is a double-layered sheath of areolar tissue that is loosely attached to the outer surface of the epitenon. The peritenon may become a synovial-filled sheath called the **tenosynovium** (or **tendon sheath**) in tendons located in the wrist and hand that are subjected to high levels of friction. The paratenon protects the tendon and enhances movement of the tendon on adjacent structures.

The bony attachment of tendon is characterized by changes in the tendon structure that occur over a length of about 1 mm. The connective tissue at the bony ends of the tendon changes first to unmineralized fibrocartilage and then to mineralized fibrocartilage and finally to bone. A tidemark exists between the unmineralized and mineralized areas. The attachment of tendon to muscle (**myotendinous junction**) is formed as collagen fibers in the tendon merge with actin filaments in the muscle's sarcomeres. In contrast to ligaments, the collagen fibers in tendons have a parallel arrangement to handle high unidirectional tensile forces.

Bursae

Bursae, which are similar in structure and function to tendon sheaths, are flat sacs of synovial membrane in which the inner sides of the sacs are separated by a fluid film. Bursae are located where moving structures are in tight approximation, that is, between tendon and bone, bone and skin, muscle and bone, or ligament and bone. Bursae located between the skin and bone, such as those found between the patella and the skin and the olecranon process of the ulna and the skin, are called **subcutaneous bursae**[1] (Fig. 2–4a). **Subtendinous bursae** lie between tendon and bone. **Submuscular bursae** lie between muscle and bone (Fig. 2–4b).

Cartilage

Cartilage is usually divided into the following types: **white fibrocartilage, yellow elastic cartilage,** and **hyaline articular cartilage.** Cartilage also may be calcified. White fibrocartilage forms the bonding cement in joints that permit little motion. This type of cartilage also forms the intervertebral disks and is found in the glenoid and acetabular labra. In contrast to the other types of cartilage, white fibrocartilage contains type I collagen in the fibrous component of the extracellular matrix. Yellow elastic fibrocartilage is found in the ears and epiglottis and differs from white fibrocartilage in that it has a higher ratio of elastin to collagen fibers than the white variety, which consists primarily of collagen fibers.[1]

Hyaline articular cartilage, which will be referred to as simply articular cartilage, forms a relatively thin (1 to 7 mm) covering on the ends of the bones in the majority of joints. It provides a smooth, resilient, low-friction surface for the articulation of one bone with another. These cartilaginous surfaces are capable of bearing and distributing weight over a person's lifetime. However, once hyaline articular cartilage is injured it has limited and imperfect mechanisms for repair. Articular cartilage has the same general structure as other connective tissues in that it is characterized by a small cellular component and a large extracellular matrix. However, the composition of both the cellular component and extracellular matrix differ somewhat from that found in tendons and ligaments. The predominant cellular component in articular cartilage contains **chondrocytes** and **chondroblasts.** Chondrocytes are specialized cells that are responsible for the development of articular cartilage and maintenance of the extracellular matrix. These cells produce aggrecan, link protein, and hyaluronan, which are extruded into the extracellular matrix and aggregate spontaneously.[27]

The fibrillar component of the extracellular matrix includes elastin and types II, VI, IX, X, XI, and XII collagen.[39] Type II collagen accounts for about 90% to 95% of the collagen content in articular cartilage. Type II collagen is the only type of collagen that has the capacity to block the deposit of hydroxypatite crystals, which are required for calcification.[40] Type XI collagen regulates the fibril size and type IX facilitates fibril interaction with proteoglycan molecules.[39] The collagen is dispersed throughout the interfibrillar component,[27] which is composed of PGs, noncollagen PGs, and between 65% and 80% water.[40]

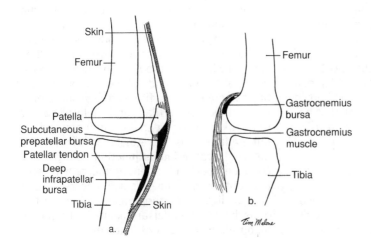

FIGURE 2–4. Bursae. (a) The subcutaneous prepatellar bursa reduces friction between the bone and the overlying skin. The subtendinous deep infrapatellar bursa reduces friction between the patellar tendon and the tibia. (b) A submuscular bursa reduces friction between the gastrocnemius muscle and the femur.

The PG content in articular cartilage is larger than that in other joint structures and the majority of PGs in articular cartilage are in the form of aggrecans, which bind with hyaluronon to form a large PG aggregate.[27] Aggrecan is the predominant PG in hyaline articular cartilage. The two major types of GAG in articular cartilage are chondroitin sulfate and keratan sulfate. The ratio of chondroitin to keratan sulfate shows variations among individuals as well as age and site variations. The higher the chondroitin sulfate concentration the better the tissue can resist compressive forces. Keratan sulfate concentration increases in aging and in joints with arthritic changes and decreases in immobilization.[40] If the proportion of keratan sulfate exceeds the chondroitin sulfate portion, the ability of the cartilage to bear loads is compromised. **Chondronectin,** a cartilage glycoprotein, plays an important role in the adhesion of chondroblasts to type II collagen fibers in the presence of chondroitin sulfate.[1]

Three distinct layers or zones of articular cartilage are found on the ends of bony components of synovial joints[41] (Fig. 2–5). In the outermost layer (zone I), the collagen fibers are arranged parallel to the surface. The smooth outermost layer of the cartilage helps to reduce friction between the opposing joint surfaces and to distribute forces. In the second and third zones they are randomly arranged and form an open latticework. The second layer with its loose-coiled fiber network permits deformation and helps to absorb some of the force imposed on the joint surfaces. In the third

layer (radiate stratum) some fibers lie perpendicular to the surface and extend across the interface between uncalcified and calcified cartilage to find a secure hold in the calcified cartilage.[1,29] The calcified layer of cartilage, sometimes referred to as the fourth zone, lies adjacent to subchondral bone and anchors the cartilage securely to the bone.[42] The interface between the calcified and uncalcified cartilage is called the **tidemark.**[1,27,32] The tidemark area of the cartilage is important because of its relation to growth, aging,[43] injury,[40] and healing.[44] Normally, replacement of the calcified layer of articular cartilage by bone occurs by **endochondral ossification.** The calcification front advances to the noncalcified area of cartilage at a slow rate, which is in equilibrium with the rate of absorption of calcified cartilage by endochondral ossification.[45] In aging, replacement of the calcified layer of cartilage by bone and subsequent advancement of the tidemark area results in the thinning of the hyaline articular cartilage. In injuries that involve microfractures to the subchondral bone, the secondary ossification center in the bone may be activated to produce new bone growth. A process similar to that which occurs in aging ensues. Bone growth expands into the calcified layer, the tidemark advances, and the noncalcified layer thins.

During joint motion or when the cartilage is compressed, some of the fluid content of the cartilage is exuded through pores in the outermost layer. The fluid flows back into the cartilage after motion or compression ceases. The rate of fluid flow is affected by the magnitude and duration of the applied force. When the applied force is increased and sustained over a long period, the permeability of the cartilage is decreased and fluid flow, either in or out of the cartilage, is decreased accordingly.[46] Because hyaline cartilage is devoid of blood vessels and nerves in the adult, its nourishment is derived solely from the back and forth flow of fluid. The free flow of fluid is essential for the survival of articular cartilage and as an aid to reducing friction. The fact that hyaline articular cartilage often undergoes degenerative changes after prolonged immobilization may be related to an interference with the nutrition of the cartilage.[47] The effects of immobilization, in which compression of joint surfaces is absent or diminished, are similar to the effects of prolonged high compressive forces in that fluid flow in and out of the cartilage is diminished,

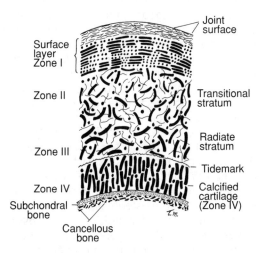

Surface layer
Zone I

Zone II

Zone III

Zone IV

Subchondral bone

Cancellous bone

Joint surface

Transitional stratum

Radiate stratum

Tidemark

Calcified cartilage (Zone IV)

t.m.

FIGURE 2–5. Structure of hyaline cartilage.

and hence cartilage nutrition is adversely affected.[47]

Bone

Bone is the hardest of all connective tissue found in the body. Like other forms of connective tissue, it consists of a cellular component and an extracellular matrix consisting of an interfibrillar component and a fibrillar component. However, bone differs from other connective tissue structures in the composition of all three components and therefore is considered to be a specialized form of connective tissue. The cellular component consists of fibroblasts, fibrocytes, osteoblasts, osteocytes, osteoclasts, and osteoprogenitor cells. The fibroblasts and fibrocytes are essential for the production of collagen. The osteoblasts are the primary bone forming cells that are responsible not only for the synthesis of bone but also for its deposition and mineralization. Osteoblasts also secrete procollagen into the surrounding matrix. When osteoblasts cease their bone-making activity, they turn into osteocytes. Osteoclasts are large polymorphous cells with multiple nuclei. Osteoclasts are responsible for bone resorption. The interfibrillar component of the extracellular matrix in bone contains minerals in addition to PGs, glycoproteins, and water. The mineral content, which consists mainly of calcium and phosphate crystals that are embedded within and between collagen fibrils, is referred to as the inorganic component of bone. The inorganic component of bone helps to give bone its solid consistency[1] and distinguishes bone from other connective tissue structures. The fibrillar component of the extracellular matrix contains reticular fibers, in addition to predominantly type I collagen fibers, and elastin fibers. Type I collagen, which is synthesized by osteoblasts, is the only type of collagen that is able to bind to mineral.

The highly calcified extracellular matrix in bones takes different forms: in both the innermost layer, called **cancellous (spongy) bone,** and in the outer layer called **compact bone.** In cancellous bone the calcified tissue forms thin plates called **trabeculae.** The trabeculae are laid down in response to stresses placed on the bone. The trabeculae undergo self-regulated modeling that not only maintains the shaft and other portions of the bone but also maintains an articular surface shape that is capable of distributing the load optimally. The loading history of the trabeculae, including loading from multiple directions, has been suggested to influence the distribution of bone density and trabecular orientation.[48] Increases in bone density in some areas and decreases in density in other areas occur in response to the loads placed on bone. The cancellous bone is covered by a thin layer of dense compact bone called **cortical bone,** which is laid down in concentric layers.

The cortical bone, which appears to be solid, is covered by a tough fibrous membrane called the **periosteum.** The inner surface of the periosteum is composed of osteoblasts, which are essential for the growth and repair of bone. The periosteum is well vascularized and contains many capillaries that provide nourishment for the bones. The terminal collagen fibers of ligaments and tendons are often imbedded in the matrix of cortical bone. In all synovial joints the periosteum at the ends of bones is replaced by hyaline articular cartilage.

At the microscopic level, two distinct types of bone organization are visible: **woven bone** and **lamellar bone.** In woven (primary) bone, collagen fibers are irregularly arranged to form a pattern of alternating coarse and fine fibers that resemble woven material. Woven bone is young bone and able to form without a scaffolding or underlying framework. In contrast, lamellar bone requires a framework to form and it is older bone that comprises most of the adult skeleton. Cortical and cancellous bone are both types of lamellar bone. In cortical bone collagen fibers are arranged in layers in which osteocytes are embedded.[1]

Bone has the capacity for remodeling, which occurs normally throughout life, as it responds to external forces (or loads), such as the pull of tendons and the weight of the body during functional activities. Internal influences such as aging or various metabolic and disease processes also affect bone remodeling. Application of external forces (or loads) repetitively or over time, causes osteoblast activity to increase and, as a result, bone mass increases. Without these forces, osteoclast activity predominates and bone mass decreases. If the osteoclasts break down or absorb the bone at a faster rate than the osteoblasts can remodel or rebuild the bone, a condition called **osteoporosis** results. In osteoporosis, the bones have a decreased density (mass per unit volume) as compared to normal bone and thus are

Table 2–4. *Composition of Selected Joint Structures*

Structure	Water Content	Principal Cell	Principal PG/GAG	Collagen Content
Bone	60%	Osteoblasts and osteocytes[2]	Chondroitin sulfate	Type I[1,2]
Capsule	70%[6]			Collagen and elastin comprise 90% of the dry weight. Type I predominates. Lesser amounts of type III[2]
Cartilage	60–85% wet weight[6,28,41]	Chondrocytes 10% wet weight[27]	Chondroitin sulfate 8–10% dry weight[2] total PGs 3–10%[27]	Total collagen 10–30%[27] Type II 90–95%. Lesser amounts of types VI, IX, X, and XI L[27,40]
Nucleus pulposus	65–90% wet weight varies with age	Chondrocytes	Total PGs make up 65% of dry weight	Total collagen ranges from 20–30% dry weight Type II predominates with lesser amounts of type IX[39] and type III
Annulus	65–70% wet weight	Fibrocytes and chondrocytes	Chondroitin sulfate and keratan sulfate 20% of dry weight	Total collagen ranges from 50–60% dry weight Types I and II predominate, with lesser amounts of types IX,[34] V, VI, and III
Ligament	70% wet weight[36]	Fibrocytes 20 % of wet weight	Dermatan sulfate < 1% of dry weight 20% of dry weight is unknown[36]	Total collagen is 75% of dry weight. Type I is 85% of total dry weight with lesser amounts of types III, VI and XII. Elastin 1–2%[36]
Menisci	70–78%	Fibrocytes and chondrocytes	Chondroitin and dermatan sulfate < 10% dry weight	Type I 60–90% dry weight Lesser amounts of types II and III
Tendon	60–75%[31]	Tenocytes[2]	Dermatan sulfate 0.2–1% of dry weight[2,31]	Type I 70–80% dry weight Lesser amounts of types III, IV, V,[31] XII, and XIII

GAG, glycosaminoglycan; PG, proteoglycan.

weaker (more susceptible to fracture) than bones with normal density. Bone is considered to be a composite material because its properties are the result of the combined properties of the different components that make up bone and these properties differ significantly from the properties of any one of its components. Bone differs from cartilage in that bone receives its nourishment from blood supplies located within the bone, whereas cartilage receives its nourishment from sources outside the cartilage.

The preceding paragraphs provided a brief overview of the composition of the various connective tissue structures that are associated with the joints. The composition of bones, capsules, cartilage, intervertebral disks, menisci, ligaments, and tendons are summarized in Table 2–4.

General Properties of Connective Tissue

All of the structures that have been discussed in the preceding section can be described as **heterogeneous** in that they are composed of a variety of solid and semisolid components including water, collagen, and other composite materials. Each of these materials has its own properties and thus the properties of the structure as a whole are a combination of the properties of the different components and the varying proportions of each component in the structure as a whole. The heterogeneous nature of connective tissue structures causes these structures to exhibit mechanical behaviors that vary according to where a force is applied to the structure. The label **anisotropic** is applied to structures demonstrating this behavior.

> EXAMPLE 1: In the case of a long bone, which is a heterogeneous composite material, the mechanical response by the bone will be different when a constant force is applied along the length of a section of bone than when forces are applied across the middle of the shaft of a bone.

Anisotropic materials differ from **isotropic** materials such as metal in that isotropic materials exhibit the same properties regardless of where the force is applied on the structure.[49]

Connective tissues also have the ability to change their structures and functions in response to either externally or internally applied forces. For example, connective tissues are able to respond to changes in applied external stresses by altering the composition of the extracellular matrix (PG content and type). This adaptive behavior illustrates the dynamic nature of connective tissue and the strong relationship between structure and function.

Viscoelasticity

Although connective tissue appears in many forms throughout the body, all connective tissue exhibits the common property of **viscoelasticity.** The behavior of viscoelastic materials is a combination of the properties of elasticity and viscosity. **Elasticity** refers to a material's ability to return to its original state following deformation (change in dimensions, i.e., length or shape) after removal of the deforming load. When a material is stretched, it has work done on it and its energy increases. An elastic material stores this energy and keeps the energy available so that the stretched elastic material can recoil immediately to its original dimensions following removal of the distractive force. The term elasticity implies that length changes or deformations are directly proportional to the applied forces or loads. **Viscosity** refers to a material's ability to dampen shearing forces. When forces are applied to viscous materials, the tissues exhibit time-dependent and rate-dependent properties.

Time-Dependent Properties (Creep and Stress-Relaxation)

Viscoelastic materials are capable of undergoing deformation under either a tensile (distractive) or compressive force and of returning to their original state after removal of the force. However, under normal conditions viscoelastic materials do not return to their original state immediately. Viscoelastic materials, unlike pure elastic materials, have time-dependent mechanical properties. In other words, viscoelastic materials are sensitive to the duration of the force application. When a viscoelastic material is subjected to either a constant compressive or tensile load, the material initially responds by rapidly deforming and then continues to deform over a finite length of time (hours, days, and months) even if the load remains constant. Deformation of the tissue continues until a state of equilibrium is reached when the load is balanced. This phenomenon is called **creep** and is attributed to different mechanisms in different materials (Fig. 2–6). In bone, at the microscopic level, creep in compression has been attributed to the slip of lamellae within the **osteons** (haversian system) and the flow of the interstitial fluid.[31] In hyaline articular cartilage subjected to a compressive force, creep is attributed to the grad-

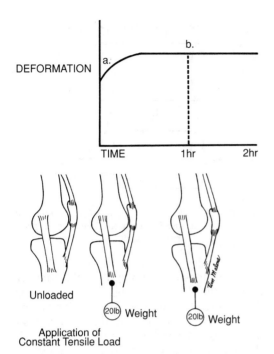

FIGURE 2–6. Creep response of a ligament or tendon when a constant load is applied. The tendon or ligament deforms rapidly at first as seen in the portion of the curve labeled (a) and then continues to deform (elongate) over time.

ual loss of fluid from the tissue. In tendons and ligaments, creep is due to motion of long GAG chains in the solid matrix.[27] Generally, the longer the duration of the applied force, the greater the deformation. Increases in the magnitude of the applied load tend to increase the rate of creep. In some tissues, an acceleration of the rate of creep occurs after a prolonged time. Changes in temperature also affect the rate of creep. High temperatures increase the rate of creep and low temperatures decrease the rate. Theoretically, if one wishes to stretch out (elongate) a connective tissue structure, one should heat it and use a large load over a long period of time to produce creep.

Stress-relaxation occurs when a viscoelastic material experiences a constant deformation. It responds initially with a high initial stress that decreases over time until equilibrium is reached and the stress equals zero.

Rate-Dependent Properties

Viscoelastic materials respond differently to different rates of loading. When viscoelastic materials are loaded rapidly, they exhibit greater resistance to deformation than the re-

sistance exhibited when they are loaded more slowly. Generally, the higher the rate of loading and the longer the duration of the applied force, the greater the deformation. Viscoelastic materials do not store all of the energy that is transferred to them when they are deformed by an applied force, and thus the transferred energy is not available for recovery. When a force is applied and then removed, some of the energy created during the stretching or compression of the material may be dissipated (lost) in the form of heat and therefore the material may not return to its original dimensions. The loss of energy (difference between energy expended and energy regained) is called **hysteresis.** Hysteresis is exhibited by viscoelastic materials when they are subjected to the application and removal of forces and is illustrated in Figure 2–7.

Mechanical Behavior

The materials used in the construction of human joints are subjected to continually changing forces during activities of daily living, and the ability of these materials to withstand these forces and thus provide support and protection for the joints of the body is extremely important. To understand how different materials and structures are able to provide support (the mechanical behavior of these structures),

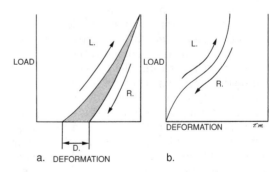

FIGURE 2–7. Hysteresis. (a) A typical curve obtained from the measurement of the elasticity of cartilage. The arrow labeled (L) represents the loading cycle, and the curve represents the energy expended during the loading cycle. The arrow labeled (R) represents the unloading cycle, and the curve represents the energy regained. The shaded area represents the loss of energy or hysteresis (difference between energy expended and energy regained). The distance between (L) and (R), which is labeled (D), represents the deformation (change in dimensions). (b) In this figure, which represents a more elastic material, the energy expended (L) and energy regained (R) are the same and, therefore, the material returns to its original dimensions following removal of the load.

the reader must be familiar with the concepts and terminology used to describe their behavior, for example **stress, strain, failure,** and **stiffness,** among others. The types of tests that are used to determine the mechanical behavior of human building materials are the same as the types of tests used for nonhuman building materials, although viscoelastic materials may respond differently.

Stress and Strain

The term **load** commonly is used to refer to an external force or forces applied to a structure. Many examples of externally applied loads are given in Chapter 1, including the forces exerted on the table by the book lying on the table, the forces exerted on the man's hand and arm by the suitcase he is carrying, and the forces exerted by a weight on the leg. The external forces exerted by the book, suitcase, and weight can all be designated as applied loads. When such loads (forces) are applied to a structure or material, forces are created within the structure or material that are called **mechanical stresses.** Stress can be expressed mathematically in the following formula, where S = stress; F = applied force; and A = area:

$$S = F/A$$

or stress equals the magnitude of the force applied to an object per unit area.[49]

In a solid or semisolid material, deformation (change in shape, length, or width) of the structure or material may accompany the stress and is referred to as **strain.** The type of stress and strain that develops in human structures, as we have already discussed, depends on the nature of the material, type of load that is applied, the point of application of the load, direction, magnitude of the load, and the rate and duration of loading. When a structure can no longer support a load, the structure is said to have failed. **Ultimate stress** is the stress at the point of failure of the material; **ultimate strain** is the strain at the point of failure. If two externally applied forces are equal and act along the same line and in opposite directions, they constitute a distractive or **tensile load** and will create **tensile stress** and **tensile strain** in the structure or material (Fig. 2–8a).

Tensile stress = tensile force/cross-sectional area (perpendicular to the direction of the applied force)

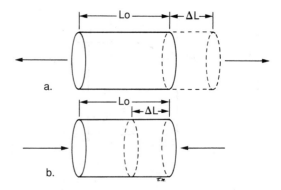

FIGURE 2–8. Strain. (a) Tensile strain in the rod is evidenced by an increase in length. (b) Compressive strain is evidenced by a decrease in length.

When a tensile load is applied, the stress can be thought of as the intensity of the force and the strain as the amount of elongation and narrowing (deformation) that the structure sustains. The deformation is defined by comparing the original dimensions (L0) of the object with change in dimensions L brought about by the application of the force (see Fig. 2–8a). Elongation of the structure produced by a tensile stress is accompanied by a proportional amount of narrowing of the material (lateral strain). Maximal (normal or principal) tensile stress occurs on a plane perpendicular to the applied load.

If two externally applied forces are equal and act in a line toward each other on opposite sides of a structure, they constitute **compressive loading** and **compressive stress** and, as a result, **compressive strain** will develop in the structure (Fig. 2–8b).

Compressive stress = compressive force/cross-sectional area (perpendicular to the direction of the force)

When a compressive load is applied, the stress can be considered to be a measurement of the intensity of the force that develops on the plane surface of the structure and the strain as the amount of deformation (shortening and widening) that occurs in the structure. Maximal compressive stress occurs on a plane perpendicular to the applied load. Shortening of the structure is accompanied by a proportional amount of widening (lateral strain).

Compressive strain = decrease in length (ΔL)/original length (L0)

Both tensile and compressive stresses and strains are created when a structure such as a

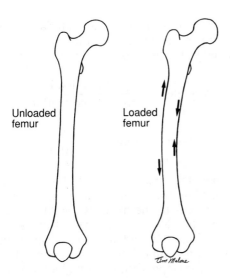

FIGURE 2–9. Stress and strain in a long bone. The arrows that point away from each other on the convex side of the bone indicate tensile stress and strain. The arrows that point toward each other on the concave side of the bone indicate compressive stress and strain in the structure.

long bone is subjected to bending moments. Tensile stress and strain develop on the convex side and compressive stress and strain develop on the concave side of the long axis of the bone (Fig. 2–9).

If two externally applied forces are equal, parallel, and applied in the opposite direction but are not in line with each other they constitute **shear loading,** which causes **shear stress** and **strain** in the structure (Fig. 2–10).

Shear stress = shear force/cross sectional area (parallel to the direction of the applied force)[49]*

Load-Deformation and Stress-Strain Curves

Load-deformation curves and stress-strain curves are used to determine the strength of

*The reader may notice the similarity between the formula for stress and the formula for pressure. Pressure is defined as force per unit area or (P = F/A) where the force is perpendicular to the area. Usually the term "pressure" is reserved for liquids and gases, but it may be used for other materials. Pressure applied to a confined liquid at rest follows Pascal's principle in that the pressure is transmitted equally to every point within the liquid.[50] The application of a uniform compression force to a confined liquid at rest produces uniform pressure in all directions and volumetric strain equals change in volume/original volume. The joint disks found between the vertebral bodies in the vertebral column have a fluid-filled central portion that behaves according to Pascal's principle.

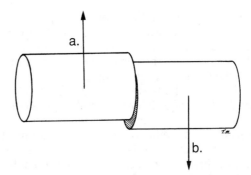

FIGURE 2–10. Shear stress and strain.

building materials, including human building materials such as bones, ligaments, tendons, joint capsules, and other structures that constitute and support human joints. The load-deformation curve in which the applied load (external force) is plotted against the deformation provides information regarding the strength properties of a particular material or structure (Fig. 2–11). The load-deformation curve can be transformed into a stress-strain curve by dividing the force by the tissue cross-sectional area and the change in length (deformation) by the original length (stress = force/cross-sectional area and strain =length increase/original length).[31] The stress-strain curve, in which stress is expressed in load per unit area and strain is expressed in deformation per unit length (or percentage of deformation),

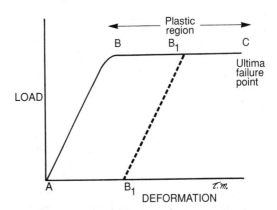

FIGURE 2–11. Load/deformation curve. The A-B area of the curve is the elastic region. Point B is the yield point. The area of the curve from B to C is the plastic region in which permanent deformation occurs. C is the ultimate failure point. The distance between A and B represents the amount of permanent deformation that would occur if the load were removed at B_1.

is used to compare the strength properties of one material with another material. Although each type of material has a unique curve, some characteristics of the curves are similar among materials that have similar properties.

The load-deformation curve depicted in Figure 2–11 provides information about the elasticity, plasticity, ultimate strength, and stiffness of the material as well as the amount of energy that the material can store before failure. The first region of the curve between point A and point B is the **elastic region.** In this region, deformation of the material will not be permanent and the structure will return to its original dimensions after removal of the load. Point B is the **yield point,** which indicates that at this point the material will no longer react elastically and some deformation will be evident after release of a load. Therefore, point B signifies the end of the elastic region or elastic limit. The next region on the curve from B to C is the **plastic region.** In this region deformation of the material will be permanent when the load is removed. If the load is removed at B_1, the amount of permanent deformation is represented by the distance from A to B_1. If loading continues in the plastic range, the material will continue to deform until it reaches the **ultimate failure point C.**

Materials are designated as *brittle*, or *ductile*, or as a combination of the two, depending on the amount of deformation that they can undergo before reaching the ultimate failure point. Brittle materials such as glass do not have a plastic region and undergo very little deformation before failure. Ductile materials such as soft metal undergo considerable deformation before failure. Materials also are designated as having **resilience** and **toughness.** The resilience of a material is its ability when loaded to absorb and store energy within the elastic range and to release that energy and then return to its original dimensions immediately following removal of the load. Toughness is the ability of a material to absorb energy within the plastic range. Toughness reflects the material's resistance to failure or ability to absorb large amounts of energy prior to failure.

Young's modulus or **modulus of elasticity** of a material under compressive or tensile loading is represented by the slope of the curve from point A to point B in Figure 2–11. A value for stiffness can be found by dividing the load by the deformation at any point in the elastic range. The modulus of elasticity defines the

mechanical behavior of the material and is a measure of the material's stiffness (resistance offered by the material to external loads).

$$\text{Modulus} = \frac{\text{stress (load)}}{\text{strain (deformation)}}$$

$$\text{Young's modulus} = \frac{F/A}{\Delta L/L_0}$$

When the first portion of the curve is a straight line, the deformation (strain) is directly proportional to the material's ability to resist the load (see Fig. 2–11). If the slope of the curve is steep and the modulus of elasticity is high, the material will exhibit a high degree of stiffness. If the slope of the curve is gradual and the modulus of elasticity is low, the material will exhibit a low degree of stiffness. Cortical bone has a high modulus of elasticity, whereas subcutaneous fat has a low modulus of elasticity.

Each type of material has its own unique curve, but a typical curve for tendons and extremity ligaments using a constant rate of loading is presented in Figure 2–12. The first region of the curve from O to A is called the **toe region,** and for tendons and ligaments is described as being the region wherein the wavy pattern (**crimp**) that exists in collagen fibers at rest is straightened out. In this region, a minimal amount of force produces a relatively large amount of deformation (elongation). The toe region may be equated to the area in which an evaluator clinically tests the integrity of a liga-

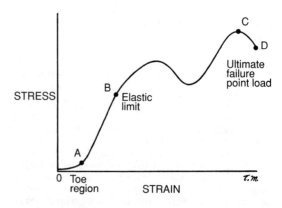

FIGURE 2–12. Load/deformation curve for a tendon or ligament. The O-A area of the curve is the toe region. The A-B area of the curve is the elastic region. The area of the curve between B and C is the plastic range. The ultimate failure point is indicated by the letter D.

ment by the application of a tensile force. The toe region also represents the slack in a tendon that must be taken up by the muscle before the muscle can apply a force to the bone through the tendon. The second linear A-B region of the curve is the elastic region in which elongation (strain) has a more or less linear relationship with the stress. The stiffness or resistance to deformation increases in this region, so more force is required to produce elongation. However, within this region, the ligament or tendon returns to its prestressed dimensions following the removal of a load although because of the viscoelasticity of the structures, the return is time dependent. This region illustrates the type of stress and strain that occurs in normal physiologic motion. In the third region, B-C (the plastic range) progressive failure of collagen fibers occurs and the ligament or tendon is no longer capable of returning to its original length. Plasticity may be considered to be a form of microfailure. When the plastic range is exceeded, overt **failure** or microfailure of the tissue occurs at D. In the case of a ligament or tendon, the failure may occur in the middle of the structures through tearing and disruption of the connective tissue fibers; this is called a **rupture.** If the failure occurs through a tearing off of the bony attachment of the ligament or tendon it is called an **avulsion.** When failure occurs in bony tissue, it is called a **fracture.**

Each type of connective tissue is able to undergo a different percentage of deformation before failure. This percentage varies not only among the types of connective tissue but also within the various types. Generally, ligaments are able to deform more than cartilage and cartilage is able to deform more than bone.

Properties of Specific Tissues

Bone

Stress-strain curves for bone demonstrate that cortical bone is stiffer than cancellous (trabecular) bone, meaning that cortical bone can withstand greater stress but less strain than cancellous bone. When cortical bone is loaded in compression, the strength of longitudinal sections of the bone have the greatest strength. In the femur, longitudinal sections have twice the modulus of elasticity of transverse sections. The compressive stress and strain that cortical bone can withstand before failure is greater than the tensile stress and strain. In other words, bone can withstand greater stress in compression than it can in tension.

The application of high loads maintained for a short period of time or low loads held for a long period of time will produce high stress and strain. Like cortical bone, the compressive strength of trabecular bone is greater than the tensile strength, whereas the modulus of elasticity is higher with tensile loads than with compressive loads. The physiologic response of trabecular bone to an increase in loading is hypertrophy. If loading is decreased or absent, the trabeculae become smaller and as a consequence less able to provide support. The rate, frequency, duration, and type of loading affect bone in that repeated loadings, either high repetition coupled with low load or low repetition with high load, can cause permanent strain and lead to bone failure. Bone loses stiffness and strength with repetitive loading as a result of creep strain. Creep strain occurs when a tissue is loaded repetitively during the time the material is undergoing creep.

Tendons

Tendons exhibit creep when subjected to either constant or uninterrupted cyclic tensile loading. Creep also occurs when a stress is applied to a tendon but the length of the tendon is held constant. If the length cannot change, there is a relaxation of tension within the tissue known as a stress-relaxation. If the muscle to which the tendon is attached contracts with a force of sufficient magnitude to just straighten out the crimp in the tendon, this straightening out of the crimp occurs in the toe region of the stress-strain curve. In this region there is little increase in stress with elongation and only 1.2% to 1.5% strain.[51] A force that stretches the already straightened fibers brings the tendon into the linear region of the curve where there is a linear relationship between the applied force and resulting tissue deformation. However, all the fibers are not perfectly parallel and therefore are not equally straightened. As a result the fibers that were already straightened will be the first to fail. Most of the normal activity of tendons occurs in the toe region and the first part of the linear region. As the loading increases beyond the linear region, the first damage is intrafibrillar slippage between molecules, then interfibrillar slippage between fibrils, and finally gross disruption of collagen fibers.

The cross-sectional area and the length of the

tendon determine the amount of force that a tendon can resist and the amount of elongation that it can undergo. The physiologic response of tendons to intermittent tension (application and release of a tensile force) is an increase in thickness and strength. Tendons are stronger when subjected to tensile stress than they are when subjected to compressive and shear forces. Generally larger tendons are able to withstand larger forces than smaller tendons. Differences in stress-strain curves among different tendons reflect differences in the proportion of type I and type II collagen, differences in cross-linking, maturity of collagen fibers, organization of fibrils, variations in ground substance concentration, and level of hydration. According to Benjamin and Ralphs, the enthesis is a common site of degenerative changes, whereas the myotendinous junction is a common site for muscle strains and pulls.[41] Therefore, under normal conditions the tendon is most vulnerable at either end rather than in the midsubstance. However, tendons rarely rupture under normal conditions and are able to withstand large tensile forces without injury. Tendons subject to immobilization show atrophy at the myotendinous junction and a decrease in collagen. Tendons subject to continual compressive forces will change their structure and function (show a decrease in tensile strength).

Ligaments

Ligament testing is similar to tendon testing in that a tensile load is applied to an isolated ligament and its behavior is graphically plotted on a load-deformation curve. The viscoelastic behavior of the ligament is exhibited by creep and stress-relaxation behavior. Ligaments exhibit creep wherein on the application of a fixed load the length of the ligament continues to increase up to either a new equilibrium or to the point of failure. Ligaments exhibit stress-relaxation when pulled to a fixed length and maintained at that length; over time, the amount of load in the ligament decreases (the ligament "relaxes"). The decrease is thought to be due to the load relaxation of the viscous component of the ligament. The load continues to decrease until a new equilibrium within the ligament is reached. Continuous adjustments between the viscous and elastic behavior allows the ligament to function within a range of loads without being damaged.[36] The physiologic response of ligaments to intermittent tension (application and

release of a tensile force) is an increase in thickness and strength. Ligaments are more variable than tendons in that they are designed to withstand both compressive and shear forces as well as tensile forces.

Cartilage

According to Cohen and Mow three forces in cartilage act to balance an applied load and are responsible for the viscoelastic behavior of cartilage. The forces are (1) stress developed in the extracellular matrix, (2) pressures developed in the fluid phase, and (3) frictional drag due to fluid flow through the extracellular matrix.[27] Compression of cartilage causes a change in the volume of the cartilage. The volumetric change leads to a pressure change that causes the flow of interstitial fluid. Fluid flow through the extracellular matrix creates a significant frictional resistance to the flow within the tissues (frictional drag). During creep caused by an applied compressive force, exudation of fluid occurs rapidly at first, causing a concomitant rapid rate of deformation. Subsequently, fluid flow and deformation gradually diminish and cease when stress in cartilage balances the applied load.[27] Magnetic resonance imaging (MRI) has made it possible to study changes in cartilage volume and thickness in joints in living subjects. In a MRI study of the knee joints of eight volunteers, Eckstein et al[52] found that up to 13% of the fluid was displaced from the patellar cartilage 3 to 7 minutes after exercise (50 knee bends).

Tensile stresses called **hoop stresses** are created in cartilage as a result of compression forces.[27] Although the tensile behavior of cartilage is similar to that of ligaments and tendons in that all of these tissues exhibit nonlinear tensile behavior, the cause of that behavior is slightly different in cartilage. The nonlinear tensile load deformation behavior of cartilage in the toe region of the curve is thought to be caused by the drag force that is needed to slide the collagen meshwork through the PGs. In ligaments and tendons the nonlinear behavior in the toe region is attributed the straightening of collagen fibers. In cartilage, as in ligaments and tendons, collagen fibers become taut in the linear region of the curve and demonstrate linear behavior. However, cartilage specimens taken from the different zones of cartilage (I, II, and III) have shown differences in tensile behavior. These differences have been attributed to differences in orientation of the collagen fibers among the zones and can be considered to represent anistropic effects.[27] Cartilage resistance to shear depends on the amount of collagen that is present because PGs provide little resistance to shear.[27] Shear stresses are apt to develop at the interface between the calcified cartilage layer and the subchondral bone.

The properties of the connective tissue structures described in the preceding section are designed to provide the reader with an introduction to the nature of the joint components and should help the reader to understand basic joint structure and function. The following two sections include the traditional classification system for human joints as well as a detailed description of synovial joint structure and function.

Human Joint Design

An appreciation of the complexities that are involved in human joint design may be gained by considering the nature of the bony components and the functions that the joints must serve. The human skeleton has about 200 bones that must be connected by joints. These bones vary in size from the pea-sized distal phalanx of the little toe to the over-a-foot-long femur of the thigh. The shape of the bones varies from round to flat, and the contours of the ends of the bones vary from convex to concave. The task of designing a series of joints to connect these varied bony components to form a stable structure would be difficult. The task of designing joints that are capable of working together to provide both mobility and stability for the total structure represents an engineering problem of considerable magnitude.

Joint designs in the human body vary from simple to complex. Although generally the designs used are complex, the same principles used in the table joints are used in human joint design. The more simple human joints usually have stability as a primary function; the more complex joints usually have mobility as a primary function. However, most joints in the human body have to serve a dual mobility-stability function and must also provide dynamic stability. The human stability joints are similar in design to the table joints in that the ends of the bones may be contoured either to fit into each other or to lie flat against each other. Bracing of human joints is accomplished through the use of joint capsules, ligaments, and tendons.

Joints designed primarily for human mobility are called **synovial joints.** These joints are constructed so that the ends of the bony components are hyaline cartilage covered and enclosed in a **synovial sheath** (joint capsule). The capsules, ligaments, and tendons located around mobility (synovial) joints not only help to provide stability for the joint but also guide, limit, and permit motion. Wedges of cartilage, called **menisci, disks, plates,** and **labrums** are used in synovial joints to increase stability, to provide shock absorption, and to facilitate motion (see Fig. 2–2). In addition, a lubricating fluid, called **synovial fluid,** is secreted at all mobility (synovial) joints to help reduce friction between the articulating surfaces.

In the traditional method of joint classification, the joints (**arthroses** or **articulations**) of the human body are divided into two broad categories based on the type of materials and the methods used to unite the bony components. Subdivisions of joint categories are based on materials used, the shape and contours of the articulating surfaces, and the type of motion allowed. The two broad categories of arthroses are **synarthroses** (nonsynovial joints) and **diarthroses** (synovial joints).[1]

Synarthroses

The material used to connect the bony components in synarthrodial joints is interosseus connective tissue (fibrous or cartilaginous). Synarthroses are grouped into two divisions according to the type of connective tissue used in the union of bone to bone: **fibrous joints** and **cartilaginous joints.** The connective tissue directly unites one bone to another creating a bone-solid connective tissue-bone interface.

Fibrous Joints

In fibrous joints, the fibrous tissue directly unites bone to bone. Three different types of fibrous joints are found in the human body: **sutures, gomphoses,** and **syndesmoses.** A suture joint is one in which two bony components are united by a collagenous sutural ligament or membrane. The ends of the bony components are shaped so that the edges interlock or overlap one another. This type of joint is found only in the skull and early in life allows a small amount of movement. Fusion of the two opposing bones in suture joints occurs later in life and leads to the formation of a bony union called a **synostosis.**

EXAMPLE 2: Coronal suture (Fig. 2–13). The serrated edges of the parietal and frontal bones of the skull are connected by a thin fibrous membrane (the sutural ligament) to form the coronal suture. At birth the fibrous membrane allows some motion for ease of passage through the birth canal. Also during infancy slight motion is possible for growth of the brain and skull. In adulthood, the bones grow together to form a synostosis and little or no motion is possible.

A gomphosis joint is a joint in which the surfaces of bony components are adapted to each other like a peg in a hole. In this type of joint the component parts are connected by fibrous tissue. The only gomphosis joint that exists in the human body is the joint that is found between a tooth and either the mandible or maxilla.

EXAMPLE 3: The conical process of a tooth is inserted in the bony socket of the mandible or maxilla. In the adult, the loss of teeth is, for the most part, due to disease processes affecting the connective tissue that cements or holds the teeth in approximation to the bone. Under normal conditions in the adult these joints do not permit motion between the components.

A syndesmosis is a type of fibrous joint in which two bony components are joined directly by an interosseous ligament, a fibrous cord, or

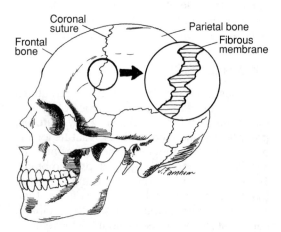

FIGURE 2–13. The coronal suture. The frontal and parietal bones of the skull are joined directly by fibrous tissue to form a synarthrodial suture joint.

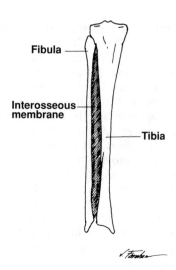

FIGURE 2–14. The shafts of the fibula and tibia are joined directly by a membrane to form a synarthrodial syndesmosis.

aponeurotic membrane. These joints usually allow a small amount of motion.

EXAMPLE 4: The shaft of the tibia is joined directly to the shaft of the fibula by an interosseous membrane (Fig. 2–14). A slight amount of motion at this joint accompanies movement at the ankle joint.

Cartilaginous Joints

The materials used to connect the bony components in cartilaginous joints are either **fibrocartilage** or **hyaline cartilage.** These materials are used to directly unite one bony surface to another creating a bone-cartilage-bone interface. The two types of cartilaginous joints are **symphyses** and **synchondroses.**

In a **symphysis joint (secondary cartilaginous joint)** the two bony components are covered with a thin lamina of hyaline cartilage and directly joined by fibrocartilage in the form of disks or pads. Examples of symphysis joints include the intervertebral joints between the bodies of the vertebrae, the joint between the manubrium and the sternal body, and the symphysis pubis in the pelvis.

EXAMPLE 5: The symphysis pubis (Fig. 2–15a). The two pubic bones of the pelvis are joined by fibrocartilage. This joint must serve as a weight-bearing joint and is responsible for withstanding and transmitting forces; therefore, under normal conditions very little motion is permissible or desirable. During pregnancy when the connective tissues are softened, some slight separation of the joint surfaces occurs to ease the passage of the baby through the birth canal. However, the symphysis pubis is considered to be primarily a stability joint with the thick fibrocartilage disk forming a stable union between the two bony components.

Synchondrosis (primary cartilaginous joint) is a type of joint in which the material used for connecting the two components is hyaline cartilage. The cartilage forms a bond between two ossifying centers of bone. The function of this type of joint is to permit bone growth while also providing stability and allowing a small amount of mobility. Some of these joints are found in the skull and in other areas of the body at sites of bone growth. When bone growth is complete some of these joints ossify and convert to bony unions (synostoses).

EXAMPLE 6: The first chondrosternal joint (Fig. 2–15b). The adjacent surfaces of the first rib and sternum are connected directly by articular cartilage.

Diarthroses

The method of joint construction in diarthrodial or synovial joints differs from that used in synarthrodial joints. In synovial joints the ends of the bony components are free to move in relation to one another because no connective tissue directly connects adjacent bony surfaces. The bony components are *indirectly connected to one another by means of a joint capsule that encloses the joint.* All synovial joints are constructed in a similar fashion and all have the following features: (1) a joint capsule that is composed of two layers; (2) a joint cavity that is enclosed by the joint capsule; (3) synovial tissue that lines the inner surface of the capsule; (4) synovial fluid that forms a film over the joint surfaces; and (5) hyaline cartilage that covers the surfaces of the enclosed contiguous bones (Fig. 2–16). In addition, synovial joints are associated with accessory structures such as fibrocartilaginous disks, plates or menisci, labrums, fat pads, and ligaments and tendons. Articular disks, menisci, and the synovial fluid

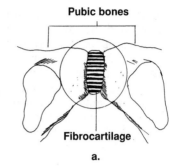

a.

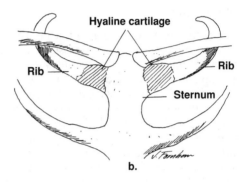

b.

FIGURE 2–15. Cartilaginous joints. (a) The two pubic bones of the pelvis are joined directly by fibrocartilage to form a symphysis joint called the **symphysis pubis.** (b) The first rib and the sternum are connected directly by hyaline cartilage to form a synchondrosis joint called the **first chondrosternal joint.**

help to prevent excessive compression of opposing joint surfaces. Articular disks and menisci often occur between articular surfaces where congruity is low. Articular disks may extend all the way across a joint and actually divide it into two separate cavities such as the articular disk at the distal radioulnar joint.

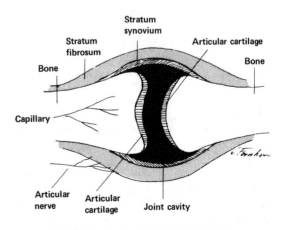

FIGURE 2–16. A typical diarthrodial joint.

Menisci usually do not divide a joint but provide lubrication and increase congruity. Ligaments and tendons associated with these joints play an important role in keeping joint surfaces together and may assist in guiding motion. Excessive separation of joint surfaces is limited by passive tension in ligaments, the fibrous joint capsule, and tendons. Active tension in muscles also limits the separation of joint surfaces.

Joint Capsule

Joint capsules vary considerably both in thickness and composition. Capsules such as the one enclosing the shoulder joint are thin, loose, and redundant and therefore sacrifice stability for mobility. Other capsules such as the hip joint capsule are thick and dense and thus favor stability over mobility. The fact that the thickness, fiber orientation, and even composition of the capsule depend to a large extent on the stresses that are placed on the joint illustrates the dynamic nature of the joint capsule. For example, in portions of the capsule that are subjected to compression forces, the capsule may become fibrocartilagenous.[3] Shoulder capsules in patients with shoulder instabilty in which the capsules are subjected to repeated tensile deformation have significantly larger mean collagen fibril diameters and increased density of elastin fibers compared with normal capsules. These changes in collagen fibrils and elastin density are interpreted as capsular adaptations oriented toward increasing capsular strength and resistance to stretching deformation.[4]

The fibrous capsule may be reinforced by and in some instances actually incorporate ligaments or tendons as a part of the capsule. For example, the capsule of the proximal interphalangeal joint of the fingers is reinforced by collateral ligaments superficially, and a central slip of the extensor tendon superficially and posteriorly.[5]

The joint capsule is composed of two layers, an outer layer called the **stratum fibrosum,** and an inner layer called the **stratum synovium** (see Fig. 2–16). The stratum fibrosum, which is sometimes referred to as the fibrous capsule, is composed of dense fibrous tissue. Collagen and elastin account for about 90% of the dry weight and water for about 70% of the wet weight.[6] The predominant type of collagen is type I, which is usually arranged in parallel

bundles. As the capsule nears its insertion to bone, initially the collagen bundles change to uncalcified fibrocartilage. Next, the uncalcified fibrocartilage changes to calcified fibrocartilage and then to bone (collagen bundles to uncalicified fibrocartilage to calcified fibrocartilage to bone). The stratum fibrosum is poorly vascularized but richly innervated by joint receptors. The receptors are located in and around the capsule.[7]

The inner layer (stratum synovium) is the lining tissue of the capsule. It also consists of two layers, the **intima** and the **subsynovial tissue.** The intima is the layer of cells that lining cells the joint space. It is composed of a layer of specialized fibroblasts known as synoviocytes that are arranged one to three cells deep and set in a fiber-free intracellular matrix.[6] Two types of **synoviocytes** are generally recognized: type A and type B.[1] Type A synoviocytes are macrophage-like cells with prominent Golgi apparatus but sparse granular endoplasmic reticulum. In contrast, type B synoviocytes have abundant granular endoplasmic reticulum and are twice as numerous as type A cells in normal synovium.[8] Type A cells are primarily responsible for the removal of debris from the joint cavity. During phagocytosis type A cells synthesize and release lytic enzymes that have the potential for damaging joint tissues. Type B cells synthesize and release enzyme inhibitors that inhibit the lytic enzymes. Type B cells are also responsible for initiating an immune response through the secretion of antigens. As part of their function in joint maintenance, both types of cells synthesize the hyaluronic acid component of the synovial fluid as well as constituents of the matrix in which the cells are embedded. Type A and B cells also secrete a wide range of cytokines including tumor necrosis factor-α, interferon-γ, fibronectin, and multiple growth factors. The interplay of the cytokines acting as stimulators or inhibitors of synoviocytes results in structural repair of synovium, response to foreign or autologous antigens, and tissue destruction.[8]

The subsynovial tissue lies outside the intima as a loose network of highly vascularized fibrous connective tissue. It attaches to the margins of the articular cartilage through a transitional zone of fibrocartilage and joins with the periosteum covering the bones that lie within the confines of the capsule. Its cells are slightly different from the intima cells in that they are more spindle shaped and more widely dispersed between collagen fibrils than the intimal cells. Also, they produce matrix collagen.[9] The subsynovial tissue provides support for the intima and merges with the fibrous capsule on its external surface. The intima is richly endowed with capillary vessels, lymphatics, and nerve fibers. The blood vessels in the subsynovial tissue transport oxygen, nutrients, and immunologic cells to the joint.

Branches of adjacent peripheral nerves and branches of nerves from muscles at the joint penetrate the fibrous joint capsule. Large-diameter sensory efferent nerves and thinly myelinated nerves are present in the fibrous capsule; nonmyelinated C-type fibers are found in the synovium. The joint receptors found in the fibrous joint capsule are sensitive to stretching or compression of the capsule, as well as to an increase in internal pressure due to increased production of synovial fluid. Most of the joint receptors in the knee are located in the subsynovial layer of the capsule in close proximity to the insertions of the anterior cruciate ligament (ACL). Mechanoreceptors (predominantly Ruffini receptors) in the subsynovial capsule and ACL respond primarily to the stretch involved in terminal extension rather than the compression involved in the movement toward flexion in the partially extended knee. Pacini receptors are reported less frequently and are thought to be activated by compression. Free nerve endings are more numerous than mechanoreceptors and function as nociceptors that react to inflammation and pain stimuli. Afferent free nerve endings in joints not only transfer information but also serve a local effector role by releasing neuropeptides.[10] Table 2–5 summarizes the receptors found in the joint capsule.

Synovial Fluid

The thin film of synovial fluid that covers the surfaces of the inner layer of the joint capsule and articular cartilage helps to keep the joint surfaces lubricated and thus reduces friction between the bony components. The fluid also provides nourishment for the hyaline cartilage covering the articular surfaces. The composition of synovial fluid is similar to blood plasma except that synovial fluid contains hyaluronate (hyaluronic acid) and a glycoprotein called **lubricin.**[19] The hyaluronate component of synovial fluid is responsible for the viscosity of the fluid and is essential for lubrication of the synovium. Hyaluronate reduces the friction between the synovial folds of the capsule and the articular surfaces.[19] Lubricin is the component of synovial fluid that is thought to be responsible for cartilage-on-cartilage lubrication.[6] Changes in the concentration of hyaluronate or lubricin in the synovial fluid will affect the overall lubrication and the amount of friction that is present. Many experiments have confirmed that articular coefficients of friction (COFs) in synovial joints are lower than those that can be produced using manufactured lubricants.[19] The lower the COF, the lower the resistance to sliding.

Normal synovial fluid appears as a clear, pale yellow viscous fluid that is present in small amounts at all synovial joints.[20] There is a direct exchange between the vasculature of the stra-

Table 2–5. ***Joint Receptors***

Type	Name	Sensitivity	Location
I	Ruffini	Stretch—usually at extremes of extension	Fibrous layer of joint capsules on flexion side of joints, periosteum, ligaments, and tendons[10]
II	Pacini or pacini-form	Compression or changes in hydrostatic pressure and joint movement[1]	Located throughout joint capsule, particularly in deeper layers and in fat pads
III	Golgi, Golgi Mazzoni	Pressure and forceful joint motion into extremes of motion	Inner layer (synovium) of joint capsules, ligaments and tendons[10]
IV	Unmyelinated free nerve endings	Nonnoxious and noxious mechanical stress or biomechanical stress	Located around blood vessels in synovial layer of capsule, and in adjacent fat pads and collateral ligaments, tendons and the periosteum.

tum synovium and the intracapsular space where nutrients can be supplied and waste products can be taken away from the joint by diffusion.[19] Usually, less than 0.5 mL of synovial fluid can be removed from large joints such as the knee.[1] However, when a joint is injured or diseased, the volume of the fluid may increase.[19]

The synovial fluid exhibits properties common to all viscous substances in that it has the ability to resist loads that produce shear.[21] The viscosity of the fluid *varies inversely* with the joint velocity or rate of shear. Thus the synovial fluid is referred to as **thixotropic.** When the bony components of a joint are moving rapidly, the viscosity of the fluid decreases and provides less resistance to motion.[21] When the bony components of a joint are moving slowly, the viscosity increases and provides more resistance to motion. Viscosity also is sensitive to changes in temperature. High temperatures decrease the viscosity, whereas low temperatures increase the viscosity.[1]

Joint Lubrication

A number of models have been proposed to explain how diarthrodial joints are lubricated under varying loading conditions. The general consensus is that no single model is adequate to explain human joint lubrication and that human joints are lubricated by two or more of the following types of lubrication used in engineering. The two basic types of lubrication are boundary lubrication and fluid lubrication.

Boundary lubrication occurs when each load-bearing surface is coated or impregnated with a thin layer of large molecules that forms a gel that keeps the opposing surfaces from touching each other (Fig. 2–17a). The molecules slide on the opposing surface more readily than they are sheared off the underlying surface. In human diarthrodial joints these molecules are composed of a special glycoprotein called lubricin, which is found in the synovial fluid. The lubricin molecules adhere to the articular surfaces.[22] This type of lubrication is considered to be most effective at low loads.[6]

Fluid lubrication models include hydrostatic (weeping) lubrication; hydrodynamic, squeeze-film lubrication; and elastohydrodynamic and boosted lubrication. Generally, fluid lubrication models include the existence of a film of fluid that is interposed between the joint surfaces. **Hydrostatic** or **weeping lubrication** is a form of fluid lubrication in which the load-bear-

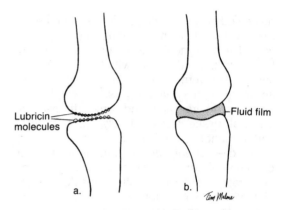

FIGURE 2–17. Joint lubrication models. (a) Schematic drawing of the lubricin molecules coating the joint surfaces in boundary lubrication. (b) Schematic drawing of the fluid film that keeps joint surfaces apart in hydrostatic lubrication.

ing surfaces are held apart by a film of lubricant that is maintained under pressure (Fig. 2–17b). In engineering, the pressure is usually supplied by an external pump. In the human body the pump action can be supplied by contractions of muscles around the joint. Compression of articular cartilage causes the cartilage to deform and to "weep" fluid, which forms a fluid film over the articular surfaces. This is possible because an impervious layer of calcified cartilage keeps the fluid from being forced into the subchondral bone.[19] When the load is removed, the fluid flows back into the articular cartilage. This type of lubrication is most effective under conditions of high loading, but it can be effective under most conditions.[6]

Hydrodynamic lubrication is a form of fluid lubrication in which a wedge of fluid is created when nonparallel opposing surfaces slide on one another. The resulting lifting pressure generated in the wedge of fluid and by the fluid's viscosity keeps the joint surfaces apart. In **squeeze-film lubrication,** pressure is created in the fluid film by the movement of articular surfaces that are perpendicular to one another.[22] As the opposing articular surfaces move closer together, they squeeze the fluid film out of the area of impending contact. The resulting pressure that is created by the fluid's viscosity keeps the surfaces separated. This type of lubrication is suitable for high loads maintained for a short duration.[5]

In the **elastohydrodynamic model,** the protective fluid film is maintained at an appropriate thickness by the elastic deformation of the articular surfaces. In **boosted lubrication** the model suggests that pools of concentrated hyaluronate molecules are filtered out of the synovial fluid and are trapped in the natural undulations and areas of elastic deformation on the articular surface just as the opposing surfaces meet.[22]

The joint lubrication models presented provide a number of possible options for explaining how diarthrodial joints are lubricated. The variety of conditions under which human joints function make it likely that more than one of the lubrication models are operating. Until a unified model of joint lubrication is proposed, proved, and accepted, the exact mechanisms involved in human joint lubrication will be subject to speculation.[1]

Subclassifications of Diarthrodial Joints

Traditionally, synovial joints have been divided into three main categories on the basis of the number of axes about which "gross visible" motion occurs. A further subdivision of the joints is made on the basis of the shape and configuration of the ends of the bony components. The three main traditional categories are uniaxial, biaxial, and triaxial. A **uniaxial joint** is constructed so that visible motion of the bony components is allowed in only one of the planes of the body around a single axis. The axis of motion usually is located near or in the center of the joint or in one of the bony components. Because uniaxial joints only permit visible motion in one plane, or around one axis, they are described as having 1° of freedom of motion.

The two types of **uniaxial diarthrodial joints** found in the human body are hinge joints and pivot (trochoid) joints. A **hinge joint** is a type of joint that resembles a door hinge.

> EXAMPLE 7: Interphalangeal joints of the fingers (Fig. 2–18a). These joints are formed between the distal end of one phalanx and proximal end of another phalanx. The joint surfaces are contoured so that motion can occur in the sagittal plane only (flexion and extension) around a coronal axis (Fig. 2–18b).

UNIAXIAL JOINTS

A **pivot (trochoid) joint** is a type of joint constructed so that one component is shaped like a ring and the other component is shaped so that it can rotate within the ring.

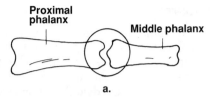

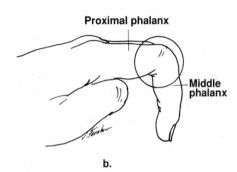

FIGURE 2–18. A uniaxial hinge joint. (a) The interphalangeal joints of the fingers are examples of simple hinge joints. The joint capsule and accessory joint structures have been removed to show the bony components in the superior view of the joint. (b) Motion occurs in one plane around one axis.

> EXAMPLE 8: The median atlantoaxial joint (Fig. 2–19). The ring portion of the joint is formed by the atlas and the transverse ligament. The odontoid process (dens) of the axis, which is enclosed in the ring, rotates within the osteoligamentous ring. Motion occurs in the transverse plane around a longitudinal axis.

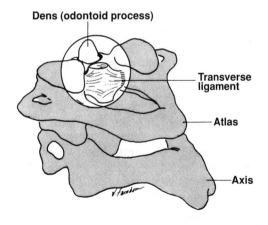

FIGURE 2–19. A pivot joint. The joint between the atlas, transverse ligament, and the dens of the axis is a uniaxial diarthrodial pivot joint called the **median atlantoaxial** joint. Rotation occurs in the transverse plane around a vertical axis.

BIAXIAL JOINTS

Biaxial diarthrodial joints are joints in which the bony components are free to move in two planes around two axes. Therefore, these joints have 2° of freedom. There are two types of biaxial joints in the body: **condyloid** and **saddle.** The joint surfaces in a condyloid joint are shaped so that the concave surface of one bony component is allowed to slide over the convex surface of another component in two directions.

EXAMPLE 9: Metacarpophalangeal joint (Fig. 2–20a). The metacarpophalangeal joint is formed by the convex distal end of a metacarpal bone and the concave proximal end of the proximal phalanx. Flexion and extension at this joint occur in the sagittal plane around a coronal axis (Fig. 2–20b). Abduction is movement away from the middle finger, whereas adduction is movement toward the middle finger. Adduction and abduction occur in the frontal plane around an anterior-posterior (A-P) axis (Fig. 2–20c).

A **saddle joint** is a joint in which each joint surface is both convex in one plane and concave in the other and these surfaces are fitted together like a rider on a saddle.

EXAMPLE 10: Carpometacarpal joint of the thumb. The carpometacarpal joint of the thumb is formed by the distal end of the carpal bone and the proximal end of the metacarpal. The motions available are flexion and extension and abduction/adduction.

TRIAXIAL JOINTS

Triaxial or **multiaxial diarthrodial joints** are joints in which the bony components are free to move in three planes around three axes. These joints have 3° of freedom. Motion at these joints also may occur in oblique planes. The two types of joints in this category are **plane joints** and **ball-and-socket joints.**
- **Plane** joints have a variety of surface configurations and permit gliding between two or more bones.

EXAMPLE 11: Carpal joints. These joints are found between the adjacent surfaces of the carpal bones. The adjacent surfaces may glide

on one another or rotate with respect to one another in any plane.

- **Ball-and-socket joints** are formed by a ball-like convex surface being fitted into a concave socket. The motions permitted are flexion/extension, abduction/adduction, and rotation.

EXAMPLE 12: Hip joint. The hip joint is formed by the head of the femur and a socket called the acetabulum (Fig. 2–21a). The motions of the flexion/extension occur in the sagittal plane around a coronal axis (Fig. 2–21b). Abduction/adduction occurs in the frontal plane around an A-P axis (Fig. 2–21c) while rotation of the femur occurs in the transverse plane around a longitudinal axis (Fig. 2–21d).

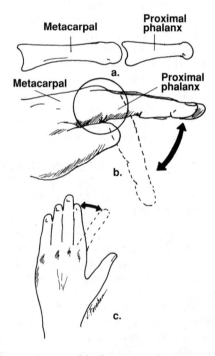

FIGURE 2–20. A condyloid joint. (a) The metacarpophalangeal joints of the fingers are biaxial condyloid joints. The joint capsule and accessory structures have been removed to show the bony components. Motion at these joints occurs in two planes around two axes. (b) Flexion and extension occur in the sagittal plane around a coronal axis. (c) Abduction and adduction occur in the frontal plane around an A-P axis.

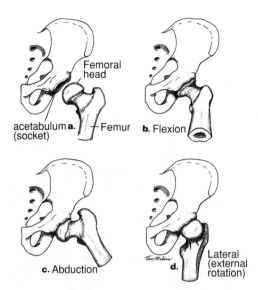

FIGURE 2–21. A ball-and-socket-joint. (a) The joint between the femoral head and the acetabulum is a triaxial diarthrodial joint called the **hip joint**. Motion may occur in three planes around three axes. (b) Flexion/extension occur in the sagittal plane around a coronal axis. (c) Abduction/adduction occur in the frontal plane around an A-P axis. (d) Rotation occurs in the transverse plane around a longitudinal axis.

Joint Function

The structure of the joints of the human body reflects the functions that the joints are designed to serve. The synarthrodial joints are relatively simple in design and function primarily as stability joints, although motion does occur. The diarthrodial joints are complex and are designed primarily for mobility, although all of these joints must also provide some variable measure of stability. Effective functioning of the total structure depends on the integrated action of many joints, some providing stability and some providing mobility. Generally, stability must be achieved before mobility if normal function is to be maintained.

Kinematic Chains

Some of the joints of the human body are linked together into a series of joints in such a way that motion at one of the joints in the series is accompanied by motion at an adjacent joint. For instance, when a person in the erect standing position bends both knees, simultaneous motion must occur at the ankle and hip joints if the person is to remain upright (Fig.

2–22a). However, when the leg is lifted from the ground, the knee is free to bend without causing motion at either the hip or ankle (Fig. 2–22b). The type of motion that occurs in the joints of the lower limb when a person is standing may be explained by using the concept of a **kinematic chain.**[23] Kinematic chains in the engineering sense are composed of a series of rigid links that are interconnected by a series of pin-centered joints. In engineering, the system of joints and links is constructed so that motion of one link at one joint will produce motion at all of the other joints in the system in a predictable manner. The kinematic chains in engineering form a closed system or **closed kinematic chain.**[23] In the human system of joints and links, the joints of the lower limbs and the pelvis function as a closed kinematic chain when a person is in the erect weight-bearing position because the ends of the limbs are fixed on the ground and the upper ends of the limbs are virtually fixed to the pelvis. However, the ends of human limbs frequently are not fixed but are free to move without necessarily causing motion at another joint. The motion of waving the hand may occur at the wrist without causing motion of the fingers distally or elbow or shoulder proximally. When the ends of the limbs or parts of the body are free to move without causing motion at another joint, the system is referred to as an **open kinematic chain.** In an open kinematic chain, motion does not occur in a predictable fashion be-

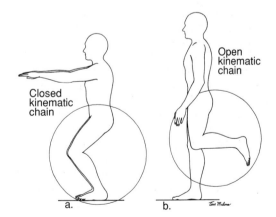

FIGURE 2–22. Closed and open kinematic chains. (a) In a closed kinematic chain, knee flexion is accompanied by hip flexion and ankle dorsiflexion. (b) Knee motion in an open kinematic may occur with or without motion at the hip and ankle. In the diagram, knee flexion is shown without simultaneous motion at the hip and the ankle.

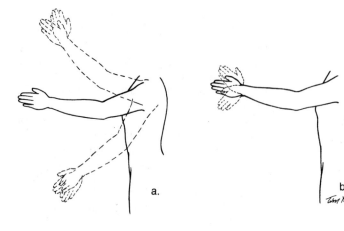

FIGURE 2–23. Open kinematic chain motion. (a) When the entire upper limb is moving at the shoulder, 9° of freedom of motion (sum of the degrees of freedom at the shoulder, elbow, and wrist) are available to the hand. (b) The hand has only the 2° of freedom at the wrist available, and the motion of the hand is limited in space.

cause joints may function either independently or in unison.

EXAMPLE 13: One may wave the whole upper limb by moving the arm at the glenohumeral joint at the shoulder (Fig. 2–23a) or one may move only at the wrist. In the first instance, all of the degrees of freedom of all of the joints from the shoulder to the wrist are available to the distal segment (hand). If the person is waving from the wrist, only the degrees of freedom at the wrist would be available to the hand, and motion of the hand in space would be more limited than in the first situation (Fig. 2–23b).

The concept of kinematic chains, which is useful for analyzing human motion and the effects of injury and disease on the joints of the body, will be referred to throughout this text. Although the joints in the human body do not always behave in a predictable fashion in either a closed or open chain, the joints are interdependent. A change in the function or structure of one joint in the system will usually cause a change in the function of a joint either immediately adjacent to the affected joint or at a distal joint. For example, if the range of motion (ROM) at the knee were limited, the hip and ankle joints would have to compensate so that the foot could clear the floor when the person was walking so he or she could avoid stumbling.

Joint Motion

Arthrokinematics

Motion at a joint occurs as the result of movement of one joint surface in relation to another.

The term **arthrokinematics** is used to refer to movements of joint surfaces. Usually one of the joint surfaces is more stable than the other and serves as a base for the motion, whereas the other surface moves on this relatively fixed base. The terms roll, slide, and spin are used to describe the type of motion that the moving part performs.[1,24] A **roll** refers to the rolling of one joint surface on another, as in a tire rolling on the road. In the knee, the femoral condyles roll on the fixed tibial surface. **Sliding,** which is a pure translatory motion, refers to the gliding of one component over another, as when a braked wheel skids. In the hand, the proximal phalanx slides over the fixed end of the metacarpal. The term **spin** refers to a rotation of the movable component, as when a top spins. Spin is a pure rotatory motion. At the elbow, the head of the radius spins on the capitulum of the humerus during supination and pronation of the forearm.

The type of motion that occurs at a particular joint depends on the shape of the articulating surfaces. Most joints fit into either an ovoid or a sellar category. In an **ovoid** joint, one surface is convex and the other surface is concave (Fig. 2–24a). In a **sellar** joint, *each* joint surface is *both* convex and concave (Fig. 2–24b). In an ovoid joint, when a convex articulating surface moves on a stable concave surface, the sliding of the convex articulating surface occurs in the *opposite direction* to the motion of the bony lever (Fig. 2–25a). When a concave articulating surface is moving on a stable convex surface, sliding occurs in the *same direction* as motion of the bony lever (Fig. 2–25b).

The sliding that occurs between articular surfaces is an essential component of joint motion and must occur for normal functioning

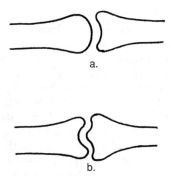

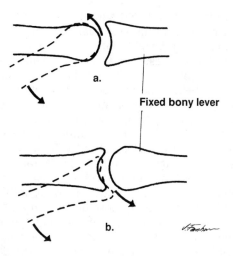

FIGURE 2–24. Ovoid and sellar joints. (a) In an ovoid joint one articulating surface is convex and the other articulating surface is concave. (b) In a sellar joint each articulating surface is concave and convex.

Fixed bony lever

FIGURE 2–25. Motion at ovoid joints. (a) When a convex surface is moving on a fixed concave surface, the convex articulating surface moves in a direction opposite to the direction traveled by the shaft of the bony lever. (b) When a concave surface is moving on a fixed convex surface, the concave articulating surface moves in the same direction as the remaining portion of the bony lever (proximal phalanx moving on fixed metacarpal).

of the joint. The distal end of a bone cannot be expected to move if the articular end of the bone is not free to move (slide) in the appropriate direction.

> EXAMPLE 14: Abduction of the distal end of the humerus must be accompanied by downward sliding (inferior movement) of the proximal convex head of the humerus on the concave surface of the glenoid fossa for the distal end to elevate without damage to the joint (Fig. 2–26a). Superior gliding of the humeral head must occur for the distal end of the humerus to be brought back downward into adduction (Fig. 2–26b).

For articular surfaces to be free to slide in the appropriate direction as the bony lever moves, the joint must have a certain amount of "**joint play.**" This movement of one articular surface on another is not usually under voluntary control and must be tested for by the application of an external force. In an optimal situation, a joint has a sufficient amount of play to allow normal motion at the joint's articulating surfaces. If the supporting joint structures are lax, the joint may have too much play and become unstable. If the joint structures are tight, the joint will have too little movement between the articular surfaces and the amount of motion of the bony lever will be restricted.

Joint motions are commonly produced as a result of a combination of sliding, spinning, and rolling. This combination of sliding and spinning or rolling produces curvilinear motion and a moving axis of motion. An axis that moves during rolling or sliding motions forms a series of successive points. The axis of rota-

tion at any particular point in the motion is called the **instantaneous axis of rotation (IAR).** IARs occur most notably when opposing articular surfaces are of unequal size. In some joints, such as the shoulder, the articulating surface of the moving bone is larger than the surface of the stabilized component. In other joints such as the metacarpophalangeal and interphalangeal joints of the fingers, the articulating surface of the moving bone is smaller than the surface of the stabilized component. When the articulating surface of a moving com-

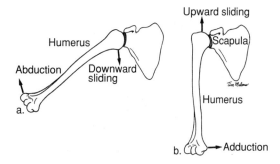

FIGURE 2–26. Sliding of joint surfaces. (a) Abduction of the humerus must be accompanied by inferior sliding of the head of the humerus in the glenoid fossa. (b) Adduction of the humerus is accompanied by superior sliding of the head of the humerus.

ponent is larger than the stabilized component (the head of the humerus is larger than the glenoid fossa of the scapula), a pure motion such as rolling will result in the larger moving component rolling off the smaller articulating surface before the motion is completed (Fig. 2–27). Therefore, combination motions, wherein a moving component rolls in one direction and slides in the opposite direction, help to increase the ROM available to the joint and keep opposing joint surfaces in contact with each other. Another method of increasing the range of available motion is by permitting both components to move at the same time. The rolling and sliding arthrokinematic movements of the articular surfaces are not usually visible and thus have not been described in the traditional classification system of joint movement. However, these motions are considered in the 6° of freedom model described by White and Panjabi.[25] These authors have suggested that motion at the intervertebral symphysis joints between the bodies of the vertebrae in the vertebral column occurs in six planes, around three axes (see Fig. 4–5a–f in Chap. 4). The implication is that motion at the joints of the body might be more thoroughly described by using a 6° of freedom model.

All synovial joints have a **close-packed** position in which the joint surfaces are maximally congruent and the ligaments and capsule are maximally taut. The close-packed position is usually at the extreme end of a ROM. In the close-packed position a joint possesses its greatest stability and is resistant to tensile forces that tend to cause distraction (separation) of the joint surfaces. The position of extension is the close-packed position for the humeroulnar, knee, and interphalangeal joints.[1,26] In the **loose-packed** position of a joint, the articular surfaces are relatively free to move in relation to one another. The loose-packed position of a joint is any position other than the close-packed position, although the term is commonly used to refer to the position at which the joint structures are more lax and the joint cavity has a greater volume than in other positions. In the loose-packed position, the joint has a certain amount of joint play. An externally applied force, such as that applied by a therapist or physician, can produce movement of one articular surface on another and enable the examiner to assess the amount of joint play that is present. Movement in and out of the close-packed position is likely to have a beneficial effect on joint nutrition because of the squeezing out of the fluid during each compression and imbibing of fluid when the compression is removed.[26]

Osteokinematics

Osteokinematics refers to the movement of the bones rather than the movement of the articular surfaces. The normal ROM of a joint is sometimes called the anatomic or physiologic ROM, because it refers to the amount of motion available to a joint within the anatomic limits of the joint structure. The extent of the anatomic range is determined by a number of factors, including the shape of the joint surfaces, the joint capsule, ligaments, muscle bulk, and surrounding musculotendinous and bony structures. In some joints there are no bony limitations to motion and the ROM is limited only by soft tissue structures. For example, the knee joint has no bony limitations to motion. Other joints have definite bony restrictions to motion in addition to soft tissue limitations. The humeroulnar joint at the elbow is limited in extension (close-packed position) by bony contact of the ulna on the olecranon fossa of the humerus.

A ROM is considered to be pathologic when motion at a joint either exceeds or fails to reach the normal anatomic limits of motion. When a ROM exceeds the normal limits the joint is hypermobile. When the ROM is less than what would normally be permitted by the structure, the joint is hypomobile. **Hypermobility** may be caused by a failure to limit motion by either the bony or soft tissues and re-

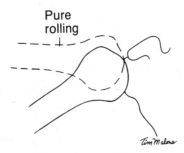

Pure rolling

FIGURE 2–27. Rolling and sliding of joint surfaces. The larger head of the humerus rolls out of the glenoid fossa when pure rolling occurs. The head of the humerus remains in contact with the glenoid fossa when a combination of rolling and sliding occurs.

sults in instability. **Hypomobility** may be caused by bony or cartilaginous blocks to motion or by the inability of the capsule, ligaments, or muscles to elongate sufficiently to allow a normal ROM. A **contracture,** which is a term used to describe the shortening of soft tissue structures around a joint, is one cause of hypomobility. Either hypermobility or hypomobility of a joint may have undesirable effects, not only at the affected joint but also on adjacent joint structures.

General Effects of Disease, Injury, and Immobilization

The design of the joints in the human body is such that each structure that is a part of a joint has one or more specific functions that are essential for the overall performance of the joint. Therefore, any process that disrupts any one of the parts of a joint will disrupt the total function of the joint. The complex joints are more likely to be affected by injury, disease, or aging than the simple joints. The complex joints have more parts and are subject to more wear and tear than stability joints. Also, the function of the complex joints depends on a number of interrelated factors. For example, the capsule must produce synovial fluid. The fluid must be of the appropriate composition and of sufficient quantity that it can lubricate and provide nourishment for the joint. The hyaline cartilage must be smooth so that the joint surfaces can move easily and must be permeable so that it can receive some of its nourishment from the joint fluid. The cartilage also must undergo periodic compressive loading and unloading to facilitate movement of the fluid. The ligaments and capsules must be able to provide sufficient support for stability and yet be flexible enough to permit normal mobility.

Disease

The general effects of disease, injury, immobilization, overuse, and aging may be postulated by using the normal function of a joint structure as a basis for analysis. For example, if the synovial membrane of a joint is affected by a collagen disease such as rheumatoid arthritis, one may assume that because the normal function of the synovial membrane is to produce synovial fluid, the production and perhaps the composition of the synovial fluid will be altered

in this disease. One could also postulate that because fluid is altered, the lubrication of the joint also would be altered. The disease process and the changes in joint structure that occur in rheumatoid arthritis actually involve more than synovial fluid alteration, but the disease does change the composition and the quantity of the synovial fluid. In another type of arthritis, osteoarthritis, which is thought to be a genetic disorder, the cartilage rather than the synovium and the soft tissue is the focus of the disease process. Based on normal cartilage function, one can assume that the cartilage in osteoarthritic joints will not be able to withstand normal stress. Actually, erosion and splitting of the cartilage occur under stress. As a result, friction is increased between the joint surfaces, thus further increasing the erosion process.

Injury

If an injury has occurred, such as the tearing of a ligament, one may assume that there will be a lack of support for the joint. In the example of the table with an unstable joint between the leg and the table top, damage and disruption of function may occur as a result of instability. If a heavy load is placed on the damaged table joint, the joint surfaces will separate under the compressive load and the leg may be angled. The once-stable joint now allows mobility and the leg may wobble back and forth. This motion may cause the screws to loosen or the nails to bend and ultimately to be torn out of one of the wooden components.

Complete failure of the joint may result in splintering of the wooden components, especially when the already weakened joint is subjected to excessive, sudden, or prolonged loads. The effects of a lack of support in a human joint are similar to that of the table joint. Separation of the bony surfaces occurs and may result in wobbling or a deviation from the normal alignment of one of the bony components. These changes in alignment create an abnormal joint distraction on the side where a ligament is torn. As a result, the other ligaments, the tendons, and the joint capsule may become excessively stretched and consequently be unable to provide protection. The supported side of the joint may also be affected and subjected to abnormal compression during weight-bearing or motion. In canine experiments in which an unstable knee joint is produced as a result of transection of the ACL of the knee, morphologic, biochemical, biomechanical, and metabolic changes occur in the articular cartilage shortly after the transection. Later, articular cartilage becomes thicker and shows fibrillation, and osteophytes are present. The cartilage also shows a much higher water content than in the opposite knee and the synovial fluid content of the knee is increased. In addition a sharp increase in bone turnover occurs as well as a thickening of the subchondral bone.[53] According to Van Osch et al, joint instability is a well-known cause of secondary osteoarthritis involving the knee joint.[54]

Immobilization (Stress Deprivation)

Generally, any process or event that disturbs the normal function of a specific joint structure will set up a chain of events that eventually affects every part of a joint and its surrounding structures. Immobilization is particularly detrimental to joint structure and function. Immobilization may be externally imposed by a cast, bed rest, weightlessness, or self-imposed as a reaction to pain and inflammation. An injured joint or joint subjected to inflammation and swelling will assume a loose-packed position in which the pressure within the joint space is minimized. This position may be referred to as the position of comfort because pain is decreased in this position. Each joint has a position of minimum pressure. For the knee and hip joints, the position of comfort is between 30° and 45° of flexion, and for the ankle joint the position is at 15° of plantar flexion.[55] If the joint is immobilized for a few weeks in the position of comfort, contractures will develop in the surrounding soft tissues. Consequently, resumption of a normal range of joint motion will be impossible.

The effects of immobilization are not confined to the surrounding soft tissues but also may affect the articular surfaces of the joint and the underlying bone. Biochemical and morphologic changes that have been attributed to the effects of immobilization include proliferation of fibrofatty connective tissue within the joint space, adhesions between the folds of the synovium, atrophy of cartilage, regional osteoporosis, weakening of ligaments at their insertion sites due to osteoclastic resorption of bone and Sharpey fibers, a decrease in the proteoglycan content and increase in the water content of articular cartilage.[27,56,57] PGs are also lost from tendons, ligaments, and the joint capsule.[8] For example, the menisci at the knee are adversely affected by immobilization. In an experiment in which the hindlegs of canines were casted for 4 weeks in a position of 90° flexion, the aggrecan gene expression and PG content in the menisci were reduced and the water content of the tissue increased. Gross atrophy of the menisci was noted.[17]

As a result of changes in joint structures brought about by immobilization, decreases may be evident in the ROM available to the joint, time between loading and failure, and the energy-absorbing capacity of the bone-ligament complex. Swelling or immobilization of a joint also inhibits and weakens the muscles surrounding the joint.[58–61] Therefore, the joint is unable to function normally and is at high risk of additional injury. A summary of the effects of prolonged immobilization is presented in Table 2–6.

Recognition of the adverse effects of immobilization has led to the development of the following strategies to help minimize the consequences of immobilization: (1) use of continuous passive motion (CPM) devices following joint surgery, (2) reduction in the duration of casting periods following fractures and sprains, and (3) development of dynamic splinting devices. The CPM is a mechanical device that is capable of moving joints passively and repeatedly through a specified portion of the physiologic ROM. In these devices the speed of the movement as well as the ROM can be controlled. The CPM devices are able to produce joint motion without the potentially deleterious compressive-tensile stresses and strains produced by active muscle contractions.

Overuse

Although immobilization is detrimental, either constant or repetitive loading of articular structures also may have adverse effects. Constant loading, such as occurs in prolonged standing, sitting, or squatting, is liable to place the joints and their supporting structures at risk for injury. When a structure that is undergoing creep is subjected to continual loading on the already deformed tissue the structure does not have time to recover and the tissues may undergo microfailure and enter the plastic range. Ligaments subjected to constant tensile loads will creep and may undergo excessive lengthening when they are loaded while undergoing

Table 2–6. ***Changes in Joint Structure and Function Following Prolonged Immobilization (Stress Reduction)***

Structure	Changes
Bone	Regional osteoporosis[55]
Cartilage	Decreased synthetic activity of chondrocytes and decrease in glycosaminoglycans and chondroitin sulfate. Decrease in proteoglycan content and increase in water content. Decrease in thickness, stiffness, permeability, and capacity to bear a load.[27]
Ligament	Osteoclastic activity at the ligament insertion site leads to weakening of ligamentous insertion.[55] Disorganization of collagen fiber arrangement and rapid deterioration of biomechanical and mechanical properties.[36] Decrease in matrix components.[36]
Menisci	Decreased proteoglycan content and aggrecan gene expression. Increased water content, atrophy, and decreased load-bearing capacity.[17]
Tendon	Protein degradation exceeds synthesis and leads to a decrease in collagen content and a decline in cross-link concentration.[31] Atrophy occurs at the myotendinous junction[31] and the size of the collagen fibrils decreases.[38]
Synovium	Proliferation of fibrofatty connective tissue into the joint space and the formation of adhesions.[3,55]

creep. Cartilage subjected to constant compressive loading will creep and may undergo excessive permanent deformation when subjected to loading during the creep phase. Cell death may occur with rigid sustained pressure at focal points on the cartilage and permeability will be decreased.[6]

Joints and their supporting structures subjected to repetitive loading may be injured and fail because they do not have time to recover their original dimensions before they are subjected to another loading cycle. Thus these structures are subjected to repeated loading while they are still deforming. An injury resulting from repetitive strain loading of connective tissues may be called **overuse injury or syndrome, repetitive motion disorder,** or **repetitive strain injury.**[7] These disorders have been identified in athletes, dancers, farmers, musicians, and factory and office workers and appear to affect a greater proportion of women than men.[18] However, the reason women have a greater incidence of these injuries than men is still under investigation. Hart et al have hypothesized that intrinsic gender differences may exist in the regulation of connective tissue structures.[18] It is well known that hormonal levels fluctuate in women during pregnancy and the menstrual cycle. Investigations of tendons in female rabbits demonstrated that type I collagen significantly decreased and collagenase significantly increased in a number of selected tendons in these rabbits during pregnancy. It would appear that the sex hormonal receptors in the tendons responded to the changed levels of hormones in the rabbits.[18] Biopsy material from tendons from human subjects undergoing surgery for repetitive motion disorders shows an inflammatory process in some tendons and a degenerative process in others. In view of the findings to date, it would appear that simple tissue fatigue is not a sufficient explanation for the cause of repetitive motion disorders and that additional research is needed to determine all of the factors involved in both the cause, effect, prevention, and treatment of repetitive motion disorders.

Summary

This chapter has presented the elementary principles of joint design, a classification system for human joints, an introduction to the material used in human joints and properties of these materials as well as the effects of disease, immobilization, and overuse on joint structures. The health and strength of joint structures and hence their function depend on a certain amount of stress and strain. Cartilage and bone nutrition and growth depend on joint movement and muscle contraction. Cartilage nutrition depends on joint movement through a full ROM to ensure that all of the articular cartilage receives the nutrients necessary for survival. Ligaments and tendons depend on a normal amount of stress and strain to maintain and increase strength. Controlled loading and motion applied early in the rehabilitation process stimulate collagen synthesis and help align collagen fibrils. Bone density and strength increase following the stress and strain created by muscle and joint activity. In contrast, bone density and strength decrease when stress and strain are absent. Therefore, micromotion and compression are recommended to promote bony union, and healing of fractures.[62]

However, because of the inadequacy of cartilage repair mechanisms and the long duration of the repair process in bones, ligaments, and tendons, the prevention of injury to joint structures is of utmost importance. In subsequent chapters the specific structure and function of each of the major joints in the body will be explored. Knowledge of the basic elements of normal joint structure and function will help the reader recognize abnormal joint function; analyze the effects of injury, disease, or aging on joint structure and function; and appreciate the complex nature of human joints, and the interrelationships between structure and function and the need for joint protection.

REFERENCES

1. Williams, PL, et al (eds): Gray's Anatomy, ed 38. Churchill Livingstone, New York, 1995.
2. Culav, EM, Clark, CH, and Merilee, MJ: Connective tissues: Matrix composition and its relevance to physical therapy. Phys Ther 79:308, 1999.
3. Ralphs, JR, and Benjamin, M: The joint capsule: Structure, composition, ageing and disease. J Anat 184:503, 1994.
4. Rodeo, SA, et al: Analysis of collagen and elastic fibers in shoulder capsule in patients with shoulder instability. Am J Sports Med 26:634, 1998.
5. Lewis, AR, et al: Distribution of collagens and glycosaminoglycans in the joint capsule of the proximal interphalangeal joint of the human finger. Anat Rec 250:281, 1998.
6. Walker, JM: Cartilage of Human Joints and Related Structures. In Zachazewski, JE, Magee, DJ, and Quillen, WS (eds): Athletic Injuries and Rehabilitation. WB Saunders, Philadelphia, 1996.
7. Grigg, P: Articular Neurophysiology. In Zachazewski, JE, Magee, DJ, and Quillen, WS (eds): Athletic Injuries and Rehabilitation. WB Saunders, Philadelphia, 1996.
8. Allan, DA: Structure and physiology of joints and their relationship to repetitive strain injuries. Clin Orthop Rel Res 352:32, 1998.
9. English, T, Wheeler, ME, and Hettinga, DL: Inflammatory Response of Synovial Joint Structures. In Malone, TR, McPoil, T, and Nitz, AJ: Orthopedic and Sports Physical Therapy. Mosby-Year Book, St. Louis, MO, 1997.
10. Hogorvost, T, and Brand, RA: Mechanoreceptors in joint function. J Bone Jt Surg 80A:1365, 1998.
11. Noyes, FR, DeLucas, JL, and Torvik, PJ: Biomechanics of anterior cruciate ligament failure: An analysis of strain-rate sensitivity and mechanisms of failure in primates. J Bone Joint Surg 56A:2, 1974.
12. Decraemer, WF, et al: A non-linear viscoelastic constitutive equation for soft biological tissues based upon a structural model. J Biomech 13:559, 1980.
13. Goldstein, SA, et al: Analysis of cumulative strain in tendons and tendon sheaths. J Biomech 20:1, 1987.
14. To, SYC, Kwan, MK, and Woo, SL-Y: Simultaneous measurements of strains on two surfaces of tendons and ligaments. J Biomech 21:511, 1988.
15. Woo, SL-Y, et al: Mechanical properties of tendons and ligaments. Biorheology 19:397, 1982.
16. Rong, G, and Wang, Y: The role of the cruciates ligaments in maintaining knee joint stability. Clin Orthop Rel Res 215:65, 1987.
17. Djurasovic, M, et al: Knee joint immobilization decreases aggrecan gene expression in the meniscus. Am J Sports Med 26:460, 1998.
18. Hart, DA, et al: Gender and neurogenic variables in tendon biology and repetitive motion disorders. Clin Othop 351:44, 1998.
19. Simkin, PA: In Schumacher, HR, Klippel, JH, and Robinson, DR (eds): Primer on the Rheumatic Diseases, ed 9. Arthritis Foundation, Atlanta, 1988.
20. Wolf, AW, et al: Current concepts in synovial fluid analysis. Clin Orthop 134:261, 1978.
21. Hettinga, DL: II Normal joint structures and their reaction to injury. J Orthop Sports Phys Ther 1:2, 1979.
22. Radin, EL, and Paul, IL: A consolidated concept of joint lubrication. J Bone Joint Surg 54A:607.
23. Lehmkuhl, D, and Smith, L: Brunnstrom's Clinical Kinesiology, ed 4. FA Davis, Philadelphia, 1984.
24. Gowitzke, BA, and Milner, M: Understanding the Scientific Basis of Human Movement, ed 3. Williams & Wilkins, Baltimore, 1988.
25. White, AA, and Panjabi MM: Clinical Biomechanics of the Spine, ed 2. JB Lippincott, Philadelphia, 1990.
26. Hertling, D, and Kessler, RM: Management of Common Musculoskeletal Disorders, ed 2. JB Lippincott, Philadelphia, 1990.
27. Cohen, NP, Foster, RJ, and Mow, VC: Composition and dynamics of articular cartilage: Structure, function and maintaining healthy state. J Othop Sports Phys Ther 28:203,1998.
28. Nimni, ME: The molecular organization of collagen and its role in determining the biophysical properties of connective tissues. Biorheology 17:51, 1980.
29. Widmann, FK: Pathobiology: How Disease Happens. Little, Brown, Boston, 1978.
30. Cailliet, R: Soft Tissue Pain and Disability, ed 2. FA Davis, Philadelphia, 1988.
31. Curwin, SL: Tendon Injuries: Pathophysiology and Treatment. In Zachazewski, JE, Magee, DJ, and Quillen, WS (eds): Athletic Injuries and Rehabilitation. WB Saunders, Philadelphia, 1996.
32. Jimenez, SA: In Schumacher, HR, Klippel, JH, and Robinson, DR (eds): Primer on the Rheumatic Diseases, ed 9. Arthritis Foundation, Atlanta, 1988.
33. Eyre, DR: In Ghosh, P (ed): The Biology of the Intervertebral Disc, Vol 1. CRC Press, Boca Raton, FL 1988.
34. Nerlich, AG: Immunolocalization of major insterstitial collagen types in lumbar intervertebral discs of various ages. Virchows Arch 432:67, 1998.
35. Hollinshead, WH: Functional Anatomy of the Limbs and Back, ed 4. WB Saunders, Philadelphia, 1976.
36. Frank, CB: Ligament Injuries: Pathophysiology and Healing. In Zachazewski, JE, Magee, DJ, and Quillen, WS (eds): Athletic Injuries and Rehabilitation. WB Saunders, Philadelphia, 1996.

37. Hettinga, DL III: Joint structures and their reaction to injury. J Orthop Sports Phys Ther 1:3, 1980.
38. Enwemeka, CS: Tendon Growth and Regeneration. In Currier, DP, and Nelson, RM (eds): Dynamics of Human Biologic Tissues. FA Davis, Philadelphia, 1992.
39. Cremar, MA, Rosloneic, EF, and Kang, AH: The cartilage collagens: A review of their structure, organization and role in the pathogenesis of experimental arthritis in animals and in human rheumatic disease. J Mol Med 76:275, 1998.
40. Walker, JM: Pathomechanics and classification of cartilage lesions, facilitation of repair. J Orthop Sports Phys Ther 28: 216, 1998.
41. Benjamin, M, and Ralphs, JR: Tendons and ligaments—An overview. Histol Histopathol 12:1135, 1997.
42. Ghadially, FH: Structure and function of articular cartilage. Clin Rheum Dis 7:3, 1980.
43. Mitchell, N, and Shepard, N: Healing of articular cartilage in intra-articular fractures in rabbits. J Bone Joint Surg 62A:4, 1980.
44. Lane, LB, and Bullough PG: Age-related changes in the thickness of the calcified zone and the number of tidemarks in adult human articular cartilage. J Bone Joint Surg 62B:3, 1980.
45. Bullough, PG, and Jagannath, A: The morphology of the calcification front in articular cartilage. J Bone Joint Surg 65:72, 1983.
46. Mansour, JM, and Mow, VC: The permeability of articular cartilage under compressive strain and at high pressures. J Bone Joint Surg 58A:4, 1976.
47. McDonough, AL: Effects of immobilization and exercise on articular cartilage—A review of literature. J Orthop Sports Phys Ther 2:5, 1981.
48. Carter, DR, Orr, TE, and Fyhrie, DP: Relationship between loading history and femoral cancellous bone architecture. J Biomech 22:231, 1989.
49. O'Dwyer, J: College Physics, ed 2. Wadsworth, Belmont, CA, 1984.
50. Buecke, F: Principles of Physics, ed 3. McGraw-Hill, New York, 1977.
51. Tillman, LJ, and Cummings, GS: Biologic Mechanisms of Connective Tissue Mutability. In Currier, DP, and Nelson, RM (eds): Dynamics of Human Biologic Tissues. FA Davis, Philadelphia, 1992.
52. Eckstein, F, et al: Effect of physical exercise on cartilage volume and thickness in vivo: MR imaging study. Radiology April: 243, 1998.
53. Brandt, KD, et al: Bone scintography in the canine cruciate deficiency model of osteoarthritis. Comparison of the unstable and contralateral knee. J Rheumatol 24:140, 1997.
54. Van Osch, GJVM, et al: Relation of ligament damage with site specific cartilage loss and osteophyte formation in collaginase induced osteoarthritis in mice. J Rheum 23:1227, 1996.
55. Perry, J: Contractures: A historical perspective. Clin Orthop Rel Res 219:8, 1987.
56. Akeson, WH, et al: Effects of immobilization on joints. Clin Orthop Rel Res 219:28–37, 1987.
57. Enneking, WF, and Horowitz, M: The intra-articular effects of immobilization on the human knee. J Bone Joint Surg 54A:973, 1972.
58. de Andrade, JR, Grant, C, and Dixon, St J: Joint distension and reflex muscle inhibition in the knee. J Bone Joint Surg 47A:313, 1965.
59. Young, A, Stokes, M, and Iles, JF: Effects of joint pathology on muscle. Clin Orthop Rel Res 219:21, 1987.
60. Spencer, JD, Hayes, KC, and Alexander, IJ: Knee joint effusion and quadriceps reflex inhibition in man. Arch Phys Med Rehabil 65:171, 1984.
61. Stokes, M, and Young, A: The contribution of reflex inhibition to arthrogenous muscle weakness. Clin Sci 67:7, 1984.
62. Buckwalter, JA: Articular cartilage: Injuries and potential for healing. J Ortho Sports Phys Ther 28:192, 1998.

Study Questions

Describe

1. The structure of a typical diarthrodial joint.
2. The type of motion that is available at a pivot joint and give at least two examples of pivot joints.
3. The composition of the interfibrillar component of the extracellular matrix in connective tissue.
4. How diarthrodial joints are lubricated.
5. The movements of the bony lever during motion at an ovoid joint.
6. What is meant by the term "toe region."

Explain

1. Creep and how it affects joint structure and function.
2. How immobilization affects joint structures.
3. What happens to a material when hysteresis occurs?
4. How an overuse injury may occur.

Compare

1. The structure and function of a synarthroses with that of diarthroses.
2. A closed chain with an open chain and give examples of each.
3. The composition, properties, and function of ligaments with those of tendons, cartilage, and bone.
4. Stress and strain. Give at least one example using a load-deformation curve.

CHAPTER 3

MUSCLE STRUCTURE AND FUNCTION

OBJECTIVES
Following the study of this chapter, the reader should be able to:

Describe
1. The structure and function of the contractile unit (sarcomere).
2. The structure and function of the functional unit (motor unit).
3. The connective tissue in a muscle.
4. The various muscle fiber types.
5. How fiber length and cross-sectional area affect excursion and force of contraction.
6. The effect of pennation angle on muscle force production.

Define
1. Muscle tension including active and passive tension.
2. Active and passive insufficiency.
3. Concentric, eccentric, and isometric muscle action.
4. Reverse action.
5. Agonists, antagonists, and synergists.

Recall
1. Factors affecting muscle tension.
2. Characteristics of different muscle fiber types.
3. Characteristics of motor units.
4. Factors affecting angular velocity and torque.
5. The effects of immobilization.

Differentiate
1. Between single-joint and multijoint muscles.

2. Among antagonists, agonists, and synergists.

3. Active from passive insufficiency.

4. Active from passive tension.

5. Concentric from eccentric.

6. Normal muscle action from reverse action.

Compare

1. The relative effect of fiber length and moment arm in determining joint torque.

2. The architecture of various muscles and suggest how the architecture may influence function of the muscle.

3. Tension development in eccentric versus concentric contractions.

4. Isokinetic exercise with dynamic constant external resistance exercise. Isoinertial exercise with dynamic constant external resistance exercise.

5. The effects of immobilization in a lengthened versus a shortened position.

Introduction

Mobility and Stability Functions of Muscles

The skeletal muscles, like the joints, are designed to contribute to the body's needs for mobility and stability. Muscle forces, like all forces that are applied to the levers of the body, have both rotatory (mobility) and translatory (usually stability) components. Muscles serve a mobility function by producing or controlling the movement of a bony lever around a joint axis; they serve a stability function by resisting extraneous movement of joint surfaces and through approximation of joint surfaces. The body is incapable of either supporting itself against gravity or of producing motion without muscle function.

A human skeleton without muscles will collapse when placed in the erect standing position. Persons with spinal cord injuries that result in a loss of muscle function in their lower extremities are unable to stand or walk without external support. The joint structures in the injured person are intact, but these structures are incapable of counteracting gravitational torques in a weight-bearing position. Therefore, when the injured person wishes to stand or walk, an external support such as a brace must be used to stabilize the joints of the lower extremities. The brace replaces some of the function of lost muscles by using a locking device that is similar to the device used in the folding table joint. When the brace is locked, it provides joint stability. Under normal conditions, the skeletal muscles of the body provide forces that help human joints move freely into and out of close-

packed and loose-packed positions. When a joint has attained a close-packed position, the stability role of the muscles is decreased. The noncontractile structures (ligaments and joint capsules) supporting the joint are taut and capable of contributing to joint stability. However, when a joint is in the loose-packed position, the muscles must assume a larger stability function because the passive supporting structures are lax and have reduced capacity for providing joint stability. The amount of force that a muscle can contribute either to joint stability or mobility is a function of its structure, contractile ability, and biomechanical characteristics. These factors must be explored to understand the interrelationships that determine human function.

Elements of Muscle Structure

The two types of materials found in skeletal muscle are muscle tissue (contractile) and connective tissue (noncontractile). The properties of these tissues and the way in which they are interrelated give muscles their unique characteristics. Muscle tissue possesses the properties of contractility and irritability. **Contractility** refers to the muscle's ability to develop tension. **Irritability** refers to a muscle's ability to respond to chemical, electrical, or mechanical stimuli.[1] Also, muscle tissue, like other biologic tissue, is viscoelastic when subjected to passive loading.[1]

Composition of a Muscle Fiber

A skeletal muscle is composed of many thousands of muscle fibers. A single muscle contains

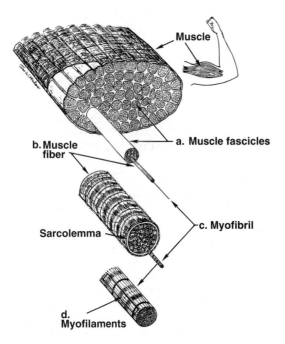

b. **Muscle fiber**

Sarcolemma

a. **Muscle fascicles**

c. **Myofibril**

d. **Myofilaments**

FIGURE 3–1. Composition of a muscle fiber. (a) Groups of muscle fibers form bundles called **fasciculi**. (b) The muscle fiber is enclosed in a cell membrane called the **sarcolemma**. (c) The muscle fiber contains myofibrillar structures called **myofibrils**. (d) The myofibril is composed of thick myosin and thin actin myofilaments.

many fasciculi, a group of muscle fibers (cells) surrounded by connective tissue (Fig. 3–1a). The arrangement, number, size, and type of these fibers may vary from muscle to muscle,[2, 3] but each fiber is a single muscle cell that is enclosed in a cell membrane called the **sarcolemma** (Fig. 3–1b). Like other cells in the body, the muscle fiber is composed of cytoplasm, which in a muscle is called **sarcoplasm.** The sarcoplasm con-

tains structures called **myofibrils** (Fig. 3–1c), which are the contractile structures of a muscle fiber and nonmyofibrillar structures such as ribosomes, glycogen, and mitochondria, which are required for cell metabolism.

The myofibril is composed of thick and thin filaments called **myofilaments** (Fig. 3–1d). The thin myofilaments are composed of the protein **actin;** the thick myofilaments are composed of the protein **myosin.** The interaction of these two myofilaments is essential for a muscle contraction to occur. The thin myofilaments are formed by two chainlike strings of actin molecules wound around each other. Molecules of the globular protein **troponin** are found in notches between the two actin strings and the protein **tropomyosin** is attached to each troponin molecule (Fig. 3–2a). The troponin and tropomyosin molecules control the binding of actin and myosin myofilaments.

The thick myofilaments are composed of large myosin molecules that are arranged to form long molecular filaments (Fig. 3–2b). The myofilaments formed by the myosin molecules are not of equal diameter throughout their length but are wider in the middle portion. Each of the myosin molecules has globular enlargements called **head groups.**[4] The head groups, which are able to swivel and are the binding sites for attachment to the actin, play a critical role in muscle contraction and relaxation. When the entire myofibril is viewed through a microscope, the alternation of thick (myosin) and thin (actin) myofilaments forms a distinctive striped pattern as seen in Figure 3–1d. Therefore, skeletal muscle is often called **striated muscle.** A schematic representation of the ordering of the myofilaments in a myofibril is presented in Figure 3–3.

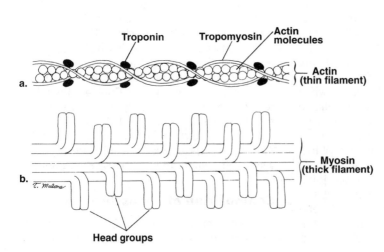

Troponin   Tropomyosin   Actin molecules

Actin (thin filament)

a.

Myosin (thick filament)

b.

Head groups

FIGURE 3–2. Myofilaments. (a) The actin molecules are shown as circles. The troponin molecules are globular and are shown located in notches between the two strands of actin molecules. The tropomyosin molecules are thin and are shown lying along grooves in the actin strands. (b) A myosin myofilament showing head groups or globular enlargements.

FIGURE 3–3. Ordering of myofibrils in a muscle at rest. The sarcomere is the portion of the myofibril that is located between the Z bands (or lines). The A band portion of the sarcomere contains an overlap of the myosin and actin filaments. The portion of the A band that contains only myosin filaments without overlap is called the H zone. The M band located in the central portion of the H zone contains transversely oriented myosin filaments that connect one myosin filament with another. The I band portion contains only actin fibers.

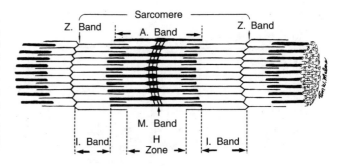

The muscle fiber also consists of several structural proteins (see Patel and Lieber[5] for a review of these proteins). Some of these proteins (**intermediate filaments**) provide a structural scaffold for the muscle fiber, whereas others (e.g., **desmin**) may be involved in the transmission of force along the fiber and to adjoining fibers. One protein, **titin,** has a particularly important role maintaining the position of the thick filament during a muscle contraction and in the development of passive tension.[6, 7] Titin is a large protein that is attached along the thick filament and spans the gap from the thick filament to the Z lines (Fig. 3–4). More will be said about titin in the discussion on the passive length-tension relationship.

The Contractile Unit

In Figure 3–3, the portion of the myofibril that is located between two Z lines is called the **sarcomere.** The Z lines, which are located at regular intervals throughout the myofibril, not only serve as boundaries for the sarcomere but also link the thin filaments together. Areas of the sarcomere called **bands** or **zones** help to identify

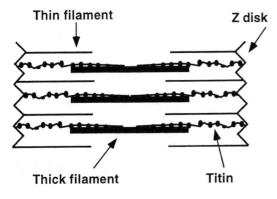

FIGURE 3–4. Sarcomere depicting the relationship between titin and the thick and thin filaments.

the arrangement of the thick and thin filaments. The portion of the sarcomere that extends over both the length of the thick filaments and a small portion of the thin filaments is called the **anisotropic** or **A band.** Areas that include only actin filaments are called **isotropic** or **I bands.**[4] The terms anisotropic and isotropic refer to the behavior of these portions of the fibers when light shines on them. The central portion of the thick filament (A band area) in which there is no overlap with the thin filaments is called the **H zone.** The central portion of the H zone, which consists of the wide middle portion of the thick filament, is called the **M band.** At the M band a small structural protein connects the central region of one thick filament with the filament above or below.

Interaction between the thick and thin filaments of the sarcomere leading to muscle contraction is initiated by the arrival of a nerve impulse at the motor end plate, which evokes an electric impulse or **action potential** that travels along the muscle fiber. The action potential initiates the release of calcium ions, and the calcium ions cause troponin to reposition the tropomyosin molecules so that receptor sites on the actin are free and the head groups of the myosin can bind with actin. This bonding of filaments is called a **cross-bridge** and is considered to be the basic unit of active muscle tension[1, 8, 9] (Fig. 3–5).

The mechanism by which active muscle tension is produced is termed the **cross-bridge cycle.** At rest the cross-bridges are not attached to the thin filament. In response to the influx of calcium causing the shift of tropomyosin, the myosin head group attaches to an open binding site on the thin filament. Myosin has a particularly high affinity for the actin in the thin filament due to the complex of **adenosine diphosphate** (ADP) and inorganic phosphate (Pi) that is bound to the head group. The myosin head group contains an en-

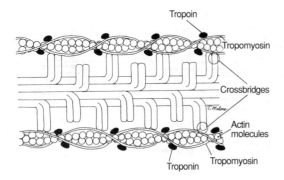

FIGURE 3–5. Cross-bridge formation. The myosin head groups attach to binding sites on the actin that have been exposed by the movement of the tropomyosin away from these binding sites. The thin actin myofilaments are pulled along past the myosin filament by movement of the head groups. Although only two cross-bridges are shown in the illustration, cross-bridges are formed at many sites during a muscle contraction.

zyme (**myosin ATPase**) that catalyses the hydrolysis of **adenosine triphosphate** (ATP) to ADP + Pi. When ADP + Pi are released from the myosin head group, the head group swivels sliding the thin filament along the thick filament. After swiveling, the myosin head group has a high affinity for ATP, and the subsequent binding of ATP to the head group causes the release of the cross-bridge. This cycling of the cross-bridges continues as long as the initiating stimulus (action potential), the supply of calcium, and the supply of ATP remain.

The sliding of the thin filaments toward and past the thick filaments accompanied by the formation and re-formation of cross-bridges in each sarcomere will result in shortening of the muscle fiber and the generation of tension. The muscle fiber will shorten (contract) if a sufficient number of sarcomeres actively shorten and if either one or both ends of the muscle fiber are free to move. The active shortening of a muscle is called a **concentric contraction** or shortening contraction. In contrast to a shortening contraction wherein the thin filaments are being pulled toward the thick filaments, the muscle may undergo an **eccentric contraction** or lengthening contraction. In a lengthening contraction, the thin filaments are pulled away from the thick filaments and cross-bridges are broken and re-formed as the muscle lengthens. Tension is generated by the muscle as cross-bridges are re-formed. Eccentric contractions occur whenever a muscle actively resists motion created by an external force (such as grav-

ity or, more rarely, by another muscle). The muscle fiber will not change length if the force created by the cross-bridge cycling is matched by the external force. The contraction of a muscle fiber without changing length is called an **isometric contraction.**

The following is a summary of the important facts about muscle contraction at the sarcomere level:

- Tension is generated whenever cross-bridges are formed.
- Calcium influx initiates the muscle contraction.
- ATP hydrolysis fuels the cross-bridge cycle.
- In a concentric contraction the thin myofilaments are pulled toward the thick myofilaments and cross-bridges are formed, broken, and re-formed.
- In an eccentric contraction the thin myofilaments are pulled away from the thick myofilaments and cross-bridges are broken, re-formed, and broken.
- In an isometric contraction the length of the muscle fiber is constant.

The Motor Unit

Although the sarcomere is the basic unit of tension in a muscle, it is actually part of a larger complex called the motor unit. The stimulus that the muscle fiber receives initiating the contractile process is transmitted through a nerve called the **alpha motor neuron** (Fig. 3–6). The cell body of the neuron is located in the anterior horn of the gray matter of the

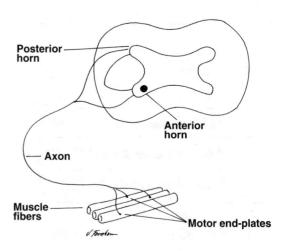

FIGURE 3–6. An alpha motor neuron. The cell body is shown as a black dot in the anterior horn.

spinal cord. The nerve cell **axon** extends from the cell body to the muscle, where it divides into either a few or as many as thousands of smaller branches. Each of the smaller branches terminates in a motor end plate that lies in close approximation to the sarcolemma of a single muscle fiber. All of the muscle fibers on which a branch of the axon terminates are part of one motor unit, along with the cell body and the axon.

The nerve impulse transmitted from the cell body along the axon to the motor end plate causes depolarization of the muscle fiber's sarcolemma and generates an action potential that spreads both along the external surface of the sarcolemma and into the interior of the fiber by way of narrow tubular invaginations called **transverse tubules (T tubules).** Two transverse tubules supply each sarcomere at the level of the junctions of the A and I bands. The **sarcoplasmic reticulum,** which has a large calcium-storage capacity, is composed of anastomosing membranous channels that fill the space between the myofibrils and form large sacs (terminal cisternae) in areas where the membranous channels are close to the T tubules. The combination of two terminal cisternae with a T tubule in the middle is called a **muscle triad,** and the junction between the terminal cisternea and T-tubule has been termed the "junctional feet."[10, 11] When the action potential sweeps down the T tubules, free calcium ions from the sarcoplasmic reticulum are released into the myofibrils. However, the exact mechanics by which the action potential in the T tubules causes the release of calcium from the sarcoplasmic recticulum is unknown. The release of the calcium ions initiates actin-myosin cross-bridge activity and causes muscle tension. When the sarcolemma becomes electrically stable after depolarization, calcium ions are pumped back into the sarcoplasmic reticulum by specialized proteins in the membrane of the sarcoplasmic reticulum (calcium activated ATPase enzyme) and the muscle fiber relaxes.[1,4,12] Motor units go through a latency or refractory period just after firing and require time to recover before the cycle of depolarization and tension generation can be repeated. Therefore, the frequency of firing of motor units is limited by the need for recovery time prior to reactivation.

The **motor unit** consists of the alpha motor neuron and all of the muscle fibers it innervates. The contraction of the entire muscle is the result of many motor units firing *asynchronously* and *repeatedly*. The magnitude of the contraction of the entire muscle may be altered by altering the number of motor units that are activated or the frequency at which they are activated. The number of motor units in a muscle as well as the structure of these units varies from muscle to muscle.

Motor units vary according to the size of the neuron cell body, diameter of the axon, number of muscle fibers, and type of muscle fibers. Each of these variations in structure affects the function of the motor unit. Some motor units have small cell bodies and others have large cell bodies. Units that have small cell bodies have small-diameter axons. Nerve impulses take longer to travel through small-diameter axons than they do through large-diameter axons. Therefore, in the small-diameter units, a stimulus will take longer to reach the muscle fibers than it will in a unit with a large-diameter axon.

The size of the motor unit is determined by the number of muscle fibers that it contains (Fig. 3–7). The number of fibers may vary from two or three to a few thousand. Muscles that either control fine movements or that are used to make small adjustments have small-size motor units. Such motor units generally have small cell bodies and small-diameter axons. Muscles that are used to produce large increments of force and large movements usually have a predominance of large-size motor units, large cell

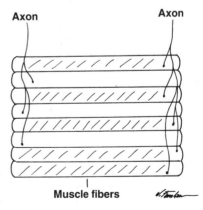

FIGURE 3–7. The size of the motor unit is determined by the number of muscle fibers it contains. Large units may contain as many as a few thousand muscle fibers, whereas small units may contain as few as three. As can be seen in the diagram, the muscle fibers innervated by a single axon are not necessarily located next to one another.

bodies, and large-diameter axons. The motor units of the small muscles that control eye motions may contain as few as six muscle fibers, whereas the gastrocnemius muscles have motor units that contain about 2000 muscle fibers.[4] Muscles with a predominantly large number of fibers per motor unit usually have a relatively smaller total number of motor units than muscles that have few fibers per motor unit. The platysma muscle in the neck has relatively small motor units consisting of approximately 25 muscle fibers, but the muscle has a total of 1000 of these motor units. The gastrocnemius, on the other hand, has relatively large motor units consisting of about 2000 muscle fibers per unit, but the muscle has a relatively small number (600) of such units. In most instances a muscle has at least some mix of small and large motor units.

Usually, when a muscle action is desired, the motor units with the small cell bodies and few motor fibers are automatically selected (recruited) first by the nervous system.[13,14] Small motor units generate less tension than large motor units and require less energy expenditure, and therefore this recruitment strategy is thought to be energy conserving. If a few small motor units are capable of accomplishing the task, the recruitment of large motor units is unnecessary. If the task demands are such that the small motor units are unable to complete the task, larger motor units can be recruited. However, the recruitment strategy may be based not only on energy conservation but also on previous experience; the nature of the task[15] (how rapidly the muscle must respond or the anticipated magnitude of the required force); type of muscle action[16] (concentric, eccentric, or isometric); and a mechanism that takes into account the actions of all muscles around a joint, including such considerations as the muscle's mechanical advantage at a particular point in the range of motion (ROM). The recruitment strategy also may involve the selection of motor units from not just one but a variety of muscles surrounding a joint to accomplish a particular task.[17] The frequency of firing of a motor unit also affects the force modulation. The contribution of recruitment or firing frequency to the development of muscle force may be different depending on the muscle. Small, distal muscles tend to rely more on increased frequency of firing and larger, proximal muscles rely more on recruitment of additional motor units.[18]

To review, tension of the whole muscle may be affected by:

- The number of muscle fibers (affects the magnitude of the response to a stimulus)
- The diameter of the axon (determines the conduction velocity of the impulse)
- The number of motor units that are firing at any one time (affects the total response of the muscle)
- The frequency of motor unit firing (affects the total response of the muscle)

In addition, the type of muscle fibers contained within a motor unit will affect the response of a muscle. All of the muscle fibers contained in a single motor unit are of one type, but the type of muscle fibers within a muscle may vary from one motor unit to another motor unit.

Muscle Structure

Fiber Types

Three principal types of muscle fibers are found in varying proportions in human skeletal muscles. These fiber types may be distinguished from one another histochemically, metabolically, morphologically, and mechanically. Because different systems of nomenclature are used in different texts,[19] Table 3–1 presents not only the characteristics of these fibers but also a few of the different names that are used to designate the fibers. In this text the three primary muscle fiber types will be referred to as: type I (slow), type IIA (intermediate), and type IIB (fast).[20] In this classification system, which is the most common system for human skeletal muscle fiber typing, the myofibrillar ATPase activity under varying acidic and alkaline conditions is used to delineate fiber types. In fact, several intermediate fiber types have been identified using this scheme. Another scheme uses the response of the muscle to metabolic enzymes. This scheme identifies three main fiber types as fast-twitch glycolytic (FG), fast-twitch oxidative glycolytic (FOG), and slow-twitch oxidative (SO).[23] This nomenclature is based on the combination of reactions of cellular enzymes with substrates to identify myofibrillar ATPase activity (fast versus slow), succinate dehydrogenase activity (oxidative potential), and α-glycerophosphate dehydrogenase activity (glycolytic potential). It is often assumed that the two schemes are interchangable; however, this may not be the case. There appears to be much overlap of metabolic enzyme activity between type IIA and type IIB.

The fact that metabolic enzyme activity levels depend on the degree of training of the muscle suggests that these two schemes may not be the same. Another scheme, using immunohistochemical analysis (identification of portions of the myosin molecule with antibodies) has found that the type I, IIA, and IIB fibers correspond to specifically different types of myosin molecules (myosin heavy chain [MHC] I, MHC IIA, and MHC IIB).[20] The combination of this scheme and the myosin ATPase system provides an estimate of the contractile properties of the muscle. Whichever classification scheme is used, it should be remembered that there is actually a continuum of fiber types without exact distinctions between types.

Each skeletal muscle in the body is composed of motor units of each of the three types of fibers, but wide variations exist among individuals in the number of motor units allocated to each fiber type in similar muscles. The variations in fiber types among individuals are believed to be genetically determined. In postmortem studies, the vastus lateralis, rectus femoris, deltoid, and gastrocnemius muscles have been found to be similar among individuals in that they contain about 50% type II and 50% type I fibers, [2] and the hamstrings contain about 55% type II and 45% type I fibers.[21] In studies using muscle biopsy samples from younger subjects, the vastus lateralis tends to be about 54% type II fibers and 46% type I fibers.[22] Although the differences may be subtle, fiber type changes with age such that there is a decrease in the number and size of the type II fibers. This may account for the differences seen in many of the studies documenting fiber type percentages.

The soleus muscle, on the other hand, contains twice as many type I fibers as type II fibers.[23] Muscles that have a relatively high proportion of type I fibers in relation to type II fibers, such as the soleus muscle, are able to carry on sustained activity because the type I fibers do not fatigue rapidly. These muscles are often called **stability, postural,** or **tonic** muscles because they help to maintain stability of the body. The relatively small, slow motor units of the soleus muscle (with small cell bodies, small-diameter axons, and a small number of muscle fibers per motor unit) are almost continually active during erect standing so as to make the small adjustments in muscle tension that are required to maintain body balance and counteract the effects of gravity. Muscles that have a higher proportion of the type II fibers, such as the biceps brachii, are sometimes designated as **mobility, nonpostural,** or **phasic** muscles. These muscles are involved in producing a large ROM of the bony components.[24] The type II fibers respond more rapidly to a stimulus but also fatigue more rapidly than type I fibers. Following intermittent bouts of high-intensity exercise, muscles with a high proportion of type II fibers, which involve a large initial response, show greater fatigue and recover more slowly than muscles with a high proportion of type I fibers.[25]

Muscle Architecture: Size, Arrangement, and Length

Many human muscles have an approximately equal proportion of fast and slow fiber types.

Table 3–1. **Characteristics of Skeletal Muscle Fibers**

	Fast-twitch Glycolytic (Type IIb)*	Fast-twitch Oxidative Glycolytic (Type IIa)†	Slow-twitch Oxidative (Type I)‡
Diameter	Large	Intermediate	Small
Muscle color	White	Red	Red
Capillarity	Sparse	Dense	Dense
Myoglobin content	Low	Intermediate	High
Speed of contraction	Fast	Fast	Slow
Rate of fatigue	Fast	Intermediate	Slow
Motor unit size	Large	Intermediate to large	Small
Axon conduction velocity	Fast	Fast	Slow

*Type IIb fibers are also referred to as fast-twitch white fibers or fast-twitch fibers.
†Type IIa fibers are also referred to as intermediate fibers or fast-twitch red fibers.
‡Type I fibers are also referred to as slow-twitch or slow-twitch red fibers.

Therefore, the determination of muscle function should not be based solely on this single characteristic. In fact, the architecture of the whole muscle may be much more important in determining muscle function than the fiber type.[26] The description of skeletal muscle architecture includes the arrangement of the fibers relative to the axis of force (amount of pennation), muscle fiber length, muscle length, muscle mass, and the **physiologic cross-sectional area** (PCSA). These structural variations affect not only the overall shape and size of the muscles but also the function of the skeletal muscles.

Each muscle fiber is capable of shortening to approximately one-half of its total length. Consequently, a long muscle fiber, with more sarcomeres in series, is capable of shortening over a greater distance than a short muscle fiber. For example, a muscle fiber that is 6 cm long is able to shorten 3 cm, whereas a fiber that is 4 cm long is able to shorten only 2 cm. The significance of the preceding example is apparent if one considers that a hypothetical muscle with long fibers has a greater potential excursion and is able to move the bony lever to which it is attached through a greater distance than a muscle with short fibers. However, the relationship between the muscle fiber length and the distance it is able to move a bony lever is not always a direct relationship. The arrangement of the muscle fibers and the length of the moment arm (MA) of the muscle affect the length-shortening relationship, and therefore, both fiber length and MA must be considered.

The amount of force that a muscle produces is directly proportional to the number of sarcomeres aligned in parallel. In other words, if the fiber increases in size (addition of myofibrils) or more fibers are packed side by side, the ability to produce force will be increased. The PCSA is a measure of the cross-sectional area of the muscle perpendicular to the orientation of the muscle fibers. It is actually calculated from several measured architectural parameters.[27]

Arrangement of fasciculi (muscle fiber groups), like the length of the muscle fibers, varies among muscles. The fasciculi may be parallel to the long axis of the muscle (Fig. 3–8a), may spiral around the long axis (Fig. 3–8b), or may be at an angle to the long axis (Fig. 3–8c). Muscles that have a parallel fiber arrangement (parallel to the long axis and to each other) are designated as **strap** or **fusiform** muscles. In strap muscles, such as the sterno-

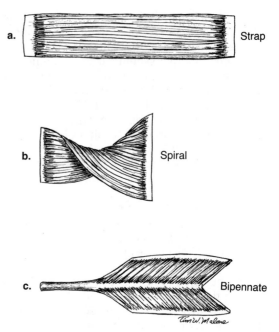

FIGURE 3–8. Arrangement of fasciculi in a muscle. (a) Parallel arrangement. (b) Spiral arrangement. (c) Bipennate arrangement.

cleidomastoid, the fasciculi are long and extend throughout the length of the muscle. However, in the rectus abdominis, which also is considered to be a strap muscle, the fasciculi are divided into short segments by fibrous intersections. In fusiform muscles, most but not all of the muscle fibers extend throughout the length of the muscle. Generally, muscles with a parallel fiber arrangement will produce a greater ROM of a bony lever than muscles with the same cross-sectional area but with a pennate fiber arrangement.

Muscles that have a fiber arrangement oblique to the muscle's long axis are called **unipennate, bipennate,** or **multipennate** muscles because the fiber arrangement resembles that found in a feather, and the word *pennate* is derived from the Latin word for feather. The fibers that make up the fasciculi in pennate muscles are usually shorter and more numerous than the fibers in many of the strap muscles. In unipennate muscles such as the flexor pollicis longus, the obliquely set fasciculi fan out on only one side of a central muscle tendon. In a bipennate muscle, such as the gastrocnemius, the fasciculi are obliquely set on both sides of a central tendon. In a multipennate muscle, such as the deltoid, the oblique fasciculi converge on several tendons. The oblique angle of the muscle fibers in a pennate muscle disrupts the direct relationship between the length of the muscle fiber and the distance that the total muscle can move a bony part and decreases the amount of force that is directed along the long axis of the muscle. Only a portion of the force of the pennate muscles goes toward producing motion of the bony lever. In fact, the more oblique a fiber lies to the long axis of the muscle, the less force the muscle is able to exert at the tendon. This decrease in muscle force is a function of the cosine of the pennation angle. Many human muscles have a pennation angle that is less than 30° at rest. Therefore, the muscle force at the tendon will be decreased by a maximum of 13% (cos 30°=.87).[28] Some recent reports suggest that with changing joint angle or during muscle contraction the pennation angle becomes much more oblique, thus potentially affecting the tendon force to an even greater degree.[29,30] This potential decreased force at the tendon, however, is offset because pennate muscles usually have a large number of muscle fibers due to increased fiber packing, thus increasing PCSA. So, despite the loss of force due to pennation, a pennated muscle, such as the gastrocnemius, is still able to transmit a large amount of force to the tendon to which it attaches.

Muscular Connective Tissue

Muscles and muscle fibers, like other soft tissues in the body, are surrounded and supported by connective tissue. The sarcolemma of individual muscle fibers is surrounded by connective tissue called the **endomysium,** and groups of muscle fibers are covered by connective tissue called the **perimysium.** The endomysium and perimysium are continuous with the outer connective tissue sheath called the **epimysium,** which envelops the entire muscle (Fig. 3–9). Continuations of the outer sheath form the tendons that attach each end of the muscle to the bony components. Tendons are attached to bones by **Sharpey fibers,** which become continuous with the periosteum.

Other connective tissues associated with muscles are in the form of fasciae, aponeuroses, and sheaths. Fasciae can be divided into two zones: superficial and deep. The zone of **superficial fasciae,** composed of loose tissue, is located directly under the dermis. This zone contributes to the mobility of the skin, acts as

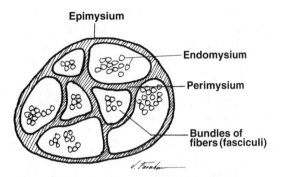

FIGURE 3–9. Muscular connective tissue. A schematic cross-sectional view of the connective tissue in a muscle shows how the perimysium is continuous with the outer layer of epimysium.

an insulator, and may contain skin muscles such as the platysma in the neck. The zone of **deep fasciae** is composed of compacted and regularly arranged collagenous fibers. The deep fasciae attach to muscles and bones and may form tracts or bands and retinacula. For example, the deep femoral fasciae in the lower extremity forms a tract known as the **iliotibial tract** or **band.** This tract transmits the pull of two of the lower-extremity muscles to the bones of the leg (Fig. 3–10). **Retinacula** are

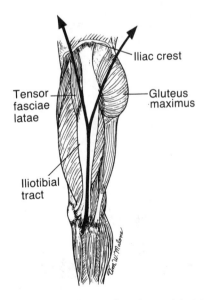

FIGURE 3–10. Iliotibial tract. A lateral view of the left lower limb showing the deep fascial iliotibial tract extending from the tubercle of the iliac crest to the lateral aspect of the knee. The right arrow represents the pull of the gluteus maximus. The left arrow represents the pull of the tensor fascia latae.

formed by localized transverse thickenings of the fasciae, which form a loop that is attached at both ends to bone (Fig. 3–11a). The tunnels or osseofibrous channels formed by retinacula retain or prevent tendons from bowing out of position during muscle action (Fig. 3–11b). Sometimes deep fasciae are indistinguishable from aponeuroses, which are sheets of dense white compacted collagen fibers that attach directly or indirectly to muscles, fasciae, bones, cartilage, and other muscles. Aponeuroses distribute forces generated by the muscle to the structures to which they are attached.[1]

All of the connective tissue in a muscle is interconnected and constitutes the passive elastic component of a muscle. The connective tissues that surround the muscle plus the sarcolemma, the elastic protein titin, and other structures (i.e., nerves and blood vessels), form the **parallel elastic component** of a muscle. When a muscle lengthens or shortens, these tissues also lengthen or shorten, because they function in parallel to the muscle contractile unit. For example, the collagen fibers in the perimysium of fusiform muscles are slack when the sarcomeres are at rest but straighten out and become taut as sarcomere lengths increase. As the perimysium is lengthened, it also becomes stiffer (resistance to further elongation increases). The increased resistance of perimysium to elongation may prevent overstretching of the muscle fiber bundles and may contribute to the tension at the tendon.[31] When sarco-

meres shorten from their resting position, the slack collagen fibers within the parallel elastic component buckle (crimp) even further. Whatever tension might have existed in the collagen at rest is diminished by the shortening of the sarcomere. Given the many parallel elastic components of a muscle, the increase or decrease in passive tension can substantially affect the total tension output of a muscle.

The tendon of the muscle is considered to function in **series** with the contractile elements. This means that the tendon will be under tension when the muscle actively produces tension. When the contractile elements in a muscle actively shorten, they exert a pull on the tendon. The pull must be of sufficient magnitude to take up the slack (compliance) in the tendon so that the muscle pull can be transmitted through the tendon to the bony lever (Fig. 3–12). Fortunately, the compliance of the tendon is relatively small (about 3% in human muscles). Thus, most of the muscle force can be used for moving the bony lever and is not dissipated stretching the tendon. The tendon is also under tension when a muscle is controlling or braking the motion of the lever in an eccentric contraction. A tendon is under reduced tension only when a muscle is completely relaxed and in a relatively shortened position.

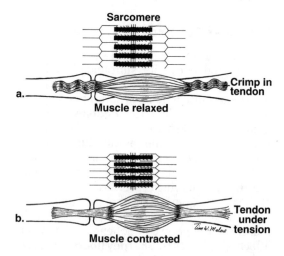

FIGURE 3–12. Series elastic component. (a) The muscle is shown in a relaxed state with the tendon slack (crimping or buckling of collagen fibers has occurred). The sarcomere shown above the muscle shows minimal overlap of thick and thin filaments and little cross-bridge formation. (b) The muscle in an actively shortened position shows that the tendons are under tension and no crimp can be observed. The sarcomere shown above the muscle shows extensive overlap of filaments and cross-bridge formation.

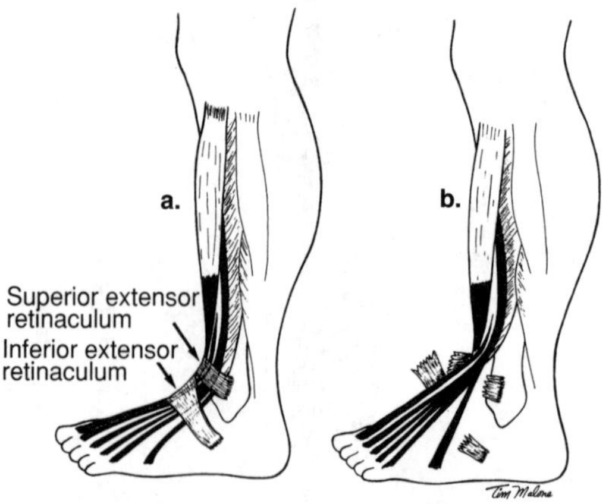

FIGURE 3–11. Retinacula. (a) The superior and inferior retinacula are shown in their normal position, in which they form a tunnel for the tendons from the extensor muscles of the lower leg. (b) When the retinacula are torn or removed, the tendons move anteriorly.

Superior extensor retinaculum
Inferior extensor retinaculum

Muscle Function

Muscle Tension

The most important characteristic of a muscle is its ability to develop tension and to exert a force on the bony lever. Tension can be either active or passive and the total tension that a muscle can develop includes both active and passive components. Total tension, which was identified in Chapter 1 as Fms, is a vector quantity that has (1) magnitude, (2) two points of application (at the proximal and distal muscle attachments), (3) an action line, and (4) direction of pull. The point of application, action line, and direction of pull were the major part of the discussion of muscle force in Chapter 1, but we now need to turn our attention to the determinants of the component called magnitude of the muscle force or the total muscle tension.

Passive Tension

Passive tension refers to tension developed in the passive noncontractile components of the muscle. Passive tension in the parallel elastic component is created by lengthening the muscle beyond the slack length of the tissues. The parallel elastic component may add to the active tension produced by the muscle when the muscle is lengthened or may become slack and not contribute to the total tension when the muscle is shortened. The total tension that develops during an active contraction of a muscle is a combination of the noncontractile (passive) tension added to the contractile (active) tension.

Active Tension

Active tension refers to tension developed by the contractile elements of the muscle. Active tension in a muscle is initiated by cross-bridge formation and movement of the thick and thin filaments. The amount of active tension that a muscle can generate depends on neural factors and mechanical properties of the muscle. The neural factors that can modulate the amount of active tension include the frequency, number, and size of motor units that are firing. The mechanical properties of muscle that determine the active tension are the isometric length-tension relationship and the force-velocity relationship.

Isometric Length-Tension Relationship

One of the most fundamental concepts in muscle physiology is the direct relationship between isometric tension development in a muscle fiber and the length of the sarcomeres in a muscle fiber.[32] The identification of this relationship was, and continues to be, the primary evidence supporting the sliding filament theory of muscle contraction. The isometric sarcomere length-tension relationship was experimentally determined using isolated single muscle fibers under very controlled circumstances. There is an optimal sarcomere length at which a muscle fiber is capable of developing maximal isometric tension (Fig. 3–13). Muscle fibers develop maximal isometric tension at optimal sarcomere length because the thick and thin filaments are positioned so that the maximum number of cross-bridges within the sarcomere can be formed. If the muscle fiber is lengthened or shortened beyond optimal length, the amount of active tension that the muscle fiber is able to generate when stimulated decreases (see Fig. 3–13). When a muscle fiber is lengthened beyond optimal length,

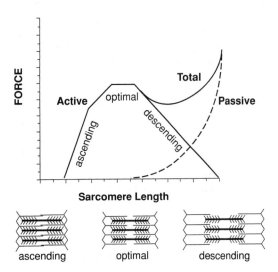

FIGURE 3–13. The skeletal muscle sarcomere length-tension relationship. Active, passive, and the total curves are shown. The plateau of the active curve signifies optimal sarcomere length where maximum active tension is developed. Isometric tension decreases as the muscle is lengthened because fewer cross-bridges are able to be formed. Tension decreases as the muscle is shortened because of interdigitation of the thin filaments. The increase in passive tension with elongation of the muscle is shown by the dashed lines. Passive plus active tension results in the total amount of tension developed by the muscles fiber.

there is less overlap between the thick and thin filaments and consequently fewer possibilities for cross-bridge formation. However, the passive elastic tension in the parallel component may be increased when the muscle is elongated. This passive tension is added to the active tension resulting in the total tension (see Fig. 3–13).

A similar loss of isometric tension or diminished capacity for developing tension occurs when a muscle fiber is shortened from its optimal sarcomere length. When the sarcomere is at shorter lengths, the distance between the Z bands is decreased and there is interdigitation of the filaments. The interdigitation of the thick and thin filaments may interfere with the formation of cross-bridges from the myosin molecules, thus decreasing the active force. The sarcomere length range in which a muscle fiber can develop maximum tension is very small, being in the vicinity of 0.2 to 0.4 μm around optimal length.

It must be remembered that the sarcomere length-tension relationship was determined using isometric contractions, and therefore should apply, in the strict sense, only to isometric muscle contraction. In addition, as we will see in the following section, the full range of sarcomere lengthening and shortening may only be possible in experiments with isolated muscle. Sarcomere length obviously changes during dynamic contractions (concentric and eccentric contractions) affecting the tension that can be developed in the muscle. However, during dynamic contractions, the length-tension relationship must be combined with the force-velocity relationship to determine the effect that both length and velocity have on the muscle tension.

APPLICATION OF THE LENGTH-TENSION RELATIONSHIP

Applying the length-tension relationship to whole muscle and ultimately to muscle-joint systems is not a simple matter. For example, sarcomere length is not homogeneous throughout the muscle, let alone between muscles with similar functions. This means that for any particular whole muscle length at a particular joint position, there may be sarcomeres at many different lengths corresponding to different points on the length-tension relationship. Also, when the muscle is acting at a joint, the torque produced is not only a function of the muscle force (which depends on muscle length), but also a function of the moment arm of the mus-

cle. This means that at a certain joint angle the muscle length may be short (suggesting that force will be low), but the moment arm may be relatively long, thus maintaining a higher torque. From these examples it is clear that the sarcomere length-tension relationship is important in our understanding of muscle physiology, but there are other important factors when considering whole muscle and joint systems.

Only a few experiments have attempted to determine the isometric sarcomere length-tension relationship in intact human muscle.[33,34] In these experiments on human wrist muscles and thigh muscles, the ranges of sarcomere lengths that are seen with normal joint motion are quite small and are located around optimal length. This design appears quite beneficial in that the muscle is not disadvantaged by being too long or too short. One empirical application of the length-tension relationship is the observation that a muscle has the diminished ability to produce or maintain isometric tension at the extremes of joint motion (**active insufficiency**). At the sarcomere level, this state may occur either when a muscle is excessively shortened or potentially when a muscle is elongated to such a degree that there is, on average, decreased overlap between the myofilaments. In many instances, as in the case of muscles crossing one joint, muscles are arranged around a joint so that the muscle cannot be excessively elongated nor excessively shortened relative to its optimal length. On the other hand, muscles that cross more than one joint (two-joint or multijointed muscles) may undergo a greater excursion of length changes during movement over the full ROM at all of the joints crossed by the muscle. A decrease in the torque produced by the muscle may be encountered when the full ROM is attempted simultaneously at all joints crossed by a multijoint muscle. Therefore, when a multijoint muscle is placed in a shortened position, the muscle may not produce maximal isometric tension.[13] A decrease in torque production due to muscle length changes also may occur in one-joint muscles, but is not as common. Although the decrease in isometric torque can be conveniently explained by the length changes in the muscle, other factors such as the change in moment arm and the passive restraint of the lengthened antagonists also play a substantial role. Sarcomere length appears to stay close to the optimal length during joint movements, so these other factors may be more important than once thought.[33,35]

EXAMPLE 1: (Fig. 3–14a). The finger flexors cross the wrist, carpometacarpal, metacapophalangeal, and interphalangeal joints. When the finger flexors shorten they will cause simultaneous flexion at all joints crossed. If all of the joints are allowed to flex simultaneously, the finger flexors will probably be shorter and as a result will develop less tension. Normally, when the finger flexors contract the wrist is maintained in slight extension by the wrist extensor muscles (Fig. 3–14b). The wrist extensors prevent the finger flexors from flexing the wrist and therefore an optimal length of the flexors is maintained.

Force-Velocity Relationship

Another factor that affects the development of tension within a muscle is the speed of internal shortening of the myofilaments. The speed of internal shortening is the rate at which the myofilaments are able to slide past one another and form and re-form cross-bridges. The force-velocity relationship describes the relationship between the velocity of the muscle contraction and the force produced, therefore providing an explanation for what happens during concentric and eccentric muscle contractions. From the experiments on isolated muscles, the force-velocity relationship states that the velocity of muscle contraction is a function of the load being lifted,[36] but, from a clinical perspective, it may also be stated with the variables reversed (the force generated is a function of the velocity of the muscle contraction, Fig. 3–15). The maximum internal shortening speed occurs when there is no resistance to the sliding, such as occurs when a muscle fiber is separated from its bony attachment. However, in this situation no tension is developed in the muscle because there is no resistance. Conversely, tension may be developed when the resistance to movement of the bony lever prevents visible shortening of the muscle such as occurs in an isometric contraction. In a concentric muscle contraction, as the shortening speed decreases, the tension in the muscle increases. In an isometric contraction the speed of shortening is zero, and tension is greater than in a concentric contraction. In an eccentric contraction, as the speed of lengthening increases, the tension increases further. Not only is this relationship seen in experimental conditions with isolated muscles lifting a load, it is also seen, to some degree, in intact muscle moving bony levers.[37,38]

Previously, it was mentioned that during dynamic contractions the length-tension relationship must be combined with the force-velocity relationship because both sarcomere

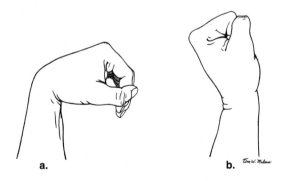

a.   **b.**

FIGURE 3–14. Decrease in active tension with muscle shortening. (a) The individual is attempting to make a tight fist but is unable to do so because the finger flexors are shortened over both the flexed wrist and fingers. In addition, the finger extensors have become lengthened, potentially restricting motion. (b) The length-tension relationship of both flexors and extensors has been improved by stabilization of the wrist in a position of slight extension. The individual, therefore, is able to form a tight fist.

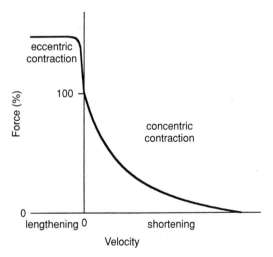

FIGURE 3–15. The skeletal muscle force-velocity curve. At maximum velocity of shortening no force is produced (in other words, maximum velocity of shortening can only be attained with no load on the muscle). As shortening velocity decreases, the force that the muscle can develop increases. At zero velocity the muscle contracts isometrically. Force increases dramatically, and then plateaus when the muscle is lengthened actively.

length and velocity of contraction affect the development of muscle tension. One cannot simply assume that as the muscle shortens, the tension developed in the muscle follows the isometric length-tension relationship. For example, at high shortening velocities the muscle tension will be low regardless of sarcomere length. The fact that most human movements do not occur at a constant velocity of contraction complicates the situation further because the force will vary with changing velocity and changing length.

In summary, active tension in the muscle can be modulated by several factors:

- Tension may be increased by increasing the frequency of firing of a motor unit or by increasing the number of motor units that are firing.
- Tension may be increased by recruiting motor units with a larger number of fibers.
- The greater the number of cross-bridges that are formed, the greater the tension.
- Muscles that have large physiologic cross-sections are capable of producing more tension than muscles that have small cross-sections.
- Tension increases as the velocity of active shortening decreases and as the velocity of active lengthening increases.

This basic understanding of the two most important mechanical properties of muscle, the length-tension relationship and the force-velocity relationship, can now be applied to clinical situations.

Types of Muscle Action

Muscle actions (or contractions) are described as isometric contraction (constant length) or dynamic contractions consisting of concentric contraction (shortening contraction) and eccentric contraction (lengthening contraction). The term *isotonic contraction* is not used here because it refers to equal or constant tension, which is unphysiologic. The tension generated in a muscle cannot be controlled or kept constant. Therefore, the types of muscle actions that will be considered in the following section are isometric, concentric, and eccentric. Two other types of muscle action, isokinetic and isoinertial, which are sometimes referred to as types of muscle contraction, will be considered in a later section of this chapter.[39]

Previously, concentric, isometric, and eccentric muscle contractions were introduced in re-

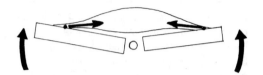

FIGURE 3–16. A concentric muscle contraction. When a muscle develops tension, it exerts a pull on both its bony attachments.

lation to the movement occurring at the sarcomere level. When muscle attaches to bones that are free to move and the force generated by the muscle can produce torque sufficient to overcome the load, then the muscle will undergo a shortening or **concentric contraction** and both bones will be pulled toward each other and toward the center of the muscle (Fig. 3–16). Usually during functional activities, one attachment of a muscle is stabilized and the other attachment is free to move. If the proximal attachment is fixed and the distal attachment is free, the muscle action will pull the distal bony component (Fig. 3–17a) toward the proximal bony component. If the distal attachment is fixed and the proximal bony component is free (Fig. 3–17b), the proximal bony component will be pulled toward the distal bony component.

During concentric contractions work is performed by the muscle as the muscle moves the

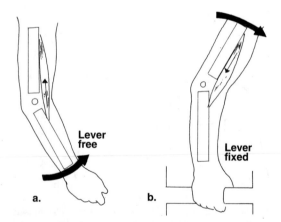

FIGURE 3–17. Normal and reverse action in a concentric contraction. (a) Motion of the free distal bony lever occurs if the proximal bony lever is fixed and the torque of the muscle force (Fms) is sufficient to overcome the torque of the gravitational resistance. (b) In reverse action, motion of the proximal bony lever occurs when the distal bony lever is fixed.

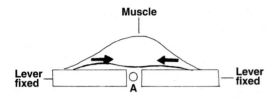

FIGURE 3–18. An isometric contraction. Both the distal and proximal bony levers are fixed and no visible motion occurs when the muscle develops active tension.

bony lever through a distance in the direction of the muscle pull. The formula for work is:

$$W = F \times d$$

When both the distal and proximal attachments of a muscle are fixed and the torque produced by a muscle is *equal to* the torque of the resistances, the visible muscle length will remain unchanged, although shortening occurs at the myofibril level. When there is no visible change in the joint angle, the muscle action is called an **isometric contraction** (Fig. 3–18). No mechanical work is performed in an isometric contraction because the force (F) has not moved the lever through a distance (d). There is no distance involved in an isometric contraction because both bony components are fixed and neither end moves during the contraction. However, energy is being expended to produce cross-bridge cycling.

When the force and resulting torque that a muscle generates is insufficient to offset an opposing torque on a lever, the muscle will undergo a lengthening or **eccentric contraction**. In this type of contraction the muscle acts as a brake as it attempts to control the movement of a bony component as the lever moves in a direction opposite to the eccentric muscle pull. When the hand holding a glass is moved from the face to the table, the flexor muscles of the elbow undergo an eccentric contraction as they control the gravity-produced descent of the hand. In this activity the two ends of the muscle move apart or away from each other (Fig. 3–19). The muscle acts as the resistance to the gravitational effort and a second-class lever is formed on the forearm/hand segment as it rotates around the elbow joint. Eccentric muscle action, like concentric muscle action, can occur as motion of either the distal or proximal bony lever. The mechanical work that is done by a muscle during an eccentric contraction is called negative work because work is done *on* the muscle rather than *by* the muscle. The energy cost of an eccentric contraction is considerably less than that of a concentric contraction when equal loads are used because fewer motor units are being activated in an eccentric contraction than a concentric contraction.

The amount of tension that can be developed in a muscle varies according to the type of contraction. A greater amount of tension can be developed in an isometric contraction than in a concentric contraction.[40] In general, the tension developed in an eccentric contraction is greater than what can be developed in an isometric contraction. However, this relationship may not hold true for all muscles at all points in a joint's ROM.[41] The reason for greater tension development in a muscle during an eccentric contraction than in a concentric contraction may be due, in part, to either mechanical factors in the attachment and detachment of cross-bridges or to alterations in the neural activation of the muscle.[42]

Angular Velocity and Torque

Velocity is a vector quantity and has direction in addition to magnitude. When an object moves

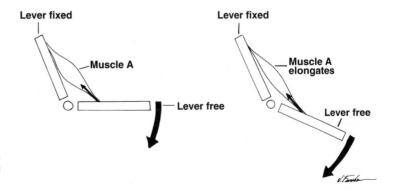

FIGURE 3–19. An eccentric contraction. The muscle elongates while continuing to produce active tension.

along a linear path in a certain direction, the velocity of the object may be calculated by determining the distance that the object travels in a certain period of time or, in other words, its rate of change of position. When an object is undergoing rotatory motion, such as occurs when a bony component moves around a joint axis, the rate of change of position of the bony component is referred to as its **rotational (angular) velocity.**

The angular velocity that a bony lever attains during a dynamic muscle contraction (eccentric or concentric) is a function of the magnitude of the net torque applied to the lever. When the total muscle force (Fms) and gravity or an external load (Fext) or both are applied in opposite directions (as they are commonly), net torque can be determined by the following equation:

$$\text{Net torque} = (\text{Fms} \times \text{MA}) - (\text{Fext} \times \text{MA})$$

The equation, however, can be seen as an oversimplification when one examines the components and subcomponents of the formula. These are:

I. Muscle torque
   A. Total muscle tension (Fms)
      1. Active tension
         a. Number of motor units recruited
         b. Fiber type of motor units recruited
         c. Type of contraction being performed
         d. Frequency of firing of motor units
      2. Passive elastic tension
         a. Parallel elastic tension
         b. Series elastic tension
   B. MA of the muscle
II. Torque of the external force
   A. Magnitude of gravitational and/or external load (R)
   B. MA of gravitational and/or external load

Note in either the simplified or conceptually expanded formula, a positive net torque is a concentric contraction, a negative net torque is an eccentric contraction, and 0 net torque is an isometric contraction.

A change in any of the components above can and will change the results of the formula and, consequently, the magnitude or direction of net torque and angular velocity. During normal activities many and sometimes all of these components are changing simultaneously. The impact of change in one component or subcomponent can be determined by holding the other components constant. In the following section only one factor will be changed at a time using the net torque formula as a reference.

The active tension component of total muscle tension is largely under the volitional control of the individual within physiologic limitations (i.e., conduction velocity of the axons and rate of sacromere shortening). By increasing the number of motor units recruited or the frequency of firing of motor units, the total force generated by the muscle can be increased. An increase in the muscle force will increase the net torque and the angular velocity, presuming a concentric contraction is occurring. If a slower motion is desired, the person can reduce the number of motor units recruited and the frequency of firing, which decreases the muscle force and the net torque. When no motion is desired, such as in an isometric contraction, the force generated by the muscle can be reduced until the muscular force balances that of gravity and the applied load. If the person wishes to lower an object with control (an eccentric contraction), the muscle force can be minimized to a point where the torque of the external load exceeds the torque produced by the muscle. In this instance the net torque will have a negative value indicating that the angular velocity is in the direction opposite to the muscle pull. The larger the negative net torque, the faster the limb will move opposite to the muscle pull.

When the magnitude of the applied load on a bony lever is increased during a concentric contraction, the torque of the external force is increased and net torque and angular velocity will decrease if other contributors remain unchanged. A decrease in the magnitude of the applied load will decrease the torque of the external force and cause an increase in angular velocity. If the magnitude of the external force increases to the point where its torque is equivalent to the torque produced by the muscle, the net torque will be zero and an isometric contraction will occur. If the torque of the external force exceeds the torque produced by the muscle force, the muscle will undergo an eccentric contraction.

In both the instance of the muscle force and the force of the external load, the MAs are generally changing as the lever moves and are position dependent. The MA of the muscle and the MA of the external load may change in the same direction (both increase or decrease) or they may change in opposite directions. For this reason, the net torque of the moving lever will vary even when all other components are kept constant. If a constant velocity is desired, the changing MAs require a constant adjustment of active muscle tension. Active tension must be modified because the passive muscle tension is not under voluntary control. Although the changing position of the joint will affect the MAs of both muscular and external forces, the muscular force also will be affected by the changes in the length of the muscle that accompany joint movement. Changing the length of a muscle will change both the active tension contribution of the muscle and the passive tension contribution.

The actual angular velocity achieved by a lever is affected by constantly changing variables. Consequently, changes in the velocity of the lever as it moves through the ROM are common.

Muscle Action Under Controlled Conditions

ISOKINETIC EXERCISE AND TESTING

Advances in technology have led to the development of testing and exercising equipment that provide for manipulation and control of some of the variables that affect muscle function. In **isokinetic exercise and testing**[43] or **isokinetic muscle contraction,**[40] the angular velocity of the bony component is preset and kept constant by a mechanical device throughout a joint ROM. The concept of an "isokinetic contraction" may not be so much a type of muscle action as it is a made-up variable. To maintain a constant velocity, the resistance produced by the isokinetic device is *directly proportional* to the torque produced by a muscle at all points in the ROM. Therefore, as the torque produced by a muscle increases, the magnitude of the torque of the resistance increases proportionately. Control of the resistance may be accomplished mechanically by using isokinetic devices such as a Biodex, Cybex, KINCOM, Orthotron, or others.

Experienced evaluators of human function may attempt to control manually the angular velocity of a bony component and apply resistance that is proportional to the torque produced by a muscle throughout the ROM. In manual muscle testing the evaluator may apply manual resistance to a concentric muscle contraction throughout the ROM produced by the subject being tested. The evaluator's resistance must adjust constantly so that it is proportional to the torque produced by the muscle being tested at each point in the ROM. If the evaluator successfully balances the torque output of the subject, a constant angular velocity is achieved. However, manually controlled angular velocity and the manually adjusted resistance required to produce it cannot be given with the same measure of precision or consistency that can be given by a mechanical device. Furthermore, manual resistance cannot be quantified as accurately as mechanical resistance.

The advantage of isokinetic exercise over free weight lifting through a ROM is that isokinetic exercise accommodates for the changing torques created by a muscle throughout the ROM. As long as the preset speed is achieved, the isokinetic device provides resistance that is proportional to the torque produced by a muscle at all points in the ROM. For example, the least amount of resistance is provided by an isokinetic device at the point in the ROM where the muscle has the least torque-producing capability. The resistance provided is greatest at the point in the ROM where the muscle has the largest torque-producing capability.[43]

The maximum isokinetic torques for concentric contractions obtained at high-angular velocities are less than the maximum isokinetic torques obtained at low-angular velocities. This decline in torque with increasing contraction velocity is expected based on the force-velocity relationship of muscle. In fact, isometric torque values are higher than isokinetic concentric torque values at any other velocity for a particular point in the joint ROM. Therefore, the closer the angular velocity of a concentric isokinetic contraction approaches zero, the greater the isokinetic torque.[44,45]

Isokinetic equipment is used extensively for determining the amount of torque that a muscle can develop at different velocities, for strength training, and for comparing the relative strength of one muscle group with another. Some isokinetic devices permit quantification for testing eccentric muscle torque. In comparisons of isometric and isokinetic testing of the strength of back and arm muscles during lifting, significant differences have been found between peak isometric and peak isokinetic lifting strength capabilities of muscles throughout the lifting range. Isometric strength was found to be significantly higher than isokinetic concentric strength, and concentric isokinetic strength was found to decline as lifting speed increased.[46] Normal on-the-job lifting is not performed isokinetically and therefore isokinetic testing or exercising for the performance of lifting and other tasks may not be appropriate. However, this is an area of concentration for current research. Some current research shows that isokinetic testing or exercising may differentiate performance in functional tasks or may enhance the training effect for functional activities and some showing that it does not.

ISOINERTIAL EXERCISE AND TESTING

Isoinertial testing and exercising has been developed to quantify dynamic muscle work. Isoinertial muscle action is defined as a type of muscle action in which muscles act against a constant load or resistance and the measured torque is determined while the constant load is accelerating or decelerating.[39] It is thought to more closely mimic the functional performance of the muscle-joint system than isokinetic testing and exercising. If the torque produced by the muscle is equal to the resistance, the muscle contracts isometrically. If the torque produced by the muscle is greater than the resistance, the muscle shortens and the muscle contracts concentrically. Conversely, if the torque produced by the muscle is less than the resistance, the muscle will contract eccentrically. Isoinertial muscle action is similar to normal muscle activity in which isometric and either accelerating or decelerating muscle contractions are used in response to a constant load.

EXAMPLE 2: When a person begins to lift a constant external load, the inertia of the load must be overcome by the lifting muscles. At the initial moment of lifting, the muscles contract isometrically as they attempt to develop the torque necessary to match inertial resistance. Once the inertial resistance is exceeded, the muscles contract concentrically as the muscle torque increases and the load begins to move (accelerate).[39] Once in motion, antagonists to the "lifting" muscle may need to contract eccentrically to decelerate the load.

The advantage of both isokinetic and isoinertial devices is that they are capable of quantifying muscle activity. The degree to which either testing method can determine accurately the performance level of the person being tested is the primary question. At this point, the answer to this question appears to be that both are able to determine the difference between those who can perform a functional task well and those who cannot, given that the testing is done in a way that is task specific.[47]

Summary of Factors Affecting Active Muscle Tension

Active muscle tension is one component of total muscle tension, and total muscle tension is one component of a muscle's ability to move a bony lever. Active tension is, however, the most variable of the components of total muscle tension.

How rapidly a muscle can develop maximal tension is affected by:

- *Recruitment order of the motor units*: Units with slow conduction velocities are generally recruited first.
- *Type of muscle fibers in the motor units*: Units with type II muscle fibers can develop maximum tension more rapidly than units with type I muscle fibers; rate of cross-bridge formation, breaking, and re-formation may vary.
- *The length of the muscle fibers*: Long fibers have a higher shortening velocity than shorter fibers.

The magnitude of the active tension is affected by:

- *Size of motor units*: Larger units produce greater tension.
- *Number and size of the muscle fibers in a cross-section of the muscle*: The larger the cross-section, the greater the amount of tension that a muscle may produce.
- *Number of motor units firing*: The greater the number of motor units firing in a muscle, the greater the tension.
- *Frequency of firing of motor units*: The higher the frequency of firing of motor units, the greater the tension.
- *Sarcomere length*: The closer the length to optimal length, the greater the amount of isometric tension that can be generated.
- *Fiber arrangement*: A pennate fiber arrangement gives a greater number of muscle fibers, and therefore a greater amount of tension may be generated in a pennate muscle than in a parallel muscle.
- *Type of muscle contraction*: An isometric contraction can develop greater tension than a concentric contraction; eccentric contraction can develop greater tension than an isometric contraction.

- *Speed*: As the speed of shortening increases, tension decreases in a concentric contraction. As speed of active lengthening increases, tension increases in an eccentric contraction.

Classification of Muscles

Individual muscles may be named according to shape (rhomboids, deltoid) or location (biceps femoris or tibialis anterior) or by a combination of location and function (extensor digitorum longus or flexor pollicis brevis). Groups of muscles are categorized on the basis of either the actions they perform or the particular role they serve during specific actions. When muscles are categorized on the basis of action, muscles that cause flexion at a joint are categorized as **flexors.** Muscles that cause either extension or rotation are referred to as **extensors** or **rotators.** When muscles are categorized according to role, individual muscles or groups of muscles are described in terms that demonstrate the specific role that the muscle plays during action. When using this type of role designation, it does not matter what action is being performed (flexion, extension) but only what role the muscle plays.

The term **prime mover (agonist)** is used to designate a muscle whose role is to produce a desired motion at a joint. If flexion is the desired action, the flexor muscles are the prime movers and the muscles (extensors) that are directly opposite to the desired motion are called the **antagonists.** The desired motion is not opposed by the antagonists, but these muscles have the potential to oppose the action.

Ordinarily when an agonist is called on to perform a desired motion, the antagonist is inhibited (**reciprocal inhibition**). If, however, the agonist and the potential antagonist contract simultaneously, then **co-contraction** occurs (Fig. 3–20). Co-contraction of muscles around a joint can help to provide stability for the joint and represents a form of synergy that may be necessary in certain situations. Co-contraction of muscles with opposing functions can be undesirable when a desired motion is prevented by involuntary co-contraction such as occurs in disorders affecting the control of muscle function.

Muscles that help the agonist to perform a desired action are called **synergists.**

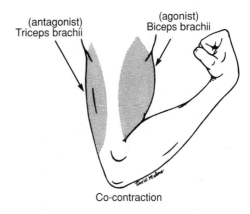

FIGURE 3–20. Co-contraction of agonist and antagonist.

EXAMPLE 3: If flexion of the wrist is the desired action, the flexor carpi radialis and the flexor carpi ulnaris are referred to as the "agonists" or "prime movers" because these muscles produce flexion. The finger flexors are the synergists that might directly help the wrist flexors. The wrist extensors are the potential antagonists.

Synergists may assist the agonist directly by helping to perform the desired action, such as in the wrist flexion example, or the synergists may assist the agonist indirectly either by stabilizing a part or by preventing an undesired action.

EXAMPLE 4: If the desired action is finger flexion, such as in clenching of the fist, the finger flexors, which cross both the wrist and the fingers, cannot function effectively (a tight fist cannot be achieved) if they flex the wrist and fingers simultaneously. Therefore, the wrist extensors are used synergistically to stabilize the wrist and to prevent the undesired motion of wrist flexion. By preventing wrist flexion, the synergists are able to maintain the joint in a position that allows the finger flexors to develop greater torque, a combination of optimizing sarcomere length and MA.

Sometimes the synergistic action of two muscles is necessary to produce a pure motion such as radial deviation (abduction) of the wrist. The radial flexor, flexor carpi radialis, of the wrist acting alone produces wrist flexion and radial deviation. The radial extensor, extensor carpi radialis brevis and longus, acting alone produces wrist extension and radial de-

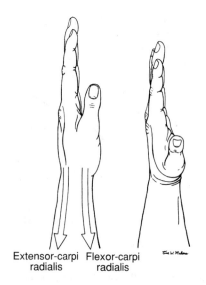

Extensor-carpi   Flexor-carpi
radialis   radialis

FIGURE 3–21. Synergistic muscle activity. When the flexor carpi radialis and the extensor carpi radialis work synergistically, they produce radial deviation of the wrist.

viation. When the wrist extensor and the wrist flexor work together as prime movers to produce radial deviation of the wrist, the flexor action of the flexor is prevented or neutralized by the extensor action of the extensors, and pure motion of radial deviation results (Fig. 3–21). In this example, the muscles that are the potential antagonists of the desired motion are the wrist extensor and flexor on the ulnar side of the wrist (extensor carpi ulnaris and flexor carpi ulnaris, respectively).

Placing muscles into functional categories

such as flexor and extensor or agonists and antagonists helps to simplify the task of describing the many different muscles and of explaining their actions. However, muscles can change roles. A potential antagonist in one instance may be a synergist in another situation. Despite this apparent change in role, muscles that have similar functions also have similar architectural characteristics. This may seem obvious, because muscle architecture plays such an important role in determining the potential force and velocity of muscle contraction. However, it was not until recently that several studies confirmed that the functional groups of muscles have similar architecture. Examples of this may be seen in experiments using both animals and humans.[26,48,49] In the lower extremity, the knee extensors have a short fiber length and large PCSA, as opposed to the knee flexors, which have a longer fiber length and smaller PCSA. The ankle plantarflexors typically have short fiber lengths and large PCSA, thus setting them apart from the ankle dorsiflexors that have longer fiber lengths and smaller PCSA. In the upper extremity, the finger flexors have longer fiber lengths and greater PCSA as opposed to the shorter and smaller finger extensors (Figs. 3–22 and 3–23).

The orientation of the muscle to the joint has also been used to classify muscles into groups. The length of the muscle MA is an important component of determining the joint torque and, in combination with the fiber length, the ROM through which the muscle can move the

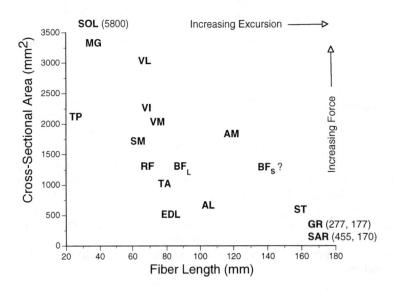

FIGURE 3–22. The relationship between PCSA and fiber length of selected muscles of the lower extremity. Note the general grouping of muscles with similar function. For example, the soleus (SOL) and medial gastrocnemius (MG); the tibialis anterior (TA) and extensor digitorum longus (EDL); and the vastus lateralis, vastus medialis, and vastus intermedius (VL,VM, VI). (Note: Data are only for fiber length of the biceps femoris short head, BFs.) (Adapted from Lieber, RL: Skeletal Muscle Structure and Function: Implications for Rehabilitation and Sports Medicine. Williams & Wilkins, Baltimore 1992, with permission.)

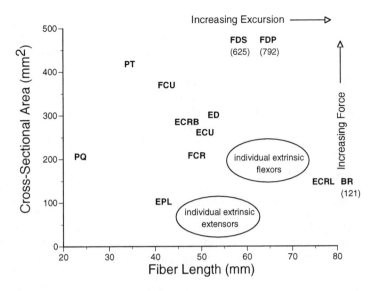

FIGURE 3–23. The relationship between PCSA and fiber length of selected muscles of the upper extremity. Note the general grouping of muscles with similar function. For example, the flexor digitorum superficialis (FDS) and profundus (FDP); the extensor carpi radialis brevis (ECRB), extensor carpi ulnaris (ECU), and extensor digitorum (ED); and the individual finger flexors and extensors. Adapted from Lieber RL: Skeletal Muscle Structure and Function: Implications for Rehabilitation and Sports Medicine. Williams & Wilkins, Baltimore 1992, with permission.)

joint.[28] The ratio of the fiber length to the MA provides a way of identifying which factor plays a greater role in the production of the joint torque and in determining the resulting ROM at the joint. For example, the fiber length to MA ratio is much higher in the wrist extensor muscles than the wrist flexor muscles suggesting that fiber length plays a greater role than MA in the wrist extensors than the wrist flexors.[33]

Although all skeletal muscles adhere to a general basic structural design, a considerable amount of variability exists among muscles in regard to the number, size, arrangement, and type of muscle fibers. Therefore, attempts to classify muscles into only a few groups may be inappropriate. Based on the evidence that subpopulations of motor units from muscles rather than groups of muscles appear to work together for a particular motor task, a more appropriate way of describing muscle action might be in terms of motor units.[17] However, more research needs to be performed in this area before a motor unit classification system can be widely used and accepted.

Factors Affecting Muscle Function

In addition to the large number of factors that affect muscle function presented previously, a few other factors need to be considered:

- Types of joints and location of muscle attachments
- Number of joints crossed by the muscle
- Passive insufficiency
- Sensory receptors

Types of Joints and Location of Muscle Attachments

The type of joint affects the function of a muscle in that the structure of the joint determines the type of motion that will occur (flexion and extension) and the ROM. The muscle's location or line of action relative to the joint determines which motion the muscle will perform. Generally, muscles that cross the anterior aspect of the joints of the upper extremities, trunk, and hip are flexors, whereas the muscles located on the posterior aspect of these joints are extensors. Muscles located laterally and medially serve as abductors and adductors, respectively, and may also serve as rotators. Muscles that have their distal attachments close to a joint axis usually are able to produce a wide ROM of the bony lever to which they are attached. Muscles that have their distal attachments at a distance from the joint axis, such as the brachioradialis, are designed to provide stability for the joint, because a large majority of their force is directed toward the joint that compresses the joint surfaces. A muscle's relative contribution to stability will change throughout a motion as the rotatory and compressive components of the muscle's force vary indirectly with each other. A muscle provides maximum joint stabilization at the point where its compressive component is greatest.

Usually one group of muscles acting at a joint is able to produce more torque than another group of muscles acting at the same joint. Disturbances of the normal ratio of agonist-antagonist pairs may create a muscle imbalance at the joint and may place the joint at risk for injury. Agonist-antagonist strength ratios for normal joints are often used as a basis for establishing treatment goals following an injury to a joint. For example, if the shoulder joint were to be injured, the goal of treatment might be to strengthen the flexors and extensors at the injured joint so that they had the same strength ratio as at the uninjured joint.

Number of Joints

Many functional movements require the coordinated movement of several joints controlled by a combination of muscles that cross one or many of the joints. To produce a purposeful movement pattern, many believe that the control of the movement is designed to minimize necessary muscle force to accomplish the task (least motor unit activity), and thus minimize muscle fatigue. These strategies of motor control attempt to ensure that movement is done efficiently.

One way of providing an efficient movement pattern is through the coordinated efforts of single-joint and multijoint muscles. In many ways, the number of joints that the muscle crosses determines the muscle function. Single-joint muscles tend to be recruited to produce force and work, primarily in concentric and isometric contractions. This recruitment strategy occurs primarily when a simple movement is performed at one joint, but may also be used during movements involving multiple joints. Multijoint muscles, on the other hand, tend to be recruited to control the fine regulation of torque during dynamic movements involving eccentric more so than concentric muscle actions.[50,51] Multijoint muscles tend to be recruited during more complex motions requiring movement around multiple axes. For example, the movement of elbow flexion with concurrent supination uses the biceps brachii (a multijoint muscle) with added contribution of the brachialis (a single-joint muscle). This may seem obvious because of the attachment of the biceps brachii to the radius allowing supination, whereas the brachialis attaches to the ulna allowing only flexion of the elbow.[52] If a single-joint motion is desired, a single-joint muscle is recruited because recruitment of a multijoint muscle may require the use of either additional muscles or motor units from additional muscles to prevent motion from occurring at the other joint(s) crossed by the multijoint muscles. For example, elbow flexion with the forearm in pronation is accomplished primarily with the brachialis and not the biceps brachii.

Single-joint and multijoint muscles may also work together in such a way that the single-joint muscle can assist in the movement of joints that it does not cross. For example, the simple movement of standing from a chair requires knee and hip extension. The hip extension is accomplished by activation of the single-joint hip extensor muscles (gluteus maximus) and the multijoint hip extensors (hamstrings). The concomitant knee extension is accomplished by activation of the single-joint knee extensor muscles (vasti) and the multijoint knee extensors (rectus femoris). An interesting corollary is that the single-joint knee extensors may actually assist in hip extension in this movement of standing from a chair. If the hamstrings are active, the knee extension (produced by the vasti) will pull on the active hamstring muscles (which act as a tie-rod) resulting in hip extension.

Passive Insufficiency

If one's elbow is placed on the table with the forearm in a vertical position and the hand is allowed to drop forward into wrist flexion, one will notice that the fingers tend to extend (Fig. 3–24a). Extension of the fingers is a result of the insufficient length of the finger extensors that are being stretched over the wrist. The insufficient length is termed **passive insufficiency.** The finger extension due to the increase in passive tension that results from the stretching of the muscle over the wrist is called the **tendon action** of a muscle or **tenodesis.** If the person moves his or her wrist backward into wrist extension, the fingers will tend to flex (Fig. 3–24b). Flexion of the fingers is a result of insufficient length of the finger flexors as they are stretched over the extended wrist.

Under normal conditions, one-joint muscles rarely, if ever, are of insufficient length to allow full ROM at the joint. Two-joint or multijoint muscles, however, frequently are of insufficient length or extensibility to permit a full ROM to be produced simultaneously at all joints crossed by these muscles. The passive tension developed in these stretched muscles is sufficient to either check further motion of the bony lever (passive resistance torque = torque of the effort force) or, if one segment of the joint is not fixed, may actually pull the bony lever in

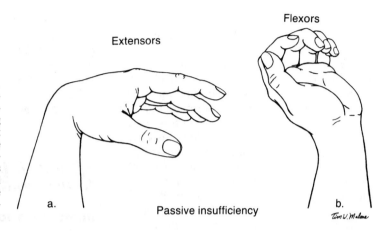

Extensors

Flexors

a.

Passive insufficiency

b.

Tim V. Malone

FIGURE 3–24. Passive insufficiency. (a) The finger extensors become passively insufficient as they are lengthened over the wrist and fingers during wrist flexion. The passive tension that is developed causes extension of the fingers (tenodesis). (b) The finger flexors become passively insufficient as they are lengthened over the wrist and fingers during wrist extension. The passive tension developed in the finger flexors causes the fingers to flex.

the direction of the passive muscle pull. If the bone is not free to move in the direction of passive muscle pull, damage to the muscle being stretched may occur. Usually pain will signal a danger point in stretching and active contraction of the muscle will be initiated to protect the muscle.

When a multijoint muscle on one side of a joint becomes excessively shortened, a multijoint muscle on the opposite side of the joint often becomes excessively lengthened.

> EXAMPLE 5: When the wrist and fingers are simultaneously flexed, the formation of a tight fist is almost impossible. If the fingers are fully flexed before flexing the wrist, the fingers have a tendency to extend when the wrist is flexed. If the wrist is flexed first, full flexion of the fingers to make a tight fist is very difficult if not impossible.

In this example, at the same time that the finger flexors are shortened, the inactive finger extensors are being passively stretched over all of the joints that they cross. The extensors are providing a passive resistance to wrist and finger flexion at the same time that the finger flexors are having difficulty performing the movement (Fig. 3–25). Insufficient length of the extensors is responsible for pulling the fingers into slight extension when the wrist is flexed prior to attempting finger flexion. The combination of excessive lengthening of passive muscle and attempted shortening of active muscle is threatening to the integrity of the muscle and such positions are not usually encountered in normal activities of daily living but may be encountered in sports activities.

Sensory Receptors

Two important sensory receptors, the **Golgi tendon organ** and the **muscle spindle,** affect muscle function. The Golgi tendon organs, which are located in the tendon at the myotendinous junction, are sensitive to tension and may be activated either by an active muscle contraction or by an excessive passive stretch of the muscle. When the Golgi tendon organs are excited, they send a message to the nervous system to inhibit the muscle in whose tendon the receptor lies.

The **muscle spindles,** which consist of 2 to 10 specialized muscle fibers (intrafusal fibers) enclosed in a connective tissue sheath, are interspersed throughout the muscle. These fibers are sensitive to the length and the veloc-

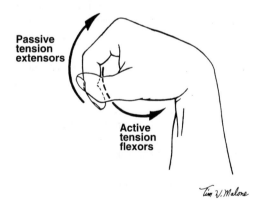

Passive tension extensors

Active tension flexors

Tim V. Malone

FIGURE 3–25. Increase in passive tension with passive muscle lengthening. When attempting to make a tight fist with the wrist fully flexed, the active shortening of the finger and wrist flexors results in passive lengthening of the finger extensors. The length of the finger flexors is insufficient to allow full range of motion at both the wrist and the fingers and therefore passively limits the ability of the finger flexors to make a tight fist.

ity of lengthening of the muscle fibers (extrafusal fibers). The spindles are activated by muscle lengthening. They send messages to the brain (cerebellum) about the state of stretch of the muscle. When the muscle fiber shortens, the spindles stop sending messages because they are no longer stretched. When the signal decreases, the higher centers send a message to the intrafusal muscle fibers in the spindle to shorten so they once again are able to respond to the length change in the muscle.

The muscle spindle is responsible for sending the message to the muscle in which it lies to contract when the tendon of a muscle is tapped with a hammer. The quick stretch of the muscle caused by tapping the tendon activates the muscle spindles, and the muscle responds to the unexpected spindle message by a brief contraction. This response is called by various names, for example, deep tendon reflex (DTR), muscle spindle reflex (MSR), or simply stretch reflex. Both the Golgi tendon organs and the muscle spindles help to protect the muscle from injury by monitoring changes in muscle length.

The presence of the stretch reflex is beneficial for preventing muscle injury but presents a problem for treatment programs or fitness programs in which stretching of a muscle is desirable for improving flexibility and restoring a full range of joint motion. Muscle contraction or reflex activation of motor units during intentional stretching of a muscle may create a resistance to the stretching procedure and makes stretching more difficult and possibly ineffective. Methods of stretching that may prevent reflex activity and motor unit activation during stretching are being investigated.[53,54] The noncontractile components of a muscle also provide resistance to stretching and need to be considered when a muscle-stretching program is implemented.

Receptors that lie in joint capsules and ligaments may have an influence on muscle activity through their signals to the central nervous system. Swelling of the joint capsule and noxious stimuli such as pinching of the capsule will cause reflex inhibition of muscles.

EXAMPLE 6: Nocioceptors and other receptors in and around the knee joint can have flexor excitatory and extensor inhibitory action. Even a small joint effusion which is undetectable to the naked eye can cause inhibition.[55–57]

The effects of the sensory receptors on muscle activity add an aspect of involuntary control of muscle function to the factors previously discussed. A review of the recent literature related to motor control or "movement science" is beyond the scope of this text, but some aspects of motor control will be presented in Chapter 13.

Effects of Immobilization, Injury, and Aging

Immobilization

Immobilization affects both muscle structure and function. The effects of immobilization depend on immobilization position (lengthened or shortened), percentage of fiber types within the muscle, and length of the immobilization period. Studies focusing on single muscle fibers and on whole muscles have found that immobilization in a shortened position produces the following structural changes:

- Decrease in the number of sarcomeres[58–60]
- Increase in sarcomere length[58,60,61]
- Increase in the amount of perimysium[61]
- Thickening of endomysium[61]
- Increase in ratio of collagen concentration
- Increase in ratio of connective tissue to muscle fiber tissue
- Loss of weight and atrophy[60,62,63]

Changes in function that result from immobilization in the shortened position reflect the structural changes. The decrease in the number of sarcomeres coupled with an increase in the length of sarcomeres brings muscle to a length wherein it is capable of developing maximal tension in the immobilized position. The loss of sarcomeres displaces the length-tension relationship of the muscle so that the maximum tension generated corresponds to the immobilized position. Therefore, the muscle is able to generate maximal tension in the shortened position. Although this altered capacity for developing tension may be beneficial while the muscle is immobilized in the shortened position, the muscle will not be able to function effectively at the joint it crosses immediately following cessation of the immobilization. The muscle that has adapted to its shortened state will resist lengthening passively, thus checking joint motion. Furthermore, the overall tension-generating capacity of the muscle is decreased. The increase in connective tissue in relation to muscle fiber tissue results in increased stiffness to passive stretch. The reason for increased fatigability of a muscle following immobilization in the shortened position is still being investigated.

Muscles immobilized in the lengthened position exhibit fewer structural and functional changes than muscles immobilized in the shortened position. The primary structural changes are an increase in the number and decrease in the length of sarcomeres, and muscle hypertrophy that may be followed by atrophy.[58,61,63] The primary functional changes in muscles immobilized in a lengthened rather than in a shortened position are an increase in maximum tension-generating capacity and displacement of the length-tension curve close to the longer immobilized position. Passive tension in the muscle approximates that of the muscle before immobilization.[60]

Recovery of a muscle from the effects of immobilization in the shortened position (development of pre-immobilization maximal tension-generating capacity, relocation of the length-tension curve, and extensibility) may take a relatively long time. However, prevention of the effects of immobilization in the shortened position may require only short periods of daily movement.[64] In summary, a word of caution concerning the interpretation of the response of muscle to immobilization: The studies on sarcomere adaptation to immobilization have all been done using specific muscles in animals. It is not clear whether these changes are apparent in all muscles and in humans.

Injury

Overuse may cause injury to tendons, ligaments, bursae, nerves, cartilage, and muscle. The common etiology of these injuries is repetitive trauma that does not allow for complete repair of the tissue. The additive effects of repetitive forces lead to microtrauma, which in turn triggers the inflammatory process and results in swelling. The tissue most commonly affected by overuse injuries is the musculotendinous unit. Tendons can fatigue with repetitive submaximal loading and are most likely to be injured when tension is applied rapidly and obliquely and the muscle group is stretched by external stimuli. Bursae may become inflamed with resultant effusion and thickening of the bursal wall as a result of repetitive trauma. Nerves can be subjected to compression injuries by muscle hypertrophy, decreased flexibility, and altered joint mechanics.[65]

Injuries to muscles may occur as a result of even a single bout of eccentric exercise. After 30 to 40 minutes of eccentric exercise (walking downhill), or as few as 15 to 20 repetitions of high-load eccentric contractions, significant and sustained reductions in maximal voluntary contractions occur. Also a loss of coordination, delayed-onset muscle soreness (DOMS), swelling, and a dramatic increase in muscle stiffness have been reported. The DOMS reaches a peak 2 to 4 days after exercise.[65–68] DOMS occurs in muscles performing eccentric exercise but not in muscles performing concentric exercise.[69] The search for a cause of DOMS is still under investigation. It is known to be related to the forces experienced by muscles and may be a result of mechanical strain in the muscle fibers or in their associated connective tissues.[70,71] Morphologic evidence shows deformation of the Z line (Z-line streaming) and other focal lesions following eccentric activity that induces soreness. Biomechanical and histochemical studies have demonstrated evidence for collagen breakdown and for other connective tissue changes.[66]

Aging

As one ages, skeletal muscle strength decreases due to changes in fiber type and motor unit distribution. After the sixth decade of life there is a loss of muscle fibers with some muscles (vastus lateralis) showing a 25% to 50% loss of fibers for those in their seventies and eighties.[72] In addition, the muscle gradually decreases the number and size of type II fibers and then is left with a relative increase in type I fibers.[73] There is also a decrease in the number of motor units, with the remaining motor units increased in the number of fibers per motor unit.[74] Aging will also increase the amount of connective tissue within the endomysium and perimysium of the skeletal muscle. It is generally assumed that the increased connective tissue results in decreased ROM and increased muscle stiffness.[75,76] Recently, there have been reports that muscle stiffness may not change or may decrease with aging.[77,78] Resistance exercise training in the elderly appears to have positive effects on aging muscles causing an increase in the size of muscle fibers and an increase in strength and functional performance.[79] However, a more limited response to resistance training occurs in the elderly than in the young.[80]

Summary

A great many factors affect the function of the muscles. A large number of the basic elements of muscle structure and their relationships to muscle function have been presented in this chapter. The interrelationships between structure and function in muscles are complex and often indistinguishable. Muscles are more adaptable than the joints that they serve and are more complex. Artificial joints have been designed and used to replace human joints, but it is as yet impossible to design a structure that can be used to replace a human muscle.

At the present time our knowledge of muscle contraction at the sarcomere level is still incomplete. However, it is known that the structural characteristics of muscle fibers change in response to functional demands. Exercises performed against high resistance with low number of repetitions (weight lifting) will cause the type II muscle fibers to increase in size.[81] Because the amount of tension a muscle can produce is determined by the total cross-sectional area of active muscle fibers, the increase in muscle fiber size results in an increase in the tension output of the muscle. Changes in a muscle fiber's oxidative capacity have been found after endurance training exercises,[82] but no evidence has been found to suggest that the contractile speed of muscle fibers can be changed in training.[83]

All skeletal muscles adhere to the general principles of structure and function that have been presented in this chapter. The muscles produce motion at the joints as well as providing joint stability. The structure and function of specific muscles and the relationship of the muscles to specific joints will be presented in the following chapters. The role that muscles play in supporting the body in the erect standing posture and in moving the body (walking) will be explored in the last two chapters of this book.

REFERENCES

1. Williams, PL, Warwick, R, Dyson, M, and Bannister, LH (eds): Gray's Anatomy, ed 37. Churchill Livingstone, London, 1989.
2. Johnson, MA, Pogar, J, Weightman, D, and Appleton, D: Data on the distribution of fibre types in thirty-six human muscles: An autopsy study. J Neurol Sci 18:111, 1973.
3. Gans, C: Fiber architecture and muscle function. Exerc Sports Sci Rev 10:160–207, 1982.
4. Netter, FH: The Ciba Collection of Medical Illustrations, Vol 8. Ciba-Geigy Corp., Summit, New Jersey, 1987.
5. Patel, TJ, and Lieber, RL: Force transmission in skeletal muscle: From actomyosin to external tendons. Exerc Sport Sci Reviews 25:321–363, 1997.
6. Horowits, R, et al: A physiological role for titin and nebulin in skeletal muscle. Nature 323:160–164, 1986.
7. Wang, K, et al: Viscoelasticity of the sarcomere matrix of skeletal muscles: The titin-myosin composite filament is a dual-stage molecular spring. Biophys J 64:1161–1177, 1993.
8. Huxley, AF: Muscle structure and theories of contractions. Prog Biophys Biophys Chem 7:225–318, 1957.
9. Huxley, AF, and Simmons, RM: Proposed mechanism of force generation in striated muscle. Nature 233:533–538, 1971.
10. Nordin, M, and Frankel, VH: Basic Biomechanics of the Musculoskeletal System, ed 2. Lea & Febiger, Philadelphia, 1989.
11. Peachey, LD, and Franzini-Armstrong, C: Structure and function of membrane systems of skeletal muscle cells. In Peachey, LD (ed): Handbook of Physiology. Bethesda, MD: American Physiological Society, 23–73, 1983.
12. Entman, ML, and Van Winkle, WB (eds): Sarcoplasmic Reticulum in Muscle Physiology. Vol 1. Boca Raton, FL, CRC Press, 1986.
13. Gowitzke, BA, and Milner, M: Scientific Basis of Human Movement, ed 3. Williams & Wilkins, Baltimore, 1988.
14. Henneman, E, et al: Functional significance of cell size in spinal motorneurons. J Neurophysiol 28:560–580, 1965.
15. Gielen, CCAM, and Denier van der Gon, JJ: The activation of motor units in coordinated arm movements in humans. News Physiol Sci 5:159–163, 1990.
16. Howell, JN, et al: Motor unit activity during isometric and concentric-eccentric contractions of the human first dorsal interosseus muscle. J Neurophysiol 74:901–904, 1995.
17. Van Zuylen, EJ, Gielen, AM, and Van Der Gon, JJD: Coordination and inhomogenous activation of human arm muscles during isometric torques. J Neurophys 60:1523–1548, 1988.
18. Kukulka, CG, and Clamann, HP: Comparison of the recruitment and discharge properties of motor units in human brachial biceps and adductor pollicis during isometric contractions. Brain Res 219:45–55, 1981.
19. Rosse, C, and Clawson, DK: The Musculoskeletal System in Health and Disease. Harper & Row, Hagerstown, MD, 1980.
20. Staron, RS: Human skeletal muscle fiber types: Deliniation, development, and distribution. Can J Appl Physiol 22:307–327, 1997.
21. Garrett, WE, Califf, JC, and Bassett, FH: Histochemical correlates of hamstring injuries. Am J Sports Med 12:98–103, 1984.
22. Staron, RS, et al: Strength and skeletal muscle adaptations in heavy-resistance-trained women after detraining and retraining. J Appl Physiol 70:631–640, 1991.
23. Saltin, B, et al: Fiber types and metabolic potentials of skeletal muscles in sedentary man and endurance runners. Ann N Y Acad Sci 301:3–29, 1977.
24. Eyzaguirre, C, and Fidone, S: Physiology of the Nervous System, ed 2. Yearbook Medical Publishers, Chicago, 1975.

25. Colliander, EB, Dudley, GA, and Tesch, PA: Skeletal muscle fiber type composition and performance during repeated bouts of maximal concentric contractions. Eur J Appl Physiol 58:81–86, 1988.

26. Lieber, RL, et al: Architecture of selected muscles of the arm and forearm: Anatomy and implications for tendon transfer. J Hand Surg 17:787–798, 1992.

27. Sacks, RD, and Roy, RR: Architecture of the hind limb muscle of cats: Functional significance. J Morphol 173:185–195, 1982.

28. Lieber, RL: Skeletal Muscle Structure and Function: Implications for Rehabilitation and Sports Medicine. Williams & Wilkins, Baltimore, 1992.

29. Maganaris, CN, et al: In vivo measurements of the triceps surae complex architecture in man: Implications for muscle function. J Physiol 512:603–614, 1998.

30. Kawakami, Y, et al: Architectural and functional features of human triceps surae muscles during contraction. J Appl Physiol 85:398–404, 1998.

31. Purslow, PP: Strain-induced reorientation of an intramuscular connective tissue network: Implications for passive muscle elasticity. J Biomech 22:21–31, 1989.

32. Gordon, AM, Huxley, AF, and Julian, FJ: The variation in isometric tension with sarcomere length in vertebrate muscle fibers. J Physiol 184:170–192, 1966.

33. Lieber, RL, Ljung, B, and Friden, J: Intraoperative sarcomere length measurements reveal differential design of human wrist extensor muscles. J Exper Biol 200:19–25, 1997.

34. Ichinose, Y, et al: Estimation of active force-length characteristics of human vastus lateralis muscle. Acta Anat 159:78–83, 1997.

35. Lutz, GJ, and Rome, LC: Built for jumping: The design of the frog muscular system. Science 263:370–372, 1994.

36. Hill, AV: First and Last Experiments in Muscle Mechanics. Cambridge: Cambridge University Press. 1970.

37. Griffin, JW: Differences in elbow flexion torque measured concentrically, eccentrically, and isometrically. Phys Ther 67:1205–1208, 1987.

38. Perrine, JJ, and Edgerton, VR: Muscle force-velocity and power-velocity relationships under isokinetic loading. Med Sci Sports 10:159–166, 1978.

39. Parnianpour, M, Nordin, M, Kahanovitz, N, and Frankel, V: The triaxial coupling of torque generation of trunk muscles during isometric exertions and the effect of fatiguing isoinertial moments on the motor output and movement patterns. Spine 13:982–990, 1988.

40. Knapik, JJ, et al: Muscle groups through a range of joint motion. Phys Ther 63:938–947, 1983.

41. Singh, M, and Karpovich, PV: Isotonic and isometric forces of forearm flexors and extensors. J Appl Physiol 21:1435–1437, 1966.

42. Enoka, RM: Eccentric contractions require unique activation strategies by the nervous system. J Appl Physiol 81:2339–2346, 1996.

43. Hislop, H, and Perrine, JJ: The isokinetic exercise concept. Phys Ther 47:114–117, 1967.

44. Murray, P, et al: Strength of isometric and isokinetic contractions. Phys Ther 60:4, 1980.

45. Knapik, JL, and Ramos, ML: Isokinetic and isometric torque relationships in the human body. Arch Phys Med Rehabil 61:64, 1980.

46. Kumar, S: Isometric and isokinetic back and arm lifting strengths: Device and measurement. J Biomech 21:35–44, 1988.

47. Murphy, AJ, and Wilson, GJ: The assessment of human dynamic muscular function: A comparison of isoinertial and isokinetic tests. J Sports Med Phys Fitness 36:169–177, 1996.

48. Burkholder, T, et al: Relationship between muscle fiber types and sizes and muscle architectural properties in the mouse hindlimb. J Morphol 221:177–190, 1994.

49. Wickiewicz TL, et al: Muscle architecture of the human lower limb. Clin Orthop Rel Res 179:275–283, 1983.

50. van Ingen Schenau, GJ, et al: The control of monoarticular muscles in multijoint leg extensions in man. J Physiol 484:247–254, 1995.

51. Sergio, LE, and Ostry, DJ: Coordination of mono- and bi-articular muscles in multi-degree of freedom elbow movements. Exp Brain Res 97:551–555, 1994.

52. van Groeningen, CJJE, and Erkelens, CJ: Task-dependent differences between mono- and bi-articular heads of the triceps brachii muscle. Exp Brain Res 100:345–352, 1994.

53. Guissard, N, Duchateau, J, and Hainaut, K: Muscle stretching and motorneuron excitability. Eur J Appl Physiol 58:47–52, 1988.

54. Entyre, BR, and Abraham, LD: Antagonist muscle activity during stretching: A paradox revisited. Med Sci Sports Ex 20:285–289, 1988.

55. Young, A, Stokes, M, Iles, JF, and Phil, D: Effects of joint pathology on muscle. Clin Orthop Rel Res 219:21–26, 1987.

56. Spencer, J, Hayes, KC, and Alexander, IJ: Knee joint effusion and quadriceps reflex inhibition in man. Arch Phys Med Rehabil 65:171–177, 1984.

57. Stokes, M, and Young, A: The contribution of reflex inhibition to arthogenous muscle weakness. Clin Sci 67:7–14, 1984.

58. Tabary, JC, et al: Physiological and structural changes in the cats soleus muscle due to immobilization at different lengths by plaster casts. J Physiol 224:231–244, 1987.

59. Wills, et al: Effects of immobilization on human skeletal muscle. Orthop Rev XI(11):57–64, 1982.

60. Williams, PE, and Goldspink, G: Changes in sarcomere length and physiological properties in immobilized muscle. J Anat 127:459–468, 1978.

61. Williams, PE, and Goldspink, G: Connective tissue changes in immobilized muscle. J Anat 138:343–350, 1984.

62. Witzman, FA: Soleus muscle atrophy induced by cast immobilization: Lack of effect by anabolic steroids. Arch Phys Med Rehabil 69:81–85, 1988.

63. Booth, F: Physiologic and biomechanical effects of immobilization on muscle. Clin Orthop Rel Res 219:15–20, 1986.

64. Williams, PE: Use of intermittent stretch in the prevention of serial sarcomere loss in immobilized muscle. Ann Rheum Dis 49:316–317, 1990.

65. Herring, SA, and Nilson, KL: Introduction to overuse injuries. Clin Sports Med 6:225–239, 1987.

66. Stauber, WT: Eccentric action muscles: physiology, injury and adaptation. Exerc Sport Sci Rev 17:157–185, 1989.

67. Howell, JN, Chleboun, GS, and Conatser, RR: Muscle stiffness, strength loss, swelling and soreness following exercise-induced injury in humans. J Physiol 464:183–196, 1993.

68. Chleboun, GS, et al: Relationship between muscle swelling and stiffness after eccentric exercise. Med Sci Sport Exerc 30:529–535, 1998.

69. Buroker, KC, and Schwane, JA: Does postexercise static

stretching alleviate delayed muscle soreness? Phys Sports Med 17:65–83, 1989.

70. Lieber, RL, and Friden, J: Muscle damage is not a function of muscle force but active muscle strain. J Appl Physiol 74:520–526, 1993.

71. Warren, GL, et al: Mechanical factors in the initiation of eccentric contraction-induced injury in rat soleus muscle. J Physiol 464:457–475, 1993.

72. Lexell, J, et al: Distribution of different fiber types in human skeletal muscle: Effects of aging studied in whole muscle cross sections. Muscle Nerve 6:588–595, 1983.

73. Lexell, J, et al: What is the cause of the ageing atrophy? Total number, size and proportion of different fiber types studied in whole vastus lateralis muscle from 15- to 83-year old men. J Neurol Sci 84:275–294, 1988.

74. Doherty, TJ, et al: Effects of aging on the motor unit: A brief review. Can J Appl Physiol 18:331–358, 1992.

75. Alnaqeeb, MA, Alzaid, NS, and Goldspink, G: Connective tissue changes and physical properties of developing and aging skeletal muscle. J Anat 139:677–689, 1984.

76. Gajdosik, R, et al: Influence of age on concentric isokinetic torque and passive extensibility variables of the calf muscles of women. Eur J Appl Physiol 74:279–286, 1996.

77. Winegard, KJ, et al: An evaluation of the length-tension relationship in elderly human plantarflexor muscles. J Gerontol 52A:B337–343, 1997.

78. Oatis, CA: The use of a mechanical model to describe the stiffness and damping characteristics of the knee joint in healthy adults. Phys Ther 73:740–749, 1993.

79. Grimby, G, et al: Training can improve muscle strength and endurance in 78- to 84-yr-old men. J Appl Physiol 73:2517–2523, 1992.

80. Brown, M: Resistance exercise effects on aging skeletal muscle in rats. Phys Ther 69:46–53, 1989.

81. Edgerton, VR: Mammalian muscle fiber types and their adaptability. Am Zool 18:113, 1978.

82. Costill, DL, et al: Adaptations in skeletal muscle following stretch training. J Appl Physiol 46:1, 1979.

83. Gollnick, PD, et al: The muscle biopsy: Still a research tool. Phys Sports Med 8:1, 1980.

Study Questions

1. Describe the contractile and noncontractile elements of muscle.

2. Explain what happens at the sarcomere level when a muscle contracts.

3. Identify the antagonists in each of the following motions: abduction at the shoulder, flexion at the shoulder, and abduction at the hip.

4. Describe action in the following muscles when the distal bony segment is fixed and the proximal bony segment moves: triceps, biceps, gluteus medius, iliopsoas, and hamstrings. Give examples of activities in which this type of action of these muscle would occur.

5. Compare the function of the quadriceps and hamstrings muscles based on the architectural characteristics of each muscle group.

6. Diagram the changes in the MA of the biceps brachii muscle from full elbow extension to full flexion. Explain how these changes will affect the function of the muscle.

7. Identify the muscles that are involved in lowering oneself into an armchair by using one's arms. Is the muscle contraction eccentric or concentric? Is the muscle acting in reverse action? Please explain your answer.

8. Describe the factors that could affect the development of active tension in a muscle. Suggest positions of the upper extremity in which each of the following muscles would not be able to develop maximal tension: biceps brachii, triceps brachii, and flexor digitorum profundus. Describe the position in which the same muscles would passively limit motion (be passively insufficient).

9. Explain how a motor unit composed of type I fibers differs from a motor unit composed of type II fibers.

10. List the factors that affect muscle function and explain how each factor affects muscle function.

11. Explain how isokinetic exercise differs from other types of exercise such as weight lifting and isometrics.

12. Explain isoinertial exercise.

13. Describe the effects of immobilization on muscles.

14. Describe the adaptations that occur in skeletal muscle to aging.

CHAPTER 4

THE VERTEBRAL COLUMN

OBJECTIVES

Following the study of this chapter, the reader should be able to:

Describe

1. The curves of the vertebral column using appropriate terminology.
2. The articulations of the vertebral column.
3. The major ligaments of the vertebral column.
4. The structural components of typical regional vertebrae.
5. The structural components of atypical regional vertebrae.
6. The structure of the intervertebral disk.
7. Motions of the vertebral column.
8. Lumbar-pelvic rhythm.
9. The neutral zone.
10. Thoracolumbar fascia.

Compare

1. The structure of typical cervical vertebra with the structure of a typical thoracic and typical lumbar vertebra.

Identify

1. Structures that provide stability for the column.
2. Muscles of the vertebral column and their specific functions.

3. Ligaments that limit specific motions (flexion-extension, lateral flexion, and rotation).

4. Forces acting on the vertebral column during specific motions.

Explain

1. The relationship between the intervertebral and zygapophyseal joints during motions of the vertebral column.

2. The role of the intervertebral disk in stability and mobility.

3. How stability of the vertebral column is maintained.

Analyze

1. The effects of deficits such as disk degeneration and muscle weakness using the model presented in this chapter.

2. The effects of an increased lumbosacral angle on the pelvis and lumbar vertebral column.

Introduction

Although the vertebral column is complex, it is positioned in the text before the extremities because of its importance as a supporting and linking structure. An understanding of the structure and function of the vertebral column forms the basis for understanding how the various elements of the musculoskeletal system are related to one another and to total functioning of the body.

General Structure and Function

The interrelationship between structure and function in the human body is clearly illustrated in a study of the vertebral column. The design of the structural elements and of the systems of linkages uniting the elements allows the column to fulfill a variety of functions. The column is able to provide a base of support for the head and internal organs; a stable base for the attachment of ligaments, bones, and muscles of the extremities, rib cage, and the pelvis; a link between the upper and the lower extremities; and mobility for the trunk. In addition, the column protects the spinal cord. Some of these functions require structural stability, whereas others require mobility. The structural requirements for stability frequently are opposite to the requirements for mobility; therefore, a structure that is capable of meeting both functions is complex. Each of the many separate but interdependent components of the vertebral column is designed to contribute to the overall function of the total unit, as well as to perform specific tasks.

Structure

The vertebral column is divided into the following five regions: cervical, thoracic, lumbar, sacral, and coccygeal (Fig. 4–1). The column is composed of 33 short bones called vertebrae and 23 intervertebral disks. The vertebrae adhere to a common basic structural design but show regional variations in size and configuration. The vertebrae increase in size from the cervical to the lumbar region and decrease in size from the sacral to coccygeal region (Fig. 4–2). Twenty-four of the vertebrae in the adult are distinct entities. Seven vertebrae are located in the cervical region, 12 in the thoracic region, and 5 in the lumbar region. Five of the

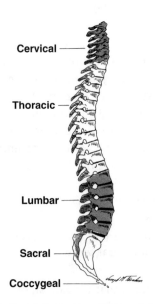

FIGURE 4–1. Five distinct regions of the vertebral column.

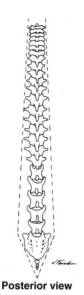

Posterior view

FIGURE 4–2. A cephalocaudal increase in the size of the vertebrae from the cervical to the lumbar region. The vertebrae show a decrease in size from the first sacral vertebra to the last coccygeal vertebrae.

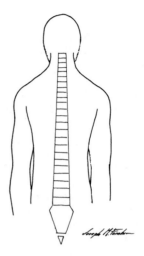

FIGURE 4–3. From the posterior aspect, the vertebral column appears as a vertical line that divides the trunk into two symmetrical parts.

remaining nine vertebrae are fused to form the sacrum, and the remaining four form the coccygeal vertebrae.

Primary and Secondary Curves

When the vertebral column is viewed from the posterior aspect, all regions together present a single vertical line that bisects the trunk (Fig. 4–3). When the column is viewed from the side, a number of curves that vary with age are evident. The vertebral column of a baby at birth exhibits one long curve that is convex posteriorly (Fig. 4–4). However, when the column of an adult is viewed from the side, four distinct anterior-posterior curves are evident (see Fig. 4–4). The two curves (thoracic and sacral) that retain the original posterior convexity throughout life are called **primary curves,** whereas the two curves (cervical and lumbar) that show a reversal of the original posterior convexity are called **secondary curves.** Curves that have a posterior convexity (anterior concavity) are referred to as **kyphotic curves;** curves that have an anterior convexity (posterior concavity) are called **lordotic curves.** The secondary or lordotic curves develop partly as a result of the accommodation of the skeleton to the upright posture. The superior secondary curve in the cervical region may occur as early as the sev-

enth week in utero as the muscles responsible for head extension develop in the fetus.[1] However, the curve continues to develop as the infant begins to hold his head up against gravity. The inferior secondary curve in the lumbar region develops as the infant begins to walk and hold his trunk upright. These curves continue to develop until growth stops somewhere between the ages of 12 and 17. The curves are interdependent, and if the head is to remain balanced over the sacrum, the region between the head and the pelvis behaves as if it were part of a closed kinematic chain. Changes in the position of any one segment will result in changes in position of adjacent superior or inferior segments.

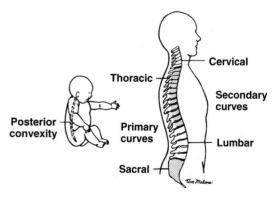

FIGURE 4–4. Primary and secondary curves. The shaded areas represent the primary curves.

Articulations

Two main types of articulations are found in the vertebral column: **cartilaginous** joints of the **symphysis** type between the vertebral bodies and the interposed disks; and **diarthrodial**, or **synovial**, joints between the zygapophyseal facets located on the superior articular processes of one vertebra and the zygapophyseal facets on the inferior articular processes of an adjacent vertebra above. The joints between the vertebral bodies and disks are referred to as the **intervertebral joints.** The joints between the zygapophyseal facets are called the **zygapophyseal (apophyseal** or **facet)** joints. All of the zygapophyseal joints, except for the joint between the first two cervical vertebrae, are plane synovial joints. Synovial joints also are present where the vertebral column articulates with the ribs (see Chap. 5), with the skull, and with the pelvis at the **sacroilac joints.**

Generally motion between any two vertebrae at the intervertebral joints is extremely limited and consists of a small amount of gliding (translation) and rotation. According to White and Punjabi,[2] one vertebra can move in relation to an adjacent vertebra in six different directions (three translations and three rotations) along and around three axes (Fig. 4–5, a–f). The compound effects of these small amounts of translation and rotation at a series of vertebrae produce a large range of motion (ROM) for the column as a whole. The motions available to the column as a whole may be likened to that of a joint with 3° of freedom, permitting flexion and extension, lateral flexion, and rotation.

However, motions in the vertebral column often are coupled motions. **Coupling** is defined as the consistent association of one motion about an axis with another motion around a different axis. For example, when the lumbar spine is axially rotated it bends in the frontal and sagittal planes (axial rotation is coupled with lateral flexion and forward flexion).[2] Another example of a coupled motion is lateral flexion, which is accompanied by axial rotation and forward flexion.[2-7] Coupling patterns as well as the types and amounts of motion that are available differ from region to region and depend on the spinal posture and curves,[8] orientation of the articulating facets, fluidity, elasticity, and thickness of the intervertebral disks and extensibility of the muscles, ligaments, and joint capsules. Lumbar lordosis and instrinsic mechanical properties of the vertebral column have about an equal effect in predicting the coupling between axial rotation and lateral bending. Lumbar lordosis alone accounts for coupled flexion associated with lateral bending.[8] Coupled motion patterns for left lateral flexion are presented in Table 4–1.

A Typical Vertebra

The structure of a typical vertebra consists of two major parts: an anterior cylindrically shaped vertebral body (Fig. 4–6a), and a posterior irregularly shaped vertebral arch (Fig. 4–6b). The vertebral body is composed of a block of trabecular or spongy bone, which is covered by a layer of cortical bone. According

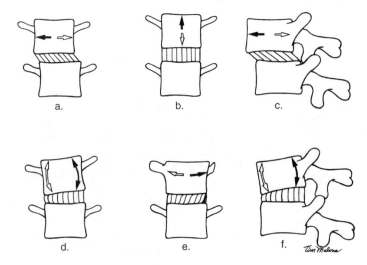

a.   b.   c.

d.   e.   f.

FIGURE 4–5. Translations and rotations of one vertebra in relation to an adjacent vertebra. (a) Side-to-side translation (gliding) occurs in the frontal plane. (b) Superior and inferior translation (axial distraction and compression) occur vertically. (c) Anterior-posterior translation occurs in the sagittal plane. (d) Side-to-side rotation (tilting) in a frontal plane occurs around an anterior-posterior axis. (e) Rotation occurs in the transverse plane around a vertical axis. (f) Anterior-posterior rotation (tilting) occurs in the sagittal plane around a frontal axis.

Table 4–1. **Coupling Patterns[2,7]**

Spinal Segment	Spinal Motion	Coupling Motion
Midcervical (C2–C5) Lower cervical (C5–T1) Upper Thoracic (T1–T4)	Left lateral flexion	Rotation to the left and forward flexion.
Midthoracic (T4–T8) Lower thoracic (T8–L1)	Left lateral flexion	Considerable individual variation and rotation may be either to the right or the left. Forward flexion.
Upper lumbar (L1–L4) Lower lumbar (L4–L5) Lumbosacral (L5–S1)	Left lateral flexion	Rotation to the right and forward flexion. Rotation to the left.

The coupling patterns presented represent average patterns. Coupling patterns may differ in both direction and degree in a normal population.

to the results of a study conducted by Wu and Chen, the stresses induced in the cortical bone shell are always much higher than in the trabecular bone. Also, stresses induced in the vertebral body are always larger at the anterior side than on the posterior side.[9] The cortical covering of the superior and inferior surfaces, or plateaus, is thickened around the rim where the epiphyseal plates are located and in the center by a layer of hyaline cartilage called the cartilaginous end-plate (Fig. 4–7).[10] Vertical, oblique, and horizontal trabecular systems that correspond to the stresses placed on the bodies are found within the spongy bone (Fig. 4–8).The vertical systems help to sustain the body weight and resist compression forces (Fig. 4–9). The other trabecular systems help to resist shearing forces. When the trabecular systems are viewed together (see Fig. 4–8), an area of weakness is evident in the anterior portion of the body, whereas areas of strength are demonstrable where the trabeculae cross each other.[11] The area of weakness is a potential site for collapse of the vertebrae (compression fracture).

The vertebral arch is a more complex structure than the body, because it has many projections, including three nonarticular processes and four articular processes (Figs. 4–10 and 4–11). The three nonarticular processes, two transverse and one spinous, provide sites for the attachment of ligaments and muscles. The two transverse processes divide the arches into anterior and posterior portions. The portions of the arch located anterior to the transverse processes are called the pedicles. The pedicles attach the arches to the right and left upper posterior walls of the vertebral body. The portions of the arches posterior to the transverse processes constitute the laminae. The posterior portions of the laminae that are located between the superior and inferior articular processes on each side are called the pars interarticularis. This is the area in which the vertically oriented lamina and horizontally oriented pedicle meet. The cortical bone in this area is usually thickened to withstand the stresses created by the change in direction of the forces that occurs in this area. The laminae join to form the peak of the arch and continue posteriorly to form the spinous process. The trabecular systems of the vertebral arch extend into the vertebral body and the area where the transverse

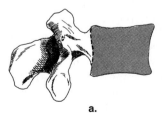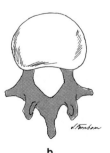

FIGURE 4–6. (a) The anterior portion of a vertebra is called the **vertebral body**. (b) The posterior portion of a vertebra is called the **vertebral arch**.

a.

b.

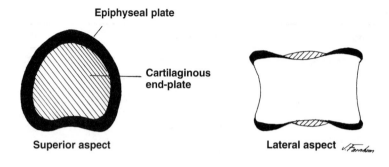

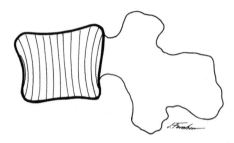

FIGURE 4–7. The cartilaginous end plates and epiphyseal plates are located on the superior and inferior vertebral plateaus.

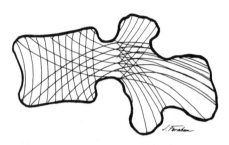

FIGURE 4–8. Schematic representation of the internal architecture of a vertebra. The various trabeculae are arranged along the lines of force transmission.

FIGURE 4–9. The vertical trabeculae of the vertebral bodies are arranged to resist compressive loading.

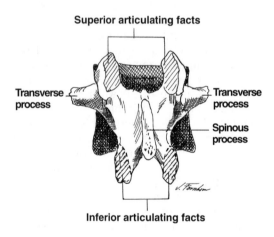

FIGURE 4–10. When a vertebra is viewed from the posterior aspect, seven projections are evident.

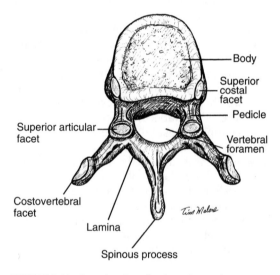

FIGURE 4–11. Superior view of a thoracic vertebra.

and articular processes arise is reinforced by many crossing trabeculae[11] (see Fig. 4–8). The paired superior and inferior zygapophyseal articular processes arise from the laminae and support articular surfaces called the zygapophyseal facets. Gender differences in structure have been identified in some vertebrae. Mclaughlin and Oldale found that by using the vertebral body diameters of T11, T12,

and L1 that they were able to predict a person's gender with an 89% accuracy rate.[12]

The Intervertebral Disk

The intervertebral disks, which make up about 20% to 33% of the length of the vertebral column, increase in size from the cervical to the lumbar region.[2] The disk thickness varies from

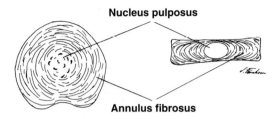

Nucleus pulposus

Annulus fibrosus

FIGURE 4–12. The nucleus pulposus is totally enclosed by the fibers of the annulus fibrosus.

approximately 3 mm in the cervical region to about 9 mm in the lumbar region.[11] Although the disks are largest in the lumbar region and smallest in the cervical region, the ratio between disk thickness and vertebral body height is greatest in the cervical and lumbar regions and least in the thoracic region.[11] The greater the ratio, the greater the mobility, and therefore the disks in the cervical and lumbar regions contribute to the greater mobility found in the cervical and lumbar regions in comparison with the thoracic region. Natural variations in disk height are associated with relatively small differences in mechanical function. However, secondary disk narrowing due to degenerative changes is associated with large changes in mechanical function.[13]

The disk is composed of two parts: a central portion called the **nucleus pulposus** and a peripheral portion called the annulus fibrosus (Fig. 4–12). The composition of the nucleus and annulus are similar in that they both are composed of water, collagen, and proteoglycans (PGs). However, the relative proportions of these substances and the types of collagen that are present differ in the two parts of the disk. Fluid and PG concentrations are highest in the nucleus and lowest in the outer annulus. Conversely, collagen concentrations are highest in the outer annulus and lowest in the nucleus pulposus. Table 4–2 provides a disk composition summary.

NUCLEUS PULPOSUS

The nucleus pulposus in healthy young adults is composed of a matrix that contains the following glycosaminoglycans: chondroitin 6-sulfate, chondroitin 4-sulfate, keratan sulfate, and hyaluronate.[7] When glycosaminoglycans are linked to proteins, they form large molecules (PGs). The PG molecules have the capacity to attract and retain water. This ability is due to the concentration of chondroitin 4-sulfate within the molecule. If the concentration of chondroitin 4-sulfate is high, the disk will have a high fluid-attracting and fluid-maintaining capacity.[7]

The fluid content and composition of the disk varies with aging. In a newborn baby, the fluid content of the nucleus pulposus accounts

Table 4–2. **Composition of the Intervertebral Disk**

Substance	Nucleus pulposus	Annulus Fibrosus
Water	70–90% varies with age,[7] 65% in 77-year-old,[14–16] 88% in newborns[2,14]	60–70%
Proteoglycans	65% dry weight	20% of dry weight
Collagen (total)	15–20% dry weight,[7] 6–25% dry weight[16]	50–60% dry weight[7] 70% dry weight[16]
Type I	Absent from central portion of the nucleus or exists in extremely small amounts[7]	Predominant type in outer annulus
Type II	15–20% dry weight [7,16–18]	Small amounts throughout inner and outer annulus[7]
Type III	Trace amounts	Small amounts in inner annulus[7]
Type V	Absent	Associated with type I found in small amounts
Type VI	Small amounts	Small amounts
Type IX	Small amounts	Small amounts
Type XI		Associated with type I and found in small amounts.
Elastin	Small number of fibers	10%[7]
Cells	Chondrocytes	Chondrocytes in inner annulus and fibrocytes in outer annulus[7]

for approximately 88% of the weight.[2,14] In a person at the age of 77, the fluid content may account for only 65% of the weight of the nucleus pulposus.[14-16] The composition (PG/collagen ratio) of the disk and the applied load affect the fluid content. Disks with a high PG/collagen ratio (young disks) will hold more fluid than older degenerated disks that have a low PG/collagen ratio. Under equal loads the percentage of fluid will be greatest in disks with the highest PG ratio. The fluid content of any disk may vary considerably during the day because the disk can lose a considerable amount of its fluid content when it is loaded continuously for a number of hours.

Seven different types of collagen have been identified in intervertebral disks; however, type I and type II collagen predominate.[16] Type I collagen typically is found in tissues that are designed to resist tensile forces, that is, skin, tendon, and ligaments. Type II collagen is present in high concentrations in tissues that are required to resist compression.[7] The total amount of collagen in the disk increases steadily from about 6% to 25% of the dry weight in the center of the nucleus pulposus to 70% in the outer annulus.[16] The types of collagen that are present also vary between the nucleus and the annulus and also in different portions of the annulus. The nucleus pulposus contains primarily type II collagen,[16-18] which constitutes about 15% to 20% of the dry weight of the nucleus pulposus in the healthy young adult.[7] The annulus fibrosus, which is subjected to both tensile and compression loading, contains collagen types I and II, but type I collagen predominates.[7]

ANNULUS FIBROSUS

The collagen fibers of the annulus fibrosus are arranged in sheets called **lamellae** (Fig. 4–13). The lamellae are arranged in concentric rings that totally enclose the nucleus. Collagen fibers in adjacent rings are oriented in opposite directions at 120° to each other.[2] Stress testing of annulus fibers taken from lumbar vertebrae has shown that the middle fibers of the lumbar annulus fibrosus are stiffer and fail at lower strains than the fibers from the outer and inner regions.[19] The testing also demonstrated that the radial tensile behavior of the annulus fibers was highly nonlinear.[19] The annulus fibers are attached to the cartilaginous end-plates on the inferior and superior vertebral plateaus of adjacent vertebrae and to the epiphyseal ring region by Sharpey fibers.

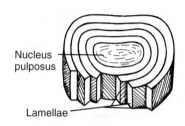

FIGURE 4–13. Schematic representation of an intervertebral disk showing arrangement of lamellae in annulus fibrosus. The collagen fibers in any two adjacent concentric bands or sheets (lamellae) are oriented in opposite directions. Anterior portions of the lamellae have been removed to show the orientation of the collagen fibers.

Maturation, aging, and disease as well as normal and abnormal stresses on the disk may affect the distribution and relative proportions of type I and type II collagen in the annulus. In adolescents and young adults, the concentration of type I collagen is greatest in the outer portion of the annulus and smallest next to the nucleus pulposus. The reverse is true for type II collagen. The concentration of type II collagen is smallest in the outer portion of the annulus and progressively increases toward the nucleus pulposus.

During maturation and aging, a greater proportion of type II relative to type I collagen has been found in the outer annulus portions of the anterior aspect of the disk, while the reverse was found for the posterior aspect of the disk. The reasons why these changes occur in the relative proportions of collagen types in lumbar vertebrae have not been determined. Changes also have been found in the distribution of the two types of collagen in annuli fibrosi located at the apices of abnormal curvatures of the vertebral column.

EXAMPLE 1: Disks of patients with an abnormal curvature of the spine show a difference in the distribution of types I and II collagen on opposite sides of the disk. The sides of the disks on the concave side of the curvature (which is subject to compression) have more type I collagen than the disks on the convex side of the curve.[17,19] The sides of disks on the convex side of the curve (which are subject to tension) show a decrease in the proportion of type I collagen in the outer portion of the annulus.[18]

These changes are the reverse of what one might expect (sides of disks subject to compression would contain more type II collagen, whereas sides of disks subject to tension would contain more type I collagen). The reason these changes occur has not been found. Investigators have hypothesized that the changes may represent remodeling of the collagen in the disk in response to altered mechanical loading.[16,18] An alternative explanation is that the changes in the distribution of collagen preceded the development of a curvature and may have led to the formation of the abnormal curvature.

INNERVATION AND NUTRITION

In the cervical and lumbar regions, the outer third of the annulus is innervated by branches from the vertebral and sinuvertebral nerves.[20] The sinuvertebral nerve also innervates the peridiskal connective tissue and specific ligaments associated with the vertebral column. Neither blood vessels[21] nor nerves[22] have been found to penetrate as far as the nucleus. Nutrition of the disk is thought to occur primarily by diffusion through the central portion of the cartilaginous end plate.[16]

Vertebral End Plates

The vertebral end plates are thin layers of cartilage that cover the superior and inferior surfaces of the vertebral bodies. Sometimes, the vertebral end plate is considered to be part of the disk.[7] The chemical composition of the end plate is similar to that found in the intervertebral disk (PGs, collagen, and water). However, the disk contains more water.[23] The center of the end plate, like the center of the disk, has a higher fluid and PG content and lower collagen content than the peripheral areas.[23] The collagen fibers in the end plate are arranged horizontally to withstand the swelling pressure of the nucleus pulposus, which occurs when the nucleus imbibes water or is subject to axial compression. In the very young (0 to 6 months) the end plates are covered by multiple small holes and depressions that are thought to represent blood vessel markings.[24] The holes and depressions disappear by the second year of life, and ridges and sulci begin to develop at the periphery of the end plates, especially in the lumbar and lower thoracic regions. The ridges and sulci elaborate up until the age of 18 and give the vertebrae a toothlike appearance. The ridges and sulci disappear when ossification of the end plate occurs. Edelson[24] has suggested that the ridges and sulci may provide

translational stability for the end plates in areas of the vertebral column in which the ribs and uncinate processes are not present to provide stability. The uncinate processes, which are found only in the cervical spine, prevent posterior translation of one cervical vertebrae on another and limit lateral bending. At around 20 to 25 years of age, osteophytes begin to appear at the periphery of the end plate plateau predominantly in areas of greatest stress in the column (C4/C5, T9/T10, and L3/L4).[24]

By the age of 50 years and with continued aging, osteolytic patches begin to appear in the end plates. These osteolytic patches are found most commonly in the cervical region and least commonly in the thoracic region.[24] Also intrusions of disk tissue into the end plate (**Schmorl's nodes**) may occur in areas of congenital weakness [25] (Fig. 4–14). These nodes weaken the end plate and may be a precursor to collapse of the end plate and disk degeneration. The nodes adversely affect the ability of the end plate to resist the swelling pressure of the nucleus.[23] If the disk ruptures and herniates, disk material may protrude through the end plate to make contact with the trabecular bone of the vertebral body, and sclerosis of the trabecular bone may occur in areas of contact.[25]

Zygapophyseal Articulations

The zygapophysial joints are composed of the articulations between the right and left superior articulating facets of a vertebra and the right and left inferior facets of the adjacent superior vertebra (Fig. 4–15). The four zygapophyseal joints are plane diarthrodial joints. In the lumbar region, rudimentary fibrous invaginations of the dorsal and ventral capsule have been identified as associated with the joints.[26] These invaginations

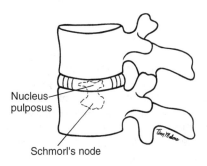

Nucleus pulposus

Schmorl's node

FIGURE 4–14. A schematic drawing of a Schmorl's node, in which nuclear material is extruded into the vertebral body.

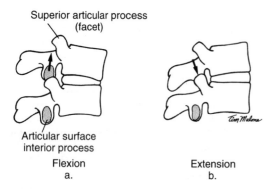

Superior articular process
(facet)

Articular surface
interior process

Flexion
a.

Extension
b.

FIGURE 4–15. Zygapophyseal joints. (a) The inferior articular process of the superior vertebra articulates with the superior process of the inferior vertebra. The shaded area on the superior vertebra represents the articular surface of the facet joint as the superior vertebra tilts anteriorly during forward flexion of the vertebral column. (b) The articular surfaces are obscured as the superior vertebra tilts posteriorly during extension of the vertebral column. Note also the approximation of the spinous processes and narrowing of foramen that occurs during extension.

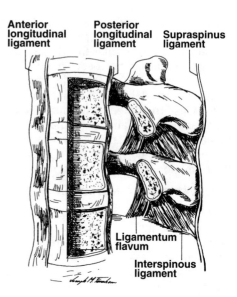

FIGURE 4–16. The anterior and posterior longitudinal ligaments are located on the anterior and posterior aspects of the vertebral body, respectively. The ligament flavum runs from lamina to lamina on the posterior aspect of the vertebral canal.

may be involved in protecting articular surfaces that are exposed during flexion and extension of the vertebral column. The capsular ligaments of the zygapophyseal joints in the lumbar spine play a dominant role in resisting flexion of the intervertebral joints.[27–29] The zygapophyseal joints protect the disks in the lumbar region by resisting a large proportion of the shear.[27,28] Maximal mineralization is found at the upper and lower edges of the articular surfaces in those areas where joint components remain in contact in extreme flexion and extension. The cancellous bone of the most lateral extended parts of the superior articular processes possess a characteristic architecture that can be recognized as an adaptation to the bending and shear forces acting on the upper lumbar motion segment.[30]

Ligaments and Joint Capsules

The ligamentous system of the vertebral column is extensive and exhibits considerable regional variability. Six main ligaments are associated with the intervertebral and zygapophyseal joints. They are the **anterior** and **posterior longitudinal ligaments;** the **ligamentum flavum;** and the **interspinous, intertransverse,** and **supraspinous ligaments** (Figs. 4–16 and 4–17). All of the individual ligaments except the anterior longitudinal ligament are oriented oblique to the long axis of the vertebral column and vary somewhat regionally.[30]

ANTERIOR AND POSTERIOR LONGITUDINAL LIGAMENTS

The anterior and posterior longitudinal ligaments are associated with the intervertebral joints. The anterior longitudinal ligament runs along the anterior and lateral surfaces of the vertebral bodies from the sacrum to the second cervical vertebra. An extension of the ligament from C2 to the occiput is called the anterior atlantoaxial ligament. The anterior longitudinal ligament has at least two layers that are made up of thick bundles of collagen fibers.[30,32] The fibers in the superficial layer are long and bridge several vertebrae, whereas the deep fibers are short and run between single pairs of vertebrae. The deep fibers blend with the fibers of the annulus fibrosus and reinforce the anterolateral portion of the intervertebral disks and the anterior intervertebral joint aspects. The ligament is well developed in the lordotic sections (cervical and lumbar) of the vertebral column but has little substance in the region of thoracic kyphosis. The anterior longitudinal ligament increases in thickness and width from the lower thoracic to L5/S1.[30] The tensile strength of the ligament is greatest at the high cervical, lower thoracic, and lumbar regions. However, when tested in axial tension, the ligament demonstrates its greatest tensile

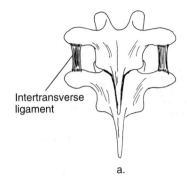
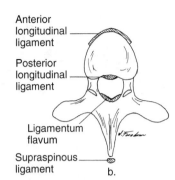

FIGURE 4–17. (a) The intertransverse ligament connects the transverse processes. (b) The relative positions of the other ligaments are shown in a superior view of the vertebra.

Intertransverse ligament

Anterior longitudinal ligament

Posterior longitudinal ligament

Ligamentum flavum

Supraspinous ligament

a.

b.

strength (676 N) in the lumbar area.[33] The ligament is compressed in flexion (Fig. 4–18a) and is stretched in extension (Fig. 4–18b). The ligament may become slack in the neutral position of the spine when the normal height of the disks is reduced, such as might occur when the nucleus pulposus is destroyed or degenerated.[34] The anterior longitudinal ligament is reported to be twice as strong as the posterior longitudinal ligament.[33]

The posterior longitudinal ligament runs within the vertebral canal along the posterior surfaces of the vertebral bodies from the second cervical vertebra to the sacrum. It consists of at least two layers, a superficial and a deep layer. In the superficial layer the fibers span several levels. In the deep layer, the fibers extend only to adjacent vertebrae interlacing with the outer layer of the annulus fibrosus and attaching to the margins of the vertebral end plates in a manner that varies from segment to segment.[30] Superiorly the ligament continues to the occiput, becoming the tectorial membrane at C2. In the lumbar region, the ligament narrows to a thin ribbon that continues down into the sacral canal. The ligament provides little support for the intervertebral joints in the lumbar region.

The posterior longitudinal ligament's resistance to axial tension in the lumbar area is only one-sixth of that of the anterior longitudinal ligament (160 N compared to 676 N).[33] The posterior longitudinal ligament is stretched in flexion (Fig. 4–19a) where maximal strain in the ligament occurs, and is slack in extension (Fig. 4–19b). However, if the axis of motion moves posteriorly, as it does when the nucleus pulposus is destroyed either experimentally or by degenerative processes, the ligament may be stretched in extension.[34]

LIGAMENTUM FLAVUM

The ligamentum flavum is a thick, elastic ligament, which is located on the posterior surface of the vertebral canal. The fibers of the ligament run within the canal from the second cervical vertebra to the sacrum, connecting laminae of adjacent vertebrae. Some fibers extend laterally to cover the articular capsules of the zygapophyseal joints. In the lumbar region the ligament is composed of superficial and deep components. The superficial component is a fibrous light yellow structure 2.5 to 3.5 mm thick that fills the interlaminar space. The deep component is a thin dark yellow structure approxi-

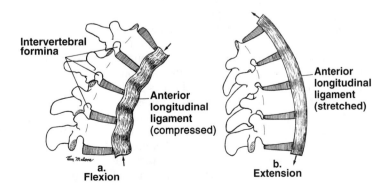

FIGURE 4–18. Anterior longitudinal ligament (ALL). (a) The ALL is slack in forward flexion of the vertebral column. (b) In extension of the vertebral column, the ligament is stretched.

Intervertebral formina

Anterior longitudinal ligament (compressed)

Anterior longitudinal ligament (stretched)

a.
Flexion

b.
Extension

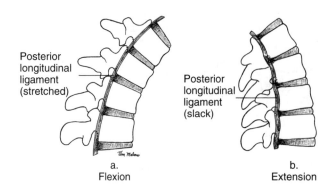

Posterior
longitudinal
ligament
(stretched)

Posterior
longitudinal
ligament
(slack)

a.
Flexion

b.
Extension

FIGURE 4–19. Posterior longitudinal ligament (PLL). (a) The PLL is stretched during forward flexion of the vertebral column. (b) The ligament is slack and may be compressed during extension.

mately 1 mm thick. It spans the interlaminar space, attaches to adjacent laminae, and contributes to the formation of the smooth dorsal wall of the spinal canal that abuts the dura.[35] Most of the anterior surface of the lumbar laminae is covered by the ligamentum flavum. The percentage of anterior surface covered increases from L1 to L5. Approximately 100% of the anterior surface of the L5 laminae are covered by the ligament. Insertions of the ligamentum flavum on its adjacent lumbar laminae vary according to segment level.[31,35] Cross-sectional areas of 80 to 110 mm have been identified in the lumbar region.[32] The ligamentum flavum is strongest in the lower thoracic and weakest in the midcervical region.[33] Although the highest strain in this ligament occurs during flexion when the ligament is stretched,[7,33] this ligament is under constant tension even when the spine is in a neutral position.[31,32] The ligamentous tension creates a continuous compressive force on the disks, which causes the intradiskal pressure to remain high. The raised pressure in the disks makes the disks stiffer and thus more able to provide support for the spine in the neutral position.[36]

INTERSPINOUS LIGAMENTS

The interspinous ligaments vary from region to region. In the cervical and upper two-thirds of the thoracic region, the ligaments connect and cover the margins of adjacent spinous processes. The parallel fibers of the ligaments run diagonally and fill up the space between the spinous processes. Longitudinal bundles of fibers some 2 to 3 mm thick bind the vertebral spines together. In the lower thoracic region and at T12/L1 no prevailing direction of the fibers can be determined. In the lumbar region, the ligaments are particularly well developed and attach to both the thoracolumbar fascia and the caudal

fibers of the joint capsules.[30] The ligaments are slack in extension and stretched in forward flexion when they resist the separation of the spinous processes that accompanies flexion. The ligaments have a tensile strength of only 24 to 185 N and thus are potentially weaker in tensile strength than the anterior longitudinal ligament, the posterior longitudinal ligament, and the ligamentum flavum.[33]

SUPRASPINOUS LIGAMENT

The supraspinous ligament is a strong cordlike structure that connects the tips of the spinous processes from the seventh cervical vertebra to L3 or L4.[1,7] The fibers of the ligament become indistinct in the lumbar area where they merge with the thoracolumbar fascia and insertions of the lumbar muscles. In the cervical region the ligament becomes the **ligamentum nuchae.** The supraspinous ligament, like the interspinous ligament, is stretched in flexion and its fibers resist separation of the spinous processes during forward flexion. During hyperflexion the supraspinous and the interspinous are maximally stretched and are the first of the posterior ligaments to fail.[27]

INTERTRANSVERSE LIGAMENTS

The structure of the paired intertransverse ligaments is extremely variable. Generally the ligaments pass between the transverse processes and attach to the deep muscles of the back. In the cervical region only a few fibers of the ligaments are found. In the thoracic region the ligaments consist of a few barely discernible fibers that blend with adjacent muscles. In the lumbar region the ligaments consist of broad sheets of connective tissue that resembles a membrane. The membranous fibers of the ligament form part of the thoracolumbar fascia. The ligaments are alternately stretched and compressed during lateral bending. The ligaments on the right side are stretched and offer resistance during lateral bending to the left while the ligaments on the left side are slack and compressed during this motion. Conversely, the ligaments on the left side are stretched during lateral bending to the right and offer resistance to this motion.

ZYGAPOPHYSEAL JOINT CAPSULES

The zygapophyseal joint capsules assist the ligaments in providing limitation to motion and stability for the vertebral column. However, the exact role that the capsules play and their strength in comparison to ligamentous supporting structures are still under investigation. The capsules are strongest in the thoracolumbar region and at the cervicothoracic junction[33] sites where the spinal configuration changes from a kyphotic to lordotic curve and from a lordotic to kyphotic curve, respectively. Therefore the potential exists for excessive stress in these areas. The joint capsules, like the supraspinous and interspinous ligaments, are vulnerable to hyperflexion, especially in the lumbar region. It has been suggested that the joint capsules in the lumbar region provide more restraint to forward flexion than any of the posterior ligaments because they fail after the supraspinous and interspinous ligaments when the spine is hyperflexed.[37] During axial loading the upper portion of the capsule is stretched because the height of the disk is reduced and the upper articular processes slide down on the lower processes. The superior portion of the capsule also is stretched during extension as one vertebra slides over another.[34] In the lumbar region the zygapophyseal joint capsules limit axial rotation.[38] Table 4–3 provides a summary of the ligaments and their functions.

Muscles

Numerous muscles contribute to stability and provide mobility for the vertebral column. Muscle attachments and functions are presented in detail in the appendix at the end of this chapter. The simplest classification of the vertebral muscles is on the basis of function, in which case there are forward flexors, lateral flexors, rotators, and extensors. Generally, the forward flexors are located anteriorly, the extensors posteriorly, and the lateral flexors and rotators on either side of the vertebral column. Muscles that attach to the pelvis and span a

maximum number of vertebrae are most efficient for providing lateral stability for the lumbar vertebral column. Efficiency increases as the muscles are positioned more laterally because of the increased moment arm (MA) of the muscle action lines.[31] In addition to the muscles and ligaments, the thoracolumbar fascia has been identified as playing a role in the stability of the vertebral column.[6,7]

Function

Stability

The stiffness of the vertebral column is the column's ability to resist an applied load. Stiffness can be represented graphically by the slope of the stress-strain curve.[7] The steeper the slope of the curve, the stiffer the structure. The complexity of the column has made accurate determinations of both the stiffness of the column as a whole and the contributions of various structures to stiffness very difficult to obtain.

Researchers investigating the spine have used small segments of the column, **motion segments,** to determine stiffness. A motion segment consists of two adjacent vertebrae and the intervening soft tissues.[36,39] By applying a specified load to a motion segment, an investigator can determine the stiffness of that particular segment. The sequential removal of ligaments, joint capsules, and portions of the disk followed by repeated measurements of stiffness yields information on how the stiffness of the segment is affected by the removal of the particular structure. Mathematical modeling, and the assessment of hysteresis and creep, also have been investigated in attempts to assess the stiffness of the spine.[40–46] Panjabi[2,47] has used the size of the **neutral zone** to provide a clinical measure of spinal stability.

The neutral zone is the ROM through which the spine can be displaced from a neutral position to the point at which elastic deformation begins when a small load is applied. In a stress-strain curve the neutral zone would be represented by the toe region of the curve. Panjabi[47] has suggested that the existence of a large neutral zone indicates instability. Instability of the vertebral column can be considered as a lack of stiffness, and an unstable structure is one that is not in an optimal state of equilibrium.[48] When the vertebral column is unstable, it exhibits a greater than normal (abnormal) ROM.

The vertebral column is subjected to axial compression, tension, bending, torsion, and

Table 4–3. **Major Ligaments of the Vertebral Column**

Ligaments	Function	Region
Annulus fibrosus (outer fibers)	Resists distraction, translation and rotation of vertebral bodies.	Cervical, thoracic, and lumbar.
Anterior longitudinal ligament	Limits extension and reinforces anterolateral portion of annulus fibrosus and anterior aspect of intervertebral joints.	C2 to sacrum but well developed in cervical, lower thoracic, and lumbar regions.
Anterior atlantoaxial (continuation of the anterior longitudinal)	Limits extension.	C2 to the occipital bone.
Posterior longitudinal ligament	Limits forward flexion and reinforces posterior portion of the annulus fibrosus.	Axis (C2) to sacrum. Broad in the cervical and thoracic regions and narrow in the lumbar region.
Tectorial membrane (continuation of the posterior longitudinal ligament)	Limits forward flexion.	Axis (C2) to occipital bone.
Ligamentum flavum	Limits forward flexion particularly in the lumbar area where it resists separation of the laminae.	Axis (C2) to sacrum. Thin, broad and long in cervical and thoracic regions and thickest in lumbar region.
Posterior atlantoaxial (continuation of the ligamentum flavum)	Limits flexion.	Atlas (C1) and axis (C2)
Supraspinous ligaments	Limit forward flexion.	Thoracic and lumbar (C7–L3 or L4). Weak in lumbar region.
Ligamentum nuchae	Limits forward flexion.	Cervical region (occipital protuberance to C-7)
Interspinous ligaments	Limit forward flexion.	Primarily in lumbar region where they are well developed.
Intertransverse ligaments	Limit contralateral lateral flexion.	Primarily in lumbar region.
Alar ligaments	Limit rotation of head to same side and lateral flexion to the opposite side.	Atlas (C1 and C2)
Iliolumbar ligament	Resists anterior sliding of L5 on S1	Lower lumbar region.
Zygapophyseal joint capsules	Resist forward flexion and axial rotation	Strongest at cervicothoracic junction and in the thoracolumbar region.

shear stress not only during normal functional activities, but also at rest.[49] The column's ability to resist these loads varies among spinal regions and depends on the type, duration, and rate of loading; the person's age and posture; the condition and properties of the various structural elements (vertebral bodies, joints, disks, muscles, joint capsules, and ligaments); and the integrity of the nervous system.[50]

AXIAL COMPRESSION

Axial compression (force acting through the long axis of the spine at right angles to the disks) occurs due to the force of gravity, ground reaction forces, and forces produced by the ligaments and muscular contractions. Most of the compressive force is resisted by the disks and vertebral bodies, but the arches and zygapophyseal joints share some of the load in certain postures and during specific motions. The compressive load is transmitted from the superior end plate to the inferior end plate through the trabecular bone of the vertebral body and the cortical shell. The cancellous body contributes 25% to 55% of the strength of a lumbar vertebra under the age of 40 years and the cortical bone carries the remainder. After age 40, the cortical bone carries a greater proportion of the load as the trabecular bone's compressive strength and stiffness decrease with decreasing bone density.[43] Depending on the posture and region of the spine, the zygapophyseal joints carry from 0% to 33% of the compression load. The spinous processes also may share some of the load when the spine is in hyperextension.

The nucleus pulposus acts as a ball of fluid that can be deformed by a compression force. The pressure created in the nucleus actually is greater than the force of the applied load.[51] When a weight is applied to the nucleus pulposus from above, the nucleus loses height as it exhibits a swelling pressure and tries to expand outward toward the annulus and the end plates (Fig. 4–20). As the nucleus attempts to distribute the pressure in all directions, stress is created in the annulus and central compressive loading occurs on the vertebral end plates. The forces of the nucleus on the annulus and the annulus on the nucleus form an interaction pair. Normally, the annulus and the end plates are able to provide sufficient resistance to the swelling pressure in the nucleus to reach and maintain a state of equilibrium. The pressure exerted on the end plates is transmitted to the superior and inferior vertebral bodies. The annulus fibrosus is under tensile stress and thus is able to better resist the compressive load. The disks and trabecular bone are able to undergo a greater amount of deformation without failure than the cartilaginous end plates or cortical bone when subjected to axial compression. The end plates are able to undergo the least deformation and therefore will be the first to fail (fracture) under high compressive loading. The disks will be the last to fail (rupture).

When the disks are subjected to a constant load by forces that are not large enough to cause permanent damage, the disks exhibit creep. Under sustained compressive loading such as incurred in the upright posture, the rise in the swelling pressure causes fluid to be ex-

pressed from the nucleus pulposus and the annulus fibrosus. The amount of fluid expressed from the disk depends both on the size of the load and the duration of its application. The expressed fluid is absorbed through microscopic pores in the cartilaginous end plate. When the compressive forces on the disks are decreased in the recumbent posture or absent in weightlessness, the disk imbibes fluid back from the vertebral body.[41] The recovery of fluid that returns the disk to its original state explains why a person getting up from bed is taller in the morning than in the evening. It also explains why an astronaut returning from weightlessness of space is taller on his return than on his departure. Running is a form of dynamic loading that decreases disk height more rapidly than static loading. The height of the vertebral column is a widely used indicator of cumulative disk compression. Ahrens in a study involving 31 men found that the men had a mean loss of 0.89 cm and 0.72 cm following a 6-mile run.[52] In the elderly the amount of creep that occurs is greater than in the young and the recovery from creep and hysteresis is slower.[41] The loss of height that occurs as people grow older is due to the fact that the nucleus loses a large proportion of its fluid-imbibing capacity with aging.

BENDING

Bending causes both compression and tension on the structures of the spine. In forward flexion the anterior structures (anterior portion of the disk, anterior ligaments, and muscles) are subjected to compression; the posterior structures are subjected to tension. The resistance offered to the tensile forces by collagen fibers in the posterior outer annulus fibrosus, zygapophyseal joint capsules, and posterior liga-

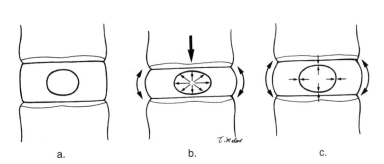

FIGURE 4–20. Compression of an intervertebral disk. (a) In this schematic representation of a disk, the nucleus is shown as a round ball in the middle of the annulus fibrosus. (b) Under compressive loading, the pressure is exerted in all directions as the nucleus attempts to expand. Tension in the annulus fibrosus rises as a result of the nuclear pressure. (c) A force equal in magnitude but opposite in direction is exerted by the annulus on the nucleus, which restrains radial expansion of the nucleus and establishes equilibrium. The nuclear pressure is transmitted by the annulus to the end-plates.

a.   b.   c.

ments help to limit extremes of motion and hence provide stability in flexion. Creep occurs when the vertebral column is subjected to sustained loading such as might occur in either the fully flexed postures commonly assumed in gardening or in the fully extended postures assumed in painting the ceiling. The resulting deformation (elongation or compression) of supporting structures such as ligaments, joint capsules, and intervertebral disks leads to an increase in the ROM beyond normal limits and places the vertebral structures at risk of injury. If the creep deformation of tissues occurs within the toe region of the stress-strain curve, the structures will return to their original dimensions in either minutes or hours following a cessation of the gardening or painting activity.

In extension the posterior structures generally are either unloaded or subjected to compression, whereas the anterior structures are subjected to tension.[53] Generally, resistance to extension is provided by the anterior outer fibers of the annulus fibrosus, zygapophyseal joint capsules, passive tension in the anterior longitudinal ligament, and possibly by contact of the spinous processes. In lateral bending, the ipsilateral side of the disk is compressed; that is, in right lateral bending the right side of the disk is compressed while the outer fibers of the left side of the disk are stretched. Therefore, the contralateral fibers of the outer annulus fibrosus and the contralateral intertransverse ligament help to provide stability during lateral bending by resisting extremes of motion.

TORSION

Torsional forces are created during axial rotation that occurs as a part of the coupled motions that take place in the spine. The torsional stiffness in flexion and lateral bending of the upper thoracic region from T1 to T6 is similar in stiffness, but torsional stiffness increases from T7/T8 to L3/L4. Torsional stiffness is provided by the outer layers of both the vertebral bodies and intervertebral disks and by the orientation of the facets.[54] The outer shell of cortical bone reinforces the trabecular bone and provides resistance to torsion.[54] When the disk is subjected to torsion, one-half of the annulus fibers resist clockwise rotations, whereas fibers oriented in the opposite direction resist counterclockwise rotations. It has been suggested that the annulus fibrosus may be the most effective structure in the lumbar region for resisting torsion.[55] However, the risk of rupture of the disk fibers is increased when torsion, heavy axial compression, and bending are combined.[44]

SHEAR

Shear forces act on the midplane of the disk and tend to cause each vertebra to undergo translation (move anteriorly, posteriorly, or from side to side in relation to the inferior vertebra). In the lumbar spine the zygapophyseal joints resist some of the shear force and the disks resist the remainder. When the load is sustained, the disks exhibit creep and the zygapophyseal joints may have to resist all of the shear force. Table 4–4 summarizes vertebral function.

Table 4–4. **Summary: Vertebral Function**

Structure	Function
Body	Resists compressive forces.
	Transmits compressive forces to vertebral end plates.
Pedicles	Transmit bending forces (exerted by muscles attached to the spinous and transverse processes) to the vertebral bodies.
Laminae	Resist and transmit forces (that are transmitted from spinous and zygapophyseal articular processes) to pedicles. Serve as attachment sites for muscles and ligaments.
Transverse processes	Serve as attachment sites for muscles and ligaments.
Spinous processes	Resist compression and transmit forces to laminae. Serve as attachment sites for ligaments and muscles.
Zygapophyseal facets	Resist shear, compression, tensile and torsional forces.
	Transmit forces to laminae.
Nucleus pulposus	Resists compression forces to vertebral end plates and translates vertical compression forces into circumferential tensile forces in annulus.
Annulus fibrosus	Resists tensile, torsional, and shear forces.

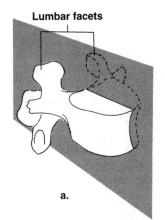

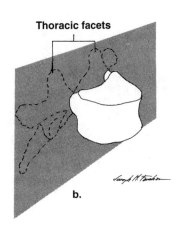

FIGURE 4–21. (a) Sagittal plane orientation of the lumbar zygapophyseal facets favors the motions of flexion and extension. (b) Coronal plane orientation of the thoracic zygapophyseal facets favors lateral flexion.

a.

b.

Mobility

Motions at the intervertebral and zygapophyseal joints are interdependent. The amount of motion available is determined primarily by the size of the disks, whereas the direction of the motion is determined primarily by the orientation of the facets. The motion that occurs between the vertebral bodies at the intervertebral joints is similar to what occurs when a rubber ball is placed between two blocks of wood. The blocks may be tilted or rotated in any direction and may glide if the ball rolls. If the size of the ball is increased or decreased, the amount of tilting possible is increased or decreased, respectively.

The motions of flexion and extension occur as a result of the tilting and gliding of a superior vertebra over the inferior vertebra. As the superior vertebra moves through an ROM, it follows a series of different arcs each of which has a different instantaneous axis of rotation.[56,57] The nucleus pulposus acts like a pivot but, unlike a ball, is able to undergo greater distortion because it behaves as a fluid.

Regardless of the magnitude of motion created by the ratio of disk height to width, a gliding motion (translation) occurs at the zygapophyseal joints as the vertebral body tilts (rotates) over the disk at the intervertebral joint. The orientation of the zygapophyseal facet surfaces, which varies from region to region, determines the direction of the tilting and gliding within a particular region. If the superior and inferior zygapophyseal facet surfaces of three adjacent vertebrae lie in the sagittal plane, the motions of flexion and extension are facilitated (Fig. 4–21a). On the other hand, if the zygapophyseal facet surfaces

are placed in the frontal plane the predominant motion that is allowed is that of lateral flexion (Fig. 4–21b).

FLEXION

In vertebral flexion the anterior tilting and gliding of the superior vertebra causes a widening of the intervertebral foramen and a separation of the spinous processes (Fig. 4–22a). Although the amount of tilting is partly dependent on the size of the disks, tension in the supraspinous and interspinous ligaments resists separation of the spinous processes and thus limits the extent of flexion. Passive tension in the zygapophyseal joint capsules, ligamentum flavum,

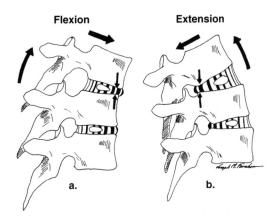

Flexion   **Extension**

a.   **b.**

FIGURE 4–22. (a) The superior vertebra tilts and glides anteriorly over the adjacent vertebra below during flexion. The anterior tilting and gliding cause compression and bulging of the anterior annulus fibrosus and stretching of the posterior annulus. (b) In extension the superior vertebra tilts and glides posteriorly over the vertebra below. The anterior annulus fibers are stretched and the posterior portion of the disk bulges posteriorly.

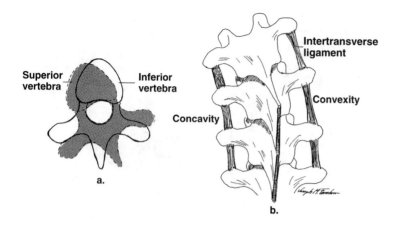

Superior vertebra **Inferior vertebra**

Concavity

a.

Intertransverse ligament

Convexity

b.

FIGURE 4–23. (a) The superior vertebra tilts laterally and rotates over the adjacent vertebra below during lateral flexion. (b) Lateral flexion and rotation of the vertebra are limited by tension in the intertransverse ligament on the convexity of the curve.

posterior longitudinal ligament, posterior annulus, and the back extensors also imposes controls on excessive flexion. Tension in the posterior ligaments can be produced by contractions of the hip extensors pulling downward on the pelvis when a person is in the standing position. Tension in the thoracolumbar fascia produced by contractions of the transversus abdominis also can limit flexion by the pull of the fascia on the spinous processes in the lumbar area. The disks influence flexion because the anterior portion of the annulus fibrosus is compressed and bulges anteriorly during flexion while the posterior portion is stretched and resists separation of the vertebral bodies.

EXTENSION

In extension, the intervertebral foramen is narrowed and the spinous processes move closer together (Fig. 4–22b). The amount of motion available in extension, in addition to being limited by the size of the disks, is limited by bony contact of the spinous processes, passive tension in the zygapophyseal joint capsules, anterior fibers of the annulus, anterior trunk muscles, and the anterior longitudinal ligament. In general, there are many more ligaments that limit flexion than there are ligaments that limit extension. The only ligament that limits extension is the anterior longitudinal ligament. The numerous checks to flexion follow the pattern of finding ligamentous checks to motion where bony limits are minimal. Few ligamentous checks to extension are necessary given the presence of numerous bony checks.

LATERAL FLEXION

In lateral flexion, the superior vertebra tilts, rotates, and translates over the adjacent vertebra

below (Fig. 4–23). The annulus fibrosus is compressed on the concavity of the curve and stretched on the convexity of the curve. Passive tension in the annulus fibers, intertransverse ligaments, and anterior and posterior trunk muscles on the convexity of the curve limit lateral flexion. The rotation that accompanies lateral flexion differs slightly from region to region because of the orientation of the facets.

All intervertebral and zygapophyseal joint motion that occurs between the vertebrae from L5 to S1 adheres to the general descriptions that have been presented. Regional variations in the structure, function, and musculature of the column are covered in the following sections. Table 4–5 summarizes the regional variations in the structure of the vertebrae.

Regional Structure and Function

The complexity of a structure that must fulfill many functions is reflected in the design of its component parts. Regional structures differ to meet different but equally complex functional requirements. Structural variations evident in the first cervical vertebra and the thoracic, fifth lumbar, and sacral vertebrae represent adaptations necessary for joining the vertebral column to adjacent structures. Differences in vertebral structure are also apparent at the cervicothoracic, thoracolumbar, and lumbosacral junctions, where a transition must be made between one type of vertebral structure and another. The vertebrae located at regional junctions are called **transitional vertebrae** and they usually possess characteristics common to two regions. The cephalocaudal increase in the size

Table 4–5. **Regional Variations in Vertebral Structure**

Part	Cervical Vertebrae	Thoracic Vertebrae	Lumbar Vertebrae
Body	The body is small with a transverse diameter greater than anterior-posterior diameter. Anterior surface of the body is convex; posterior surface is flat. The superior surface of the body is saddle-shaped due to the presence of uncinate processes on the lateral aspects of the superior surfaces.	The transverse and anterior-posterior diameters of the bodies are equal. Anterior height is greater than posterior. Two demifacets for articulation with the ribs are located on the postero-lateral corners of the vertebral plateaus.	The body is massive with a transverse diameter greater than the anterior-posterior diameter and height.
Arches	**Cervical Vertebrae**	**Thoracic Vertebrae**	**Lumbar Vertebrae**
Pedicles	Project posterolaterally.	Variable in shape and orientation	Short and thick
Laminae	Project posteromedially and are thin and slightly curved.	Short, thick, and broad	Short and broad
Superior zygapophyseal facets	Face superiorly and medially.	Thin and flat and face posteriorly, superiorly, and laterally.	Vertical and concave and face posteromedially. Support mamillary processes on posterior borders.
Inferior zygapophyseal facets.	Face anteriorly and laterally.	Face anteriorly, superiorly, and medially.	Vertical, convex, and face anterolaterally.
Transverse processes	Possess foramen for vertebral artery, vein, and venous plexus. Also have a gutter for spinal nerve.	Processes are large with thickened ends. Possess paired oval facets for articulation with the ribs. Show a caudal decrease in length.	Processes are long, slender, and extend horizontally. They support accessory processes on the posterior inferior surfaces of the root.
Spinous processes	Short, slender, and extend horizontally. Have bifid tips.	T1–T10 slope inferiorly. T11 and T12 have a triangular shape.	Broad, thick, and extend horizontally.
Vertebral foramen	Large and roughly triangular	Small and circular	Triangular. It is larger than the thoracic but smaller than the cervical.

of the vertebral bodies reflects the increased proportion of body weight that must be supported by the lower thoracic and lumbar vertebral bodies. Fusion of the sacral vertebrae into a rigid segment reflects the need for a firm base of support for the column. In addition to the above variations, a large number of minor alterations in structure occur throughout the column. However, only the major variations are discussed here.

Structure of the Cervical Region

The first two cervical vertebrae, C1 and C2, or respectively the **atlas** and **axis,** are atypical vertebrae. The seventh cervical vertebra is a transitional vertebra and therefore has characteristics of both the cervical and thoracic regions. The rest of the cervical vertebrae, C3 to C6, conform to the general basic structural design of all vertebrae with the following regional variations.

Typical Cervical Vertebrae

BODY

The body (Fig. 4–24) of the cervical vertebra is small, with a transverse diameter greater than anterior-posterior diameter and height. The upper and lower end plates from C2 to C7 also have transverse diameters (widths) that are greater than the corresponding anterior-posterior diameters. The transverse and anterior-posterior diameters increase from C2 to C7 with a significant increase in both diameters in the upper end plate of C7.[58] The lateral margins of the upper surfaces of the vertebral bodies from C3 to C7 support **uncinate processes** that give the upper surfaces of these vertebrae a saddle-shaped form. The uncinate processes are present prenatally and after birth gradually enlarge from 9 to 14 years of age.[59]

ARCHES

Pedicles. The pedicles project posterolaterally and are located halfway between the superior and inferior surfaces of the vertebral body.

Laminae. The laminae are thin and slightly curved. They project posteromedially.

Zygapopyseal articular processes (superior and inferior). The processes support paired superior facets that are flat, oval shaped, and face superoposteriorly. The width and height of the superior zygapophyseal facets gradually increase from C3 to C7. The paired inferior facets face anteriorly and lie closer to the frontal plane than the superior facets.[1]

Transverse processes. A foramen is located in the transverse processes bilaterally for the vertebral artery, vein, and venous plexus. Also, there is a groove for the spinal nerves.

Spinous processes. The cervical spinous processes are short, slender, and extend horizontally. The tip of the spinous process is bifid (split into two portions). The length of the spinous processes decreases slightly from C2 to C3, remains constant from C3 to C5, and undergoes a significant increase at C7.[58]

Vertebral foramen. The vertebral foramen is relatively large and triangular shaped.

Atlantoaxial Complex

The first two cervical vertebrae are markedly atypical vertebrae. The **atlas** (C1) is different from other vertebrae in that it has no body or spinous process and is shaped like a ring (Fig. 4–25). It has four articulating facets, two superior and two inferior, on the thickened lateral portions of the ring. The superior zygapophyseal facets are slightly concave and are designed to articulate with the slightly convex surface of the occipital bone. The inferior zygapophyseal facets are slightly convex, flattened, and directed inferiorly for articulation with the superior zygapophyseal facets of the axis (C2). The atlas also possesses a facet on the internal surface of the anterior arch for articulation with the dens (**odontoid process**) of the axis. The **axis** is atypical in that the anterior portion of the body extends inferiorly and a vertical projection called the dens arises from the superior surface of the body (Fig. 4–26). The dens has an anterior facet for articulation with the anterior arch of the atlas and a posterior groove for articulation with the transverse (cruciform) ligament. The arch of the axis has inferior and superior zygapophyseal facets for articulation with the adjacent inferior vertebra and the atlas, respectively. The spinous

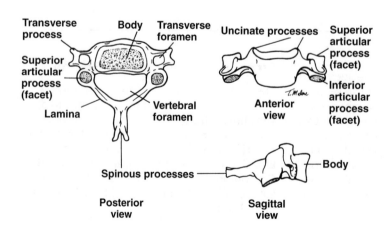

Transverse process

Body

Transverse foramen

Uncinate processes

Superior articular process (facet)

Superior articular process (facet)

Inferior articular process (facet)

Lamina

Vertebral foramen

Anterior view

Spinous processes

Body

Posterior view

Sagittal view

FIGURE 4–24. The body of a typical cervical vertebra is small and supports uncinate processes on the posterolateral superior and inferior surfaces.

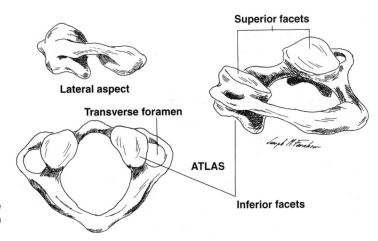

FIGURE 4–25. The atlas is a markedly atypical vertebra. It lacks a body and a spinous process.

process of the axis is large and elongated with a bifid tip. The superior zygapophyseal facets of the axis, which have the largest surface area (width and height) of all the cervical vertebrae, face upward and laterally. The inferior zygapophyseal facets, which have the same surface area dimensions as the inferior zygapophyseal facets of C3, face anteriorly.[60]

The **atlanto-occipital joint** is a plane synovial joint and is composed of the two concave superior zygapophyseal facets of the atlas that articulate with the two convex occipital condyles of the skull. The atlantoaxial joint is composed of three separate joints: the **median atlantoaxial (atlanto-odontoid)** joint between the dens and the atlas and two lateral joints between the superior zygapophyseal facets of the axis and the inferior zygapophyseal facets of the atlas (Fig. 4–27). The median joint is a synovial trochoid (pivot) joint in which the

dens of the axis rotates in an osteoligamentous ring formed by the anterior arch of the atlas and the **transverse atlantal (cruciform) ligament.** The two lateral joints are plane synovial joints.

Ligaments

Besides the ligaments mentioned earlier in the chapter, a number of other ligaments are specific to the cervical region. Many of these ligaments attach to the axis, atlas, or skull and reinforce the articulations of the upper two vertebrae. Four of the ligaments are continuations of the longitudinal tract system; the four remaining ligaments are specific to the cervical area. The posterior **atlantoaxial,** the anterior

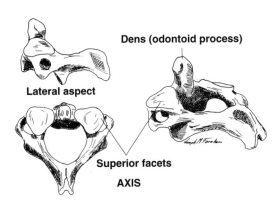

FIGURE 4–26. The dens (odontoid process) arises from the anterior portion of the body of the axis. The superior articulating facets are located on either side of the dens.

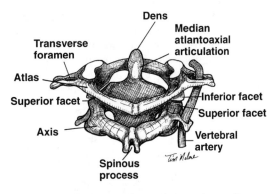

FIGURE 4–27. Atlantoaxial articulation. The median atlantoaxial articulation is shown with the posterior portion (transverse ligament) removed to show the dens and the anterior arch of the atlas. The two lateral atlantoaxial joints between the superior facets of the axis and the inferior facets of the atlas can be seen on either side of the median atlantoaxial joint.

atlantoaxial, the **tectorial membrane,** and the **ligamentum nuchae** are continuations of the ligamentum flavum, anterior longitudinal ligament, posterior longitudinal ligament, and the supraspinous ligament, respectively.

TRANSVERSE ATLANTAL LIGAMENT

The **transverse atlantal ligament** stretches across the ring of the atlas and divides the ring into a large posterior section for the spinal cord and a small anterior space for the dens. The transverse length of the ligament is about 21.9 mm.[61] The transverse atlantal ligament has a thin layer of articular cartilage on its anterior surface for articulation with the dens. Longitudinal fibers of transverse ligament extend superiorly to attach to the occipital bone and inferior fibers descend to the posterior portion of the axis. The transverse atlantal ligament and its longitudinal bands are sometimes referred to as the **atlantal cruciform ligament** (Fig. 4–28). The transverse portion of the ligament holds the dens in close approximation against the anterior ring of the atlas and therefore plays a critical role in maintaining stability at the median atlantoaxial joint. Although the transverse portion of the ligament serves as an articular surface for the dens, its primary function is to prevent anterior displacement of C1 on C2. The superior and inferior longitudinal bands of the transverse ligament provide some assistance in providing stability. The transverse atlantal ligament is very strong and the dens will fracture before the ligament will tear.[1]

ALAR LIGAMENTS

The two **alar ligaments** are also specific to the cervical region (Fig.4–28). These paired ligaments arise from the axis on either side of the dens and extend laterally and superiorly to attach to roughened areas on the medial sides of the occipital condyles[62] and to the lateral masses of the atlas[61] The ligaments are approximately 1 cm in length and about a pencil width in diameter and consist mainly of collagen fibers arranged in parallel.[62] These ligaments are relaxed with the head in midposition and taut in flexion.[62] Axial rotation of the head and neck tightens both alar ligaments.[62] The right upper and left lower portions of the alar ligaments limit left lateral flexion of the head and neck.[2] These ligaments also help to prevent distraction of C1 on C2. The alar ligaments are weaker than the transverse atlantal ligament. The **apical ligament** of the dens connects the axis and the occipital bone of the skull. It runs in a fan shaped arrangement from the apex of the dens to the anterior margin of the foramen magnum of the skull.[1]

Function of the Cervical Region

Stability

The cervical region differs from the thoracic and lumbar regions in that the cervical region bears less weight and is generally more mobile. Although the cervical region demonstrates the most flexibility of any of the regions of the vertebral column, stability of the cervical region, especially of the atlanto-occipital and atlantoaxial joints, is essential for support of the head and protection of the spinal cord and vertebral arteries. The design of the atlas is such that it provides more free space for the spinal cord than any other vertebra. The extra space helps to ensure that the spinal cord is not impinged on during the large amount of motion that occurs here. The bony configuration of the atlanto-occipital articulation confers some stability, but the application of small loads produces large rotations across the occipito-atlantoaxial complex[63,64] and also across the lower cervical spine.[63] The neutral zone across the occipital-atlantoaxial complex has been estimated to be 50% larger than in the lower

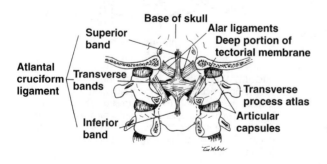

FIGURE 4–28. The transverse atlantal ligament. This is an aposterior view of the vertebral column in which the posterior portion of the vertebrae (spinous processes and portion of the arches) has been removed to show the atlantal cruciform and alar ligaments.

cervical spine.[63] The existence of a large neutral zone implies that the ligaments and joint capsules are lax and that the muscles play an important role in providing stability for the occipito-atlantoaxial complex.[65] The muscles responsible for providing stability are the **multifidus, interspinalis, semispinalis capitis,** and **semispinalis cervicis.**[65] If these muscles are cut during surgery or torn during injury, the stability of the complex will be severely compromised.

No disks are present at either the atlanto-occipital or atlantoaxial articulations. Therefore, the weight of the head (compressive load) must be transferred directly through the atlanto-occipital joint to the articular facets of the axis. These forces are then transferred through the pedicles and laminae of the axis to the inferior surface of the body and to the two inferior zygapophyseal articular processes. Subsequently the forces are transferred to the adjacent inferior disk. The laminae of the axis are large, which reflects the adaptation in structure that is necessary to transmit these compressive loads. The trabeculae show that the laminae of both the axis and C7 are heavily loaded, whereas the intervening ones are not. Loads diffuse into the lamina as they are transferred from superior to inferior articular facets.[66]

The loads imposed on the cervical region vary with the position of the head and body and are minimal in a well-supported reclining body posture. In the cervical region from C3 to C7 compressive forces are transmitted by three parallel columns: a single anterocentral column formed by the vertebral bodies and disks and two rodlike posterolateral columns composed of the left and right zygapophyseal joints. The compressive forces are transmitted mainly by the bodies and disks with a little over one-third transmitted by the two posterolateral columns.[64,66,67] Compressive loads are relatively low during erect stance and sitting postures and high during the end ranges of flexion and extension.[36] Cervical motion segments tested in bending and axial torsion exhibit lower stiffness than lumbar motion segments but exhibit similar stiffness in compression.[68] Combinations of sagittal loads in vitro demonstrated that the midcervical region from C2 to C5 is significantly stiffer in compression and extension than the lower region C5 to T1.[69] Also, specimens that were axially rotated before being tested in flexion and compression failed at a lower flexion angle (17°) than the mean angle (25°) of nonaxially rotated specimens. The implication is that the head should be held in a nonrotated position during flexion/extension activities to reduce the risk of injury.[69] Stability of the remainder of the cervical column is provided for by the same structures that were presented previously and that are summarized in Table 4–6. The joint capsules in

---

Table 4–6. *Cervical Region: Mobility/Stability Summary*

Region	Factors Affecting Mobility and Stability
Cervical atlanto-occipital	Forward flexion is limited by bony contact of the anterior ring of the foramen magnum on the dens and passive tension in the tectorial membrane.
Atlantoaxial	Forward flexion is limited by passive tension in the posterior atlantoaxial ligament and tectorial membrane.
	Extension is limited by passive tension in the anterior atlantoaxial ligament.
	Lateral flexion and lateral rotation of the head are limited by the alar ligaments.
	The transverse atlantal ligament prevents anterior dislocation of C1 on C2.
C-2–C-7	Forward flexion is limited by the posterior longitudinal ligament, ligamentum flavum, and the ligamentum nuchae.
	Excessive extension is limited by contact of the spinous processes and tension in the anterior longitudinal ligament and anterior neck muscles.
	Lateral flexion and posterior translation of the vertebral bodies are limited by the uncinate processes.
	Rotation and anteroposterior and medial/lateral tilting of the vertebrae are limited by the fibers of the annulus fibrosus.
	A large range of motion is permitted by the laxity of the zygapophyseal joint capsules.
	Zygapophyseal facet orientation favors forward flexion and extension and causes rotation to occur with lateral flexion.

the cervical region are lax and therefore provide less restriction to motion than in the thoracic and lumbar regions. The uncinate processes often enlarge with increasing age, and constitute a bony block to motion laterally and posterolaterally. The uncinate processes provide additional stability by reinforcing the posterolateral aspects of the disks.[59]

Mobility

The cervical spine is designed for a relatively large amount of mobility. Normally the neck moves 600 times every hour whether we are awake or asleep.[59] The motions of flexion and extension, lateral flexion, and rotation are permitted in the cervical region. These motions are accompanied by translations that increase in magnitude from C2 to C7.[70] However, the predominant translation occurs in the sagittal plane during flexion and extension.[71,72] Excessive anterior-posterior translation is associated with damage to the spinal cord.[71]

It is generally agreed that the atlanto-occipital joint permits primarily a nodding motion of the head (flexion and extension in the sagittal plane around a coronal axis)[73-75]; however, some axial rotation and lateral flexion are possible.[64] There is less agreement about the ROM. The combined ROM for flexion-extension reportedly ranges from 10° to 30°.[63,73-75] Maximum rotation at the atlanto-occipital joint reportedly ranges from 2.5% to 5 % of the total cervical spine rotation.[62,76] Flexion at the atlanto-occipital joint is limited by osseous contact of the anterior ring of the foramen magnum of the skull on the dens. Extension is checked by the tectorial membrane.

Motion at the atlantoaxial joint includes rotation, lateral flexion, flexion, and extension. Approximately 55% to 58% of the total rotation of the cervical region occurs at the atlantoaxial joint.[62,76] The atlas pivots about 45° to either side or a total of about 90°. Rotation at the atlantoaxial joint is limited by the alar ligaments. The remaining 40% of total rotation available to the cervical spine is distributed evenly in the lower joints.[76] However, a considerable amount of variation is found in the rotatory ROM within a population and gender differences have been identified. Dumas and colleagues found a significant gender difference between mean maximum rotation in the lower spine (C5 to T1) in that women, aged 20 to 50 years, had a much greater mean ROM in rotation than men aged 20 to 50 years.[76]

The ROM in lateral flexion and rotation is greater in the cervical region than in any other region. Lateral flexion and rotation are coupled below the level of C2 due to the configuration of the zygapophyseal articulating facets.

The site of maximum motion in flexion and extension occurs between C4 and C6 and the minimum amount of flexion and extension occurs at C2/C3. Dvorak and associates found a statistically significant difference in the average passive ROM in flexion-extension at C5/C6 between men and women.[70] Generally, motion is limited by tension in the ligaments, and annulus fibrosus, and by zygapophyseal facet orientation. Lateral flexion is limited by the uncinate processes, whereas hyperextension is limited by bony contact of the spinous processes. The height in relation to the diameter of the disks also plays an important role in determining the amount of motion available in the cervical spine. The height is large in comparison to the anterior-posterior and transverse diameters of the cervical disks. Therefore a large amount of flexion, extension, and lateral flexion may occur at each segment, especially in the young when there is a large amount of water in the disks. The laxity of the zygapophyseal joint capsules also promotes mobility.

In persons older than 45 years, Bland found no evidence of a gel-like nucleus pulposus in cervical disks. The disks appeared ligamentous and dry with little PG content present.[59] In a magnetic resonancÂ imaging (MRI) study of 2480 cervical disks from (C3/C4, C4/C5, and C5/C6) in 497 asymptomatic subjects (262 men and 235 women), Matsumoto and colleagues[77] found disk degeneration in 17% of the disks in men and 12% of the disks in women in their twenties. The percentage of disk degeneration increased to 86% in men and 89% in women over 60 years of age. The frequency of each degenerative finding (disk degeneration, disk protrusion, and narrowing of the disk space) increased linearly with age, with disk degeneration being the most prevalent finding in each age group. The MRI signs of disk degeneration were rare at C2/C3 and C3/C4. The frequency of degenerative MRI findings was highest at C5/C6 followed by C6/C7 and C4/C5. Posterior disk protrusions and compression of the spinal cord were most common at C5/C6.[77] Milne found that the anterior and lateral margins of the vertebral bodies of C5/C6 had the highest levels of pathology in the cervical spine[72] (Fig.

4–29). The disk at C5/C6 may be subject to a greater amount of stress than other disks because C5/C6 is the area which has the greatest range of flexion-extension and where the mechanical strain is greatest.[70] Joosab and associates performed a study to determine the effects of carrying heavy loads on the head (head loading) on the structural integrity of the cervical spine. They found that head loading appears to straighten the normal cervical lordosis and to create a shift from the location of degenerative changes observed in non-headloaders at the C5/C6 intervertebral disk space to the disk between C2 and C3. The degenerative changes observed in headloaders at C2/C3 were the same as observed in aged non-headloaders at C5/C6.[78]

Muscles

Flexion of the head at the atlanto-occipital joint is produced by the **longus capitis** and **rectus capitis anterior** muscles. The **sternocleidomastoid** muscles when acting bilaterally also will flex the head and neck. Extension at the atlanto-occipital joint is produced by the **recti capiti posteriores major and minor,** the **oblique capitis superior, semispinalis capi-** **tis, splenius capitis** and cervical portion of the **trapezius.** The muscles that act at the atlanto-occipital joint to produce lateral flexion of the head on the neck are the **rectus capitis lateralis, semispinalis capitis, splenius capitis, sternocleidomastoid** and the cervical part of the **trapezius**. Rotation at the atlanto-occipital joint is produced by the oblique capitis superior, rectus capitis posterior minor, splenius capitis and sternocleidomastoid. Flexion of the lower cervical region is produced by the action of the **longus colli.** The **scalene muscles** acting bilaterally may either flex the neck on the thorax or elevate the upper ribs when the cervical spine is stabilized.[79]

The primary extensors of the head and neck are numerous, and most of these muscles are also capable of producing rotation. Extensors that produce rotation to the opposite side are the **multifidus, rotators,** and **semispinalis.** The extensor muscles that cause rotation to the same side are the **oblique capitis** and **erector spinae.**

Structure of the Thoracic Region

The majority of the thoracic vertebrae adhere to the basic structural design of all vertebrae

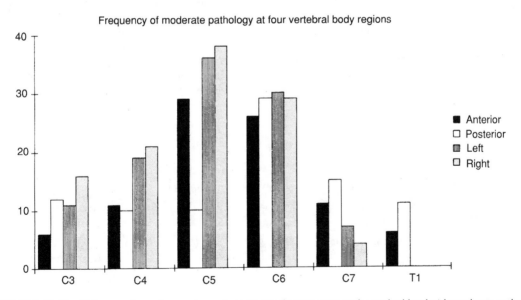

Frequency of moderate pathology at four vertebral body regions

FIGURE 4–29. The histogram shows the numbers of specimens (frequency) at each vertebral level with moderate pathology at the margins of the vertebral bodies. The frequency of findings of moderate pathology affecting the anterior, medial, and lateral margins of the C5 and C6 vertebral bodies was found to be significantly higher than at the other levels. A high incidence of pathology can also be seen at the posterior margins of C5 and C6, but it was not significantly higher than the incidence found at other levels. (From Milne, N: The role of zygapophyseal joint orientation and uncinate processes in controlling motion in the cervical spine. J Anat 178:189, 1991; with permission of the Cambridge University Press.)

except for some minor variations. The 1st and 12th thoracic vertebrae are transitional vertebrae and therefore possess characteristics of the cervical and lumbar vertebrae, respectively. The first thoracic vertebra has a typical cervical shaped body with a transverse diameter practically twice the anteroposterior diameter. The 12th thoracic vertebra has thoracic-like superior zygapophyseal articular facets that face posterolaterally. The inferior zygapophyseal facets have convex surfaces that face anterolaterally to articulate with the vertical, concave, posteromedially facing superior zygapophyseal facets of the first lumbar vertebra. The pedicles in the thoracic region exhibit considerable variations in shape and orientation throughout the region and Panjabi and colleagues found it impossible to quantify the numerous complex shapes exhibited.[80] The laminae are short, thick, and broad. The end plates show a gradual increase in transverse and anteroposterior diameters from T1 to T12. The inferior end plate width increases by 55% and the superior end plate anteroposterior diameter increases by 75%. Increase in width for both superior and inferior end plates is greatest at T11/T12.[81]

Typical Thoracic Vertebrae

BODY

The body of a typical thoracic vertebra has equal transverse and anteroposterior diameters (Fig. 4–30). In a study of 144 vertebrae Panjabi and coworkers found that the posterior height of each vertebra increased from approx-imately 14.3 mm at T1 to 22.7 mm at T12 representing an increase of 60% or a 0.8-mm increase per vertebral level.[81] **Demifacets** for articulation with the heads of the ribs are located on the posterolateral corners of the vertebral plateaus.

ARCHES

Pedicles. Exhibit variations in orientation and shape throughout the thoracic region but the majority of the pedicles are teardrop or kidney shaped with a laterally directed concavity and a medial convexity.[81]

Laminae. The laminae are short thick and broad.

Zygapophyseal articular processes. The superior zygapophyseal facets are thin and almost flat and face posteriorly and slightly superolaterally. The inferior zygapophyseal facets face anteriorly and slightly superomedially. The orientation of the facets changes at either T10 or T11 so that the superior facets face posterolaterally and the inferior facets face anterolaterally.

Transverse processes. The transverse processes have thickened ends that support paired large oval facets (**costotubercular facets**) for articulation with the tubercles of the ribs. The relationship of the transverse process to the pedicle changes from a position approximately 5.45 mm rostral to the pedicle to a position approximately 6.6 mm caudal to the pedicle. The crossover consistently occurs in the region of T6/T7.[82]

Spinous processes. The spinous processes slope inferiorly and from T5 to T8 overlap

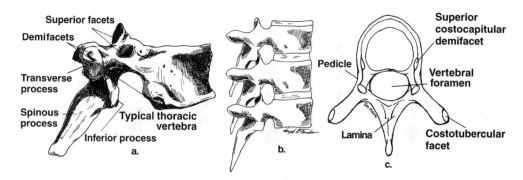

FIGURE 4–30. (a) Lateral view of the thoracic vertebra shows the superior and inferior facets of the zygapophyseal joints and the demifacets for articulation with the ribs. (b) Overlapping of spinous processes in thoracic region. (c) A superior view of a thoracic vertebra showing the small circular shape of the vertebral foramen, the costotubercular facets for articulation with the tubercles of the ribs, and the superior costocapitular facets for articulation with the heads of the ribs.

the spinous process of the adjacent inferior vertebra. The spinous processes of T11 and T12 have a triangular shape and project horizontally.

Vertebral foramen. The vertebral foramen is small and circular.

Function of the Thoracic Region

Stability and Mobility

The thoracic region is less flexible and more stable than the cervical region because of the limitations imposed by structural elements such as the rib cage, spinous processes, zygapophyseal joint capsules, the ligamentum flavum, and the dimensions of the vertebral bodies. Each thoracic vertebra articulates with a set of paired ribs by way of two joints: the **costovertebral** and the **costotransverse** joints. The vertebral components of the costovertebral joints are the demifacets located on the vertebral bodies. The vertebral components of the costotransverse joints are the oval facets on the transverse processes. These joints are discussed in detail in Chapter 5. The ligaments associated with the thoracic region are the same as those described previously for the vertebral column, except that the ligamentum flavum and anterior longitudinal ligaments are thicker in the thoracic region than in the cervical region. The zygapophyseal facet joint capsules are tighter than in the cervical region.

All motions are possible in the thoracic region, but the range of flexion and extension is extremely limited in the upper thoracic region (T1 to T6), by the rigidity of the rib cage and by the zygapophyseal facet orientation in the frontal plane. In the lower part of the thoracic region (T9 to T12), the zygapophyseal facets lie more in the sagittal plane, allowing an increased amount of flexion and extension. Lateral flexion and rotation are free in the upper thoracic region. The ROM in lateral flexion is always coupled with some axial rotation. The amount of accompanying axial rotation decreases in the lower part of the region due to the change in orientation of the zygapophyseal facets at T10 or T11. In the upper part of the thoracic region, rotation is accompanied by movement of the spinous process toward the convexity of the lateral flexion curve, whereas rotation in the lower region may be accompanied by rotation of the spinous process toward the concavity of the lateral flexion curve.[32] However, the direction of coupled rotation may vary among individuals.[2]

Flexion in the thoracic region is limited by tension in the posterior longitudinal ligament, the ligamentum flavum, the interspinous ligaments, and the capsules of the zygapophyseal joints. Extension of the thoracic region is limited by contact of the spinous processes, laminae, and zygapophyseal facets and by tension in the anterior longitudinal ligament, zygapophyseal joint capsules, and abdominal muscles. Lateral flexion is restricted by impact of the zygapophyseal facets on the concavity of the lateral-flexion curve and by limitations imposed by the rib cage.[71] Rotation in the thoracic region also is limited by the ribcage. When a thoracic vertebra rotates, the motion is accompanied by distortion of the associated rib pair (Fig. 4–31). The posterior portion of the rib on the side to which the vertebral body rotates becomes more convex as the anterior portion of the rib becomes flattened. The reverse occurs for the rib on the side opposite to the vertebral rotation. The amount of rotation that is possible depends on the ability of the ribs to undergo distortion and the amount of motion available in the costovertebral and costotransverse joints. As a person ages, the costal cartilages ossify and allow less distortion. This results in a reduction in the amount of rotation available with aging.

Muscles

The muscles that produce movement of the thoracic region also produce motion at the lumbar region and therefore the anterior, lateral, and posterior trunk muscles are discussed following the sections on the lumbar and sacral

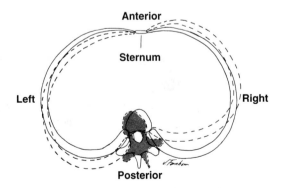

FIGURE 4–31. Rotation of a thoracic vertebral body to the left produces a distortion of the associated rib pair that is convex posteriorly on the left and convex anteriorly on the right.

regions. The other muscles specific to the thoracic region are muscles of respiration. These muscles are discussed in Chapter 5.

Structure of the Lumbar Region

The first four lumbar vertebrae are similar in structure. The fifth lumbar vertebra has structural adaptations for articulation with the sacrum.

Typical Lumbar Vertebrae

BODY

The body (Fig. 4–32a) of the typical lumbar vertebra is massive with a transverse diameter that is greater than anterior diameter and height.

ARCHES

Pedicles. The pedicles are short and thick.
Laminae. The laminae are short and broad.
Zygapophyseal articular processes. According to *Gray's Anatomy* the superior zygapophyseal facets are vertical and concave and face medially and posteriorly.[1] However, according to Bogduk, both the superior and inferior zygapophyseal facets vary considerably in shape and orientation (Fig. 4–32b). **Mamillary processes,** which appear as a small bumps, are located on the posterior edge of each superior zygapophyseal facet[7] (Fig. 4–32c). The mamillary processes serve as attachment sites for the multifidus and medial intertransverse muscles.[1] The inferior zygapophyseal facets are vertical, convex, and face slightly anteriorly and laterally.[1]

Transverse process. The transverse process is long, slender, and extends horizontally.
Accessory processes, which are small and irregular bony prominences, are located on the posterior surface of the transverse process near its attachment to the pedicle[7] (see Fig 4–32c). The accessory processes serve as attachment sites for the multifidus and medial intertransverse muscles.
Spinous process. The spinous process is broad and thick and extends horizontally.
Vertebral foramen. The vertebral foramen is triangularly shaped, larger than the thoracic vertebral foramen but smaller than the cervical vertebral foramen.

The fifth lumbar vertebra is a transitional vertebra and differs from the rest of the lumbar vertebrae in that it has a wedge-shaped body wherein the anterior portion of the body is of greater height than the posterior portion. The L5/S1 lumbosacral disk also is wedge shaped. The superior diskal surface area of L5 is about 5% greater than the areas of disks at L3 and L4. The inferior diskal surface area of L5 is smaller than the diskal surface area at other lumbar levels. Also the spinous process is smaller than other lumbar spinous processes and the transverse processes are large and directed superiorly and posteriorly.

The **lumbosacral articulation** is formed by the fifth lumbar vertebra and first sacral segment. The first sacral segment, which is inclined slightly anteriorly and inferiorly, forms an angle with the horizontal called the **lumbosacral angle**[83] (Fig. 4–33). The size of the angle varies with the position of the pelvis and affects the superimposed lumbar curvature. An

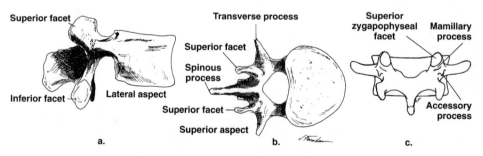

FIGURE 4–32. (a) A lateral view of a typical lumbar vertebra shows the large body and facets. (b) A superior view of a typical lumbar vertebra shows transverse and spinous processes. (c) A posterior view of a lumbar vertebra shows the location of the mamillary and accessory processes. The mamillary processes appear as small smooth bumps on the posterior edges of each zygapophyseal facet. The accessory processes are easily recognizable as the bony prominences on the posterior surfaces of the transverse processes close to the attachment of the transverse processes to the pedicles.

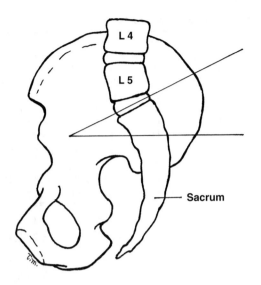

FIGURE 4–33. The lumbosacral angle is determined by measuring the angle formed by a line drawn parallel to the superior aspect of the sacrum and a horizontal line.

increase in this angle will result in an increase in the anterior convexity of the lumbar curve and will increase the amount of shearing stress at the lumbosacral joint.

Ligaments and Fascia

The majority of the ligaments associated with the lumbar region are the same ligaments described previously (ligamentum flavum, posterior longitudinal ligament, anterior longitudinal ligament, interspinous and supraspinous ligaments, and joint capsules). However, a few of these ligaments have variations specific to the lumbar region and need to be mentioned here before introducing the **iliolumbar ligaments** and the **thoracolumbar fascia.** The supraspinous ligament is well developed only in the upper lumbar region and may terminate at L3 although the most common termination site appears to be at L4. The ligament is almost always absent at L5/S1. The deep layer of the supraspinous ligament is reinforced by tendinous fibers of the multifidus muscle. The middle fibers of the supraspinous ligament blend with the dorsal layer of the thoracolumbar fascia. The intertransverse ligaments lack some features of true ligaments in the lumbar area and are replaced by the iliolumbar ligament at L4.[7] In a study of 132 ligaments of the lumbar spine, Pintar found that the ligamentum flavum had the largest cross-sectional area (84.2 ±

17.9 mm²) while the posterior longitudinal ligament had the smallest (5.2 ± 2.4mm²).[84] The interspinous ligament had the least overall stiffness and the joint capsules the highest. Pintar and coworkers also found that the anterior longitudinal ligament and supraspinous ligaments were able to absorb the most energy before failure in contrast to the posterior longitudinal ligament which was able to absorb the least energy prior to failure[84] (Table 4–7).

ILIOLUMBAR LIGAMENTS

The iliolumbar ligaments consist of five bands that extend from the tips and borders of the transverse processes of L4 and L5 to attach bilaterally on the iliac crests of the pelvis (see Fig.4–38). The liliolumbar ligaments as a whole are very strong and play a significant role in stabilizing the fifth lumbar vertebra (preventing the vertebra from anterior displacement) and in resisting flexion, extension, axial rotation, and lateral bending of L5 on S1.[7,85–87]

THORACOLUMBAR FASCIA

The thoracolumbar fascia consists of three layers (anterior, middle, and posterior) that arise from the transverse and spinous processes of the lumbar vertebrae. The thoracolumbar fascia completely surrounds the muscles of the lumbar spine (Fig. 4–34). The anterior layer of the thoracolumbar fascia is derived from the fascia of the quadratus lumborum muscle and blends with the intertransverse ligaments.[7] The middle layer is not as well defined as the other two layers, but is thought to lie posterior to the quadratus lumborum muscle. It attaches medially to the tips of the transverse processes and like the anterior layer it is continuous with the intertransverse ligaments. The posterior layer consists of two laminae, a superficial lamina with fibers oriented caudomedially and a deep lamina with fibers oriented caudolaterally. The posterior layer covers the back muscles from the sacrum throughout the thoracic region to the ligamentum nuchae. The posterior layer's superficial lamina is continuous with the following muscles: **latissimus dorsi, gluteus maximus** and indirectly with the external oblique abdominis, and the **trapezius.** Most of the fibers of the superficial lamina derive from the aponeurosis of the latissimus dorsi and attach to the interspinous ligaments and spinous processes cranial to L4. Caudal to L4/L5 the superficial lamina is generally only loosely (or not at all) attached to midline structures. Fibers

Table 4–7. **Biomechanical Parameters of Human Lumbar Ligaments**

Parameter	Ligament	T12–L1	L1–L2	L2–L3	L3–L4	L4–L5	L5–S1
Stiffness	ALL	32.9±20.9	32.4±13.0	20.8±14.0	39.5±20.3	40.5±14.3	13.2±10.2
(N mm^{-1})	PLL	10.0±5.5	17.1±9.6	36.6±15.2	10.6±8.5	25.8±15.8	21.8±16.0
	JC	31.7±7.9	42.5±0.8	33.9±19.2	32.3±3.3	30.6±1.5	29.9±22.0
	LF	24.2±3.6	23.0±7.8	25.1±10.9	34.5±6.2	27.2±12.2	20.2±8.4
	ISL	12.1±2.6	10.0±5.0	9.6±4.8	18.1±15.9	8.7±6.5	16.3±15.0
	SSL	15.1±6.9	23.0±17.3	24.8±14.5	34.8±11.7	18.0±6.9	17.8±3.8
Energy to	ALL	3.30±2.01	3.88±2.34	5.31±1.98	5.35±4.54	8.68±7.99	0.82±0.54
failure (J)	PLL	0.22±0.15	0.22±0.21	0.33±0.11	0.11±0.04	0.07±0.05	0.29±0.27
	JC	1.55±0.55	4.18±2.15	3.50±1.61	2.35±1.88	2.05±0.99	2.54±1.31
	LF	2.18±1.89	1.58±0.93	0.56±0.46	2.63±2.09	3.31±1.20	2.47±0.60
	ISL	0.72±0.47	2.65±0.25	1.06±0.73	0.59±0.29	1.13±0.91	0.78±0.56
	SSL	3.75±2.78	4.09±2.00	4.72±5.77	11.65±5.39	3.40±2.59	3.18±1.94
Stress at	ALL	9.1±0.6	13.4±3.9	16.1±6.2	12.8±7.0	15.8±1.9	8.2±2.5
failure	PLL	7.2±4.1	11.5±10.0	28.4±11.3	12.2±1.9	20.6±7.3	19.7±7.1
(MPa)	JC	13.2±1.1	10.3±2.9	14.4±1.4	7.7±1.6	3.5±1.2	5.6±2.5
	LF	4.0±1.2	2.5±0.8	1.3±0.4	2.9±1.7	2.9±1.4	4.1±0.5
	ISL	4.2±0.2	5.9±1.8	1.8±0.1	1.8±0.3	2.9±1.9	5.5±0.1
	SSL	8.9±3.2	15.5±5.1	9.9±5.8	12.6±2.7	12.7±7.1	14.0±1.7
Strain at	ALL	31.9±24.5	44.0±23.7	49.0±31.7	32.8±23.5	44.7±27.4	28.1±18.3
failure (%)	PLL	16.2±9.3	15.7±7.4	11.3±0.2	15.8±3.7	12.7±6.3	15.0±8.4
	JC	78.2±24.3	90.4±17.7	70.0±27.5	52.7±7.2	47.9±5.4	53.8±28.8
	LF	61.5±11.9	78.6±6.7	28.8±8.2	70.6±13.6	102.0±12.9	83.1±19.3
	ISL	59.4±36.1	119.7±14.7	51.5±2.9	96.5±35.8	87.4±6.7	52.9±22.3
	SSL	75.0±7.1	83.4±21.4	70.6±45.0	109.4±2.5	106.3±9.7	115.1±49.1

cross to contralateral sides where they attach to the sacrum, posterior superior iliac spines, and iliac crest.

At sacral levels, the superficial lamina is continuous with the fascia of the gluteus maximus. Deep lamina fibers are continuous with the sacrotuberous ligament and connected to the posterior superior iliac spines, iliac crests, and posterior longitudinal ligament.[88] The two laminae of the posterior layer fuse with the middle layer to form a dense raphe to which the **transversus abdominis** muscle is attached. This connection provides the transversus abdominis muscle with an indirect attachment to the lumbar spinous processes.[87] The internal oblique muscles also are indirectly attached to the fascia through the dense raphe. Gracovetsky has designated the anterior layer of the thoracolumbar fascia as the "passive part" and the posterior layer as the "active part."[89] According to Gracovetsky, the passive part serves to transmit tension produced by a contraction of the hip extensors to the spinous processes. The active portion is activated by a contraction of the transversus abdominis muscle, which

tightens the fascia. The fascia transmits tension longitudinally to the tips of the spinous processes of L1/L4 and may help the spinal extensor muscles to resist an applied load.[89] Vleeming found that both the gluteus maximus and contralateral latissimus dorsi tensed the superficial layer and provided a pathway for the mechanical transmission of forces between the pelvis and the trunk.[88]

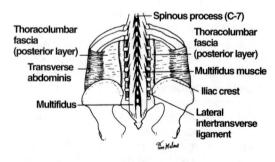

FIGURE 4–34. The thoracolumbar fascia. The anterior and middle layers of the fascia have been partially removed to show the posterior layer fusing with the transversus abdominis-muscle.

Function of the Lumbar Region

Stability

During flexion the anterior translation of the vertebra is resisted by direct impaction of the inferior zygapophyseal facets of the superior vertebra against the superior zygapophyseal facets of the adjacent vertebra below. The orientation of the lumbar zygapophyseal joints and the shape (curved or flat) of the articulating surfaces are extremely variable.[7] According to convention, the orientation of the lumbar zygapophyseal joints is defined by the angle made by the average plane of the joint with respect to the sagittal plane. The effectiveness of the zygapophyseal joint in providing resistance to anterior translation during flexion depends on the extent to which the inferior vertebra's superior facets face posteriorly. The more that the superior zygapophyseal facets of an adjacent inferior vertebra face posteriorly, the greater the resistance they are able to provide to forward displacement because the posteriorly facing facets lock against the inferior facets of the adjacent superior vertebra. The effectiveness of the zygapophyseal joints in resisting axial rotation depends on the extent that the superior facets face medially. The greater the medial orientation of the joint surfaces the greater the resistance to axial rotation.

One of the primary functions of the lumbar region is to provide support for the weight of the upper part of the body in static as well as in dynamic situations. The increased size of the lumbar vertebral bodies and disks in comparison to their counterparts in the other regions helps the lumbar structures to support the additional weight. Experimental testing of 10 cadaver spines subjected to 1000-N compressive loading demonstrated that load sharing of lumbar facet joints in axial compression was 20% of the total load.[90] The compressive load that must be sustained by the lumbar structures is altered by changes in the lumbar curvature or arrangement of body segments. Changes in the position of body segments will change the location of the body's center of gravity and thus change the forces acting on the lumbar spine. In the normal standing posture the line of gravity passes through the combined axis for the lumbar vertebrae and therefore no net gravitational torque exists. Any deviation of the line of gravity will lead to torque production. The muscle contractions required to oppose the gravitational torque create additional compression on the vertebrae as well as torsional and shear stresses.

EXAMPLE 2: In a situation in which a person is standing holding an object in the right hand with arm extended, two torques will be created: a forward flexion moment and a right lateral flexion moment. The muscles of the lumbar and trunk regions will have to contract to exert an opposing moment (countertorque) to maintain equilibrium of the spine in the static upright position and prevent motion of the trunk in the direction of the external moments.[91]

Wilke and associates studied simulated muscle action of the erector spinae, psoas major, multifidus, and rotatores on the L4/L5 segment. They found that muscle action stiffened the motion segment in that the ROM and the neutral zone were decreased.[92] The decrease was most evident for flexion-extension. The multifidus muscle was responsible for more than two-thirds of the stiffness increase. Khoo and colleagues compared lumbosacral loads (ground reaction forces and accelerations plus forces generated by erector spinae and rectus abdominis muscle groups) at the center of the L5/S1 joint in static versus dynamic situations in 10 men. Lumbosacral loads in the erect standing posture were in the range of 0.82 to 1.18 times body weight, whereas lumbosacral loads during level walking were in the range of 1.41 to 2.07 times body weight (an increase of 56.3%). The shear forces acted anteriorly in standing static posture and posteriorly in the dynamic situation.[93]

Goel and coworkers[94] used a combined three-dimensional finite element model and optimization approach to study the effects of muscle action on the translation of L3, disk bulge, interdiskal pressure, and facet loading among other variables and to compare predicted muscle responses from active muscles to a ligamentous finite element model. The optimization model was developed to predict muscles and disk forces across the L3/L4 segment when a person had the spine flexed to 30° and was standing with knees straight holding a 90-N weight in his hands. The addition of muscle forces to the ligamentous model resulted in a decrease in the anteroposterior translation of the L3 vertebra and flexion rotation displacements in the sagittal plane of the L3/L4 lumbar segment compared to ligamentous predictions. Muscles imparted stability to the ligamentous

L3/L4 segment, decreased stresses in the vertebral body and did not cause an increase in intradiskal pressure. However, load bearing of the facets increased in the muscle model in comparison to the ligamentous model. The force carried by the facets in the muscle model was 385 N compared to no force in the ligamentous model.[94] Gardner-Morse and associates found that muscles played a significant role in maintaining the stability of the lumbar spine during loading and motion and that they appear to act as "stabilizing springs."[95]

Mobility

The orientation of the zygapophyseal facets from L1 to L4 limits lateral flexion and rotation. However, a considerable amount of variation exists in the degree of axial rotation of lumbar vertebrae. In addition to being affected by facet orientation, the amount of rotation available at each vertebral level appears to be affected by the position of the lumbar spine. When the lumbar spine is flexed, the ROM in rotation is less than when the lumbar spine is in the neutral position. The posterior annulus fibrosus and the posterior longitudinal ligament seem to play an important role in limiting axial rotation when the spine is flexed. The zygapophyseal joint capsules limit rotation both in the neutral and flexed positions of the spine.[38]

The orientation of the lumbar zygapophyseal facets favors flexion and extension. Flexion of the lumbar spine is more limited than extension and, normally, it is not possible to flex the lumbar region to form a kyphotic curve. The amount of flexion varies at each interspace of the lumbar vertebrae, but most of the flexion takes place at the lumbosacral joint. In a study of 42 lumbar motion segments, Adams and Dolan found that the average range of flexion was 8° degrees at L1/L2 , 9° at L2/L3, and 12° at L3/L4 and L5/S1.[96] Panjabi in a study of nine cadaveric lumbar spines found that the ROM in flexion and extension clearly increased from L1/L2 to L5/S1.[97] During flexion and extension the greatest mobility of the spine occurs between L4 and S1, which is the area that must support the most weight. In a radiographic study of 46 men and 40 women, Lin and colleagues also found that the ROM in flexion-extension increased from L1 to L5 but that the ROM decreased at L5/S1. They found that the mean values of anteroposterior translation in flexion and extension tended to increase from L1 to L5 but decreased at L5/S1 (L1/L2=1.4; L2/L3=1.5; L3/L4=2.2; L4/L5=2.0; L5/S1=0.4).[98] During everyday bending and lifting tasks, the flexion moment acting on the lumbar spine at L5/S1 has been estimated to be about 18 Nm. However, it may be much higher when lifting heavy weights. In an erect standing posture, pressures on the lower disks are much greater than the weight of the body, and these pressures increase with movement and muscle contraction.

Cailliet described a specific instance of coordinated, simultaneous activity of lumbar flexion and anterior tilting of the pelvis in the sagittal plane during trunk flexion and extension. He called the combined lumbar and pelvic motion, **lumbar-pelvic rhythm.** The activity of bending over to touch one's toes with knees straight depends on lumbar-pelvic rhythm.[99] According to Cailliet, the first part of bending forward consists of lumbar flexion (Fig. 4–35a). This is followed by anterior tilting

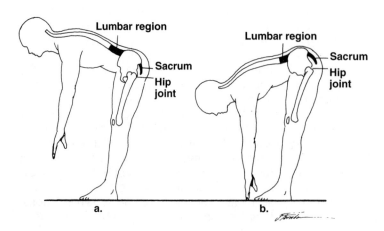

FIGURE 4–35. Lumbar-pelvic rhythm. (a) The lumbar spine flexes and (b) the pelvis rotates anteriorly in the sagittal plane.

of the pelvis at the hip joints (Fig. 4–35b). A return to the erect posture is initiated by posterior tilting of the pelvis at the hips followed by extension of the lumbar spine. The initial pelvic motion delays lumbar extension until the trunk is raised far enough to shorten the moment arm of the external load thus reducing the load on the erector spinae. Nelson and coworkers studied lumbar-pelvic motion in 30 healthy women, aged 19 to 35 years, who lifted and replaced a 9.5-kg weight on the floor. They found that lumbar and pelvic motion was variable among these individuals and tended to occur simultaneously during trunk flexion and more sequentially during trunk extension.[100] The use of a weight may have affected the lumbar-pelvic rhythm, but this study raises questions about exactly when and how trunk and pelvic motion occurs. However, the integration of motion of the pelvis with motion of the vertebral column not only increases the ROM available to the total column but also reduces the amount of flexibility required of the lumbar region. The contribution to motion from multiple areas to produce a larger ROM is similar to what is found at the shoulder in scapulohumeral rhythm. A restriction of motion at either the lumbar spine or at the hip joints may disturb the rhythm and prevent a person from reaching her toes. Restriction of motion at one segment also may result in hypermobility of the unrestricted segment.

Lateral flexion and axial rotation of the lumbar vertebrae are most free in the upper lumbar region and progressively diminish in the lower region. The largest lateral flexion ROM and axial rotation occurs between L2 and L3.[97] Rotation of the vertebrae in the upper area is accompanied by movement of the spinous process toward the concavity of the lateral flexion curve, which is similar to rotation in the lower thoracic region. Little or no lateral flexion or rotation is possible at the lumbosacral joint because of the most common orientation of the zygapophyseal joints at 45° to the sagittal plane.[7] Table 4–8 provides a stability-mobility summary for the thoracic and lumbar regions.

Structure of the Sacral Region

Five sacral vertebrae are fused to form the triangular or wedge-shaped structure that is called the sacrum. The base of the triangle, which is formed by the first sacral vertebra, supports two articular facets that face posteriorly for articulation with the inferior facets of the fifth lumbar vertebra. The apex of the triangle, formed by the fifth sacral vertebra, has a small facet for articulation with the coccyx.[101]

Sacroiliac Articulations

The two **sacroiliac joints** consist of the articulations between the left and right articular surfaces on the sacrum (which are formed by fused portions of the first, second, and third sacral segments) and the left and right iliac bones (Fig. 4–36). The sacroiliac joints are unique in that both the structure and function of these joints change significantly from birth through adulthood.

ARTICULATING SURFACES ON THE SACRUM

The articulating surfaces on the sacrum are auricular- (C-) shaped[102] and are located on the sides of the fused sacral vertebrae lateral to the sacral foramina. The fetal and prepubertal surfaces are flat and smooth; the postpubertal surfaces are marked by a central groove or surface depression that extends the length of the articulating surfaces.[102,106] The articular surfaces are covered with hyaline cartilage. The overall mean thickness of the sacral cartilage is greater than the iliac cartilage, the sacral cartilage being 1.5:1 to 3:1 thicker.[103–105] This difference in thickness exists in fetal specimens[103,105] and a greater thickness has been found in females as compared to males.

ARTICULATING SURFACES ON THE ILIA

The articular surfaces on the ilia are also C-shaped. In the first decade of life, the iliac joint surfaces are smooth and flat, and covered with fibrocartilage. The type of cartilage covering the iliac articular surfaces in the adult continues to be a matter of debate. The cartilage is different in gross appearance and is thinner than the sacral articular cartilage. Usually it was described as fibrocartilage.[102,107] However, more recently, type II collagen, which is typical of hyaline cartilage, has been identified in the iliac cartilage[108] and the iliac cartilage is described as being hyaline cartilage in the 38th edition of *Gray's Anatomy*.[1] After puberty, the joint surfaces develop a central ridge that extends the length of the articulating surface and corresponds to the grooves on the sacral articulating surfaces.[103,109]

The smooth sacroiliac joint surfaces in early childhood permit gliding motions in all direc-

Table 4–8. **Thoracic and Lumbar Regions: Mobility/Stability Summary**

Region	Factors Affecting Mobility and Stability
Thoracic	Forward flexion is limited by the rib cage, costotransverse joints, orientation of the zygapophyseal facets and by passive tension in the posterior longitudinal ligament, ligamentum flavum, supraspinous and interspinous ligaments, and zygapophyseal joint capsules.
	Extension is limited by passive tension in the anterior longitudinal ligament and anterior trunk musculature. Bony contact of the spinous processes and the orientation of the zygapophyseal facets also limit extension.
	Zygapophyseal facet orientation favors lateral flexion, which is limited by tension in contralateral annulus fibrosus fibers and unilateral portion of the rib cage.
T12–L1	Forward flexion is limited by passive tension in the posterior longitudinal ligament, ligamentum flavum, supraspinous and interspinous ligaments, posterior annulus fibrosus fibers, and zygapophyseal joint capsules.
	Extension is limited by contact between zygapophyseal facets and laminae and between adjacent spinous processes.
	Lateral flexion is limited by contralateral annulus fibrosus fibers, zygapophyseal joint capsules, intertransverse ligaments, and passive tension in lateral trunk musculature.
	Zygapophyseal facet orientation favors rotation and causes rotation to be accompanied by a slight amount of lateral flexion.
L1–L4	Forward flexion is limited primarily by the ligamentum flavum, posterior fibers of the annulus fibrosus, and the zygapophyseal joint capsules. The supraspinous and interspinous ligaments have a lesser contribution.
	Extension is limited by the anterior longitudinal ligament, anterior fibers of the annulus fibrosus, anterior trunk musculature, and contact of the spinous processes. However, the range of motion in extension is greater than the range of motion in forward flexion.
	Rotation is limited by the zygapophyseal joint capsules, fibers of annulus fibrosus, impaction of the inferior zygapophyseal facets of an upper vertebra on the zygapophyseal facets of the adjacent vertebra below. The supraspinous and interspinous ligaments offer slight resistance.
	Lateral flexion is limited by the intertransverse and iliolumbar ligaments, zygapophyseal joint capsules, and contralateral annulus fibrosus fibers.
	Facet orientation favors flexion/extension and limits rotation and lateral flexion.
L5–S1	Zygapophyseal facet orientation limits lateral flexion and rotation.

tions, which is typical of a synovial plane joint.[102] However, after puberty, the joint surfaces change their configuration and according to Walker, motion in the adult is restricted to a very few millimeters of translation and or rotation.[103] However, a considerable amount of controversy exists regarding both the type and amount of motion available at the sacroiliac joints. **Nutation** is the commonly used term to refer to movement of the sacral promontory of the sacrum anteriorly and inferiorly while the coccyx moves posteriorly in relation to the ilium (Fig. 4–37a). **Counternutation** refers to the opposite movement in which the anterior tip of the sacral promontory moves posteriorly and superiorly while the coccyx moves anteriorly in relation to the ileum (Fig.4–37b). The change in position of the sacrum during nutation and counternutation affects the diameter of the pelvic brim and pelvic outlet. During nutation, the anteroposterior diameter of the pelvic brim is reduced and the anteroposterior diameter of the pelvic outlet is increased. During counternutation, the reverse situation occurs. The anteroposterior diameter of the pelvic brim is increased and the diameter of the pelvic outlet is decreased.[11] These changes in diameter are of particular importance during pregnancy and childbirth, and it is possible that the most motion that occurs at the sacroiliac joints may occur in pregnancy and childbirth when the joint structures are under hormonal influence and ligamentous structures are softened. Accurate descriptions of the sacroiliac joints and the motions that occur at these joints have been difficult to obtain because the planes of the joint surfaces are oblique to the angle of an x-ray beam used to make a standard anteroposterior radiograph of the pelvis.[108]

Accessory or **axial sacroiliac joints** have

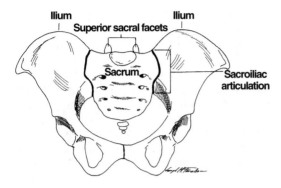

FIGURE 4–36. The sacroiliac joints consist of the articulations between the first three sacral segments and the two ilia of the pelvis.

been found in anywhere from 8% to 40% of adult samples, with a higher incidence in men. No accessory or axial joints have been reported in fetuses or in children. Accessory joints are considered to occur sporadically at the level of the sacral crest, at the first and second posterior foramina, on the ilium at the medial surface of the posterior superior iliac spines and on the iliac tuberosity.[1] Axial joints are considered to occur regularly and most joint surfaces appear to be covered with fibrocartilage.[106] Speculation exists that these joints may be aquired as a result of the stress of weight bearing developing behind the articular surface between the lateral sacral crest and posterior iliac spine and the iliac tuberosity.

Ligaments

The **anterior, interosseous,** and **posterior sacroiliac ligaments** are directly associated with the sacroiliac joints. A separate portion of the posterior sacroiliac ligament is called either the **long posterior sacroiliac ligament**[1] or the **long dorsal sacroiliac ligament**.[110] The **iliolumbar ligaments,** which connect the fifth lumbar vertebra to the sacrum and the **sacrospinous ligaments,** and the **sacrotuberous ligaments,** which connect the sacrum to the ischium, are indirectly associated with the sacroiliac joints (Fig. 4–38).

SACROILIAC LIGAMENTS

The sacroiliac ligaments as a whole extend from the iliac crests to attach to the tubercles of the first four sacral vertebrae. The sacroiliac ligaments, which are reinforced by fibrous expansions from the quadratus lumborum, erector spinae, gluteus maximus, gluteus minimus, piriformis, and iliacus muscles, contribute to the joint's stability. The fascial support is greater posteriorly than anteriorly because more muscles are located posteriorly.[106] The anterior sacroiliac ligaments are considered by *Gray's Anatomy* to be capsular ligaments because of the ligaments' intimate connections to the anteroinferior margins of the joint capsules.[1] According to Bogduk, the anterior sacroiliac ligaments cover the anterior aspects of the sacroiliac joints and join the ilia to the sacrum.[7] The interosseous sacroiliac ligaments, which constitute the major bonds between the sacrum and the ilia, are considered to be the most important ligaments directly associated with the sacroiliac joints.[1,7] The ligaments are composed of superficial and deep portions, which are divided into superior and inferior bands. The superficial bands unite the superior articular processes and lateral crests of the first two sacral segments to the ilia. This portion of the interosseous ligament is referred to as the **short posterior sacroiliac ligament**.[1,7]

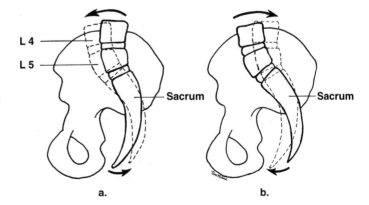

FIGURE 4–37. (a) Nutation. The solid lines indicate the neutral position of the sacrum. The dotted lines indicate the movement of the sacrum in nutation. The arrow at the top of the sacrum indicates the anterior-inferior motion of the anterior tip of the sacral promontory during nutation. The arrow just below the coccyx indicates the posterior-superior movement of the coccyx. (b) Counternutation. The sacral promontory moves posteriorly and superiorly in counternutation and the coccyx moves anteriorly and inferiorly.

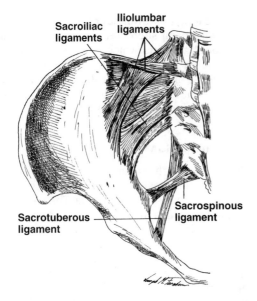

FIGURE 4–38. The sacroiliac and iliolumbar ligaments reinforce the sacroiliac and lumbosacral articulations, respectively. The sacrospinous ligament forms the inferior border of the greater sciatic notch and the sacrotuberous ligament forms the interior border of the lesser sciatic notch.

The deeper portions of the interosseous sacroiliac ligament extend from depressions posterior to the sacral articular surface to depressions on the iliac tuberosities. The posterior sacroiliac ligaments connect the lateral sacral crests to the posterior superior iliac spines and iliac crests.

The paired long dorsal sacroiliac ligaments have superior attachments to the posterior sacroiliac spine and adjacent parts of the ilium. Inferiorly the ligaments are attached to the lateral crest of the third and fourth sacral segments. The medial fibers are connected to the deep lamina of the posterior layer of the thoracolumbar fascia and the aponeurosis of the erector spinae.[110] The sacrospinous ligaments connect the ischial spines to the lateral borders of the sacrum and coccyx. The sacrotuberous ligaments connect the ischial tuberosities to the posterior spines at the ilia and the lateral sacrum and coccyx. The sacrospinous ligament forms the inferior border of the greater sciatic notch; the sacrotuberous ligament forms the inferior border of the lesser sciatic notch.[111,112]

ILLI'S LIGAMENT

Evidence for the existence of a superior **intracapsular ligament (Illi's ligament),** first described by Illi in 1950, has been presented by Freeman, Fox, and Richards, who found Illi's ligament in 75% (31) of cadavers examined. The authors described the ligament as a dense fibrous band of connective tissue that coursed from a posterosuperior attachment on the ilium to an anteroinferior attachment directly into the hyaline articular cartilage on the sacrum. The width of the ligament varied from 2 to 8 mm and was located about 2 mm below the interosseous ligament. Because of its small size the ligament probably has a limited biomechanical role.[112]

Symphysis Pubis Articulation

The symphysis pubis is a cartilaginous joint located between the two ends of the pubic bones. The end of each pubic bone is covered with a layer of articular cartilage and the joint is formed by a fibrocartilaginous disk that joins the hyaline cartilage-covered ends of the bones. The disk has a thin central cleft,[11] which in women may extend throughout the length of the disk.[5] The three ligaments that are associated with the joint are the **superior pubic ligament,** the **inferior pubic ligament,** and the **posterior ligament.**[11] The superior ligament is a thick and dense fibrous band that attaches to the pubic crests and tubercles and helps to support the superior aspect of the joint. The inferior ligament arches from the inferior rami on one side of the joint to the inferior portion of the rami on the other side and thus reinforces the inferior aspect of the joint. The posterior ligament consists of a fibrous membrane that is continuous with the periosteum of the pubic bones.[11] The anterior portion of the joint is reinforced by aponeurotic expansions from a number of muscles that cross the joint (Fig 4–39). Kapandji describes the muscle expan-

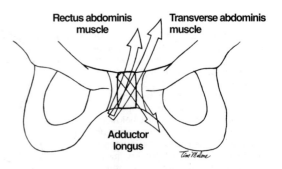

FIGURE 4–39. The aponeurotic extensions of the muscles crossing the anterior aspect of the symphysis pubis.

sions as forming an anterior ligament consisting of expansions of the transversus abdominis, rectus abdominis, internal obliquus abdominis, and the adductor longus.[11]

Function of the Sacral Region

Stability and Mobility

Stability of the sacroiliac joints is extremely important because these joints must support a large portion of the body weight. In normal erect posture the weight of head, arms, and trunk (HAT) is transmitted through the fifth lumbar vertebra and lumbosacral disk to the first sacral segment. The force of the body weight creates a nutation torque on the sacrum. Concommittantly, the ground reaction force creates a posterior torsion on the ilia. The countertorques of nutation and counternutation of the sacrum and posterior torsion of the ilia are prevented by the ligamentous tension and fibrous expansions from adjacent muscles that reinforce the joint capsules and blend with the ligaments.[103] Tension developed in the sacrotuberous, sacrospinous, and anterior sacroiliac ligaments counteract the nutation of the sacrum although the sacrotuberous and sacrospinous ligaments have not been found to play a major role in pelvic stability.[113] However, the sacrotuberous and interosseous ligaments compress the sacroiliac joint during nutation.[110] The long dorsal sacroiliac ligament is under tension in counternutation and relaxed in nutation.[110] The interosseous sacroiliac ligament binds the ilia to the sacrum.[7] Surface irregularities and texture of the sacroiliac joints also contribute to stability of the joint in the adult. In a study of sacroiliac joints, the highest coefficients of friction were found in sample joints with ridges, depressions, and coarse-textured cartilage. Sample joints with ridges, depressions, and smooth cartilage showed higher coefficients of friction than samples without ridges and depressions. These findings suggest that the complimentary ridges and depressions as well as the coarse surface textures found in the adult reflect a dynamic, normal development of the sacroiliac joints. Vertical load bearing is facilitated by these changes but motion is limited by the changes.[103,112,114,115]

The sacroiliac joints permit a small amount of motion that varies among individuals. Both the amount and type of motion available at these joints has been and continues to be a matter of controversy. At most it appears as if the motion available is very slight and not easily defined. The sacroiliac joints are linked to the symphysis pubis in a closed kinematic chain, and therefore any motion occurring at the symphysis pubis is accompanied by motion at the sacroiliac joints and vice versa.[116] During pregnancy, **relaxin**, a polypeptide hormone is produced by the corpus luteum and decidua. This hormone is thought to activate the collagenolytic system, which regulates new collagen formation and alters the ground substance by decreasing the viscosity and increasing the water content. The action of relaxin is to decrease the intrinsic strength and rigidity of collagen and is thought to be responsible for the softening of the ligaments supporting the sacroiliac joints and the symphysis pubis. Consequently, the joints become more mobile and less stable and the likelihood of injury to these joints is increased. The combination of loosened posterior ligaments and an anterior weight shift caused by a heavy uterus may allow excessive movement of the ilia on the sacrum and result in stretching of the sacroiliac joint capsules.

The sacroiliac joints and symphysis pubis are closely linked functionally to the hip and joints and therefore affect and are affected by movements of the trunk and lower extremities. For example, weight shifting from one leg to another is accompanied by motion at the sacroiliac joints. Fusions of the lower lumbar vertebrae have been found to cause compensatory increases in motion at the sacroiliac joints.[117] Shearing forces are created at the symphysis pubis during the single-leg-support phase of walking as a result of lateral pelvic tilting. In a normal situation, the joint is capable of resisting the shearing forces and no appreciable motion occurs. If, however, the joint is dislocated, the pelvis becomes unstable during gait with increased stress on the sacroiliac and hip joints as well as the vertebral column. The joints of the pelvis are linked to the hip and vertebral column in nonweight-bearing as well as in weight-bearing postures. Hip flexion in a back-lying position tilts the ilia posteriorly in relation to sacrum. This pelvic motion causes nutation at the sacroiliac joints, which increases the diameter of the pelvic outlet. During the process of birth, the increase in the diameter of the pelvic outlet facilitates delivery of the fetal head. Counternutation is brought about by hip extension in the supine position and enlarges the pelvic brim. Therefore, a hip-extended position is favored early in the birthing process to facilitate the descent of the fetal head into the pelvis, whereas the hip-flexed position is used during delivery.[12]

Muscles of the Vertebral Column

Flexors

Muscles that flex the trunk are located anteriorly and laterally with attachments on the ribs, sternum, and pelvis. These muscles act indirectly on the vertebral column by exerting a pull on the adjacent structures. Contractions of the flexor muscles cause compression forces on the vertebral column. When the pelvis and ribs are free to move, a shortening contraction of the flexors will pull these structures closer together and as a consequence flex the total spine, as in a sit-up. If the ribs are fixed, a shortening contraction of the rectus abdominis muscle will exert an upward pull on the anterior pelvis. The resulting posterior rotation of the pelvis in the sagittal plane (posterior pelvic tilt) will flex the contiguous lumbar spine.

The internal and external oblique abdominal muscles turn and twist the lumbar spine into axial rotation. However, because these muscles are oblique rather than transverse, they exert a flexion moment in addition to causing axial rotation.[118] Forward flexion of the trunk from the erect standing posture does not require any action of the trunk flexors because the gravitational force will pull the trunk forward. However, any activity that involves pushing, pulling, or lifting will initiate an immediate isometric contraction of the flexors to stabilize the ribs and pelvis and, indirectly, the vertebral column.

The flexor muscles are not active during normal erect standing. However, they are considered essential for balancing the pull of the back extensor and the hip flexor muscles in dynamic situations and for keeping the pelvis in a normal position. When either the back extensor or hip flexor muscles act unopposed, they cause an anterior tilting of the pelvis in the sagittal plane (anterior pelvic tilt) and an increase in extension in the contiguous lumbar spine. In any motion that involves flexion of the trunk against gravity, the abdominal muscles will be required to produce the flexion motion. Also, the abdominal muscles perform the function of protecting and supporting the viscera. During

pregnancy, especially in the second and third trimesters and immediately postpartum, the **rectus abdominis** muscle may separate or relax along the linea alba (**diastasis recti abdominis**). This condition may have adverse effects on the ability of the flexors to function as static or dynamic stabilizers and movers of the vertebral column.[119]

The **psoas major** muscle has been described as a flexor, as a stabilizer, and as an extensor of the lumbar spine.[120] When the spine is in the flexed position, the psoas fibers cross anterior to the axis of rotation of the lumbar intervertebral joints and thus, the muscle has a flexion moment and a concentric contraction can produce flexion. When the lumbar spine is extended, most of the fibers are posterior to the axis of rotation and produce an extension moment. During the activity of lifting, the psoas is active in stabilization of the lumbar spine.[120]

Sit-ups are often performed in a bent-knee position to reduce lumbar load and activity of the psoas. However, McGill found little difference in load as a result of bending the knees. Sit-ups with bent knees caused a compression force of 3410 N, whereas sit-ups with straight knees caused a compression force of 3230 N. Shear forces with bent knees were 300 N, whereas the same forces with knees straight were 260 N. McGill suggested that because of the high compression forces involved in sit-ups that perhaps sit-ups should not be used as an exercise.[121]

Rotators and Lateral Flexors

Rotation of the trunk is usually coupled with some degree of lateral flexion. Anterior muscles that produce rotation and lateral flexion are the **external** and **internal oblique abdominals.** Rotation of the trunk to the left requires a simultaneous contraction of the right external oblique and the left internal oblique. Rotation of the trunk to the right requires a simultaneous contraction of the left external oblique and the right internal oblique. The posterior muscles that rotate the trunk may be divided into two groups: muscles that produce rotation and lateral flexion to the *same side* and muscles that produce rotation to the *opposite side*. Rotation and lateral flexion to the *same side* are a function of the iliocostalis, longissimus, spinalis muscles, quadratus lumborum, and serratus posterior superior. Muscles that produce rotation to the *opposite side* are the semispinalis thoracis, multifidus, rotatores, and intertransversarii thoracis. The lateral flexors of the trunk are the quadratus lumborum and the iliopsoas. When either of these muscles contracts unilaterally, it causes lateral flexion of the trunk ipsilaterally if the pelvis and femur are fixed. If lateral flexion occurs, from erect standing, the force of gravity will continue the lateral flexion movement and the contralateral muscles will be required to balance the gravitational moment and control the movement by contracting eccentrically. A unilateral contraction of the quadratus lumborum will "hike the hip" or laterally tilt the pelvis in the frontal plane if the pelvis is free to move (Fig.4–40a and b) but will laterally flex the trunk if the pelvis is fixed (Fig.4–40c). The psoas muscle, when acting bilaterally in a closed kinematic chain with the femurs fixed, will pull the lumbar spine anteriorly and thus extend the lumbar spine and increase the lordosis. The psoas muscle also acts to flex the hip when either the femur or the pelvis and lumbar vertebrae are fixed. See the Appendix to Chapter 4 for a complete listing of the muscles of the vertebral column.

Extensors

Muscles that extend the vertebral column are located posteriorly (Fig. 4–41). The sacrospinalis muscles (erector spinae), which consist of three divisions (lateral, medial, and intermediate), represent the largest portion of the posterior musculature (Fig.4–42). This group of muscles extends from the sacrum to the occipital portion of the skull, attaching to the transverse and spinous processes of all vertebrae and the angles of the ribs by various divisions. The most lateral division that attaches to the ribs is called the **iliocostalis group** and consists of the **iliocostalis cervicis, thoracis,** and **lumborum.** The most medial division of the erector spinae muscle attaches to the spinous processes and is called the **spinalis group,** which includes the **spinalis cervicis, capitis,** and **thoracis.** The intermediate division that attaches to the transverse processes is called the **longissimus.** The longissimus consists of the **longissimus capitus, cervicis,** and **thoracis.** Other muscle groups that lie deep to the erector spinae include the **semispinalis capitis, cervicis** and **thoracis, multifidus, rotatores cervicis, thoracis** and **lumborum,** and the **interspinales** and **intertransversarii.** These muscles attach to the transverse, spinous, or articular processes of the vertebrae.

A higher percentage of type I fibers (slow twitch, high oxidative, low glycolytic capacity that are resistant to fatigue) has been found in the longissimus and multifidus muscles at thoracic levels in comparison to the same muscles in the lumbar region.[122] This finding is related

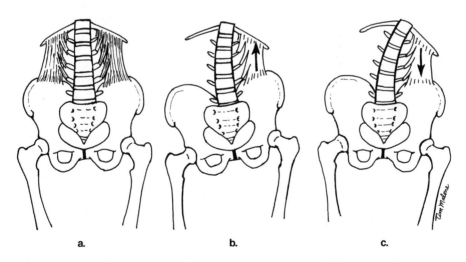

a.   **b.**   **c.**

FIGURE 4–40. (a) The illustration shows the attachments of the right and left quadratus lumborum muscles. (b) A unilateral contraction of the left quadratus lumborum muscle will lift and tilt the left side of the pelvis and hike the hip when the trunk is fixed and the pelvis and leg are free to move. (c) A unilateral contraction of the left quadratus lumborum muscle when the pelvis and left leg are fixed will cause ipsilateral lateral trunk flexion.

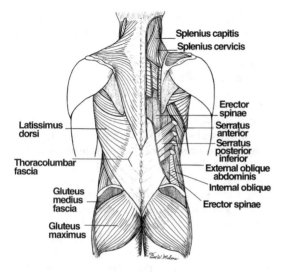

FIGURE 4–41. Posterior back muscles. The superficial muscles have been removed on the right side to show the erector spinae. The anterior layer of the thoracolumbar fascia is intact on the left side of the back.

to the need for more or less continual low level of activity in the thoracic muscles to counteract the flexion moment that exists in the thoracic region during erect stance (line of gravity falls anterior to thoracic spine and either through or posterior to the lumbar spine). Also researchers have found gender differences in the muscle fiber composition of the back muscles. Roy and coworkers, using surface electromyog-

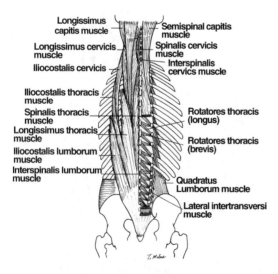

FIGURE 4–42. Erector spinae and deep back muscles. The erector spinae muscle has been removed from the right side of the back to show the deep back muscles.

raphy to measure fatigue in the iliocostalis lumborum, longissimus thoracis, and multifidus at L1, L2, and L5, found that subjects with low back pain had more fatigable muscles than their pain-free cohorts.[123]

All of the posterior trunk muscles can produce extension of the spine and can increase the lumbar curve. Conversely, a contraction of the flexor muscles decreases the lumbar curve. The extensor muscles are responsible for controlling forward flexion of the vertebral column in the standing position. The gravitational moment will produce forward flexion, but the extent and rate of flexion is controlled partially by eccentric contractions of the extensors and partially by the thoracolumbar fascia and posterior ligamentous system. The thoracic and lumbar extensors act eccentrically until approximately two-thirds of maximal flexion has been attained, at which point they become electrically silent.[7,87,89] This is called the **flexion-relaxation phenomenon,** which is thought to occur at the point when stretched and deformed passive tissues are able to generate the required moment. However, the extensor muscles may be only relaxed in the electrical sense because they may be generating force elastically through passive stretching[124] (Table 4–9). According to Gracovetsky,[89] control of flexion becomes the responsibility of the passive elastic response of the thoracolumbar fascia and posterior ligamentous system. The posterior ligaments (supraspinous and interspinous ligaments) have longer moment arms than the extensor muscles and thus have a mechanical advantage over the extensors. The longissimus thoracis and iliocostalis thoracis control movement of the thorax on the lumbar spine, whereas the multifidus, longissimus thoracis, and iliocostalis lumborum control flexion of the lumbar spine. The latter two muscles also help to prevent anterior translation of the lumbar vertebrae that may accompany flexion.

The extensors lie parallel to the vertebral column and thus, like the abdominals, exert a compression force on the column during contractions. MacIntosh, Pearcy, and Bogduk modeled the action of 49 fascicles of the following muscles—lumbar portion of the longissimus thoracis, the iliocostalis thoracis, and the lumbar multifidus—using radiographs of nine young male subjects in erect stance and in full lumbar flexion. The authors found that in the erect posture a maximal axial torque of only 4

Table 4–9. **Muscle Passive Elastic Forces During "Relaxation"**

Muscle	Length (l/l_0)	Length Coefficient	Passive Elastic Force (N)
Pars lumborum			
(L-1)	1.30	0.73	5.9
(L-2)	1.31	0.72	7.5
(L-3)	1.34	0.68	8.9
(L-4)	1.28	0.75	8.6
(L-5)	1.12	0.93	4.6
Iliocostalis lumborum	1.26	0.77	15.1
Longissimus thoracis	1.25	0.79	23.4
Quadratus lumborum	1.18	0.87	5.4
Latissimus dorsi (L-5)	1.17	0.88	4.2

When the extensor muscles are said to be "relaxed," they are actually stretched passively in full flexion. The passive elastic force is calculated (for selected muscles on the right side of the body) from the normalized length (l/l_0) used to calculate a length coefficient and a passive elastic force.

Reprinted from Spine, 19(19), 1994, McGill, SM, and Kippers, V, Transfer of Loads Between Lumbar Tissues During Flexion-Relaxation Phenomenon, pp. 2190–2196, with permission of Lippincott William & Wilkins.

Nm was exerted by these muscle fascicles on the L4 vertebra. The fascicles of these muscles exerted little or no lateral or posterior force because the fibers are parallel to the long axis of the vertebral column.[125] The MA of the lumbar extensors is considerably decreased when the trunk is in a forward flexed position and increased when the lumbar lordotic curvature is increased.[126,127]

Exercises to increase the strength of the back extensors are often performed in the prone position to take advantage of the resistance provided by gravity to back, leg, and arm extension. Callaghan and colleagues assessed loading of the L4/L5 segment in 13 male volunteers during commonly prescribed exercises. The authors found that the lowest compression forces at the L4/L5 segment were found in single leg extension in the quadraped position (on hands and knees) Fig. 4–43a). Raising an arm and leg simultaneously (right arm and left leg) increased compression forces by 1000 N and upper erector spinae muscle activity levels by 30% in comparison to single-leg extension in the hands and knees position (Fig. 4–43b). The right erector spinae and contralateral abdominal muscles were activated during single right leg extension to maintain a neutral pelvis and spine posture and to balance internal moments and lateral shear forces. The authors recommended that only single-leg extension exercises be performed because the lumbar posture is more neutral and the compression forces are relatively low (approximately 2500 N). The authors recommend that

the exercise in which the subject raises the upper body and legs from a prone lying position never be prescribed for anyone at risk of low back injury or reinjury to the lumbar spine because during this exercise lumbar compression forces of approximately 4000 to 6000 N are incurred. The extremely high compression forces are a result of bilateral muscle activity when the spine is hyperextended. In this posture the facets are subjected to high loads and the interspinous ligament is in danger of being crushed.[128]

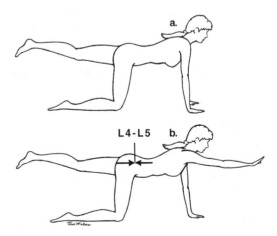

FIGURE 4–43. (a) Single leg extension in the quadriped position creates low compression forces at the L4 to L5 segment. (b) Raising the opposite leg and arm simultaneously increases compression forces at the L4 to L5 segment by 1000 N and upper erector spinae muscle activity by 30% compared to single leg raising.

Role of Flexors and Extensors in Lifting

The extensor muscles are at a disadvantage in the fully flexed position of the spine because of shortened MAs in this position and the possibility of passive insufficiency due to the elongated state of the muscles. The diminished capacity of the extensors in the forward flexed position is one reason why lifting in this position is discouraged. However, the primary reason for not lifting in the forward flexed position is because of the increase in intradiskal pressures in the lumbar area.[129] Even standing with the trunk in a fully flexed position with a small load in one's hand creates a substantial lumbar joint load. Eight subjects who held an 8-kg weight symmetrically in their hands while standing in full trunk flexion generated an average low back extensor moment of 154 Nm, which resulted in an average compressive load of 2859 N on the L4 to L5 segment and a shear load of 755 N. Externally generated anterior shear (tendency of the superior vertebra to shear anteriorly on the adjacent inferior vertebra) was created by the action of gravity on the body mass of the trunk while internally generated shear appeared to be due to interspinous ligament and posterior longitudinal strain. The compressive load in the studied flexed position approached the safety limit of 3433 N established by the Institute for Occupational Safety and Health.[124]

The critical factors in lifting in the flexed posture appear to be the distance from the body of the object to be lifted from the body,[7] the velocity of the lift, and the degree of lumbar flexion.[130] The farther away the load is from the body, the greater the gravitational moment acting on the vertebral column. Greater muscle activity is required to perform the lift, and consequently greater pressure is created in the disk. The higher the velocity of the lift, the greater the amount of weight that can be lifted, but the higher the load on the lumbar disks. The relative spinal load and applied erector spinae force increase significantly with the velocity of trunk extension[131] (Fig. 4–44). A possible reason for the high load is because collagenous tissue is viscoelastic and resists rapid deformations more strongly than slow ones. Laboratory experiments have demonstrated that a motion segment's resistance to bending increases by 8% if the duration of the loading cycle decreases from 10 to 3 seconds and by an additional 2% if the loading cycle lasts only 1 second.[130] Dolan and colleagues in a study of 149 men and women who pulled upward with steadily increasing force on a floor-mounted load cell found that the passive extensor moment (which was determined when all parts of the erector spinae muscles (up to T1) were electrically silent) increased with lumbar flexion. From the lordotic standing posture to 80% flexion the increase was slight but above 80% the passive extensor moment rose to about 120 Nm for men and 77 Nm for women. The authors concluded that the reason for the increase in the passive extensor moment was due to the stretching of the noncontractile tissue in muscles, tension in ligaments and fascia, and raised intra-abdominal pressure.[130]

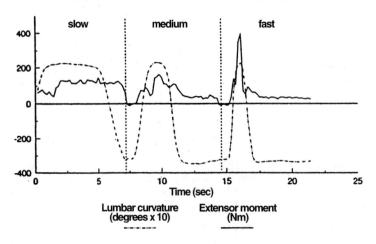

THE EFFECT OF LIFTING SPEED ON SPINAL LOADING

slow   medium   fast

Lumbar curvature (degrees x 10)

Extensor moment (Nm)

Time (sec)

FIGURE 4–44. Changes in the extensor moment during a series of three lifts. The subject lifted a 10-kg weight at three different speeds. Lumbar curvature is also shown to indicate the time course of the lifts. (Reprinted from Dolan, P, and Adams, MA: The relationship between EMG activity and extensor moment generation in the erector spinae muscles during bending and lifting activities. J Biomech 26:513–522, 1993; copyright 1993 with permission from Elsevier Science.)

The prevalence of back problems in the general population and the difficulties of resolving these problems has generated a great deal of research both to explain the mechanisms involved in lifting and to determine the best method of lifting so that back injuries can be prevented. The intra-abdominal pressure theory that was proposed to explain how the forces needed to perform a heavy lift are generated and the compressive forces on the disks are reduced. In 1957, Bartelink postulated that a contraction of the abdominal muscles (transversus abdominis and internal oblique muscles) in the presence of a closed glottis raises the intra-abdominal pressure, supporting the thorax and thus assisting the back muscles in raising the weight.[132] This theory has been challenged on the basis of calculations that demonstrate that the intra-abdominal pressure would have to exceed systolic aortic blood pressure to provide the required upward force on the thorax. Furthermore, it has been calculated that the force of the contraction necessary to generate this pressure exceeds the maximum possible hoop tension of the abdominal muscles.

The questions raised about the viability of the intra-abdominal pressure theory have led investigators to develop new theories to explain how lifting is accomplished. Gracovetsky[89] proposed a theory that includes intra-abdominal pressure as a component, but he has ascribed a different role for intra-abdominal pressure than was proposed in the original theory. He suggests that the back extensor muscles are assisted in lifting a large weight by extension moments generated by passive tension in the posterior ligamentous system and passive and active tension in the thoracolumbar fascia (TLF). According to Gracovetsky, tension is created by forward flexion of the trunk, which stretches the posterior ligamentous system, including the zygapophyseal joint capsules, posterior longitudinal, supraspinous, and ligamentum flavum, and interspinous ligaments. Contractions of the hip extensors in a closed kinematic chain exert a posterior tilting force on the pelvis, which places tension along the posterior ligamentous system. MacIntosh and coworkers suggest that the passive extensor moment is due predominantly to the passive elastic elements in the multifidus, iliocostalis lumborum, and lumbar portion of the longissimus thoracis, which experience a 15% to 59% increase in muscle belly length during full flexion from the erect posture.[118]

Using a finite element model of lifting tasks, Kong found that at both higher loads or at higher flexed postures muscles played a more critical role in stabilizing the spine than the passive structures. Muscle dysfunction destabilized the spine, increased the role of the facet joints in transmitting load, and shifted loads to ligaments and disks. The stress and strain in the posterior ligament increased significantly with a 10% decrease in muscle strength leading to a 65% increase in strain in the posterior ligament.[133]

Passive tension in the TLF is created by forward flexion of the spine and posterior tilting of the pelvis. Active tension in the TLF is created by contractions of the latissimus dorsi, internal oblique muscles, and transversus abdominis muscles. Also, contractions of the transversus abdominis and internal oblique muscles are thought to be responsible for increasing the intra-abdominal pressure in the presence of a closed glottis.[120] The intra-abdominal pressure adds tension to the TLF and thus increases the force of the extension moment that the TLF can generate. The TLF requires an appropriate amount of intra-abdominal pressure to function properly and a degree of spinal flexion to function efficiently.[89] When the intra-abdominal pressure is low, tension on the TLF is reduced and consequently the extension moment generated is decreased. Granata and Marras, using a biomechanical model, determined that during lifting activities the rectus abdominis and external oblique muscle groups contribute a significant flexion moment, which may approach 47% of the extension moment. Therefore, the moment produced by the back extensors in lifting must offset the flexor muscles' moment as well as the applied gravitational trunk moment. The total moment generated by the extensor muscles must be greater than the gravitational moment by as much as 47%. Flexor muscle activity also increases the compression and anterior shear on the lumbar spine.[131]

Gracovetsky's theory, which includes a role for the central nervous system (CNS), has not been proven, but the theory provides a direction for future research efforts. According to the theory, the CNS acts as a controlling computer that monitors the amount of stress acting at each intervertebral joint and adjusts the amount of stress to minimize stress and protect the joint structures. Stress minimization can be accomplished through reduction in muscle contraction, switching to ligamentous support, switching the relative contributions made by the muscles and ligaments, changing the posture of the spine, or by aborting the lift.[89] The use of ligamentous rather than muscle support also conserves energy. Ladin and associates found that muscles appear to function to conserve energy in that they have periods of activity and inactivity in response to an applied load. Furthermore, they found that the loading threshold required for a muscle or group of muscles to respond can be predicted.[91]

Squat lifting has been proposed as a way of lifting that offers protection for the low back. In squat lifting, a person bends primarily at the knees and the trunk is only slightly flexed compared to stoop lifting in which a person bends primarily at the trunk with the knees either straight or slightly flexed. Povin investigated the contributions of muscles and ligaments in both types of lifts in 15 men lifting loads from 5.8 to 32.4 kg. As might be expected, compression forces increased significantly for both squat and stoop lifts as the load increased. Squat lifting resulted in higher compression forces than stoop lifting. However, shear forces at L4/L5 were two to four times higher for the stoop lift compared to the squat lift. The anterior shear in the stoop lift was attributed to the external oblique abdominal muscles and the interspinous and supraspinous ligaments. Posterior shear was attributed to the erector spinae. Abdominal muscles and the latissimus dorsi showed relatively low activity (below 20% of maximum) for all lifts. The extensor musculature contributed most to the compression force increase with increasing load. The authors concluded that based on the dominance of muscle moment over ligamentous moment that the ligaments had a neglible role in generating extensor moments. However, there was an interplay between muscle and passive tissues. Muscle activation was reduced in lifts where ligamentous moments were highest.[134]

Changes in the velocity of the lift also have been proposed as a means of increasing the ability of a person to lift a large load. When lifting is performed slowly or when a weight is held continuously and the ligamentous system and TLF are providing most of the force for the activity, the ligaments are subjected to creep. The ligamentous elongation during creep imposes a limit on the maximum weight that can be lifted slowly because the ligaments must remain taut to balance the external moments.

Only about one-quarter of the amount of weight can be lifted at slow speed in comparison to the amount that can be lifted at a high speed.[89] However, during fast-speed lifting higher moments may occur at the L5/S1 levels than during slower-speed lifting.[135]

Muscles of the Pelvic Floor

Structure

Although the **levator ani** and **coccygeus** muscles neither play a major supporting role for the vertebral column nor produce movement of the column, these muscles are mentioned here because of their proximity to the column and possible influence on the linkages that form the pelvis. The levator ani muscles comprise two distinct parts, the iliococcygeus and the pubococcygeus, which help to form the floor of the pelvis and separate the pelvic cavity from the perineum. The left and right broad muscle sheets of the levator ani form the major portion of the floor of the pelvis. The medial borders of the right and left muscles are separated by the visceral outlet though which pass the uretha, vagina, and anorectum. The pubococcygeal part of the muscle arises from the posterior aspect of the pubis and has attachments to the sphincter, urethrae, walls of the vagina (in the female), and to the pineal body and rectum in both genders. The iliococcygeal portion, which arises from the obturator fascia, is thin. Its fibers blend with the fibers of the anococcygeal ligament, form a raphe, and attach to the last two coccygeal segments. The coccygeus muscle arises from the spine of the ischium and attaches to the coccyx and lower portion of the sacrum. The gluteal surface of the muscle blends with the sacrospinous ligament (Fig. 4–45).

Function

Voluntary contractions of the levator ani muscles help to constrict the openings in the pelvic floor (urethra and anus) and prevent unwanted micturition and defecation (stress incontinence). Involuntary contractions of these muscles occur during coughing or holding one's breath when the intra-abdominal pressure is raised. In women, these muscles surround the vagina and help to support the uterus. During pregnancy the muscles can be stretched or traumatized and result in stress incontinence whenever the intra-abdominal pressure is

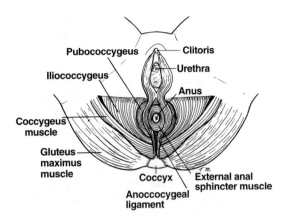

Pubococcygeus — Clitoris

Iliococcygeus — Urethra

— Anus

Coccygeus muscle

Gluteus maximus muscle — Coccyx — External anal sphincter muscle

Anoccocygeal ligament

FIGURE 4–45. Muscles of the pelvic floor.

raised. In men, damage to these muscles may occur after prostate surgery. The coccygeus muscle assists the levator ani in supporting the pelvic viscera and maintaining intra-abdominal pressure.

General Effects of Aging and Injury

The vertebral column, like other structures in the body, is subject to aging, injury, disease processes, and development deficits. Any one or more of the structural components may be affected by these conditions, but injuries and degenerative diseases are more likely to occur in those areas that are subjected to the greatest stress. Normally the spine is able to withstand large amounts of stress, but when the stresses are unexpected, prolonged, or excessive, the likelihood of injury is increased. Even relatively minor stresses may cause damage when the integrity of the structure has been previously compromised.

Aging

Aging causes changes in the structure of the disks and, consequently, in the function of the disk and related structures. According to Beattie, degeneration of the intervertebral disk begins with tears in the annulus, which leads to a loss of restraint on the nucleus pulposus, The nucleus becomes less hydrated and more fibrous, which reduces its height and narrows the disk space.[136] Consequently, the load-bearing capacity of the motion segment is reduced, as well as the stabilizing capacity of the annu-

lus, which can lead to segmental instability. Osteophytes may form on the margins of the vertebral bodies. The decrease in disk height brings the vertebrae closer together and alters the relationships of the zygapophyseal joints. The narrowed intervertebral spaces between vertebrae cause more compressive stress to be applied to these joint surfaces. The posterior ligamentous system also is affected by the loss in vertebral height and becomes slack. The lack of tension in the posterior ligaments permits more motion in flexion and increases the extent of the neutral zone, thus decreasing the stability of the spine. These age-related changes in disk structure affect men and women differently. For example, Miller and colleagues[137] studied 600 lumbar spine disks from subjects aged 0 to 90 years. Disks from men showed signs of degeneration (presence of osteophytes and loss of disk height) earlier than disks from women. For men, the signs of degeneration first occurred in the 11 to 19 year age group, whereas in women, signs of degeneration did not occur until a decade later.[137] It is possible that the reasons for the gender difference may be due to the variations in activity levels and amount of lifting performed by men in comparison to women or to differences in vertebral structures between men and women.

Magnetic resonance imaging provides for a reliable classification of disk abnormalities and detection of anatomic variations associated with degenerative disk disease.[138] Beattie, in a study using MRIs of lumbar intervertebral disks, found that some form of multilevel degeneration or disk bulge was visible on the MRIs of between 25% and 85% of an adult male and female population whose lumbar back pain was not severe enough to limit activity. The prevalence of these findings increased significantly in the elderly population with the two lower lumbar segments substantially more involved than the upper three segments. Abnormal MRI findings were more prevalent in people with symptoms than in people without symptoms. In fact, abnormal findings are rarely absent in patients with symptoms. The degree of disk herniation was not as important as the location of the herniation in relation to the size of the spinal canal and effect on the stability of the motion segment.[136]

In an investigation of 2480 cervical disks, Matsumoto and colleagues found that positive MRI findings increased significantly with age. The highest level of disk degeneration was found at C5/C6 followed by C6/C7 and C4 and C5.[77]

Injury

The lumbar region in particular is susceptible to injuries but injuries are frequent in other regions as well. Injury or failure occurs when the applied load exceeds the strength of a particular tissue. Repetitive strain causes injury by either the repeated application of a relatively low load or by application of a sustained load for a long duration (prolonged sitting or stooped posture). Vertebral body injury (end plate fracture and underlying trabeculae damage) is usually due to compression of the spine in the neutral position. Compression fractures generally cause a collapse of the anterior aspect of the vertebral body where there is an area of weakness (see Fig. 4–8). Subsequently, the loss of height, and disturbed relationships may cause tension failure of the posterior elements. Stress or fatigue fractures of the pars interarticularis result in weakened laminae. The shear forces acting on the affected vertebra may cause it to slip forward (Fig 4–46). This condition called **spondylolisthesis,** is described as the slippage of all or part of one vertebra on another (*spondylos* = vertebra and *olisthesis* = slip or slide down an incline). Spondylolisthesis may be due to a wide variety of causes, and although it is common in the lumbar area, it may also occur in other regions of the spine. The altered location of the slipped vertebra changes its relationship to adjacent structures and creates excessive stress on associated supporting ligaments and joints. Overstretched ligaments may lead to the lack of stability or **hypermobility** of the segment. Narrowing of the posterior joint space, which occurs with forward slippage of a vertebra, may cause stress to nerve roots. The slipped vertebrae may even create a shear stress on the spinal cord and result in a paralysis. Pain in spondylolisthesis may arise from excessive stress on any of the following pain-sensitive structures: anterior and posterior longitudinal ligaments, interspinous ligament, nerve roots, vertebral bodies, zygapophyseal joint capsules, synovial linings, or the muscles.

Spinal stenosis (narrowing of the spinal canal) in the lumbar spine may be caused by bone hypertrophy of the lamina, disk bulging, osteophytes over the posterior margins of the vertebral body, and enlargement of the inferior zygapophyseal facets. Degenerative changes in the ligamentum flavum in which the ligament loses much of its elasticity and becomes fibrotic can cause the ligament to bulge into the canal.[140] Spinal stenosis in the cervical region appears to be associated with aging. Matsumoto and associates[77] found that 23% of patients over age 64 years had MRI evidence of spinal cord involvement in the cervical area. However, the reduction in spinal cord cross-sectional area never exceeded 16%.

Disk herniation is usually the result of either cyclic loading in flexion and torsion or prolonged sustained loading in flexed and rotated positions. Ligamentous injury in the lumbar region is often the result of a fall in a sitting position with the spine flexed.[139] In the cervical region ligamentous injury often occurs as a result of an automobile accident in which the injured person's car is hit from behind. As a result of the unexpected acceleration, the person's head and neck are forced into extremes of flexion and extension.

Model for Determining Effects of Deficits

The hypothetical effects of an injury, aging, disease, or development deficit on the vertebral column may be analyzed by taking the following points into consideration:

1. The normal function that the affected structure is designed to serve
2. The stresses that are present during normal situations
3. The anatomic relationship of the structure to adjacent structures

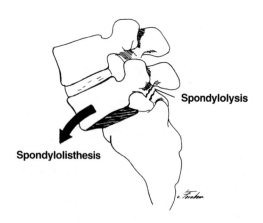

FIGURE 4–46. Shearing forces on the fifth lumbar vertebra may cause spondylolisthesis when spondylolysis is present.

4. The functional relationship of the structure to other structures

Normal Structure and Function

We will consider the posterior longitudinal ligament as an example. (1) The normal function of this ligament is to reinforce the posterior aspect of the intervertebral joints and to limit flexion of the vertebral column. (2) During flexion of the column, the ligament normally is subjected to tension. Under *normal conditions* the ligament elongates during flexion, provides resistance to flexion, and provides stability at the intervertebral joints. When the spine returns to neutral position, the ligament returns to its normal state. (3) Anatomically, the ligament is adjacent to the spinal cord on one side and the disks and vertebral bodies on the other. (4) Functionally, the ligament works in conjunction with the supraspinous, interspinous, and ligamentum flavum to limit flexion of the column and provide stability of the joints.

Hypothetical Effects of Injury

If one uses the background knowledge of normal function and structure of the ligament as a foundation, then it is possible to offer a number of hypotheses regarding the effects of ligamentous damage due to injury or disease (Table 4–10). (1) If the posterior longitudinal ligament is stretched there will be a lack of support for the intervertebral joint, which may lead to excessive tilting of the vertebra during flexion. (2) The excessive tilting combined with lack of support for the posterior annulus may lead to the possibility of tearing the annulus fibers. (3) Under compression forces, the posterior part of the annulus may bulge excessively into the spinal canal as a result of the lack of normal reinforcement provided by the posterior longitudinal ligament and resulting damage to its own fibers. The bulging annulus may cause pressure on the spinal cord or nerve roots and result in disturbed functioning of structures supplied by the spinal cord or affected nerve roots. (4) Other structures that are

Table 4–10. **Injury—Posterior Disk Herniation at L-4 to L-5 Caused by Rupture of Posterior Annulus Fibrosus**

Normal Intervertebral Disk	Hypothetical Effects of Injury
Normal Function 1. Shock absorption 2. Distribution of forces 3. Pivot of motion 4. Stability-joint integrity	**Loss of Normal Function** 1. Loss of shock-absorbing capability. 2. Abnormal concentration of forces on vertebral bodies. 3. Decreased motion—disturbance of normal tilting action. 4. Decreased stability initially, but subsequent replacement of damaged tissue by fibrocartilaginous tissue.
Normal Stress 1. Compression 2. Tension	**Abnormal Stresses** 1. Increased compression due to loss of shock absorbing capability and ability to distribute forces. Also initial spasm of surrounding muscles may increase compression. 2. Increased tension on any remaining posterior annulus fibrosus fibers and on posterior longitudinal ligament during flexion.
Anatomic Relationships 1. Posterior longitudinal 2. Spinal cord	**Disrupted Anatomic Relationships** 1. Pressure exerted on the posterior longitudinal ligament when nuclear material extrudes posteriorly. 2. Possible pressure on spinal cord or nerve roots due to either nuclear protusion or narrowing of foramen.
Functional Relationships 1. Intevertebral joints 2. Spinous processes	**Disrupted Functional Relationships** 1. The diminished joint space at the intervertebral joint caused by the loss of the hydrostatic pressure in the nucleus may cause compression at the facet joints during extension of the column. 2. Impingement of one spinous process on another may occur in extension as a result of the diminished joint space at the intervertebral joint.

functionally related, such as the supraspinous ligaments and the joint capsules of the facet joints, will be under increased stress due to the diminished stability at the intervertebral joints. These structures may be excessively stretched during flexion of the column, resulting in further instability.

Summary

The model for analyzing the effects of alterations in structure, which was presented in the preceding paragraphs, can be used throughout this text. The hypotheses and Table 4–10 represent just a sampling of the type of theoretical reasoning one can apply to analyze the effects of injury and disease on any structure. Normal function, functional relationships, and specifics regarding particular injuries or diseases can be determined by referring to the references included in this chapter as well as a perusal of the current literature. The reader is encouraged to follow this method of analysis, using a variety of structures both in this chapter and in subsequent chapters.

REFERENCES

1. Williams, PL et al (eds): Gray's Anatomy, ed 38. Churchill Livingstone, New York, 1995.
2. White, AA, and Panjabi, MM: Clinical Biomechanics of the Spine, ed 2. JB Lippincott, Philadephia, 1990.
3. Panjabi, M: Symposium on the lumbar spine 11. Orthop Clin North Am 8:169–179, 1977.
4. Panjabi, M, Yamamoto, I, Oxland, T, and Crisco, J: How does posture affect coupling in the lumbar spine? Spine 14:1002–1011, 1989.
5. Palastanga, N, Field, D, and Soames, R: Anatomy and Human Movement: Structure and Function, Heinemann Medical Books, Halley Court, Jordan Hill, Oxford, 1989.
6. Gracovetsky, S, and Farfan, H: The optimum spine. Spine 11:543–573, 1986.
7. Bogduk, N: Clinical Anatomy of the Lumbar Spine and Sacrum, ed 3. Churchill Livingstone, New York, 1997.
8. Cholewicki, J, et al: Effects of posture and structure on three-dimensional coupled rotations in the lumbar spine. Spine 21:2421, 1996.
9. Wu, JSS, and Chen, JH: Clarification of the mechanical behavior of spinal motion segments through a three-dimensional poroelastic mixed finite element model. Med Eng Phys 18:215, 1996.
10. Jensen, GM: Biomechanics of the lumbar intervertebral disk: A review. Phys Ther 60:4, 1980.
11. Kapandji, IA: The Physiology of the Joints 3, ed 2. Churchill Livingstone, Edinburgh, 1974.
12. MacLaughlin, SM, and Oldale, KNM: Vertebral body diameters and sex prediction. Ann Human Biol 19:285, 1992.
13. Lu, MY, and Hutton, WC: 3-D finite element model of L2-L3 disc body unit. Spine 21:2208,1996.
14. Twomey, LT, and Furniss, BI: The life cycle of the intervertebral disc: A review. Aust J Physiol 24:4, 1978.
15. Urban, JPG, and McMullin, JF: Swelling pressure of the lumbar intervertebral discs: Influence of age spinal level, composition and degeneration. Spine 13: 179–186, 1988.
16. Ghosh, P: The Biology of the Intervertebral Disc. Vol. 1. CRC Press, Boca Raton, Florida, 1988.
17. Adam, M, and Deyl, Z: Degenerated annulus fibrosus of the intervertebral disk contains collagen type III. Ann Rheum Dis 43:258–263, 1984.
18. Brickley-Parsons, D, and Glimcher, MJ: Is the chemistry of collagen in the intervertebral disc an expression of Wolff's law? Spine 9:148–182, 1984.
19. Fujita, Y, and Lotz, JC: Radial tensile properties of the lumbar annulus fibrosus are site and degeneration dependent. J Ortho Res 15:814, 1997.
20. Bogduk, N, Windsor, M, and Inglis, A: The innervation of the cervical intervertebral discs. Spine 13:2–7, 1988.
21. Finneson, B: Low Back Pain, ed 2. JB Lippincott, Philadelphia, 1980.
22. Lamb, DW: The neurology of spinal pain. Phys Ther 59:8, 1979.
23. Roberts, S, Menage, J, and Urban, JPG: Biochemical and structural properties of the cartilage end-plate and its relation to the intervertebral disc. Spine 14: 166–173, 1989.
24. Edelson, JG, and Nathan, H: Stages in the natural history of the end-plates. Spine 13:21–26, 1988.
25. McFadden, KD, and Taylor, JR: End-plate lesions of the lumbar spine. Spine 14:867–869, 1989.
26. Bogduk, N, and Engel, R: The menisci of the lumbar zygapophyseal joints. Spine 9:454–460, 1984.
27. Adams, MA, and Hutton, WC: The mechanical function of the lumbar apophyseal joints. Spine 8: 327–330, 1983.
28. Ghosh, P: The Biology of the Intervertebral Disc, Vol 11. CRC Press, Boca Raton, Florida, 1988.
29. Cyron, BM, and Hutton, WC: The tensile strength of the capsular ligaments of the apophyseal joints. J Anat 132:145–150, 1981.
30. Putz, R: The detailed functional anatomy of the ligaments of the vertebral column. Ann Anat 174:40,1992.
31. Crisco, JJ, Panjabi, MM, and Dvorak, J: A model of the alar ligaments of the upper cervical spine in axial rotation. J Biomech 24:607, 1991.
32. Maiman, DJ, and Pintar, FA: Anatomy and clinical biomechanics of the thoracic spine. Clin Neurosurg 38:296, 1992.
33. Myklebust, JB, et al: Tensile strength of spinal ligaments. Spine 13:526–531, 1988.
34. Hedtmann, A, et al: Measurements of human spine ligaments during loaded and unloaded motion. Spine 14:175–185, 1989.
35. Olszewski, AD, Yaszemski, MJ, and White, A: The anatomy of the human lumbar ligamentum flavum. Spine 21:2307, 1996.
36. Nordin, M, and Frankel, VH: Basic Biomechanics of the Musculoskeletal System, ed 2. Lea & Febiger, Philadelphia, 1989.
37. Twomey, LT, and Taylor, JR: Sagittal movements of the human vertebral column: A qualitative study of the role of the posterior vertebral elements. Arch Phys Med Rehabil 64:322–324, 1983.
38. Gunzberg, R, et al: Role of the capsulo-ligamentous

structures in rotation and combined flexion/rotation of the lumbar spine. J Spinal Disorders 5:1, 1992.

39. Adams, MA, Dolan, P, and Hutton, WC: The lumbar spine in backward bending. Spine 13:1019–1026, 1988.
40. Twomey, L, and Taylor, J: Flexion creep deformation and hysteresis in the lumbar vertebral column. Spine 7:116, 122, 1982.
41. Twomey, LT, Taylor, JR, and Oliver, MJ: Sustained flexion loading, rapid extension loading of the lumbar spine, and the physical therapy of related injuries. Physiother Pract 4:129–138, 1988.
42. Hansson, TH, Keller, TS, and Punjabi, M: A study of the compressive properties of lumbar vertebral trabeculae: Effects of tissue characteristics. Spine 12: 56–62, 1987.
43. Keller, TS, et al: Regional variations in the compressive properties of lumbar vertebral trabeculae: Effects of disc degeneration. Spine 14: 1012–1019, 1989.
44. Shirazi-Adl, A: Strain in fibers of a lumbar disc. Spine 14:98–103, 1989.
45. Adams, MA, and Hutton, WC: Gradual disc prolapse. Spine 10:524–531, 1985.
46. Panjabi, M, et al: Intrinsic disk pressure as a measure of integrity of the lumbar spine. Spine 13:913–917, 1988.
47. Panjabi, M, et al: Spinal stability and intersegmental muscle forces: A biomechanical model. Spine 14:194–199, 1989.
48. Pope, M, and Panjabi, M: Biomechanical definitions of spinal stability. Spine 10:255–256, 1985.
49. Gracovetsky, SA: The resting spine: A conceptual approach to the avoidance of spinal reinjury during rest. Phys Ther 67:549–553, 1987.
50. Parnianpour, M, Nordin, M, Frankel, VH, and Kahanovitz, N: The effect of fatigue on the motor output and pattern of isodynamic trunk movement. Isotechnol Res Abstr, April 1988.
51. Nachemson, AL: The lumbar spine: An orthopedic challenge. Spine 1:1, 1976.
52. Ahrens, SF: The effect of age on intervertebral disc compression during running. J Otohp Sports Phys Ther 20:17, 1994.
53. Klein, JA, and Hukins, DWL: Relocation of the bending axis during flexion-extension of lumbar intervertebral discs and its implications for prolapse. Spine 8:1776–1781, 1983.
54. Klein, JA, and Hukins, DWL: Functional differentiation in the spinal column. Eng Med 12:83–85, 1983.
55. Haher, TR, et al: Contribution of the three columns of the spine to rotational stability: A biomechanical model. Spine 14:663–669, 1989.
56. Bogduk, N, Amevo, B, and Pearcy, M: A biological basis for instantaneous centers of rotation of the vertebral column. Proc Inst Mech Engrs 209:177, 1995.
57. Haher, TR, et al: Instantaneous axis of rotation as a function of three columns of the spine. Spine 17:S149, 1992.
58. Panjabi, MM, et al: Cervical human vetebrae: Qualitative three dimensional anatomy of the middle and lower regions. Spine 16:86,1991.
59. Bland, JH, and Boushey, DR: Anatomy and physiology of the cervical spine. Semin Arthritis Rheum 20:1, 1990.
60. Panjabi, MM, et al: Articular facets of the human spine. Spine 18:1298, 1993.
61. Panjabi, MM, Oxland, TR, and Parks, H: Quantitative anatomy of the cervical spine ligaments. J Spinal Disord 4:270, 1991.
62. Crisco, JJ, Panjabi, MM, and Dvorak, J: A model of the

alar ligaments of the upper cervical spine in axial rotation. J Biomech 24:607, 1991.
63. Goel, VK, et al: Moment-rotation relationships of the ligamentous occipito-atlanto-axial complex. J Biomech 8:673–680, 1988.
64. Panjabi, M, et al: Three dimensional movements of the upper cervical spine. Spine 13:726–730, 1988.
65. Nolan, JP, and Sherk, HH: Biomechanical evaluation of the extensor musculature of the cervical spine. Spine 13:9–11, 1988.
66. Pal, GP, and Routal, RV: The role of the vertebral laminae in the stability of the cervical spine. J Anat 188:485, 1996.
67. Pal, GP, and Sherk, HH: The vertical stability of the cervical spine. 13:447–449, 1988.
68. Maroney, SP, Schultz, AB, Miller, JAA, and Andersson, GBJ: Load-displacement properties of lower cervical spine motion segments. J Biomech 21:769–779, 1988.
69. Shea, M, et al: Variations in stiffness and strength along the cervical spine. J Biomech 24:95, 1991.
70. Dvorak, J, et al: In vivo flexion/extension of the normal cervical spine. J Orthop Res 9:828, 1991.
71. Oda, I, et al: Biomechanical role of the posterior elements, costovertebral joints, ribcage in the stability of the thoracic spine. Spine 21:1423, 1996.
72. Milne, N: The role of the zygapophyseal joint orientation and uncinate processes in controlling motion in the cervical spine. J Anat 178:189, 1991.
73. Kent, BA: Anatomy of the trunk: A review. Part 1. Phys Ther 54:7, 1974.
74. Basmajian, JV: Primary Anatomy, ed 7. Williams & Wilkins, Baltimore, 1976.
75. Cailliet, R: Neck and Arm Pain, ed 3. FA Davis, Philadelphia, 1991.
76. Dumas, JL, et al: Rotation of the cervical spinal column. A computed tomography in vivo study. Surg Radiol Anat 15:33, 1993.
77. Matsumoto, M, et al: MRI of cervical intervertebral discs in asymptomatic subjects. J Bone Joint Surg 80-B:19, 1998.
78. Joosab, M, Torode, M, and Rao, PV: Preliminary findings on the effect of load-carrying on the structural integrity of the cervical spine. Surg Radiol Anat 16:393, 1994.
79. Brunnstrom, S: Clinical Kinesiology, ed 3. FA Davis, Philadelphia, 1972.
80. Panjabi, MM, et al: Complexity of the thoracic spine pedicle anatomy. Eur Spine J 6:19, 1997.
81. Panjabi, MM, et al: Thoracic human vertebrae: Quantitative three-dimensional anatomy. Spine 16:888, 1991.
82. McCormack, BM, et al: Anatomy of the thoracic pedicle. Neurosurgery 37:303, 1995.
83. Cailliet, R: Low Back Pain Syndrome, ed 5. FA Davis, Philadelphia, 1995.
84. Pintar, FA, et al: Biomechanical properties of human lumbar spine ligaments. J Biomech 25:1351, 1992.
85. Basadonna, P-T, Gasparini, D, and Rucco, V: Iliolumbar ligament insertions. Spine 21:2313, 1996.
86. Rucco, V, Basadonna, P-T, and Gasparini, D: Anatomy of the iliolumbar ligament: A review of its anatomy and a magnetic resonance study. Am J Phys Med Rehabil 75:451, 1996.
87. Macintosh, JE, and Bogduk, N: The morphology of the lumbar erector spinae. Spine 12:658–668, 1987.
88. Vleeming, A, et al: The posterior layer of the thoracolumbar fascia. Spine 20:753, 1995.

89. Gracovetsky, S: The Spinal Engine. Springer-Verlag, New York, 1988.

90. Haher, TR, et al: The role of the lumbar facet joints in spinal stability. Spine 19:2667, 1994.

91. Ladin, Z, Kurukundi, RM, and DeLuca, CJ: Mechanical recruitment of low-back muscles. Spine 14:927–938, 1989.

92. Wilke, H-J, et al: Stability increase of the lumbar spine with different muscle groups: A biomechanical in vitro study. Spine 20:192, 1995.

93. Khoo, BCC, et al: A comparison of lumbosacral loads during static and dynamic activities. Australas Phys Eng Sci Med 17:55, 1994.

94. Goel, VK, et al: A combined finite element and optimization investigation of lumbar spine mechanics with and without muscles. Spine 18:1531, 1993.

95. Gardner-Morse, M, Stokes, IA, and Laible, J: Role of muscles in lumbar spine stability in maximum extension efforts. J Orthop Res 13:802, 1995.

96. Adams, MA, and Dolan, P: A technique for quantifying the bending moment on the lumbar spine in vivo. J Biomech 24:117,1991.

97. Panjabi, MM, et al: Mechanical behavior of the human lumbar and lumbosacral spine as shown by three-dimensional load-displacement curves. J Bone Joint Surg 76-A:413, 1994.

98. Lin, R-M, et al: Lumbosacral kinematics in the sagittal plane: A radiographic study in vivo. J Formos Med Assoc 92:638, 1993.

99. Cailliet, R: Soft Tissue Pain and Disability, ed 3. FA Davis, Philadelphia, 1996.

100. Nelson, JM, Walmsley, RPO, and Stevenson, JM: Relative lumbar and pelvic motion during loaded spinal flexion/extension. Spine 20:199,1995.

101. Hollinshead, WH: Functional Anatomy of the Limbs and Back. WB Saunders, Philadelphia, 1976.

102. Bowen, V, and Cassidy, JD: Macroscopic and microscopic anatomy of the sacroiliac joint from embryonic life until the eighth decade. Spine 6:620–627, 1981.

103. Walker, JM: The sacroiliac joint: A critical review. Phys Ther 72:903, 1992.

104. Salsabili, N, Valojerdy, MR, and Hogg, DA: Variations in thickness of articular cartilage in the human sacroiliac joint. Clin Anat 8:388,1995.

105. Cassidy, JD: The pathoanatomy and clinical significance of the sacroiliac joints. J Manipulative Physiol Ther 15:41, 1992.

106. Mierau, DR, et al: Sacroiliac joint dysfunction and low back pain in school aged children. J Manipulative Physiol Ther 7:81–84, 1994.

107. DonTigny, RL: Function and pathomechanics of the sacroiliac joint: A review. Phys Ther 65:35–44, 1985.

108. Reilly, JP, et al: Disorders of the sacroiliac joint in children. J Bone Joint Surg 1:40, 1988.

109. Bernard, TN, and Cassidy, JD: The sacroiliac joint syndrome. Pathophysiology, diagnosis, and management. First Interdisciplinary World Congress on Low Back Pain and Its Relation to the Sacroiliac Joint. (Eds) Vleeming, A et al. San Diego, 1992.

110. Vleeming, A, et al: The function of the long dorsal sacroiliac ligament. Spine 21:556, 1996.

111. Gould, JA, and Davies, GJ (eds): Orthopaedics and Sports Physical Therapy. CV Mosby, St. Louis, 1985.

112. Freeman, MD, Fox, D, and Richards, T: The superior intracapsular ligament of the sacroiliac joint: Presumptive evidence for confirmation of Illi's ligament. J Manipulative Physiol Ther 13:384, 1990.

113. Vrahas, M, et al: Ligamentous contributions to pelvic stability. Orthopedics 18:271, 1995.

114. Vleeming, A, et al: Relation between form and function in the sacroiliac joint. Part 1: Clinical anatomical aspects. Spine 15:130, 1990.

115. Vleeming, A: Relation between form and function in the sacroiliac joint. Part 2: Biomechanical aspect. Spine 15:11, 1990.

116. Coventry, MB, and Taper, EM: Pelvic instability. J Bone Joint Surg 54A:83, 1972.

117. Grieve, GP: The sacro-iliac joint. Physiotherapy 62:8, 1979.

118. MacIntosh, JE, Bogduk, N, and Pearcy, MJ: The effects of flexion on the geometry and actions of the lumbar erector spinae. Spine 18:884, 1993.

119. Bartelink, DL: The role of abdominal pressure in relieving the pressure on the lumbar intervertebral disc. J Bone Joint Surg 39B:718–725.

120. Sullivan, MS: Back support mechanisms during manual lifting. Phys Ther 69:52–59, 1989.

121. McGill, SM: Low back exercises: Evidence for improving exercise regimens. Phys Ther 78:754, 1998.

122. Ng, JK-F, et al: Relationship between muscle fiber composition and functional capacity of back muscles in healthy subjects and patients with back pain. J Othop Sports Phys Ther 27:389, 1998.

123. Roy, SH, et al: Classification of back muscle impairment based upon the surface electromyographic signal. J Rehabil Res Dev 34:405, 1997.

124. McGill, SM, and Kippers, V: Transfer of loads between lumbar tissues during flexion-relaxation phenomenon. Spine 19:2190, 1994.

125. MacIntosh, JE, Pearcy, MJ, and Bogduk, N: The axial torque of the lumbar back muscles and trunk. Australas N Z J Surg 63:205, 1993.

126. Edgar, M: Pathologies associated with lifting. Physiotherapy 65:8, 1979.

127. Troup, JDG: Biomechanics of the vertebral column. Physiotherapy 65:8, 1979.

128. Callaghan, JP, Gunning, JL, and McGill, SM: The relationship between lumbar spine load and muscle activity during extensor exercises. Spine 23:2097.

129. Nachemson, A: The load on lumbar discs in different positions of the body. Clin Orthop 45:107, 1966.

130. Dolan, P, Mannion, AF, and Adam, MA: Passive tissues help the muscles to generate extensor moments during lifting. J Biomech 27:1077, 1994.

131. Granata, KP, and Marras, WS: The influence of trunk muscle coactivity on dynamic spinal loads. 20:913,1995.

132. Bissonault, JS, and Blaschak, MJ: Incidence of diastasis recti abdominis during the childbearing years. Phys Ther 68:1082–1086, 1988.

133. Kong, WZ, et al: Effects of muscle dysfunction on lumbar spine mechanics: A finite element study based on a two motion segment model. Spine 21:2197,1996.

134. Potvin, JR, McGill, SM, and Norman, RW: Trunk muscle and lumbar ligament contributions to dynamic lifts with varying degrees of trunk flexion. Spine 16:1099, 1991.

135. Buseck, M, et al: Influence of dynamic factors and external loads on the moment at the lumbar spine in lifting. Spine 13:918–920, 1988.

136. Beattie, P: The relationship between symptoms and abnormal magnetic resonance images of lumbar intervertebral discs. Phys Ther 76:601, 1998.

137. Miller, JAA, Schmatz, C, and Schultz, AB: Lumbar disc

degeneration: Correlation with age, sex, and spine level in 600 autopsy specimens. Spine 13:173–178, 1988.

138. Beattie, PF, and Meyers, SP: Magnetic resonance imaging in low back pain: General principles and clinical issues. Phys Ther 78:738, 1998.

139. McGill, SM: The biomechanics of low back injury: Implications on current practice in industry and the clinic. J Biomech 30:465, 1997.

140. Postacchini, F, et al: Ligamentum flava in lumbar disc herniation and spinal stenosis. Spine 19:917, 1994.

Study Questions

1. Which region of the vertebral column is most flexible? Explain why this region has greater flexibility.

2. Describe the relationship between the zygapophyseal joints and the intervertebral joints.

3. What is the zygapophyseal facet orientation in the lumbar region? How does this orientation differ from that of other regions? How does the facet joint orientation in the lumbar region affect motion in that region?

4. How would a tear in the supraspinous ligament affect function at the intervertebral joints? How would this injury affect the interspinous, intertransverse, and posterior longitudinal ligaments? Would any other structures be affected?

5. Which structures would be affected if a person has an increased anterior convexity in the lumbar area? Describe the type of stress that would occur, where it would occur, and how it would affect different structures.

6. Explain how a limitation of motion at the hip joints affects motion at the lumbar spine.

7. Describe the function of the intervertebral disk during motion and in weight bearing.

8. During rotation of the spine, in which area will you find the spinous processes rotating to the opposite side (convexity) of the curve? In which area do they rotate to the same side as the direction of the vertebral body?

9. Identify the factors that limit rotation and lateral flexion in the thoracic spine. Explain how the limitations occur.

10. Which muscles cause extension of the lumbar spine? In which position of the spine are they most effective?

11. Explain how the Valsalva maneuver may help to provide stability for the lumbar spine.

12. Describe the forces that act on the spine during motion and at rest.

13. Explain how "creep" may adversely effect the stability of the vertebral column.

14. Describe how muscles and ligaments interact to provide stability for the vertebral column.

15. What role has been attributed to the thoracolumbar fascia in lifting?

16. How does the position of hip flexion in the supine position assist in childbirth?

APPENDIX

*Muscles of the Lumbar Vertebral Column**

Muscles	Description	Attachments	Action
Psoas major (PM)	Fibers originating from higher lumbar levels form the outer surface of the muscle. Fibers from lower levels form the deep substance of the muscle. Fibers run inferiorly and laterally following the iliacus m. and pelvic brim.	Proximal attachments are on the bodies of two adjacent vertebrae and interposed disk from T12–L5 and on the transverse processes of L1–L5. The distal attachment is to the lesser trochanter of the femur.	Primary unilateral action is hip flexion. Bilaterally, assists in flexion of the lower lumbar spine with the thigh fixed and with extension of the upper lumbar spine.
Intertransversarii lateralis (IL)	Two parts: ventrales (ILV) and dorsales (ILD). Small muscles that are located between the transverse processes. According to *Gray's Anatomy* these muscles are not well developed in the cervical region.	ILV connects margins of consecutive transverse processes of the lumbar vertebrae. ILD connects the accessory processes of one vertebra to the transverse processes of the adjacent inferior vertebra.	Thought to act with the QL in lateral flexion of trunk, but according to Bogduk, actual actions are unknown. According to *Gray's Anatomy* the IL also provides posture control, but actual action is unknown.
Quadratus lumborum (QL)	The muscle is complex with many oblique and longitudinal fibers that connect the lumbar transverse processes, ilium, and also the 12th rib where the majority of fibers are connected.	Proximal attachments are to the inferior border of the 12th rib, and to the transverse processes of L1–L4 by four small tendons. Distal attachments include the superior and anterior iliolumbar ligaments, and iliac crests.	Fixes 12th rib during respiration and helps to stabilize the lower attachments of the diaphragm in inspiration. Acts on the vertebral column to produce ipsilateral lateral flexion when the pelvis is fixed.
Interspinales (Int)	Four pairs of short muscles located on either side of the interspinous ligament between L1 and L5.	Spinous process to spinous process of adjacent lumbar vertebrae.	Assigned a role in lumbar extension and postural control. According to Bogduk, actual actions are unknown.
Intertransversarii mediales (IM)	Small, short paired muscles that according to Bogduk may have a proprioceptive function. The muscles may provide feedback that affects action of surrounding muscles.	Extend between the accessory process of one vertebra and the mamillary process of the adjacent inferior vertebra.	Feedback for posture control. *Gray's Anatomy* suggests IM couples with MULT in lateral flex of trunk but actual action is unknown.
Multifidus (MULT)	Largest and most medial of the lumbar spine muscles. Lumbar MULT consists of large fascicles arranged segmentally that radiate from spinous processes. Each of the five groups of fascicles arise from a common tendon at the caudal tip of each lumbar spinous process (L1–L5). Fascicles split caudally	Fasciculi arise from the posterior sacrum at the fourth sacral foramen, aponeurosis of the erector spinae, posterior superior iliac spines, dorsal sacroliliac ligaments and L1–L5 mamillary processes, T1–T12 transverse processes and the zygapophyseal facets from C3–C7. Varying in	Theoretically, the MULT causes lumbar spine extension and opposes or stabilizes against the flexion effect of the abdominal muscles as they produce spinal rotation. In addition, deep fibers attached to the zygapophyseal joints protect the joint capsules from becoming caught inside the joint

	to assume separate attachments to mamillary processes, iliac crest, and sacrum. Deeper fibers are attached to the zygapophyseal joints.	length, the fascicles attach along the entire spinous processes at one, two, or even three levels above.	during spinal movements.
Longissimus thoracis (LONG.T.)	Bogduk describes the lumbar portion of this muscle as the longissimus thoracis pars lumborum. *Gray's Anatomy* does not use a separate designation for the thoracic and lumbar portions of the muscle. According to Bogduk, the L5 fascicles lie deep to other fascicles that lie progressively more superficially so that the L1 fascicle is the most superficial.	In the lumbar region the muscle is composed of five fascicles. Each one arises from accessory processes and adjacent medial end of the dorsal surfaces of the transverse processes of the lumbar vertebrae. L1 through L4 fascicles form tendons that converge and form the intermuscular aponeurosis of the lumbar spine which attaches on the ilium. The L5 fascicle attaches to the superior iliac spine.	Action depends on whether the muscle contracts unilaterally, or bilaterally. Contracting unilaterally, the longissimus produces lateral flexion of the vertebral column. Bilateral contraction produces posterior sagittal rotation and posterior translation.
Iliocostalis lumbro (L.ILIO)	*Gray's Anatomy* refers to L.ILIO as attaching to the angles of the lower six or seven ribs. Bogduk refers to the muscle as consisting of four fascicles attached to the lumbar vertebrae and iliac crests.	According to Bogduk, L.ILIO consists of four overlapping fascicles that arise from the tips of the transverse processes of L1 through L4 and from the middle layer of the thoracolumbar fascia. All of the fascicles attach on the iliac crest.	Bilateral contraction causes extension of vertebral column. Unilaterally, contraction causes same side lateral flexion and cooperates with the MULT to oppose the flexion effect of abdominal muscles when they act to rotate the trunk.

Muscles of the Thoracic Vertebral Column

Muscles	Description	Origin and Insertion	Action
Longissimus thoracis (T.LONG)	Thoracic fibers consist of 11–12 pairs of small fascicles.	According to both Bogduk and *Gray's Anatomy*, in the thoracic region, fascicles are attached to the transverse processes from T1–T12 and between the tubercles and angles of the 4th to 12th ribs. According to Bogduk each fascicle forms a caudal tendon that extends to one of the spinous processes of L1–L5.	Bilateral through pull on the erector spinae aponeurosis. Unilateral contraction causes lateral flexion of the thoracic and lumbar regions.
Iliocostalis thoracis (ILIO.T)	According to Bogduk this muscle represents the thoracic component of	According to Bogduk the muscle arises from the angles of lower six or	Causes an increase in lordotic curve and aids in derotating the

		the muscle known as the iliocostalis lumborum	eight ribs, and attaches to the posterior superior iliac spine.	thoracic cage and lumbar spine.
Spinalis thoracis (SPIN)		Considered to be the medial part of erector spinae. Blends with the longissimus thoracis and semispinalis muscles.	Proximal attachments are to the spinous processes of the upper thoracic vertebrae. Distal attachments are to the spinous processes of T11–L2.	Extension of thoracic vertebral column.
Semispinalis thoracis (SEMI)			Proximal attachments are the spinous processes of C6–T4. Distal attachments are the transverse processes of T6–T10.	Extension and contra-lateral rotation of cervical and thoracic regions.
Rotatores thoracis (ROT)		Eleven pairs of muscles that lie deep to the MULT.	These muscles connect the upper posterior part of a transverse process to the lower lateral surface of T1–T12 lamina.	Rotation of vertebral column.

Muscles of the Head and Cervical Vertebral Column

Muscles	Description	Origin and Insertion	Action
Trapezius (TRAP)	Flat, triangular, paired muscles that extend over the dorsum of the neck and upper thoracic area between the scapulae.	Attachments include the medial third of the superior nuchal line, external occipital protuberance, ligamentum nuchae, and tips of spinous processes from C7–T12. Superior fibers descend to attach at the posterior border of the lateral clavicle. Middle fibers extend horizontally to attach at the medial acromion process and superior lip of scapular spine. Inferior fibers ascend to attach at the medial end of the scapular spine.	Stabilizes scapula during arm movements; with shoulder fixed, TRAP may bend the neck and head posterolaterally. Combined with the levator scapula, rhomboids, and serratus anterior the TRAP produces various scapular rotations.
Sternocleido-mastoid (SCOM)	The paired muscles form two large bands (sternal and clavicular) that run obliquely forward and downward to the antero-lateral aspect of the neck.	Fibers in the sternal head extend from the occiput to attach to the upper anterior surface of the manubrium of the sternum. Fibers in the clavicular head extend from the mastoid process to attach on the medial one-third of the clavicle.	Unilateral contraction: contralateral rotation, ipsilateral lateral flex-ion and extension. Bilateral contraction: accentuates cervical lordosis and produces neck flexion and extension. With head fixed helps to elevate thorax in forced inspira-tion.
Scalenus (A.SCAL, M.SCAL, P.SCAL)	The SCAL consists of three pairs of muscles (anterior,	The proximal attachment for the A.SCAL and	Bilateral contraction; anterolateral flexion;

	medius, and posterior) located on the antero-lateral aspect of the cervical vertebral column.	M.SCAL is the first rib. The distal attachments for A.SCAL and M.SCAL are the transverse processes of C2–C7. P.SCAL is attached to the second rib and the transverse processes from C2–C7. The proximal attachments are the first rib and transverse processes of C4–C6.	unilateral contraction: lateral flexion to same side. All muscles elevate ribs when acting in reverse action and all muscles are active during inspiration.
Spinalis cervicis (SPIN)	According to *Gray's Anatomy*, this muscle is not always present.	The proximal attachment is to the spine of the axis. Distally, the muscle has attachments to the lower ligamentum nuchae and spinous process of C7.	The spinales muscles are extensors of the vertebral column.
Spinalis capitis (SPIN)	According to *Gray's Anatomy*, the muscle is often difficult to distinguish from the semispinalis capitis.	See semispinalis capitis.	Extension of cervical vertebral column.
Semispinalis cervicis (SEMI)	Cervical portion of SEMI.	Proximally the muscle attaches to the spine of C2–C5. Distally the muscle attaches to the transverse processes of T1–T6.	The SEMI cervicis extends and contralaterally rotates the cervical spine.
Semispinalis capitis (SEMI)	This muscle is deep to SPL and medial to the longissimus cervicis and capitis. The medial portion of this muscle is called the spinalis capitis.	The proximal attachment is the area between the superior and inferior nuchal lines on the occipital bone. Distally the muscle is attached to the C7–T7 transverse processes and zygapophyseal facets from C4–C6.	The SEMI capitus extends the thoracic and cervical spine and head, and rotates the head to the contralateral side.
Splenius cervicis		Proximal attachments are to the transverse processes of C2–C3. Distal attachments are to the spinous processes of T3–T6.	Works with splenius capitis to produce retraction of the head.
Splenius capitis (SPL CAP)	These paired muscles are deep to the trapezius and the rhomboids.	Proximal attachments are to the mastoid process and the occipital bone just below the lateral nuchal line. The distal attachments are to the lower ligamentum nuchae and spinous processes of C7–T4.	Retraction of the head and flattens the cervical spine. Works synergistically with the sternocleidomastoid muscle to tilt and rotate the head.
Longus colli (L.COL)	Composed of tendinous slips that have attachments to cervical and thoracic vertebrae. The muscle has three parts	The inferior oblique extends from the anterior surface of the bodies of T1–T3 and attaches to the anterior	Bilateral action: forward flexion of cervical region. Unilateral action: lateral flexion and contralateral rotation.

	(inferior and superior oblique and vertical).	tubercles of the transverse processes of C5 and C6. The superior oblique extends from the tubercles of the transverse processes of C3–C5 to attach to the anterior arch of the atlas. Arises from the anterior aspects of T1–T3 and inserts into the antero-lateral surface of the atlas. The vertical portion of the muscle extends from the anterior surface of the bodies of C5–C7 and T1–T3 to attach on the anterior surfaces of the bodies of C2–C4.	
Longus capitis (L.CAP)	Forms a broad and thick attachment to the occipital bone but is composed of tendinous slips in its attachments to the vertebrae.	Proximal attachment is to inferior surface of the occipital bone. Distal attachments are to the transverse processes of C3–C6.	Flexion of head.
Rectus capitis anterior (RCA)	Short and flat muscles deep to the L.CAP.	Proximally, muscles insert on the inferior surface of the occipital bone. Distally muscles attach on the anterior surface and base of transverse process of atlas.	Presumed to produce flexion of head at the atlanto-occipital joint.
Rectus capitis lateralis (RCL)	Short and flat muscles that overlie the anterior surfaces of the atlanto-occipital joint.	Proximal attachment is the occipital bone. Distal attachment is to the upper surface of C1 transverse process.	Presumed to produce lateral flexion of the head to the same side at the atlanto-occipital joint. However, according to *Gray's Anatomy*, actual action is unknown.
Ilio-costalis cervicis (ILIO.C)	Medial to the tendons of the ILIO.T.	Arises from costal angles of the third through sixth ribs. Attaches to the posterior tubercles of transverse processes of C4–C6.	Aids in extension and lateral flexion of vertebral column.
Long-issimus cervicis (LONG. Cerv)	Located medial to the LONG.T.	Proximal attachments to the posterior tubercles of C2–C6. Distal attachments to transverse processes from T1–T5.	Aids in extension and lateral flexion of vertebral column.
Long-issimus capitis (LONG. Cap)	Located between the LONG.Cerv and SEMI.Cap muscles.	Proximal attachment at the posterior margin of the mastoid process. Distal attachments to transverse process T1–T5 and zygapoph-yseal facets from C4–C7.	Aids in head extension and rotation to the same side.

Rectus capitis posterior major (RCP major)	Deep to SEMI capitis.	Proximal attachment is on the occipital bone. Distal attachment is to the spinous process of the axis (C1).	Head extension and rotation to the same side.
Rectus capitis posterior minor	Deep to RCP major.	Proximal attachment is on the occipital bone. Distal attachment is on the posterior arch of the atlas (C2).	Extension of the head.
Obliquus capitis inferior (OCI).	Deep to SEMI capitis.	Extends laterally from the spine and lamina of axis to the transverse process of atlas.	Same side rotation of the head.
Obliquus capitis superior (OCS)	Deep to SEMI capitis.	Extends from the transverse process of atlas going superiorly to attach to the occipital bone.	Posterolateral flexion of the head.

*Descriptions of the muscles of the vertebral column are based on Bogduk[6], and Williams, PL, et al.[1]

CHAPTER 5

THE THORAX AND CHEST WALL

OBJECTIVES

Following the study of this chapter, the reader should be able to:

Describe

1. The articulations of the ribs with the thoracic vertebrae.
2. The articulations of the ribs and clavicle with the manubriosternum.
3. The structure and function of the manubriosternal and interchondral joints.
4. The shape and functions of the diaphragm.
5. The roll of the abdominal compliance in ventilation.
6. The functions of the parasternals and scalenes.
7. The functions of the accessory muscles of ventilation.
8. The motions of the chest wall and abdomen during ventilation.

Identify

1. Functions of the abdominal muscles in inspiration and expiration.
2. The primary muscles of ventilation.
3. The structures that provide shape, motion, and stability of the chest wall/thorax.
4. Thorocoabdominal coordination in health and in hyperinflation.

Explain

1. The relationship between the parasternal and scalene muscles during ventilation.
2. The relationship between the diaphragm and abdominal muscles during ventilation.

Compare

1. The relationship between abdominal and thoracic pressures during ventilation.
2. Thoracic structural and functional differences between an infant and an elder.

Analyze

1. The effects of pregnancy as a normal functional alteration of rib cage and diaphragmatic structure and function.
2. How structural scoliosis alters normal structure and function of ventilation.
3. The effects of hyperinflation on the chest wall and on the efficiency of respiratory muscle function.

. . . .

Introduction

The thorax and chest wall have a variety of important functions. Probably the two most important functions are ventilation of the lungs and protection of the heart, lungs, and viscera. Another important function is the provision of a stable base for the attachment of muscles of the upper extremities, the head and neck, the vertebral column, and the pelvis. As optimal ventilation of the lungs is of vital importance, the following chapter will focus on the ventilatory mechanism.

General Structure and Function

Optimal ventilation of the lungs is essential to the functioning of the human body. The process of inspiration and expiration depends on the extraordinary and complex set of musculoskeletal and kinesiologic interrelationships of the chest wall. The ventilatory bellows, as the entire mechanism is sometimes called, involves some 88 joints and more than 46 muscles.[1]

The ventilatory mechanism in humans has three parts: the rib cage, the muscles of ventilation, and the abdomen[2,3] (Fig. 5–1). The coupling and interaction of these three components to produce ventilation will be examined in detail in this chapter. Examples of abnormal structure and function of ventilation will also be presented to illustrate how altered conditions can affect the biomechanics of the ventilatory system.

Rib Cage

The rib cage consists of 12 pairs of ribs, the **costal cartilages,** the thoracic vertebral mobile segments, and the **sternum.** The first through the seventh ribs are known as "true"

ribs because their cartilages attach directly to the sternum (Fig. 5–2). The 8th to 10th ribs articulate with the sternum via the costal cartilages above them. The 11th and 12th ribs are "floating" ribs; that is, they have no attachment to the sternum at all.[5] Posteriorly, the ribs articulate with the bodies and the transverse processes of the thoracic vertebrae. Anteriorly the ribs join the sternum via the costal cartilages. The sternum provides an osseous protective plate for the heart and is composed of the **manubrium,** the body, and the **xiphoid process.** The primary function of the thoracic spine and ribs and sternum is to provide protection to the vital organs. That protective role is enhanced by the limited mobility available to the thoracic spine.[4]

Articulations of the Rib Cage

The articulations that comprise the rib cage include the **manubriosternal (MS), xiphisternal**

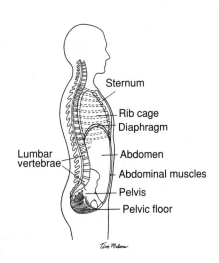

FIGURE 5–1. The chest wall.

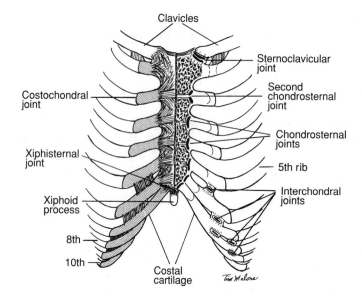

Clavicles

Costochondral joint

Xiphisternal joint

Xiphoid process

8th

10th

Costal cartilage

Tim Malone

Sternoclavicular joint

Second chondrosternal joint

Chondrosternal joints

5th rib

Interchondral joints

FIGURE 5–2. An anterior view of the articulations of the rib cage. The shaded areas indicate costal cartilage. The costal cartilages join the ribs at the CC joints. The costal cartilages of the first through the seventh ribs articulate directly with the sternum via the CS joints. The costal cartilages of the eighth through the 10th ribs articulate indirectly with the sternum through the costal cartilages of the adjacent superior rib at the interchondral joints. Interchondral joints may also exist between the fifth through the ninth costal cartilages. The MS joint has a fibrocartilaginous disk between the hyaline cartilage-covered joint surfaces of the manubrium and sternum.

(XS), **costovertebral (CV)**, **costotransverse (CT)**, **costochondral (CC)**, **chondrosternal (CS)**, and the **interchondral** joints (see Fig. 5–2).

Manubriosternal and Xiphisternal Joints

The MS joint is a synchondrosis; that is, a joint with a fibrocartilaginous disk between the hyaline cartilage-covered articulating ends of the manubrium and sternum. The MS joint is so similar to the symphysis pubis of the pelvis that some authors refer to it as the "symphysis sterni."[6] Ossification of the joint occurs in approximately 10% of older adults. In approximately one-third of adult women and elderly adults, a synovial-lined joint cavity is present secondary to resorption of the central portion of the disk.[6,7] This phenomenon has been linked to involvement of the MS joint in rheumatoid arthritis.[6] The XS joint is also a synchondrosis articulating the body of the sternum with the xiphoid process. This joint tends to ossify by 40 to 50 years of age.[4]

Costovertebral Joint

The typical CV joint is a synovial joint formed by the head of the rib, two adjacent vertebral bodies, and the corresponding intervertebral disk. Typical CV joints include those of the second to ninth ribs.[8,9] The head of each typical rib has two articular facets, or so-called **demifacets** that are separated by a ridge called the crest of the head.[10] The costal facets are small,

oval-shaped, and slightly convex. These demifacets are called the **superior** and **inferior costovertebral facets.** The vertebrae have corresponding facets; a **superior facet** on the inferior portion of the superior vertebra and an **inferior facet** on the thoracic vertebra that is numbered similarly to the rib. The articular surfaces of the head of the 2nd to 10th ribs fit snugly into the "angle" formed by the vertebral facets and the disk. The vertebral facets of T10 to T12 are located more posteriorly on the pedicle.[10] The 1st, 10th, 11th, and 12th ribs are atypical ribs and form articulations only with their corresponding vertebra.[4,5,7,8]

A fibrous capsule surrounds the entire articulation of each CV joint. The joint of the second to ninth ribs is divided into two cavities by the **interosseous or intra-articular ligament**.[4,7,8] This ligament extends from the crest of the head of the rib to attach to the annulus fibrosus of the intervertebral disk.[8,9] The **radiate ligament** is located within the capsule, with firm attachments to the anterolateral portion. The radiate ligament (Fig. 5–3) has three bands: the superior band that attaches to the superior vertebra, the intermediate band that attaches to the intervertebral disk, and the inferior band that attaches to the inferior vertebra.[4,5,8–11] Posteriorly, the capsular ligament merges with the posterior longitudinal ligament of the vertebral column.

The atypical CV joints of ribs 1st and 10th to 12th are more mobile than the typical CV joints because they form attachments with only one

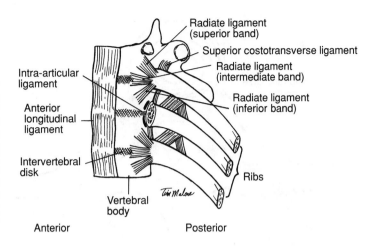

FIGURE 5–3. A lateral view of the CV joints and ligaments. The three bands of the radiate ligament reinforce the CV joints. The superior and inferior bands of the radiate ligament attach to the capsular ligament (removed) and to the vertebral body. The intermediate band attaches to the intervertebral disk. In the middle of the figure, the CV joint is shown with the radiate ligament bands removed to demonstrate the intra-articular ligament that attaches the head of the rib to the annulus.

vertebra. The interosseous ligament is absent in these joints; therefore, they have only one cavity.[8] The radiate ligament is present in these joints, however, and has a superior band that attaches to the superior vertebra. Both rotation and gliding motions occur at all of the CV joints.[11,12]

Costotransverse Joint

The CT joint is formed by the articulation of the costal tubercle of the rib with a costal facet on the transverse process of the corresponding vertebra[8] (Fig 5–4). The CT joints are present from the T1 to T10 vertebrae and the 1st to 10th ribs. The CT is a synovial joint and is surrounded by a thin, fibrous capsule. The upper CT joints contain a slightly concave costal facet and a slightly convex costal tubercle. This

provides for slight rotation movements between these segments. From approximately T7 through T10, both articular surfaces are flat, and gliding motions predominate. Three major ligaments support the CT joint capsule: the **lateral costotransverse ligament,** the **costotransverse ligament,** and the **superior costotransverse ligament** (Fig 5–5). The lateral costotransverse ligament is a short, stout band located between the lateral portion of the costal tubercle and the tip of the corresponding transverse process.[8,9,12] The costotransverse ligament is comprised of short fibers that run within the costotransverse foramen between the neck of the rib posteriorly and the transverse process at the same level.[8,9] The superior costotransverse ligament runs from the crest of the neck of the rib to the inferior border of the cranial transverse process.

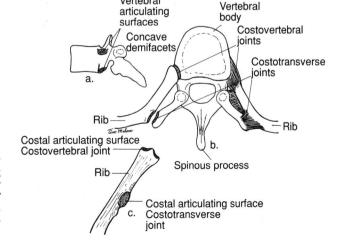

FIGURE 5–4. CV and CT joints. (a) Lateral view of a thoracic vertebra showing the articulating surfaces of the CV joints. (b) Posterior-superior view of a vertebra showing paired CV and CT joints. Joint capsules and ligaments have been removed on the left to show the articulating surfaces. (c) The articulating surfaces on the rib.

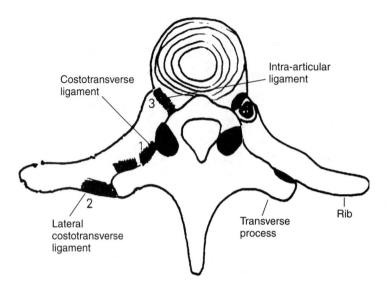

FIGURE 5–5. Ligaments supporting the costotransverse joint, including (1) the costotransverse ligament, (2) the lateral costotransverse ligament, and (3) the interosseous ligaments. (Reprinted with permission from Dos Winkel: Diagnosis and Treatment of the Spine, Figure 5-5, p 398, ©1996, Aspen Publishers, Gaithersburg, Md.)

Costochondral and Chondrosternal Joints

The first through seventh ribs articulate anteriolaterally with costal cartilages forming the CC joints. The CC joints are synchondroses surrounded by periosteum.[10] The CC joints have no ligamentous support.

The costal cartilages of ribs attach anteriorly to the sternum forming the CS joint. The costal cartilages of the first, sixth, and seventh ribs attach to the sternum via a synchondrosis. The cartilage of each of the second to fifth ribs attaches to the sternum via a synovial joint. A capsule continuous with the periosteum supports the connection of the cartilage of the first through seventh ribs as a whole.[8] Ligamentous support for the capsule includes anterior and posterior radiate ligaments.[11] Grieve also describes a **costoxiphoid ligament** of the CS joints.[4] An intra-articular ligament similar to the intra-articular ligament of the CV joint (see Fig. 5–2) always divides the second CS joint.[4,8,11] This ligament may or may not be present in other CS connections.[8] The CS joint may be obliterated with aging.[5]

In summary, the 1st to 10th ribs articulate posteriorly with the vertebral column by two synovial joints (the CV and CT joints) and anteriorly through the costocartilage with the manubriosternum. The joints, therefore, form a closed kinematic chain where the segments are interdependent and motion is restricted. The 11th and 12th ribs, however, form an open kinematic chain and the motion is less restricted.

Interchondral Joints

The 6th through the 10th (and sometimes 11th) costal cartilages articulate with the cartilage immediately above them. For the 8th to 10th ribs, this articulation forms the only connection to the sternum, albeit indirect (see Fig. 5–2). The interchondral joints are synovial joints and are supported by a capsular ligament and interchondral ligament.[8] The interchondral articulations, like the CS joints, tend to become fibrous and fuse in old age.

Kinematics of the Ribs and Manubriosternum

The movements of the ribs are an amazing combination of complex geometrics governed by the types and angles of the articulations, the movement of the manubriosternum, and the contribution of the elasticity of the costal cartilages. A controversy exists in the literature regarding the mechanisms and types of motions that are actually occurring for each rib, especially regarding the axis of motion at the CV and CT joints.[12,13]

Investigators generally agree regarding the structure and motion of the first rib. The first costal cartilage is stiffer than the rest. Also, the first CS joint is cartilaginous, not synovial, and therefore is firmly attached to the manubrium and permits relatively little movement there. The first rib articulates at the CV joint with a single facet, increasing mobility of that joint. During inspiration, the first rib elevates, moving superiorly and posteriorly at the CV joint.

The major controversy regarding rib motion centers on the types of motion at the CV articulations and whether or not the ribs can be deformed during inspiration/expiration. Kapandji and others believe the CV and CT joints are mechanically linked with a single axis passing through the center of both joints.[3,4,8,12] Saumarez argues that the rib is rigid and, therefore, cannot rotate about a single fixed axis but rather moves as successive rotations about a shifting axis.[13] The functional relevance of the controversy is unclear.

Following the more popular theory, the axis of motion for the 1st to 10th ribs is a common one through the center of the CV and CT joints. This axis lies nearly in the frontal plane for the upper ribs and nearly in the sagittal plane for the lower ribs (Fig. 5–6). The axis of motion for the 11th and 12th ribs passes through the CV joint only, because there is no CT joint present.

During inspiration, the ribs elevate. This elevation, when occurring in the upper ribs, causes a movement that simulates a "pump handle" due to the axis of motion lying nearly in the frontal plane. Most movement of the rib occurs at the anterior end of the rib. This "pump handle" motion with elevation increases the anteroposterior diameter of the thorax. When elevation occurs in the lower ribs, the movement of the rib simulates a "bucket handle" due to the axis of motion lying nearly in the sagittal plane.

Most of the movement of the lower ribs occurs at the lateral aspect. This "bucket handle" motion increases the transverse diameter of the thorax in the lower ribs. There is a gradual shift in the orientation of the axes of motion when moving from cephalad to caudal, therefore the intermediate ribs demonstrate qualities of both types of motion (see Fig. 5–6).[4,5,8,12,14] The 11th and 12th ribs have only one articulation with the vertebra and no anterior articulation to the sternum. This allows a significant difference in the motion that occurs at these two ribs. During ventilation, the quadratus lumborum muscle depresses and fixes these ribs to provide adequate diaphragmatic muscle tension.[4,11]

During inspiration, the sternum also rises and the costocartilage becomes more horizontal.[8] The sternum is pushed by the movement of the ribs, also increasing the anteroposterior diameter of the chest wall during inspiration. As the first rib is much shorter than the rest, the excursion of the manubrium is less than the sternum, causing movement at the manubriosternal joint.[9]

Muscles Associated with the Rib Cage

The muscles that act on the rib cage are generally referred to as the **ventilatory muscles** (Fig. 5–7).

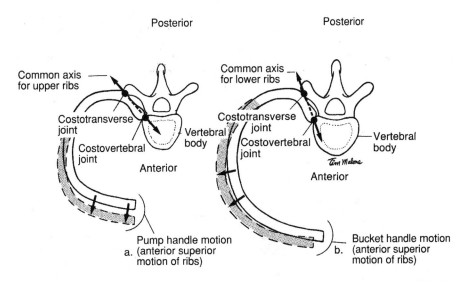

FIGURE 5–6. Axes and motions. (a) The arrow represents the common axis of motion for the upper ribs. It lies nearly in the frontal plane and passes through the centers of the CV and CT joints. The upper ribs move upward and forward in a pump handle motion. (b) The axis for the lower ribs lies closer to the sagittal plane. The upward and lateral motion of these ribs is referred to as "bucket handle motion."

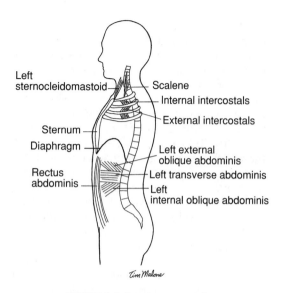

FIGURE 5–7. Respiratory muscles.

The ventilatory muscles are striated skeletal muscles that differ from other skele-tal muscles in a number of ways. The muscles of ventilation have increased fatigue resist-ance and greater oxidative capacity. They contract rhythmically throughout life rather than episodically. The ventilatory muscles work primarily against the elastic properties of the lungs and airway resistance rather than against gravitational forces. Neurologic control of these muscles is both voluntary and involuntary. Finally, the actions of these muscles are life sustaining.[2,15,16]

Any muscle that attaches to the chest wall has the potential to contribute to ventilation. The recruitment of muscles for ventilation is related to the type of breathing being performed. In quiet breathing, which occurs at rest, only the primary inspiratory muscles are needed for ventilation. During active or forced breathing, which occurs during exercise or with pulmonary pathologies, accessory muscles of both inspiration and expiration are recruited to perform the increased demand for ventilation.

The ventilatory muscles are most accurately classified as either primary or accessory muscles of ventilation. A muscle's action during the ventilatory cycle, especially the action of an accessory muscle, is neither simple nor absolute, making the categorizing of ventilatory muscles as either inspiratory muscles or expiratory muscles inaccurate and misleading.

Primary Muscles of Ventilation

The primary muscles are those recruited for quiet ventilation. These include the **diaphragm,** the **intercostals (parasternals),** and the **scalenes**.[17,18] These muscles all act on the rib cage to promote inspiration. There are no primary muscles for expiration because expiration at rest is passive.

Diaphragm

The diaphragm is the primary muscle of ventilation, accounting for approximately 70% to 80% of the inspiration during quiet breathing.[17] The diaphragm is a circular set of muscle fibers that arise from the sternum, ribs, costocartilages and vertebral bodies, and travel cephally to insert into a central tendon.[19,20] The lateral leaflets of the boomerang-shaped central tendon form the tops of the domes of the right and left hemidiaphragms (Fig. 5–8), which are innervated and supplied with blood from right and left sources, respectively. The nervous in-

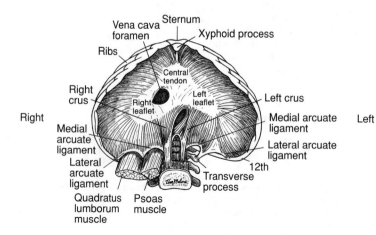

FIGURE 5–8. The diaphragm. An inferior view of the diaphragm looking up into the dome from below. The muscles (quadratus lumborum and psoas major) have been removed on the left side of the diagram to show the attachments of the medial and lateral arcuate ligaments to the transverse processes.

nervation comes from the right and left **phrenic nerves.** The blood supply comes from the right and left **internal mamillary, intercostal,** and **superior** and **inferior phrenic arteries.** Functionally, the muscular portion of the diaphragm is divided into the **costal portion,** which arises from the sternum, costocartilage and ribs, and the **crural portion,** which arises from the vertebral bodies.[21]

The costal portion of the diaphragm attaches by muscular slips to the posterior aspect of the xiphoid process and inner surfaces of the lower six ribs and their costal cartilages (Fig. 5–9).[19,20] The crural portion of the diaphragm arises from the anterolateral surfaces of the bodies and disks of L1 to L3 and from the **aponeurotic arcuate ligaments.** The **medial arcuate ligament** arches over the upper anterior part of the psoas muscles and extends from the L1 or L2 vertebral body to the transverse process of L1, L2, or L3. The **lateral arcuate ligament** covers the quadratus lumborum muscles and extends from the transverse process of L1, L2, or L3 to the 12th rib.[19,22]

The thoracoabdominal movement during quiet inspiration is a result of the pressures that are generated by the contraction of the diaphragm, the shape of the diaphragm, and angle of pull of its fibers. During **tidal breathing,** the muscle fibers of the diaphragm shorten, causing the central tendon to descend. The resultant increase in thoracic size causes a decrease in pleural pressure. This negative pleural pressure causes a decrease in intrapulmonary pressure that is responsible for inspiration. If unopposed by the scalenes and the parasternals, this negative pleural pressure and the resultant decreased intrapulmonary pressure are strong enough to cause the upper chest to collapse inward during inspiration.

The costal fibers of the diaphragm run vertically from their origin, in close apposition to the ribcage, before curving to insert into the central tendon. That portion of the diaphragm, which is close to the inner wall of the lower rib cage, is called the **zone of apposition.**[3] During tidal breathing, the descent of the dome of the diaphragm causes only a slight change in its shape, maintaining most of the zone of apposition. As the diaphragm descends, it compresses the abdominal contents, increasing intra-abdominal pressure.[22] The increased abdominal pressure is transmitted laterally via the zone of apposition causing the lower rib cage to expand (Fig. 5–10). Continued shortening of the costal fibers of the diaphragm with deeper inhalation will decrease the zone of apposition because the superior border of the zone is pulled away from the ribs toward the central tendon. As the diaphragm descends, the fibers become more horizontally aligned and further contraction no longer lifts the lower rib cage. With hyperinflation, which occurs with obstructive pulmonary disease, the fibers of

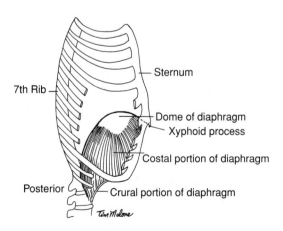

FIGURE 5–9. The diaphragm is shown in a lateral view with the intermediate ribs removed to show the dome of the diaphragm and costal attachments to the inner surfaces and costal cartilages of the lower six ribs and the xiphoid process. (Adapted from Kapandji, IA: The Physiology of the Joints, ed. 2. Churchill Livingstone, New York, 1974.)

7th Rib

Sternum

Dome of diaphragm
Xyphoid process

Costal portion of diaphragm

Posterior

Crural portion of diaphragm

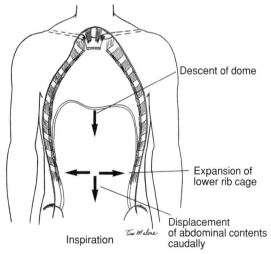

Descent of dome

Expansion of lower rib cage

Inspiration

Displacement of abdominal contents caudally

FIGURE 5–10. An anterior view of the diaphragm with the ribs removed to show the lateral motion of the ribs that accompany the descent of the diaphragm during inspiration.

the diaphragm may become so horizontally aligned that contraction of the fibers may pull the ribs inward in an expiratory direction.[23]

During diaphragmatic contraction, the abdomen becomes the fulcrum to lift the lower rib cage and rotate it outward.[2,24–26] Therefore, the compliance of the abdomen is a factor in the inspiratory movement of the thorax. Increased compliance of the abdomen, as in spinal cord injury, decreases thoracic lateral expansion during tidal breathing because there is no fulcrum available to lift the lower rib cage. Decreased compliance of the abdomen, as in pregnancy, limits diaphragmatic excursion and enhances the lateral and upward lift of the rib cage.

The crural portion of the diaphragm has a less direct inspiratory effect on the lower rib cage than the costal portion.[3,21] Indirectly, the action of the crural portion results in a descending of the central tendon, increasing intra-abdominal pressure. This increased pressure is transmitted across the apposed diaphragm to help expand the lower rib cage.[3,21]

Intercostal Muscles

The **external** and **internal intercostal muscles** are categorized as ventilatory muscles. However, only the parasternal portions of the internal intercostals are considered primary muscles of ventilation. To provide a coordinated discussion of ventilatory musculature, the entire group of intercostal muscles will be described together in this section.

The intercostal muscles connect adjacent ribs to one another and are termed **internal** or **external** intercostals depending on their anatomic orientation. The internal intercostals arise from a ridge on the inner surfaces of the 1st through 11th ribs and insert into the superior border of the rib below. The fibers of the internal intercostals lie deep to the external intercostals and run caudally and posteriorly. The external intercostals originate on the inferior borders of the 1st through 11th ribs and insert into the superior border of the rib below. The external intercostal fibers run caudally and at an oblique angle to the internal intercostals.[3,27]

The internal intercostals begin anteriorly at the chondrosternal junctions and continue dorsally to the angles of the ribs where they become the **posterior intercostal membrane.** The external intercostals begin posteriorly at the tubercles of the ribs and extend anteriorly to the costochondral junctions where they form the **anterior intercostal membrane.** Therefore, anteriorly, only the internal intercostals are present from the chondrosternal junctions to the costochondral joints. These portions of the internal intercostals are referred to as the **parasternal muscles.** Posteriorly, there are only external intercostals present from the tubercle of the ribs to the angle of the ribs. There are two layers of muscles laterally, both internal and external intercostals, which may be referred to as the **interosseous** or **lateral intercostals.**

The functions of the intercostal muscles during ventilation are intricate and controversial. In 1749, Hamberger proposed a simplistic theory that the external intercostals tend to raise the lower rib up to the higher rib, which is an inspiratory motion, and the internal intercostals tend to lower the higher rib onto the lower rib, which is an expiratory motion.[5] Recent electromyographic (EMG) studies have shown that though the external intercostals contract phasically during inspiration and the internal intercostals contract phasically during exhalation,[28] both sets of intercostal muscles may be activated during both phases of respiration as minute ventilation increases.[29] Either set of intercostal muscles can raise the rib cage from a low lung volume or lower the rib cage from a high lung volume.[30] The activation of the intercostals during the ventilatory cycle is from cephalad to caudal, meaning that the recruitment of fibers begins in the higher intercostal spaces early in inspiration and moves downward as inspiration progresses. Activation of the lower intercostals appears to occur only during deep inhalation.[31]

The parasternals, the most anterior portion of the internal intercostals, are considered primary inspiratory muscles during quiet breathing.[3,32] The action of the parasternals appears to be a rotation of the CS junctions, resulting in elevation of the ribs and descent of the sternum. The primary function of the parasternals appears to be stabilization of the ribcage.[33–35] This stabilization opposes the negative pleural pressure generated during diaphragmatic contraction, preventing a paradoxical, or inward, movement of the upper chest wall during inspiration.[35]

The kinesiology of the **interosseous intercostals** involves both ventilation and trunk rotation.[3,36,37] The interosseous intercostals, though active during the respiratory cycle, have a relatively small amount of activity compared to the parasternals and the diaphragm.[38] The interosseous intercostals play a major role in the axial rotation of the thorax. The right external intercostals and the left internal intercostals are recruited for left thoracic rotation, but are not active in right thoracic rotation. The left internal intercostals and the right external intercostals are also recruited for left thoracic rotation, but are not active in right thoracic rotation.[38]

Scalenes

The scalenes are primary muscles of quiet ventilation.[18] The scalenes attach on the transverse processes of C3 to C7 and descend to the upper borders of the first rib (scalenus anterior and medius) and second rib (scalenus posterior). Activity of the scalene muscles begins at the onset of inspiration and increases as in-spiration gets closer to total lung capacity. The length tension relationship of the scalenes allows them to generate a greater force late into the respiratory cycle when the force from the diaphragm is decreasing. Their action lifts the sternum and the first two ribs in the "pump handle" motion, an upward and outward expansion of the upper rib cage[18,24,32] The scalenes are also rib cage stabilizers. The scalenes counteract the downward pull of the parasternals on the sternum as well as the paradoxical movement of the upper chest by the negative pleural pressure of the diaphragm's contraction.

Accessory Muscles of Ventilation

The muscles that attach the rib cage to the shoulder girdle, head, or vertebral column may be classified as **accessory muscles** of ventilation. These muscles assist with inspiration or expiration in situations of stress such as exercise or disease.

When the thorax is fixed, the accessory muscles of inspiration move the vertebral column, arm, or head on the trunk. During times of increased ventilation, the latter can be fixed and the rib cage becomes the mobile segment. The accessory muscles of inspiration, therefore, increase the thoracic diameter by moving the rib cage upward and outward with reverse muscle action.[24] Some of the more commonly described accessory muscles are reported below. However, there are many more possible accessory muscles of ventilation. Many of these accessory muscles are discussed in greater detail elsewhere in this text in the context of the muscle's primary function.

The **sternocleidomastoid** runs from the manubrium and superior medial aspect of the clavicle to the mastoid process of the temporal bone. The usual bilateral action of the sternocleidomastoid is flexion of the cervical vertebrae. With a fixed cervical spine, bilateral action of the sternocleidomastoid muscles moves the rib cage superiorly, which expands the upper rib cage in the pump handle motion.

The **pectoralis major** can elevate the upper rib cage when the shoulders and the humerus are fixed. The clavicular head of the pectoralis major can be both an inspiratory or expiratory in action, depending on the position of the upper extremity. With the humeral insertion of the pectoralis major below the level of the clavicle, the muscle is an expiratory muscle, pulling the manubrium and upper ribs down. With the insertion of the pectoralis major above the level of the clavicle, such as when the arm is raised, the muscle becomes an inspiratory muscle, pulling the manubrium and upper ribs up and out.

The **pectoralis minor** can help raise the third, fourth, and fifth ribs during a forced inspiration. The **trapezius** can be helpful during active inspiration by fixing the head so that the sternocleidomastoid can function as a muscle of inspiration. The **subclavius,** a muscle between the clavicle and the first rib, usually pulls the clavicle anteriorly and caudally. With reverse action, the subclavius can assist in raising the upper chest for inspiration.

The following four muscles of the abdomen are also considered to be accessory muscles of ventilation. The **transversus abdominis** muscle attaches to the inner surface of the posterior aspect of the lower six ribs and runs circumferentially to insert in an anterior aponeurosis forming the rectus sheath. The **internal abdominal oblique** begins at the iliac crest and the inguinal ligament, running superiorly and medially to attach to the costal margin and the rectus sheath. The **external abdominal oblique** attaches to the external surfaces of the lower eight ribs with fibers running inferiorly and medially to the iliac crest, inguinal ligament, and the linea alba. The **rectus abdominis** extends from the anterior surfaces of the fifth to seventh costal cartilages and the xiphoid process to attach inferiorly to the pubis.[3,27]

The abdominals have long been considered expiratory muscles as well as trunk flexors and rotators. The major function of the abdominals with respect to ventilation is to assist with forced expiration. The muscle fibers pull the ribs and costocartilage caudally, into a motion of exhalation. By increasing intra-abdominal pressure, the abdominals can push the diaphragm upward into the thoracic cage, increasing both the volume and speed of exhalation.

The abdominals have a significant role to play in inspiration as well. The increased intra-abdominal pressure created by the abdominal muscles during exhalation forces the diaphragm cranially and exerts a passive stretch on the costal fibers of the diaphragm.[3] These changes ready the system for an optimal inspiration by optimizing the length-tension relationship of the muscle fibers of the diaphragm. During inspiration, the abdominals assist with lateral chest wall expansion by providing anterior stability to the abdomen so it may act as a fulcrum for the diaphragm action thereby maintaining the zone of apposition. In the supine position, gravity provides the anterior stability of the abdominal wall.[39] In the supine position, the abdominals are not needed and in fact, are silent on the EMG. The muscular activity of the abdominals increases during exercise as increased ventilation is needed.[3,20]

The **quadratus lumborum,** which is normally thought of as a lateral flexor of the vertebral column and a hip hiker, is an accessory muscle of expiration. The quadratus lumborum, which attaches to the 12th rib, stabilizes the diaphragm as it eccentrically contracts during phonation.[10,27,40]

The **levatores costarum** are paravertebral muscles functionally associated with the intercostal muscles. The levatores costarum lie between C7 through T11. Fibers run from the transverse processes of a vertebra to the posterior external surface of the next lower rib between the tubercle and the angle. The levatores costarum muscles assist with inspiration in the upright position as well as lateral trunk flexion.[10,27,41]

The **triangularis sterni or transversus thoracis** is a flat layer of muscle that runs deep to the parasternals. The triangularis sterni originates from the posterior surface of the caudal half of the sternum and runs cranially and laterally inserting into the inner surface of the costal cartilages of the third through the seventh ribs.[3,27] This muscle is recruited for ventilation along with the abdominals to pull the rib cage caudally. Recent studies have shown that this muscle is primarily an expiratory muscle, especially when expiration is active, as in talking, coughing, laughing or exhalation into functional residual capacity.[3,42] This muscle is inactive during rest in the supine position. The triangularis sterni muscle is active during quiet expiration in older subjects in the standing position.[43]

Coordination and Integration of Ventilatory Motions

The coordination and integration of the skeletal and muscular chest wall components during breathing are not easily understood or measured. More recent studies have used EMG techniques, electrical stimulation, and sophisticated computerized motion analysis techniques. Some analyses and descriptions of chest wall motion and muscular actions published in the 18th century are only now being questioned.[28,36,44] The intricacy of the coordinated actions of the many muscle groups involved even in quiet breathing should be apparent at this point, but the complexities have only been touched on in the above discussions. Many of the ventilatory muscles participate in activities other than ventilation, including speech, defecation, and the maintenance of posture. A high and complex level of coordination is necessary for these muscles to carry out these alternate activities while continuing to perform the necessary function of ventilation.

Normal Sequence of Chest Wall Motions During Breathing

When one observes the abdomen and chest wall of a normal, healthy person during quiet breathing, the following sequence of motion usually occurs. First, the diaphragm contracts and the central tendon moves caudally. Intra-abdominal pressure increases and abdominal contents are displaced such that the anterior epigastric abdominal wall is pushed outward. Once the central tendon is "fixed" or stabilized on the abdominal organs, the appositional, vertical fibers pull the lower ribs upward and outward resulting in lateral movement of the lower chest. Following lateral expansion, with continued inspiration, the parasternals, scalenes, and levatores costarum actively rotate the upper ribs and elevate the manubriosternum, resulting in an anterior motion of the upper chest.

The lateral and anterior motions of the chest can occur simultaneously. Expiration during quiet breathing is passive, with recoil of the elastic components of the lungs and chest wall.

Developmental Aspects of Structure and Function

Differences Associated with the Neonate

The compliance, configuration, and muscle action of the chest wall changes significantly from the infant to the elder. The healthy newborn has an extremely compliant chest wall because it is primarily cartilaginous. The cartilaginous ribs allow the distortion necessary for the infant's thorax to travel through the birth canal. The increased compliance of the rib cage is at the expense of thoracic stability, making the infant's chest wall muscles primarily stabilizers of the thorax to counteract the negative pleural pressure of the diaphragm during inspiration. Complete ossification of the ribs does not occur for several months after birth.

The rib cage of an infant shows a more horizontal alignment of the ribs, rather than the elliptical shape of an older child or adult. This configuration of the infant's rib cage alters the angle of insertion of the costal fibers of the diaphragm, the orientation being more horizontal than vertical. There is an increased tendency for these fibers to pull the lower ribs inward, thereby decreasing efficiency of ventilation and increasing distortion of the chest wall.[45–47] Only 20% of the muscle fibers of the diaphragm are fatigue-resistent fibers in the healthy newborn compared to 50% in adults. This discrepancy predisposes infants to earlier diaphragmatic fatigue.[48]

Accessory muscles of ventilation are also at a disadvantage in the infant. Until infants can stabilize their upper extremities, head, and spine, it is difficult for the accessory muscles to produce the reverse action needed to be helpful in ventilation.

Differences Associated with the Elderly

Skeletal changes that occur with aging may affect pulmonary function. The costal cartilages ossify, which interferes with their axial rotation.[12] Many of the articulations of the chest wall undergo fibrosis with advancing age. The interchrondral and costochondral joints fibrose with increasing age, the chondrosternal joints may be obliterated with age, and the xiphosternal junction usually ossifies after approximately age 40. Other chest wall articulations, which are true synovial joints, can undergo morphologic changes associated with aging resulting in reduced mobility. Overall chest wall compliance is significantly reduced with age. Reduction in diaphragm-abdomen compliance has also been reported and is at least partially related to the decreased rib cage compliance, especially the lower ribs which are part of the zone of apposition.[49]

The resting position of the thorax depends on the balance between the elastic recoil properties of the lungs pulling inward and the outward pull of the rib cage. With increased age, the lung tissue decreases in elasticity. The reduced recoil property of the lung tissue allows the thorax to rest in a more inspiratory position; that is, an increased anteroposterior diameter of the rib cage. An increased kyphosis is often observed in older individuals, decreasing the mobility of the thoracic spine and rib cage.

The results of these skeletal and tissue changes are an increase in the functional residual capacity and a decrease in inspiratory capacity of the thorax. Functionally, the changes result in more air being left in the thorax at the end of a resting exhalation, a decreased capacity for "new" air for gas exchange, and a decrease in the ventilatory reserve available during times of need, such as during an illness or exercise.

Skeletal muscles of ventilation of the elder have a documented loss of strength, fewer muscle fibers, a lower oxidative capacity, decrease in the number or the size of fast-twitch type II fibers, and a lengthening of the time to peak tension.[50–52] The ventilatory muscles become more energy expensive with age. The resting position of the diaphragm becomes less domed with a decrease in abdominal tone in aging.[12] In summary, there is a decreased compliance of the bony rib cage, an increased compliance of the lung tissue, and an over-all decreased compliance of the respiratory system.

Changes in Normal Structure and Function

This section will briefly present examples of how the structure and function of the healthy chest wall are altered by various conditions.

The examples represent problems of the musculoskeletal and respiratory systems.

Pregnancy

Pregnancy is not considered a pathologic state, but pregnancy results in an alteration of every organ system within the woman's body.[53] The effects of pregnancy on the biomechanics of the chest wall are apparent during the second half of the pregnancy, especially during the last trimester. Progressive uterine distension repositions the diaphragm cephalad with a resultant increased chest circumference. Research to date supports the theory that the augmented rib cage measurements occur due to (1) an enhanced diaphragmatic contraction secondary to an improved length-tension relationship and (2) an increased area of diaphragmatic apposition to the lower rib cage created by the elevation of the diaphragm. The increased intra-abdominal pressure that is created during the enhanced diaphragmatic contraction is then transmitted through the zone of apposition to increase the lateral expansion and elevation of the lower rib cage.[54,55] During pregnancy, there is a measurable decrease in functional residual capacity, although vital capacity does not change.

Scoliosis

Structural scoliosis is an example of a musculoskeletal abnormality that can affect chest wall biomechanics and, therefore, ventilation. Although cervical and lumbar curves may cause some changes in ventilation, thoracic curves can result in a marked limitation to ventilation. The amount of ventilatory compromise is related to the severity of the curve.

In scoliosis, the bodies of the thoracic vertebrae rotate. On the side of the convexity, the transverse processes of the vertebrae move posteriorly carrying the ribs with them. This causes the classic posterior rib hump of scoliosis. As the ribs are torsioned posteriorly, the intercostal space is widened. On the concave side of the scoliotic curve, the effects are just the opposite. The transverse processes of the vertebrae move anteriorly, bringing the articulated ribs forward. The ribs are now approximated with each other, narrowing intercostal spaces (see Fig. 4–31). If these changes are severe enough, the axes of rotation of the ribs will move as well, affecting the efficiency of the in-

tercostal muscles and other ventilatory muscles, and will reduce rib cage compliance. These abnormalities will restrict lung function and can eventually lead to decreased lung volumes and capacities.[11]

Chronic Obstructive Pulmonary Disease

A major manifestation of chronic obstructive pulmonary disease (COPD) is hyperinflation of the lungs due to destruction of the alveolar walls. The resting position of the thorax depends on the balance between the elastic recoil properties of the lungs pulling inward and the outward pull of the rib cage. As tissue destruction occurs with disease, the elastic recoil property of the lung is lessened. More air (hyperinflation) is now housed within the lungs at the end of exhalation. The resting position of the thorax has changed from the usual position of exhalation to a position more characteristic of the inspiratory cycle. A more barreled shape of the thorax is seen at rest. Hyperinflation affects not only the bony components of the chest wall, but also the muscles of the thorax. The resting position of the diaphragm changes to a more flattened configuration, again changed from the usual position of exhalation; that is, highly domed, to a position in the inspiratory cycle or flattened. The angle of pull of the diaphragm fibers becomes more horizontal with a decreased zone of apposition and decreased strength and range of contraction. In severe cases of hyperinflation, the fibers of the diaphragm will be aligned horizontally. Contraction of this very flattened diaphragm will pull the lower rib cage inward, actually working against lung inflation[23] (Fig. 5–11).

In hyperinflation, the barreled elevated thorax puts the sternocleidomastoids in a shortened position, making them much less efficient. In the severely hyperinflated chest, the diaphragm has very little available range of motion. The majority of inspiration is now performed by accessory muscles, particularly the parasternals and the scalenes. These muscles are able to generate a greater force as the lungs approach total lung capacity, therefore, hyperinflation has a far less dramatic effect on them.[56] The upper rib cage is pulled upward and outward. The diaphragm has a very limited ability to push the abdominal contents down so the forceful cranial pull of the upper rib cage effectively pulls the diaphragm and the ab-

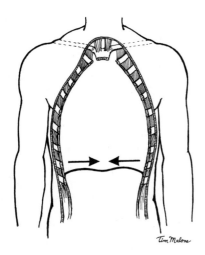

FIGURE 5–11. Contraction of the diaphragm flattened by hyperinflation pulls the lower rib cage inward.

dominal contents upward, under the rib cage.[57] This paradoxical thorocoabdominal breathing pattern (the abdomen is pulled inward and upward during inspiration and is pushed out and down during exhalation) is a reflection of the maintained effectiveness of the upper inspiratory rib cage musculature and the reduced effectiveness of the diaphragm.[58]

The disadvantages of these biomechanical alterations of hyperinflation are compounded by the increased demand for ventilation in COPD. More work is required of a less effective system. The energy cost of ventilation, or the work of breathing, in COPD is markedly increased.

Summary

In this chapter, comprehensive coverage of the structure and function of the bony thorax and the ventilatory muscles has been provided. Additional information on the structure and function of accessory muscles of ventilation will be presented in Chapter 7. Scoliosis is presented in greater depth in Chapter 13.

REFERENCES

1. Hoppenfeld, S: Physical Examination of the Spine and Extremities. Appleton-Century-Crofts, New York, 1976.
2. Derenne, JPH, Macklem, PT, and Roussos, CH: State of the art: The respiratory muscles: Mechanics, control and pathophysiology. Am Rev Respir Dis 118:119–133, 1978.
3. DeTroyer, A, and Estenne, M: Functional anatomy of the respiratory muscles. Clin Chest Med 9:175–193, 1988.
4. Grieve, GP: Common Vertebral Joint Problems, ed 2. Churchill Livingstone, New York, 1988, pp 32–39, 110–129.
5. Williams, PL, and Warwick, R (eds): Gray's Anatomy, ed 37. Churchill Livingstone, New York, 1989, pp 496–499, 591–595.
6. Kormano, M: A microradiographic and histological study of the manubriosternal joint in rheumatoid arthritis. Acta Rheum Scand 16:47–59, 1970.
7. Fam, AG, and Smythe, HA: Musculoskeletal chestwall pain. Can Med Assoc J 133:379–389, 1985.
8. Winkel, D: Diagnosis and Treatment of the Spine. Aspen, Gaithersburg, MD, 1996, pp 393–401.
9. Stockwell, RA: Joints. In Romanes, GJ (ed): Cunningham's Textbook of Anatomy, ed 12, Oxford University Press, Oxford 1981, pp 226–228.
10. Harrison, RJ: Bones. In Romanes, GJ (ed): Cunningham's Textbook of Anatomy, ed 12, Oxford University Press, Oxford, 1981, pp 103–108.
11. Schafer, RC: Clinical Biomechanics: Musculoskeletal Actions and Reactions. Williams & Wilkins, Baltimore, 1983, pp 328–374.
12. Kapandji, IA: The Physiology of the Joints, ed 2. Churchill Livingstone, New York, 1974, pp 130–163.
13. Saumarez, RC: An analysis of possible movements of human upper rib cage. J Appl Physiol 60:678–689, 1986.
14. Wilson, TA, et al: Geometry and respiratory displacement of human ribs. J Appl Physiol 62:1872–1877, 1987.
15. Rochester, DF, and Braun, NM: The respiratory muscles. Basics Respir Dis 6:1–6, 1978.
16. Edwards, RHT: The diaphragm as a muscle: Mechanisms underlying fatigue. Am Rev Respir Dis 119:81–84, 1979.
17. Tobin, MJ: Respiratory muscles in disease. Clin Chest Med 9:263–286, 1988.
18. DeTroyer, A, and Estenne, M: Coordination between rib cage muscles and diaphragm during quiet breathing in humans. J Appl Physiol 57:899–906, 1984.
19. Panicek, DM, et al: The diaphragm: Anatomic, pathologic and radiographic considerations. Radiographics 8:385–425, 1988.
20. Celli, BR: Clinical and physiologic evaluation of respiratory muscle function. Clin Chest Med 10:199–214, 1989.
21. DeTroyer, A, et al: The diaphragm: Two muscles. Science 217:237–238, 1981.
22. Deviri, E, Nathan, H, and Luchansky, E: Medial and lateral arcuate ligaments of the diaphragm: Attachment to the transverse process. Anat Anz 166:63–67, 1988.
23. Reid, WD, and Dechman, G: Considerations when testing and training the respiratory muscles. Phys Ther 75:971–982, 1995.
24. Celli, BR: Respiratory muscle function. Clin Chest Med 7:567–584, 1986.
25. Epstein, S: An overview of respiratory muscle function. Clin Chest Med 15: 619–638, 1994.
26. DeTroyer, A, et al: Action of the costal and crural parts of the diaphragm on the rib cage in dog. J Appl Physiol 53:30–39, 1982.
27. Gardner, E, Gray, DJ, and O'Rahilly, R: Anatomy: A Regional Study of Human Structure, ed 3. WB Saunders, Philadelphia, 1969, pp 286–297.
28. DeTroyer, A, Kelly, S, and Zin, WA: Mechanical action of the intercostal muscles on the ribs. Science 220:87–88, 1983.
29. LeBars, P, and Duron, B: Are the external and internal intercostal muscles synergistic or antagonistic in the cat? Neurosci. Lett 51:383–386, 1984.

30. Van Luneren, E: Respiratory muscle coordination. J Lab Clin Med 112:285–300, 1988.
31. Keopke, GH, et al: Sequence of action of the diaphragm and intercostal muscles during respiration. I. Inspiration. Arch Phys Med Rehabil 39:426–430, 1958.
32. DeTroyer, A: Actions of the respiratory muscles or how the chest wall moves in upright man. Bull Eur Physiopathol Respir 20:409–413, 1984.
33. DeTroyer, A, and Heilporn, A: Respiratory mechanics in quadraplegia. The respiratory function of the intercostal muscles. Am Rev Respir Dis 122:591–600, 1980.
34. Macklem, PT, Macklem, DM, and DeTroyer, A: A model of inspiratory muscle mechanics. J Appl Physiol 55:547–557, 1983.
35. Cala, SJ, et al: Respiratory ultrasonography of human parasternal intercostal muscles in vivo. Ultrasound Med Biol 24:313–326, 1998.
36. DeTroyer, A, et al: Mechanics of intercostal space and actions of external and internal intercostal muscles. J Clin Invest 75:850–857, 1985.
37. Rimmer, KP, Ford, GT, and Whitelaw WA: Interaction between postural and respiratory control of human intercostal muscles. J Appl Physiol 79:1556–1561, 1995.
38. Whitelaw, WA, et al: Intercostal muscles are used during rotation of the thorax in humans. J Appl Physiol 72:1940–1944, 1992.
39. Massery, M: The patient with neuromuscular or musculoskeletal dysfunction. In Frownfelter, DL, and Dean, E (eds): Principles and Practice of Cardiopulmonary Physical Therapy. Mosby, St Louis, 1996, pp 679–702.
40. Basmajian, JV: Muscles Alive: Their Functions by Electromyograph, ed 2. Williams & Wilkins, Baltimore, 1967, p 303.
41. Goldman, MD, Loh, L, and Sears, TA: The respiratory activity of human levator costal muscle and its modification by posture. J Physiol 362:189–204, 1985.
42. DeTroyer, A, et al: Triangularis sterni muscle use in supine humans. J Appl Physiol 62:919–925, 1987.
43. Estenne, M, Ninane, V, and DeTroyer, A: Triangularis sterni muscle use during eupnea in humans: Effect of posture. Respir Physiol 74:151–162, 1988.
44. Hamberger, GE: De respirationis mechanismo et usu genuino. Jena, Germany, 1749.
45. Crane, LD: Physical therapy for the neonate with respiratory dysfunction. In Irwin, S, and Tecklin, JS (eds): Cardiopulmonary Physical Therapy, ed 2. CV Mosby, St Louis, 1990, pp 389–415.
46. Muller, NL, and Bryan, AC: Chest wall mechanics and respiratory muscles in infants. Pediatr Clin North Am 26:503, 1979.
47. Krumpe, PE, et al: The aging respiratory system. Clin Geriatr Med 1:143–175, 1985.
48. Davis, GM, and Bureau, MA: Pulmonary and chest wall mechanics in the control of respiration in the newborn. Clin Perinatol 14:551–579, 1987.
49. Estenne, M, Yernault, JC, and DeTroyer, A: Rib cage and diaphragm-abdomen compliance in humans: Effects of age and posture. J Appl Physiol 59:1942–1848, 1985.
50. Grimby, G, et al: Morphology and enzymatic capacity in arm and leg muscles in 78–81 year old men and women. Acta Physiol Scand 115:125–134, 1982.
51. Makrides, L, et al: Maximal short-term exercise capacity in healthy subjects aged 15–70 years. Clin Sci 69:197–205, 1985.
52. Grimby, G, and Saltin, B: The aging muscle. Clin Physiol 3:209–218, 1983.
53. Wilder, E (ed): Obstetrics and gynecologic physical therapy. Clin Phys Ther 20:1–225, 1988.
54. Artal, R, and Wiswell, RA (eds): Exercise in Pregnancy. Williams & Wilkins, Baltimore, 1986, pp 147–148.
55. Gilroy, RJ, Mangura, BT, and Lavetes, MH: Ribcage and abdominal volume displacements during breathing in pregnancy. Am Rev Respir Dis 137:668–672, 1988.
56. Decramer, M: Hyperinflation and respiratory muscle interaction. Eur Respir J 10:934–941, 1997.
57. Camus, P, and Desmeules, M: Chest wall movements and breathing pattern at different lung volumes (abstract). Chest 82:243, 1982.
58. De Troyer, A: Respiratory muscle function in chronic obstructive pulmonary disease. In Cassabury, R, and Petty, T (eds): Principles and Practice of Pulmonary Rehabilitation. WB Saunders, Philadelphia, 1995.

Study Questions

1. Describe the articulations of the chest wall and thorax, including the CV, CT, CC, CS interchondral, and MS joints.
2. What is the normal sequence of chest wall motions during breathing? Explain why these motions occur.
3. What is transdiaphragmatic pressure?
4. What is the role of the following during breathing: the diaphragm, the intercostal muscles, and the abdominal muscles?
5. Describe the "accessory" muscles and explain their functions.
6. Compare the action of the paravertebral muscles with that of the scalene muscles.
7. What effect does COPD have on the inspiratory muscles?
8. How does the aging process affect the structure and function of the chest wall?

CHAPTER 6

THE TEMPOROMANDIBULAR JOINT

OBJECTIVES
Following the study of this chapter, the reader should be able to:

Describe
1. The articular surfaces of the temporomandibular (TM) joint.
2. The structure and function of the disk.
3. The structure and function of the ligaments of the TM joint.
4. The movement available at the TM joint.
5. The motions of the disk and condyle necessary for normal mouth opening and closing.
6. The significance of two articulations of the mandible.
7. The muscular control necessary for normal TM joint motion.
8. The joint structures that provide stability for the TM joint.
9. The characteristics of the cartilage covering the articular surfaces of the mandible and temporal bone.
10. The normal rest position of the mandible.
11. The effect of dentition on the function of the TM joint.
12. The effect of symmetrical and asymmetrical condylar motion on mandibular deviation during mouth opening and closing.

Locate
1. The attachments of selected muscles of the TM joint.

Differentiate
1. Between the motions available in the upper and lower joint compartments of the TM joint.

2. Between structures that have a passive effect on the function of the TM joint and those that have an active or elastic effect on the joint.

Predict

1. The deviations of the jaw that would be present with various internal derangements of the joint structures.

Introduction

The **temporomandibular (TM) joint** is unique in the body. The mandible is a horseshoe-shaped bone that has an articulation with the temporal bone at each end, giving it two completely separate but solidly connected joints. In addition to the two separate articulations, each TM joint has a disk that separates the TM joint into an upper and a lower joint. Therefore, mandibular movement affects four distinct joints with any motion.

Each TM joint is formed by the articulation of the **condyle** (or **head**) **of the mandible** with the **articular eminence of the temporal bone** and an interposed **articular disk.** The joint formed by the mandibular condyle and the inferior surface of the disk is a hinge joint. The joint formed by the articular eminence and the superior surface of the disk is a plane or gliding joint. Sicher[1] and Hylander[2] describe the joint as a hinge joint with movable sockets. The TM joint is a synovial joint, although there is no hyaline cartilage covering the articular surfaces. Rather, the surfaces are covered by dense collagenous tissue that is considered to be fibrocartilage.

Functionally the TM joint is also unique. Few other joints are moved as often as the TM joint. In addition to the motions of eating or chewing that can create great force within the joint, speaking and swallowing require TM joint motion that is finely controlled and requires little force. The TM joint exhibits a combination of complexity, close-to-continuous use, and capacity for force and finesse that is remarkable.

Structure

Articular Surfaces

The mandible is the "distal" or moving segment of the TM joint. It is divided into a body and two rami (Fig. 6–1). The angle of the jaw is where the body and the ramus join. The mandibular condyles are located at the end of the ramus at its most posterosuperior aspect. Each condyle protrudes medially 15 to 20 mm from the ramus[1–4] (Fig. 6–2). The portion of the condyle that can be palpated just in front of the external auditory meatus of the ear is the lateral pole. The medial pole is deep and cannot be palpated. However, the condyles can be palpated if you put your finger tips into the external auditory meatus of the ear and push anteriorly.[5] If you open and close your jaw, you will feel the movement of the mandibular condyles in front of your fingers. Lines following the axis of medial-lateral poles of each condyle will intersect just anterior to the foramen magnum.[1,6] The anterior portion of the condyle is composed of trabecular bone and is the articular portion of the condyle.[7,8]

Also on the mandible is another projection located anterior to the condyle. This is the **coronoid process** (see Fig. 6–1). In the closed-mouth position, the coronoid process sits under the zygomatic arch, but it can be palpated below the arch when the mouth is open. The coronoid process serves as an attachment for the **temporalis muscle.**

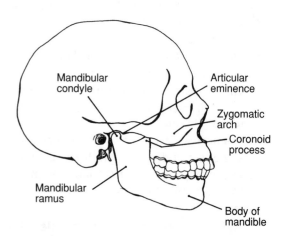

FIGURE 6–1. Lateral view of cranium and mandible. (Modified from Perry, JF, Rohe, DA, and Garcia, OA: The Kinesiology Workbook. FA Davis, Philadelphia, 1991, p 162, with permission.)

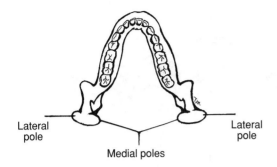

FIGURE 6–2. A superior view of the mandible (removed from the skull) shows the medial and lateral poles of the mandibular condyles.

The "proximal" or stationary segment of the TM joint is the temporal bone. The condyles of the mandible sit in the **glenoid fossa** of the temporal bone. The glenoid fossa is located between the **posterior glenoid spine** and the **articular eminence** of the temporal bone (Figs. 6–1 and 6–3). The glenoid fossa, on superficial inspection, looks like the articular surface for the TM joint. On closer inspection, the bone in that area is thin and translucent and not at all appropriate for an articular surface.[1,2,4,5] The articular eminence, however, has a major area of trabecular bone and serves as the primary articular surface for the TM joint.[8]

The articular surfaces of the condyle and the articular eminence of the temporal bone are covered with dense, avascular collagenous tissue that contains some cartilaginous cells.[1,3–5,7–9] Because some of the cells are cartilaginous, the covering is often referred to as fibrocartilage.[3–5,7] The greatest amount of fibrocartilage is found on the articular eminence and the anteriosuperior aspect of the condyle, providing further evidence that these are the primary areas of articulation.[3,5,6,8] The articular collagen fibers are aligned perpendicular to the bony surface in the deeper layers to withstand stresses. The fibers near the

surface of the articular covering are aligned in a parallel arrangement to facilitate gliding of the joint surfaces.[3] The presence of fibrocartilage rather than hyaline cartilage is significant because fibrocartilage can repair and remodel.[3,5,6] Typically, fibrocartilage is present in areas that are intended to withstand repeated and high-level stress. The repetitive stress of jaw motions is added to the tremendous bite forces that have been measured at 597 N for women and 847 N for men.[10] The fibrocartilage TM joint surfaces help withstand stress and are amenable to some degree of repair. The articular disk of the TM joint, however, does not possess this capability.[11]

Articular Disk

The articular disk of the TM joint is biconcave; that is, both its superior and inferior surfaces are concave. The disk of the TM joint allows the convex surface of the condyle and the convex surface of the articular eminence (see Fig. 6–3) to remain congruent throughout the motion available to the joint.[3,11] The disk is firmly attached to the medial and lateral poles of the condyle of the mandible, but not to the joint capsule medially or laterally.[1–3,5,11] This allows the disk to rotate around the condyle quite freely in an anterior-posterior direction. Anteriorly, the disk is attached to the joint capsule and to the tendon of the **lateral pterygoid muscle** (see Fig. 6–3). The anterior attachments restrict posterior translation of the disk. Posteriorly, the disk is attached to a complex structure, the components of which are collectively called the **bilaminar retrodiskal pad.** The two bands (or laminae) of the bilaminar retrodiskal pad are each attached anteriorly to the disk (Fig. 6–4c). The superior lamina is attached posteriorly to the tympanic plate (at the posterior glenoid fossa).[3,12] The superior lamina is made of elastic fibers that allow the superior band to

FIGURE 6–3. Lateral view of TM joint showing attachments of capsule and disk. (Modified from Perry, JF, Rohe, DA, and Garcia, OA: The Kinesiology Workbook. FA Davis, Philadelphia, 1991, p 163, with permission.)

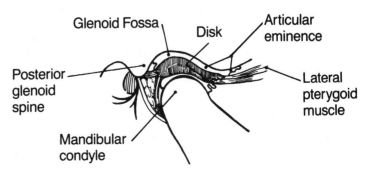

Glenoid Fossa

Disk

Articular eminence

Posterior glenoid spine

Lateral pterygoid muscle

Mandibular condyle

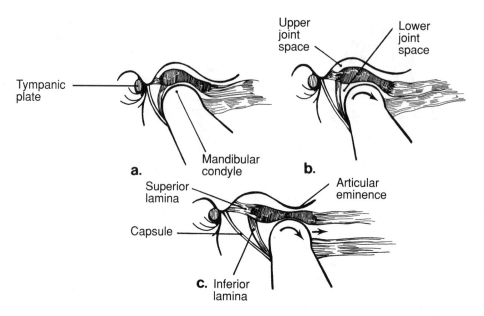

FIGURE 6–4. Lateral view of TM joint. (Modified from Perry, JF, Rohe, DA, and Garcia, OA: The Kinesiology Workbook. FA Davis, Philadelphia, 1991, p 163, with permission.)

stretch. The superior lamina allows the disk to translate anteriorly along the articular eminence during mouth opening; its elastic properties assist in repositioning the disk posteriorly during mouth closing. The inferior lamina is attached to the neck of the condyle and is inelastic. The inferior lamina simply serves as a tether on the disk, limiting forward translation, but does not assist with repositioning the disk during mouth closing.[3,11] Neither of the lamina of the retrodiskal pad are under tension when the TM joint is at rest. Between the two lamina is loose areolar connective tissue rich in arterial and neural supply.[1–5,8,11]

The articular disk varies in thickness from 2 mm anteriorly to 3 mm posteriorly to 1 mm in the middle[3] (Fig. 6–4a). This arrangement allows the disk to adapt to the bony surfaces with which it articulates and creates greater congruence of the joint surfaces.[3] The anterior and posterior portions of the disk are vascular and innervated; the middle band, however, is avascular and not innervated.[3,7,9,11] The lack of vascularity and innervation is consistent with the observation that the middle portion is the force-accepting surface of the disk.

Capsule and Ligaments

The TM joint capsule is not as well defined as many joint capsules. According to *Gray's*

Anatomy,[9] the joint is supported by short capsular fibers running from the temporal bone to the disk and from the disk to the neck of the condyle. The portion of the capsule above the disk is quite loose, whereas the portion of the capsule below the disk is tight.[9] Consequently, the disk is more firmly attached to the condyle below and freer to move on the articular eminence above. The capsule is quite thin and loose in its anterior, medial, and posterior aspects, but the lateral aspect is stronger and is reinforced with long fibers (temporal bone to condyle)[9] (Fig. 6–4c). The lack of strength of the capsule anteriorly and the incongruence of the bony articular surfaces predisposes the joint to anterior dislocation of the mandibular condyle.[1] The capsule is highly vascularized and innervated, allowing it to provide a great deal of information about position and movement.

The primary ligaments of the TM joint are the **temporomandibular (TM) ligament,** the **stylomandibular ligament,** and the **sphenomandibular ligament.** The TM ligament is a strong ligament that is composed of two parts (Fig. 6–5). The outer oblique portion attaches to the neck of the condyle and the articular eminence. It serves as a suspensory ligament and limits downward and posterior motion of the mandible, as well as limiting rotation of the condyle during mouth opening.[3,7] The inner portion of the ligament is attached to the lat-

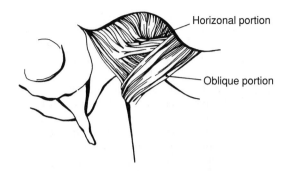

FIGURE 6–5. Temporomandibular ligament.

eral pole of the condyle and posterior portion of the disk and to the articular eminence. Its fibers are almost horizontal and resist posterior motion of the condyle. Limitation of posterior translation of the condyle protects the retrodiskal pad.[3] Neither of the bands of the TM ligament limit forward translation of the condyle or disk, but they do limit lateral displacement.[12]

The stylomandibular ligament is a band of deep cervical fascia that runs from the styloid process of the temporal bone to the posterior border of the ramus of the mandible (Fig. 6–6). It inserts between the **masseter** and the **medial pterygoid** muscles.[3] Abe and colleagues[13] state that the stylomandibular ligament also has continuity with the disk medially. Its function is uncertain[9] with some authors indicating that it limits protrusion of the jaw,[2,3,7] another indicating that it draws the disk posteriorly during closing,[13] and others stating that it has no function.[1,14,15]

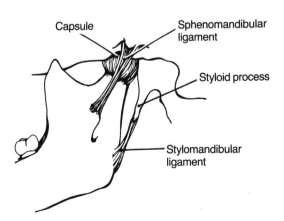

FIGURE 6–6. Capsule, sphenomandibular, and stylomandibular ligaments.

The sphenomandibular ligament attaches to the spine of the sphenoid bone and to the middle surface of the ramus of the mandible (see Fig. 6–6). Some authors state that it serves to suspend the mandible[16] and to check the mandible from excessive forward translation.[2,7,11] Other authors, however, state that it has no function.[9,14,15]

Joint Articulation

The disk divides the TM joint into two separate joint spaces (see Fig. 6–4b). The upper joint is the larger of the two. Each joint has its own synovial lining. The nutrition of the fibrocartilage covering the joint surfaces and the avascular middle portion of the disk is provided by the synovial fluid. Intermittent pressure on these collagenous structures during joint motion causes the synovial fluid to be pumped in and out of them, providing their nutrition.

Lower Joint

The lower joint of the TM joint, a hinge joint, is formed by the anterior surface of the condyle of the mandible and the inferior surface of the articular disk. The condyle and disk are firmly attached at the medial and lateral poles of the condyle. These attachments allow free rotation of the disk on the condyle or the condyle under the disk around an axis through both poles of the condyle. Although the condyle of the mandible is free to rotate anteriorly on the disk (or the disk to rotate posteriorly on the condyle), the firm medial and lateral attachments between the disk and condyle cause the two to translate forward (glide) together as a unit, with minimal translation available between the two structures.

Upper Joint

The upper joint of the TM joint, a gliding joint, is formed by the articular eminence of the temporal bone and the superior surface of the articular disk. The loose attachment of the disk to the temporal bone allows translatory movement between the two structures.

Disk Function

The biconcave shape of the disk provides three advantages to the TM joint. First, it provides increased congruence of the joint surfaces through a wide range of positions.[3,16] Second, the shape of the disk (thin in the center and wider anteriorly and posteriorly) allows greater flexibility of the disk so that it can conform to the articular surfaces of the condyle and the temporal bone as the condyle first rotates and then translates over the articular eminence.[3,11] Finally, the thick-thin-thick arrangement provides a self-centering mechanism for the disk on the condyle.[3,11] As pressure between the condyle and the articular eminence increases, the disk rotates on the condyle so that the thinnest portion of the disk is between the articulating surfaces. When less pressure is exerted between the joint surfaces and they separate, the disk is free to rotate to place a wider portion of the disk between the surfaces.

Mandibular Motions

The motions available to the TM joint are mouth opening (**mandibular depression**), mouth closing (**mandibular elevation**), jutting the chin forward (**mandibular protrusion**), sliding the teeth backward (**mandibular retrusion**), and sliding the teeth to either side (**lateral deviation** of the mandible). These motions are created by various combinations of rotation and gliding in the upper and lower joints.

The functional movements of the mandible are obtained by combinations of intra-articular movements that are controlled by the delicate interplay of many muscles. The functions that the TM joints support are chewing, talking, and swallowing.[3] For purposes of this chapter, we will only describe the movements of the mandible that occur without resistance (empty-mouth movements).

Mandibular Elevation and Depression

In normally functioning TM joints, mandibular elevation and depression are relatively symmetrical motions. The motion at each TM joint follows a similar pattern. Two distinct and somewhat conflicting descriptions of the movement of mouth opening are in the literature. The first describes two sequential phases: rotation and glide.[2,6,8,14] In the rotation phase of mouth opening, there is pure anterior rotation (spin) of the condyle on the disk (see Fig. 6–4a and b). This motion occurs in the lower joint between the disk and the condyle. The position at the end of the rotation phase can be described as either a posterior rotation of the

disk on the condyle or anterior rotation of the condyle on the disk. The second phase involves translation of the disk-condyle complex anteriorly and inferiorly along the articular eminence (see Fig. 6–4b and c). This motion occurs in the upper joint between the disk and the articular eminence and accounts for the remainder of the opening. Normal mouth opening is considered to be 40 to 50 mm.[5,8,16] Of that motion, between 11 mm[9,17] and 25 mm[3] is gained from rotation of the condyle in the disk, whereas the remainder is from translation of the disk and condyle along the articular eminence.

The second model, based on more recent research, argues that the components of rotation and gliding are present, but occur concomitantly rather than sequentially.[17–19] That is, rotation and gliding are both present throughout the range of mandibular depression and elevation starting at the initiation of mouth opening. Isberg and coworkers[17] also note that the amount of rotation has a positive correlation with the steepness of the articular eminence.

For a quick and rough, but useful, estimate of function, an individual may use the proximal interphalangeal (PIP) joints to assess opening. If two PIP joints can be placed between the central front incisors, the amount of opening is functional although three PIP joints is considered normal.[8] Dijkstra and associates[20] have demonstrated a positive correlation between the amount of mouth opening and the length of the mandible. This should be considered in determining what is normal for each patient.

Mandibular elevation (mouth closing) is the reverse of depression. It consists of translation posteriorly and superiorly and rotation of the condyle posteriorly on the disk (or the disk anteriorly on the condyle).

Mandibular Protrusion and Retrusion

This motion occurs when all points of the mandible move forward the same amount. The condyle and disk together translate anteriorly and inferiorly along the articular eminence. No rotation occurs in the TM joint during protrusion. The motion is all translation and occurs in the upper joint alone. The teeth are separated when protrusion occurs. During protrusion, the posterior attachments of the disk (the bilaminar retrodiskal tissue) stretch 6 to 9 mm to allow the motion to occur.[3] Protrusion should be adequate to allow the upper and lower teeth to touch edge-to-edge.[5]

Retrusion occurs when all points of the mandible move posteriorly the same amount. The TM ligament limits this motion, as does the soft tissue present in the retrodiskal area between the condyle and the posterior glenoid spine. The TM ligament limits motions by becoming taut, the retrodiskal tissue limits movement by occupying the space into which the condyle would move during retrusion. Although rarely measured, this range is limited to 3 mm of translation.[3]

Mandibular Lateral Deviation

The mandible can move asymmetrically either around a vertical or around an anterior-posterior axis at one of the condyles. In lateral deviation of the chin to one side, one condyle spins around a vertical axis while the other condyle translates forward[3,9] (Fig. 6–7). For example, deviation to the right would involve the right condyle spinning and the left condyle translating or gliding forward. The result is movement of the center of the mandible (or chin) to the right. Normally, the amount of lateral excursion of the joint is about 8 mm.[5,8] A functional measurement of lateral motion of the mandible involves the use of the width of the two upper central incisors. If the mandible can move the full width of one of the central incisors in each direction, motion is considered normal.[5,8]

Another asymmetrical movement of the mandible involves rotation of one condyle around an anterior-posterior axis.[3] As one condyle spins around an anteroposterior axis,

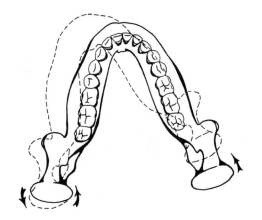

FIGURE 6–7. Demonstration of lateral deviation of the mandible to the left. (Modified from Perry, JF, Rohe, DA, and Garcia, OA: The Kinesiology Workbook. FA Davis, Philadelphia, 1991, p 171, with permission.)

the other condyle depresses. This results in a frontal plane motion of the mandible where the center of the mandible moves downward and deviates from the midline slightly toward the condyle that is spinning. This motion typically occurs when biting on one side of the teeth. Although these motions were just described separately, they are commonly combined into one complex motion used in chewing and grinding food.[16]

Function

The TM joint is one of the most frequently used joints in the body. It is involved in chewing, talking, and swallowing.[3,14,16] Most TM joint movements are empty-mouth movements;[11] that is, they occur with no resistance from food or contact between the upper and lower teeth. The joint is well designed for this intensive use. The cartilage covering the articular surfaces is designed to tolerate repeated and high-level stress. In addition to a joint structure that supports the high level of usage, the musculature is designed to provide both power[10,11] and intricate control.[11] Speech requires fine control, and the ability to chew requires great strength. Both are available through the musculature of the TM joint.

Control of the Disk

The articular disk is controlled both actively and passively. The passive control is exerted by the capsuloligamentous attachments of the disk to the condyle and has already been examined. Active control of the disk may be exerted through the attachments of the lateral pterygoid muscle, although evidence suggests that these attachments may not be consistently present.[13,21] Bell[11] also proposed two muscles that may assist with maintaining the disk position. These two muscles are derived from the masseter muscle and are attached to the anterolateral portion of the disk. They help overcome the medial pull of the anteromedially attached lateral pterygoid.

Now let us look at how the active and passive forces interact to control the disk during function. These forces will be at play whether you consider the sequential or the concomitant models of mouth opening. When TM joint rotation is occurring, all of the rotation occurs between the disk and the condyle in the lower joint compartment. The medial and lateral attachments of the disk to the condyle limit the motion of the disk on the condyle to the motion of rotation. During translation, the biconcave shape of the disk allows it to follow the condyle; no other force is necessary. The inferior retrodiskal lamina limits forward excursion of the disk. The superior portion of the lateral pterygoid is *not* active during mouth opening.[5,11]

During mouth closing, the elastic character of the superior retrodiskal lamina applies a posterior tractive force on the disk. In addition, the superior portion of the lateral pterygoid applies a force that controls the posterior movement of the disk through an *eccentric* contraction. Abe and colleagues[13] suggest that the sphenomandibular ligament also assists this action. Again, the medial and lateral attachments of the disk to the condyle limit the motion to rotation of the disk around the condyle.

Muscular Control of the TM Joint

The primary muscle responsible for mandibular depression is the **digastric** muscle (Fig. 6–8).[1,11] Some classify the lateral pterygoid muscles as depressors,[9] but Bell[11] cites evidence that the superior portion of the lateral pterygoid is not active during mouth opening,

although the lower portion is active. Bell states that the upper and lower portions of the lateral pterygoids function independently. Note that gravity is also a mandibular depressor.

Mandibular elevation is primarily accomplished by the temporalis (Fig. 6–9), masseter (Fig. 6–10), and **medial pterygoid** muscles (Fig. 6–11).[1,3,5,7,16] The superior portion of the lateral pterygoid is also active during elevation of the mandible. The purpose of this activity is to rotate the disk anteriorly on the condyle.[3,5,11,22] This can also be viewed as maintaining the disk in a forward position as the condyle begins to rotate posteriorly. The superior portion of the lateral pterygoid contracts eccentrically to allow the disk-condyle complex to translate upward and posteriorly, and then maintains the disk in a forward position until the condyle has completed its posterior rotation to return to its normal rest position.

Mandibular protrusion results from bilateral action of the masseter, medial pterygoid,[3,16] and lateral pterygoid muscles.[1,3,16,23] **Retrusion** or retraction is obtained through the bilateral action of the posterior fibers of the temporalis muscles[9,16] with assistance from the digastric and **suprahyoid** muscles.[16]

Lateral deviation, or movement of the chin or the center of the mandible away from the midline, is caused by unilateral action of various muscles. Both the medial and lateral pterygoid muscles deviate the mandible to the opposite side.[3,9] The temporalis muscle can deviate the mandible to the same side. An ex-

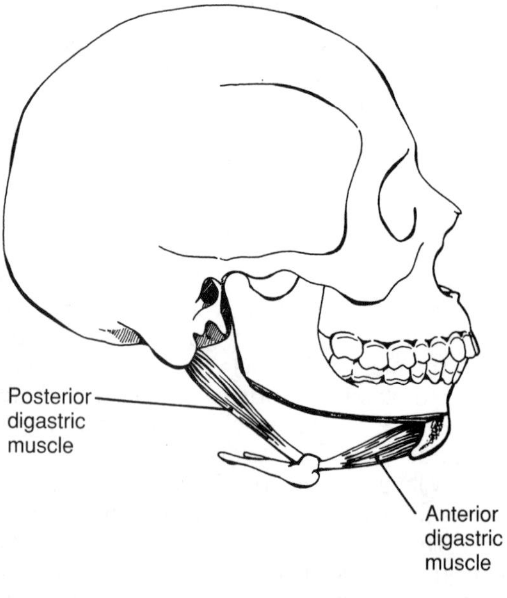

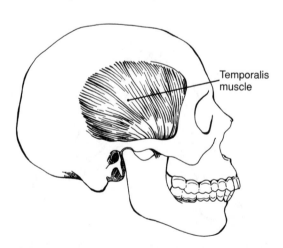

FIGURE 6–8. Digastric muscle. (Modified from Perry, JF, Rohe, DA, and Garcia, OA: The Kinesiology Workbook. FA Davis, Philadelphia, 1991, p 168, with permission.)

Posterior digastric muscle

Anterior digastric muscle

FIGURE 6–9. Temporalis muscle. (Modified from Perry, JF, Rohe, DA, and Garcia, OA: The Kinesiology Workbook. FA Davis, Philadelphia, 1991, p 166, with permission.)

Temporalis muscle

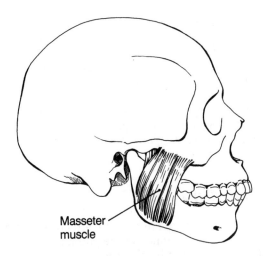

FIGURE 6–10. Masseter muscle. (Modified from Perry, JF, Rohe, DA, and Garcia, OA: The Kinesiology Workbook. FA Davis, Philadelphia, 1991, p 165, with permission.)

ception to this is the combined action of the lateral pterygoid and temporalis on the same side. These two muscles can function as an effective force couple.[16] For example, the left lateral pterygoid is attached to the medial pole of the condyle and pulls the condyle forward. The left temporalis is attached to the lateral pole of the condyle and pulls it posteriorly. Together they effectively spin the condyle to create deviation of the mandible to the left. Acting alone,

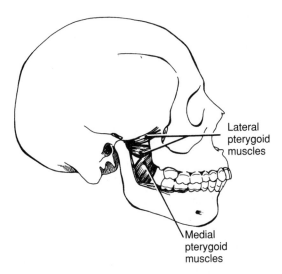

FIGURE 6–11. Medial and lateral pterygoid muscles. (Modified from Perry, JF, Rohe, DA, and Garcia, OA: The Kinesiology Workbook. FA Davis, Philadelphia, 1991, p 167, with permission.)

the left lateral pterygoid would tend to deviate the mandible to the right. Because the temporalis is also an elevator of the mandible, this combination of muscular activity is particularly useful in chewing.

Relationship with the Cervical Spine

The cervical spine and the TM joint are intimately connected. Muscles that attach to the mandible also have attachments to the head (cranium), to the hyoid bone and to the clavicle. Consequently, muscles may act not only on the mandible, but also on the atlanto-occipital joint and cervical spine. Conversely, head and neck position may also affect the tension in muscles that may affect the position or function of the mandible. Many of the symptoms of TM joint dysfunction are similar to symptoms of cervical spine problems. With the intimate relationship of these two areas, any client being seen for complaints in one area should have the other examined as well.

Dentition

The teeth are intimately involved in the function of the TM joint. Not only is chewing one of the functions of the TM joint, but the contact of the upper and lower teeth limits motion of the TM joint during empty-mouth movements. The presence and position of the teeth are critical to normal TM joint function. Normal adult dentition includes 32 teeth divided into four quadrants. The only teeth we will refer to by name are the upper and lower central incisors. These are the two central teeth of the maxilla and the two central teeth of the mandible.[24] When the central incisors are in firm approximation, the position is called **maximal intercuspation**[4] or the **occlusal position.**[9] This is not, however, the normal resting position of the mandible. Rather, 1.5 to 5 mm of **"freeway" space** between the upper and lower teeth is normally maintained.[3,11] This freeway space is particularly important. By maintaining this space, the intra-articular pressure within the TM joint is decreased, the stress on the articular structures is reduced, and the tissues of the area are able to rest and repair.[3]

Dysfunctions

Many dysfunctions of the TM joint occur. Some are caused by direct trauma such as motor vehicle accidents or falls. Others are the result of years of poor postural or oral habits such as forward head posture or **bruxism** (teeth grinding). Only two problems will be described here, reciprocal click and osteoarthritis.

Reciprocal Click

A patient who has an anteriorly dislocated disk will have an audible click from the TM joint on opening and a second when the mouth is closing. This is called a **reciprocal click.**[8] In this situation, the condyle of the mandible is in contact with the retrodiskal tissue at rest, rather than with the disk. On mouth opening, the condyle slips forward and under the disk to obtain a normal relationship with the disk. When the condyle slips under the disk, an audible click is often present. Once the condyle is in the proper relationship with the disk, motion continues normally through opening and closing until the condyle again slips out from under the disk, when another click is heard. One would expect a click to signify that the condyle and disk have lost a normal relationship. In the case of an anteriorly dislocated disk, however, the initial click signals regaining a normal relationship. When the click occurs early in opening and late in closing, the amount of anterior displacement of the disk is relatively limited. The later the click occurs in the opening phase, the more severe the disk dislocation.[8] Some evidence exists that the timing of the clicks during opening and closing can determine treatment prognosis.[25]

Osteoarthritis

Kessler and Hertling[16] state that 80% to 90% of the population over 60 years of age have some symptoms of osteoarthritis of the TM joint. According to Mahan,[12] osteoarthritis usually occurs unilaterally (unlike rheumatoid arthritis, which is usually bilateral). The primary cause of osteoarthritis is repeated minor trauma to the joint, particularly trauma that creates an impact between the articular surfaces.[12,16] Loss of posterior teeth may lead to degenerative changes because simple occlusion of the remaining teeth causes impact between the TM joint surfaces.[12,16]

The primary symptoms of osteoarthritis are pain on translation of the condyle on the articular eminence with almost pain-free rotation of the condyle, flattening of the condyle and the articular eminence, and narrowing of the TM joint space. In more advanced stages of the disease, perforation of the disk and lipping around the articular surfaces can also occur.[12,16] Persons with osteoarthritis may limit their mouth movements. Typically, the symptoms decrease over time, with most pain disappearing after approximately 8 months and apparently normal function (with crepitus, however) returning within 1 to 3 years.[12,26]

Summary

The TM joints are unique both structurally and functionally. The magnitude and frequency of jaw movement, the daily resistance encountered during chewing and muscle balance issues around this joint make this joint complex particularly vulnerable to problems. As we proceed in subsequent chapters to examine the joint complexes of the appendicular skeleton, it will be seen that each complex has its own unique features. We will not see again, however, the complexity of intra-articular and diskal motions seen at the TM joints.

REFERENCES

1. Sicher, H: Functional anatomy of the temporomandibular joint. In Sarnat, BG (ed): The Temporomandibular Joint, ed 2. Charles C Thomas, Springfield, IL, 1964.
2. Hylander, WL: Functional Anatomy. In Sarnat, BG, and Laskins, DM (eds): The Temporomandibular Joint: A Biological Basis for Clinical Practice. WB Saunders, Philadelphia, 1992.
3. Bourbon, BM: Anatomy and biomechanics of the TMJ. In Kraus, SL: TMJ Disorders: Management of the Craniomandibular Complex. Churchill Livingstone, New York, 1988.
4. Ermshar, CB: Anatomy and neuroanatomy. In Morgan, DH, House, LR, Wall, WP, and Vamvas, SJ, (eds): Diseases of the Temporomandibular Apparatus: A Multidisciplinary Approach, ed 2. CV Mosby, St Louis, 1982.
5. Kraus, SL: Temporomandibular joint. In Saunders, HD (ed): Evaluation, Treatment, and Prevention of Musculoskeletal Disorders, ed 2. Viking Press, New York, 1985.
6. Kraus, SL: Temporomandibular joint. In Saunders, HD, and Saunders, R (eds): Evaluation, Treatment, and Prevention of Musculoskeletal Disorders, Vol. 1: Spine, ed. 3. Educational Opportunities, Bloomington, MN, 1993.
7. Eggleton, TM, and Langton, DM: Clinical Anatomy of the TMJ Complex. In Kraus SL (ed): Temporomandibular Disorders, ed 2. Churchill Livingstone, New York, 1994.
8. Rocabado, M: Course notes, 1988.
9. Williams, PL (ed.): Gray's Anatomy, ed 35. Churchill Livingstone, New York, 1995.
10. Waltimo A, and Kononen, M: A novel bite force recorder and maximal isometric bite force values for

healthy young adults. Scand J Dent Res 101:171–175, 1993.

11. Bell, WE: Temporomandibular Disorders: Classification, Diagnosis, Management, ed 3. Yearbook Medical Publishers, Chicago, 1990.

12. Mahan, PE: The temporomandibular joint in function and pathofunction. In Solberg, WK, and Clark, GT (eds): Temporomandibular Joint Problems: Biologic Diagnosis and Treatment. Quintessence, Chicago, 1980.

13. Abe, S, et al: Perspectives on the role of the lateral pterygoid muscle and the sphenomandibular ligament in temporomandibular joint functions. Cranio 15: 203–207, 1997.

14. Helland, MM: Anatomy and function of the temporomandibular joint. J Orthop Sports Phys Ther 1:145–152, 1980.

15. Loughner, BA, et al: The medical capsule of the human temporomandibular joint. J Oral Maxillofac Surg 55: 363–369, 1997.

16. Kessler, RM, and Hertling, D: Management of Common Musculoskeletal Disorders: Physical Therapy Principles and Methods, ed 3. Lippincott-Raven, Philadelphia, 1996.

17. Isberg, A, and Westesson, PL: Steepness of articular eminence and movement of the condyle and disk in asymptomatic temporomandibular joints. Oral Sur Oral Med Oral Pathol Oral Radiol Endodon 86: 152–157, 1998.

18. Lindauer, SJ, et al: Condylar movement and mandibular rotation during jaw opening. Am J Orthodon Dentofac Orthop 107:573–577, 1995.

19. Ferrario, VF, et al: Open-close movements in the human temporomandibular joint: Does a pure rotation around the intercondylar hinge axis exist? J Oral Rehab 23:401–408, 1996.

20. Dijkstra, PU, et al: Influence of mandibular length on mouth opening. J Oral Rehab 26:117–122, 1999.

21. Naidoo, LC: Lateral pterygoid muscle and its relationship to the meniscus of the temporomandibular joint. Oral Sur Oral Med Oral Pathol Oral Radiol Endodon 82:4–9, 1996.

22. Bade, H, et al: The function of discomuscular relationships in the human temporomandibular joint. Acta Anat 151:258–267, 1994.

23. Murray, GM, et al: Electromyographic activity of the human lateral pterygoid muscle during contralateral and protrusive jaw movements. Arch Oral Biol 44:269–285, 1999.

24. Brand, RW, and Isselhard, DE: Anatomy of Orofacial Structures, ed 2. CV Mosby, St Louis, 1982.

25. Kirk, WS, and Calabrese, DK: Clinical evaluation of physical therapy in the management of internal derangement of the temporomandibular joint. J Oral Maxillofac Surg 47:113–119, 1989.

26. Nickerson, JW, and Boering, G: Natural course of osteoarthritis as it relates to internal derangement of the temporomandibular joint. Oral Maxillofac Surg Clin North Am 1:1, 1989.

Study Questions

1. *Describe the articulating surface of the TM joint.*
2. *What is the significance of the differing thicknesses and the differing vascularity of the disk?*
3. *How do the superior and inferior lamina of the retrodiskal area differ?*
4. *Describe the motions in the upper and lower joints during mouth opening and closing.*
5. *What limits posterior motion of the condyle? How is the motion limited?*
6. *What would be the consequences of having a left TM joint that could not translate?*
7. *What would be the consequences of having a right disk that could not rotate freely over the condyle?*
8. *Describe the control of the disk in moving from an open-mouth to a closed-mouth position.*

CHAPTER 7

THE SHOULDER COMPLEX

. . . .

. . . .

OBJECTIVES

Following the study of this chapter, the reader should be able to:

Define

1. The terminology unique to the shoulder complex.

Describe

1. The articular surfaces of the joints of the complex.
2. The function of the ligaments of each joint.
3. Accessory joint structures and the function of each.
4. Motions and ranges of motion available at each joint and movement of articular surfaces within a joint.
5. The normal mechanism of dynamic stabilization of the glenohumeral joint, using principles of biomechanics.
6. The normal mechanism of glenohumeral stabilization in the dependent arm.
7. Scapulohumeral rhythm, including contributions of each joint.
8. The extent of dependent or independent function of each joint in scapulohumeral rhythm.
9. How restrictions in the range of elevation of the arm may occur.
10. One muscular force couple at a given joint and its function.
11. The effect a given muscular deficit may have on shoulder complex function.

Compare

1. The advantage and disadvantages of the coracoacromial arch.
2. The structural stabilization of these joints, including the tendency toward degenerative changes and derangement.

Draw

1. Action lines of muscles of the shoulder complex and the moment arm for each and resolve each into components.

. . . .

Introduction

The shoulder complex is composed of the scapula, clavicle, humerus, and the joints that link these bones into a functional entity. These components constitute one-half of the weight of the entire upper limb.[1] The shoulder complex is connected to the axial skeleton by a single anatomic joint (the **sternoclavicular joint**) and is suspended by muscles that serve as the primary mechanism for securing the shoulder girdle to the rest of the body. The precarious arrangement between the upper extremity and the trunk promotes a wide range of motion (ROM) for the hand, but conflicts with the need for a stable base of operation and the need to move the hand and arm against large resistances. The contradictory mobility/stability requirements are met through **dynamic stabilization,** a concept for which the shoulder complex is the classic example and within which shoulder complex function can best be understood. In essence, dynamic stability exists when a segment or set of segments is limited very little by joint structure and relies instead on dynamic muscular control. Dynamic stabilization results in a wide range of mobility for the complex that works well under usual conditions but is susceptible to problems that may arise from any of the structures that mediate the mobility/stability compromise.

Components of the Shoulder Complex

The scapula, clavicle, and humerus that form the shoulder complex are responsible for movement of the hand through space. The three segments are controlled by four interdependent linkages: a functional articulation known as the **scapulothoracic (ST) joint** and three anatomic joints, including the **sternoclavicular (SC) joint,** the **acromioclavicular (AC) joint,** and the **glenohumeral (GH) joint.** A fifth functional articulation is commonly described as part of the complex and is formed by the coracoacromial arch and the head of the humerus. The **coracoacromial arch,** or so-called **suprahumeral joint,** plays an important role in shoulder function and dysfunction, but we will not consider it a separate linkage.

The joints that compose the shoulder complex together contribute as much as 180° of elevation to the upper extremity. **Elevation** of the upper extremity refers to the combination of scapular, clavicular, and humeral (**scapulohumeral**) motion that occurs when the arm is either raised *forward* or *to the side* (including flexion, abduction, and all the motions in between). The ST joint normally contributes approximately 60° to elevation of the arm, whereas the GH joint contributes as much as 120°. Both joints contribute lesser amounts of motion to other motions of the arm. Although integrated scapulohumeral function is of primary interest, each of the articulations and components of the shoulder complex must be examined individually before integrated dynamic function can be appreciated.

Scapulothoracic Joint

The ST joint is formed by the articulation of the scapula with the thorax on which it sits. It is not a true anatomic joint because it has none of the usual joint characteristics (union by fibrous, cartilaginous, or synovial tissues). In fact, the articulation of the scapula with the thorax depends on the anatomic AC and SC joints. The SC and AC joints are interdependent with the scapulothoracic joint because the scapula is attached by its acromion process to the lateral end of the clavicle via the AC joint; the clavicle, in turn, is attached to the axial skeleton at the manubrium of the sternum via the SC joint. Any movement of the scapula on the thorax must result in movement at either the AC joint, the SC joint, or both. That is, the functional ST joint is part of a true closed chain with the AC and SC joints. To understand the structure and function of the AC and SC joints, however, it is useful to first look at the scapular segment they serve, including how the scapula sits on the thorax and what motions can be performed.

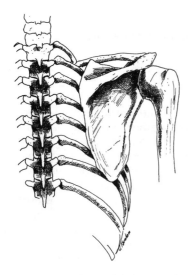

FIGURE 7–1. Resting position of the scapula on the thorax.

Scapulothoracic Position and Motions

Normally, the scapula rests at a position on the posterior thorax approximately 2 inches from the midline, between the second through seventh ribs[2] (Fig. 7–1). The scapula also lies 30° to 40° forward of the frontal plane and is tipped anteriorly approximately 10° to 20° from vertical with a good deal of individual variability [3,4] (Fig. 7–2). The motions of the scapula from this reference position are **elevation/depression, protraction/retraction** (also known as abduction and adduction, respectively), and **upward/downward rotation** (also known as lateral and medial rotation, respectively). Scapular motions are typically described as if they occur independently of each other. The linkage of the scapula to the AC and SC joints, however, actu-

ally prevents such isolated motions from occurring. Instead, for example, elevation may be associated with concomitant protraction and upward rotation. To facilitate understanding, we will describe the scapular motions separately. The more complex (and realistic) explanation of scapular motion can be best appreciated when integrated function of the shoulder complex is presented.

Elevation and depression of the scapula are described as translatory motions in which the scapula moves upward (cephalad) or downward (caudally) along the rib cage from its resting position (Fig. 7–3). Protraction and retraction of the scapula are described as translatory motions of the scapula away from or toward the vertebral column, respectively (Fig. 7–4). Upward and downward rotation are rotatory motions that tilt the glenoid fossa upward or downward, respectively. Upward and downward rotation can also be described by referencing movement of the inferior angle away from the vertebral column (upward rotation) or movement of the inferior angle toward the vertebral column (downward rotation) (Fig. 7–5).

The scapula has two other motions that are less commonly described but are still critical to its movement along the curved rib cage. These motions, known by a wide variety of other terms, will be referred to here as **medial/lateral rotation of the scapula** and **anterior/posterior tipping** of the scapula. Medial/lateral rotation and anterior/posterior tipping are typically not obvious movements of the scapular segment but are unobtrusive motions necessary to maintain the scapula relative flush with the curved rib cage. These motions of the scapula can and will occur overtly when the

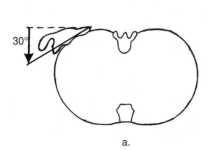

a.

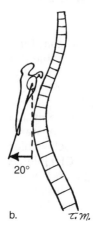

b.

FIGURE 7–2. At rest, the scapula typically lies (a) 30° to 40° forward of the frontal plane (reference line) and (b) is tipped anteriorly approximately 10° to 20° from vertical (reference line).

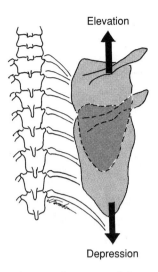

FIGURE 7–3. Elevation/depression of the scapula at the scapulothoracic joint.

range of scapular motion is exhausted or in certain pathologic conditions. Medial/lateral rotation and anterior/posterior tipping of the scapula can best be understood in the context of the AC joint at which they occur and will be discussed in that section.

Scapulothoracic Stability

Stability of the scapula on the thorax is provided by the structures that maintain integrity of the linked AC and SC joints. The muscles

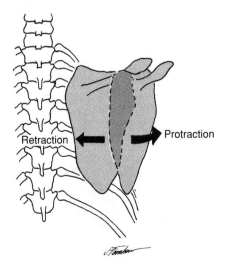

FIGURE 7–4. Protraction and retraction of the scapulothoracic joint.

that attach to both the thorax and scapula maintain contact between these surfaces while producing the movements of the scapula.

The ultimate function of scapular motion is to orient the glenoid fossa for optimal contact with the maneuvering arm, to add range to elevation of the arm, and to provide a stable base for the controlled rolling and sliding of the articular surface of the humeral head. The scapula, with its associated muscles and linkages, performs these mobility and stability functions so well that it must serve as the premier example of dynamic stabilization in the human body.

Sternoclavicular Joint

The SC joint might be considered the "base of operation" for the scapula because, via the interposed clavicle, it is the only structural attachment of the scapula to the rest of the body. Movement of the clavicle at the SC joint inevitably produces movement of the scapula. Similarly, scapular motions must produce motion at the SC joint. The SC joint is a plane synovial joint with 3° of freedom of motion. It has a joint capsule, three major ligaments, and a joint disk.

Sternoclavicular Articulating Surfaces

The SC articulation consists of two saddle-shaped surfaces, one at the sternal end of the clavicle and one at the notch formed by the manubrium of the sternum and first costal cartilage (Fig. 7–6). Although tremendous individual differences exist in each of the components of the shoulder complex, the sternal end of the clavicle and the manubrium are invariably incongruent; that is, there is little contact between the articular surfaces at this joint. The superior portion of the medial clavicle does not contact the manubrium at all; instead it serves as the attachment for the joint disk and the interclavicular ligament. At rest, the SC joint space is wedge-shaped (open superiorly).[5] Movements of the SC joint result in changes in the areas of contact between the clavicle, the joint disk, and the manubriocostal cartilage.

Sternoclavicular Disk

When two bony articular surfaces are incongruent, as is true at the SC joint, frequently an accessory joint structure contributes to the overall

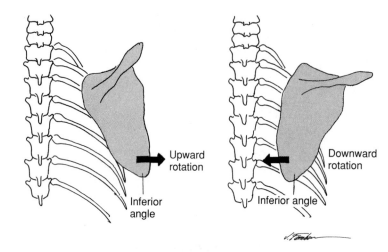

FIGURE 7–5. Upward-downward rotation of the scapula at the scapulothoracic joint.

contact of the surfaces. At the SC joint a fibrocartilage **joint disk,** or meniscus, is interposed between the articular surfaces. The upper portion of the disk is attached to the superior clavicle and lower portion to the manubrium and first costal cartilage, diagonally transecting the SC joint space (Fig. 7–7). In this way the disk actually divides the joint into two separate cavities.[1] Given the attachments of the disk, it acts like a hinge or pivot point during SC motion. In elevation and depression, the medial clavicle moves on the relatively stationary disk, with the upper attachment of the disk serving as a pivot point. In protraction/retraction, the disk and clavicle together move on the manubrial facet, with the lower attachment of the disk serving as a pivot point.[1] The disk, therefore, is part of the manubrium in elevation/depression and part of the clavicle in protraction/retraction. As the disk switches its participation from one segment to the other during clavicular motions, mobility

between the segments is maintained while stability is enhanced. The resultant movement of the clavicle in both elevation/depression and protraction/retraction is a fairly complex set of motions with the mechanical axis for these two movements located at the costoclavicular ligament while the clavicle intra-articularly pivots about the SC disk.

The SC disk also serves an important stability function by increasing joint congruence and absorbing forces that may be transmitted along the clavicle from its lateral end. Referring again to Figure 7–7, it can be seen that the unique diagonal attachment of the SC disk positions the disk to check medial movement of the clavicle that might otherwise cause the large clavicle to override the shallow manubrial facet. The disk also has substantially more contact with the medial clavicle, permitting it to dissipate the medially directed forces more effectively than the small manubrial facet. Although it might seem that medially directed forces on the clavicle are rare, we shall see that

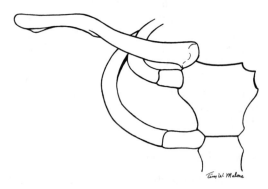

FIGURE 7–6. The clavicular and sternal segments of the SC joint.

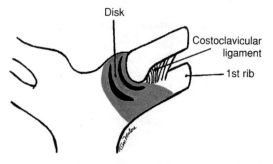

FIGURE 7–7. The SC disk and costoclavicular ligament.

this is not the case when we examine the function of the AC joint and the coracoclavicular ligament.

Sternoclavicular Joint Capsule and Ligaments

The SC joint is surrounded by a fairly strong capsule but must depend on three ligaments for the majority of its support: the **sternoclavicular ligaments,** the **costoclavicular ligaments,** and the **interclavicular ligament** (Fig. 7–8). The anterior and posterior SC ligaments reinforce the capsule. The SC ligaments serve primarily to check anterior and posterior movement of the head of the clavicle. The costoclavicular ligament is a very strong ligament found between the clavicle and the first rib below. The costoclavicular ligaments has two segments or lamina. The anterior lamina has medially directed fibers, whereas the fibers of the posterior lamina are directed laterally (see Fig. 7–7).[6] Both segments check elevation and, when the limits of the ligament are reached, may contribute to the downward gliding of the medial clavicle that occurs with SC elevation.[7] The costoclavicular ligament is also positioned to counter the superiorly directed forces applied to the clavicle by some of the muscles of the head and neck. The fibers of the medially directed posterior lamina will check medial movement of the clavicle,[8] absorbing some of the force that would otherwise be imposed on the SC disk. The interclavicular ligament checks excessive depression or downward glide of the clavicle. The limitation to clavicular depression is critical to protecting structures like the brachial plexus and subclavian artery that pass under the clavicle and over the first rib. In fact, when the clavicle is depressed and the interclavicular ligament and superior capsule are taut, the tension in these structures can support the weight of the upper extremity.[9]

The bony segments of the SC joint, its capsuloligamentous structure, and the SC disk combine to produce a joint that meets its dual functions of mobility and stability well. The SC joint serves its purpose of joining the upper limb to the axial skeleton, while contributing to mobility and withstanding imposed stresses. Although the SC joint is considered incongruent, the joint does not undergo the degree of degenerative change common to the other joints of the shoulder complex.[10,11] Strong force-dissipating structures like the SC disk and the costoclavicular ligament minimize articular stresses while also preventing excessive intra-articular motion that might lead to subluxation or dislocation. Dislocations of the SC joint represent only 1% of joint dislocations in the body, and when they occur, produce little discomfort or dysfunction.[12]

Sternoclavicular Motions

The motions that occur at the SC joint are elevation/depression, protraction/retraction, and anterior/posterior rotation of the clavicle. Motions of any lever are always described osteokinematically by the movement of the distal segment of the lever. The horizontal alignment of the clavicle (rather than the vertical alignment of most of the appendicular levers of the skeleton) can sometimes create confusion and impair visualization of the clavicular motions. The motions of elevation/depression and protraction/retraction should be visualized by referencing movement of the lateral end of the clavicle. Clavicular rotation is a rolling motion of the entire clavicle and does not seem to create the same visualization problems that may occur with the other motions.

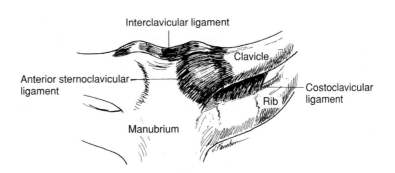

FIGURE 7–8. SC ligaments.

ELEVATION AND DEPRESSION OF THE CLAVICLE

The motions of elevation and depression occur around an anterior-posterior axis between a convex clavicular surface and a concave surface formed by the manubrium and first costal cartilage. The cephalocaudal shape of the articular surfaces and the location of the axis indicate that the convex surface of the clavicle must slide on the concave manubrium and first costal cartilage in a direction opposite to movement of the lateral end of the clavicle. Arthrokinematically, therefore, elevation of the clavicle results in downward sliding of the medial clavicular surface on the manubrium and first costal cartilage. When movement of the clavicle is plotted, the SC joint axis appears to lie lateral to the joint at the costoclavicular ligament. The location of this functional (rather than anatomic) axis so far from the joint reflects a relatively large intra-articular motion; a longer lever arm will swing through a wider arc. The range of clavicular elevation averages about 45°,[13] while there is about 15° of depression.[5] Elevation and depression of the *clavicle* are invariably associated with elevation and depression of the *scapula* because the acromion of the scapula is attached to the lateral end of the clavicle. The elevation of the scapula that occurs with clavicular elevation is not a pure motion but is associated with concomitant upward rotation of the scapula. The scapular upward rotation that accompanies clavicular elevation plays a significant role in increasing the range of elevation of the arm.

PROTRACTION AND RETRACTION OF THE CLAVICLE

Protraction and retraction of the clavicle occur at the SC joint around a vertical axis that also appears to lie at the costoclavicular ligament. The configuration of joint surfaces in this plane is the opposite of that for elevation/depression; the medial end of the clavicle is concave and the manubrial side of the joint is convex. Arthrokinematically, the clavicular surface will now slide on the manubrium and first costal cartilage in the same direction as the lateral end of the clavicle. That is, protraction of the clavicle is expected to be accompanied by anterior sliding of the medial clavicle on the manubrium and first costal cartilage. There is about 15° protraction and 15° retraction of the clavicle. Protraction and retraction of the *clavicle* are invariably associated with protraction and retraction of the *scapula* because the scapula is attached to the distal end of the clavicle.

ANTERIOR-POSTERIOR ROTATION OF THE CLAVICLE

Rotation of the clavicle occurs as a spin between the saddle-shaped surfaces of the clavicle and manubriocostal facet. Unlike many joints that can rotate in either direction from resting position of the joint, the clavicle rotates in only one direction from its resting position. The clavicle rotates posteriorly from neutral, bringing the inferior surface of the clavicle to face anteriorly (Fig. 7–9). From its fully rotated position, the clavicle can rotate anteriorly again to return to neutral. The axis for rotation runs longitudinally through the clavicle, intersecting the SC joint. The range of clavicular rotation is cited to be anywhere from 30° to as much as 55°.[5,7,10] Posterior rotation of the clavicle produces the final 30° of upward rotation of the scapula that occurs with elevation of the arm. The mechanism by which clavicular rotation causes scapular upward rotation will be presented with integrated function of the shoulder complex.

Acromioclavicular Joint

The AC joint attaches the scapula to the clavicle. It is a plane synovial joint with 3° of freedom. It has a joint capsule and two major ligaments; a joint disk may or may not be present. The primary function of the AC joint is to maintain the relation between the clavicle and the

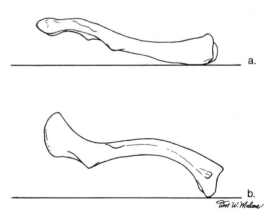

FIGURE 7–9. (a) Neutral position of the clavicle. (b) Position of the clavicle after the clavicle has rotated posteriorly, exposing the clavicle's inferior surface (as during flexion and abduction of the upper extremity).

scapula in the early stages of elevation of the upper limb and to allow the scapula additional range of rotation on the thorax in the latter stages of elevation of the limb.

Acromioclavicular Articulating Surfaces

The AC articulation consists of the articulation between the lateral end of the clavicle and a small facet on the acromion of the scapula (Fig. 7–10). The articular facets, considered to be incongruent, vary in configuration. They may be flat, reciprocally concave-convex, or reversed (reciprocally convex-concave).[6] The inclination of the articulating surfaces varies from individual to individual. Depalma[10] described three joint types in which the angle of inclination of the contacting surfaces varied from 16° to 36° from vertical. The closer the surfaces were to the vertical, the more prone the joint was to the wearing effects of shear forces. Given the variable articular configuration, arthrokinematics for this joint are not predictable.

Acromioclavicular Joint Disk

The disk of the AC joint is variable in size and differs among individuals, at various times in the life of the same individual, and between sides of the same individual. Through 2 years of age, the joint is actually a fibrocartilaginous union. Over time a joint space develops at either end that may leave a "meniscoid" fibrocartilage remnant within the joint.[11]

Acromioclavicular Capsule and Ligaments

The capsule of the AC joint is weak and cannot maintain integrity of the joint without reinforcement of the **superior** and **inferior acromioclavicular** and the **coracoclavicular ligaments** (Fig. 7–11). The superior acromioclavicular ligament assists the capsule in apposing articular surfaces and in controlling horizontal joint stability. The fibers of the superior AC ligament are reinforced by aponeurotic fibers of the trapezius and deltoid, making the superior joint support stronger than the inferior.[8]

The **coracoclavicular ligament,** although not belonging directly to the anatomic structure of the AC joint, provides much of the joint's stability and firmly unites the clavicle and scapula. This ligament is divided into a lateral portion, the **trapezoid ligament,** and a medial portion, the **conoid ligament.** The trapezoid ligament is quadrilateral in shape and is nearly horizontal. The conoid ligament is more triangular and vertically oriented (medial and slightly posterior to the trapezoid).[6] The two ligaments are separated by adipose tissue and a large bursa.[9] Although the AC capsule and ligament can restrain small AC motions, restraint of larger displacements is credited to the coracoclavicular ligament.[3]

Both portions of the coracoclavicular ligament prevent upward rotation of the scapula at the AC joint. If the scapula were to upwardly rotate around an anteroposterior axis through

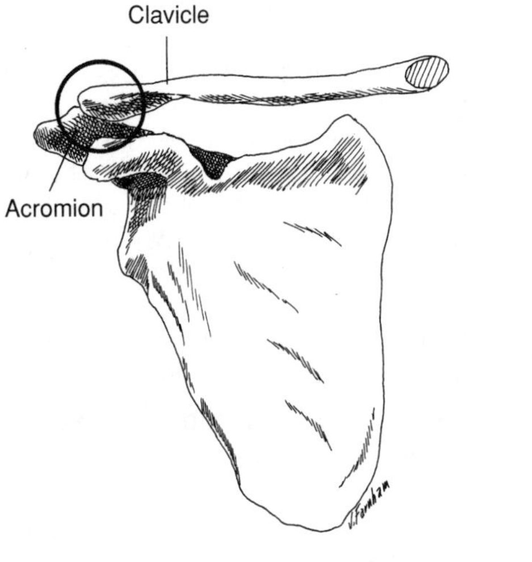

FIGURE 7–10. AC joint. Articulation between acromion of the scapula and the clavicle is shown.

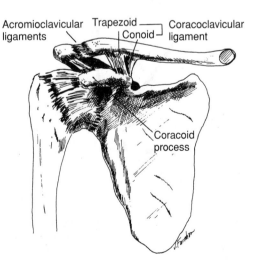

FIGURE 7–11. AC ligaments.

the AC joint, the coracoid process would drop away from the clavicle (Fig. 7–12). This cannot happen as long as the coracoclavicular ligament is intact. The extremely strong bands of the coracoclavicular ligament also assist in transferring to the clavicle medially directed forces applied to the scapula. The potentially large external forces that push the humerus into the glenoid fossa and medially directed muscles of the scapula would displace the scapula medially on the thorax. The small AC joint and its relatively weak capsule and ligament would not be able to resist such large forces; the clavicle would override the acromion and the joint would dislocate. Medial displacement of the scapula (and its coracoid process) is prevented by tension in the coracoclavicular ligament (especially the horizontal trapezoid portion) that then transfers the medially directed force to the clavicle and on to the very strong SC joint. The most critical role played by the coracoclavicular ligament, as shall be seen later, is in producing the longitudinal rotation of the clavicle necessary for a full ROM in elevation of the upper extremity.

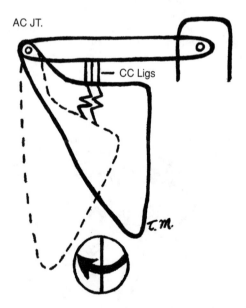

FIGURE 7–12. In this schematic diagram of the clavicle and the scapula, the coracoclavicular (CC) ligament ties the clavicle to the scapula, maintaining a relatively fixed scapuloclavicular angle. Upward rotation of the scapula at the AC joint around an A-P axis cannot normally occur because it would require substantial stretching of the relatively inelastic coracoclavicular ligament.

Acromioclavicular Motions

The articular facets of the AC joint are small, afford limited motion, and have a wide range of individual differences. For these reasons studies are inconsistent in identifying the movement and axes of motion for this joint. The primary motions that take place at the AC joint are **anterior/posterior tipping** of the scapula and **medial/lateral rotation** of the scapula (although terminology for these motions varies widely). The AC joint must also permit rotation of the clavicle around its long axis. Despite documentation that little movement occurred at the AC joint,[3] it was previously thought that half the range of upward/downward rotation of the scapula took place around an anteroposterior axis at the AC joint. The coracoclavicular ligament, however, normally prevents upward/downward rotation from occurring at the AC joint.[3,11]

MEDIAL AND LATERAL ROTATION OF THE SCAPULA

Medial/lateral rotation of the scapula occurs around a vertical axis through the AC joint. Medial and lateral rotation bring the glenoid fossa medially (or anteriorly) and laterally (or posteriorly), respectively. These motions must occur to maintain the contact of the scapula with the horizontal curvature of the thorax as the scapula slides around the thorax in protraction and retraction (Fig. 7–13). If protraction of the scapulothoracic joint occurred as a pure translatory movement, the scapula would move directly away from the vertebral column and the glenoid fossa would face laterally. Only the vertebral border of the scapula would remain in contact with the rib cage. In reality, full scapular protraction results in the glenoid fossa facing anteriorly with the full scapula in contact with the rib cage. The scapula follows the contour of the ribs by rotating about a vertical axis at the AC joint, with the vertebral border of the scapula moving posteriorly and the glenoid fossa moving anteriorly. The anterior orientation of the glenoid fossa is also important in flexion of the arm to keep the fossa behind the humeral head and prevent posterior dislocation.

ANTERIOR AND POSTERIOR TIPPING OF THE SCAPULA

The second AC motion is anterior/posterior tipping of the scapula around a coronal axis through the joint. Anterior tipping moves the superior border of the scapula anteriorly and

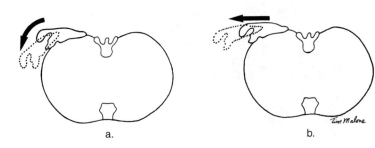

FIGURE 7–13. (a) Protraction of the scapula is normally accompanied by medial rotation of the scapula around a vertical axis at the AC joint, resulting in an anterior orientation of the glenoid fossa when the motion is complete. (b) If medial rotation of the scapula did not accompany scapular protraction, only the vertebral border of the scapula would remain on the rib cage and the glenoid fossa would maintain its lateral orientation.

a.   b.

the inferior angle posteriorly. Posterior tipping is, of course, the opposite motion. Scapular tipping, like medial/lateral rotation of the scapula, occurs to maintain the contact of the scapula with the contour of the rib cage. As the scapula moves upward or downward on the rib cage in elevation or depression, the scapula must adjust its position to maintain full contact with the vertical curvature of the ribs. Elevation of the scapula requires anterior tipping (Fig. 7–14). More significant anterior tipping of the scapula occurs during posterior rotation of the clavicle. If the clavicle and scapula were

one piece (no AC joint), attempted posterior rotation of the clavicle at the SC joint would force the inferior angle of the scapula into the rib cage and the motion would be stopped. Instead, the AC joint absorbs the clavicular rotation, effectively allowing the scapula to remain in place by counter-rotating (anteriorly tipping). Anterior tipping can also be appreciated in pathologic situations such as a round-shouldered posture, where the inferior angle of the scapula projects posteriorly off the rib cage.

Unlike the stronger SC joint, the AC joint is extremely susceptible to both trauma and degenerative change. This is likely to be due to its small and incongruent surfaces that result in large forces per unit area. Degenerative change occurs from the second decade on,[11] with the joint space itself commonly narrowed by the sixth decade.[14] Treatment of sprains, subluxations, and dislocations of this joint occupy a large amount of the literature on the shoulder complex. Controversy centers on description and classification of subluxations and dislocations and on both nonsurgical and surgical management.[15–17] This relatively unstable joint, however, appears to do reasonably well after injury despite periarticular structures that may be loose and plastic or overstabilized through some form of internal fixation. These observations have been used to support the hypothesis that the AC joint is not critical to scapular motion.[3]

Glenohumeral Joint

The GH joint is a ball-and-socket synovial joint with 3° of freedom. It has a capsule and several associated ligaments and bursae. The articulation is made up of the large head of the humerus and the small glenoid fossa (Fig. 7–15). Because the glenoid fossa of the scapula is the proximal segment of the GH joint, any motions of the scapula (and its interdependent

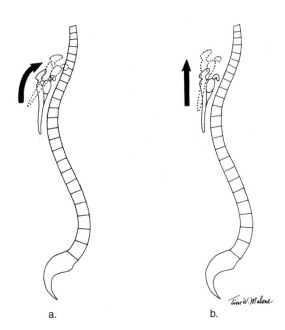

a.   b.

FIGURE 7–14. (a) Elevation of the scapula is accompanied by anterior tipping of the scapula around a coronal axis at the AC joint. The superior border of the scapula moves anteriorly to hug the changing contour of the rib cage. (b) If anterior tipping of the scapula did not occur with scapular elevation, the scapula would lose close contact with the rib cage.

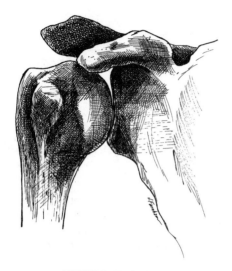

FIGURE 7–15. GH joint.

SC and AC linkages) may affect GH joint function. The GH joint has sacrificed congruency to serve the mobility needs of the hand. It is, according to Fenlin,[18] a "sloppy arrangement," susceptible both to degenerative changes and to derangement. There are substantial individual differences in almost all aspects of GH structure and function, leading Bigliani and colleagues[19] to comment on "a surprising lack of consensus as to even the most fundamental aspects of shoulder function." Consequently, the description of shoulder biomechanics that follows should be considered as a conceptual framework rather than predictable findings for any given patient.

Glenohumeral Articulating Surfaces

The glenoid fossa of the scapula serves as the proximal articular surface for this joint. The orientation of the shallow concavity of the glenoid varies with the resting position of the scapula on the thorax (see Scapulothoracic Position and Motions) and with the form of the scapula itself. The glenoid fossa may be tilted slightly upward or downward when the arm is at the side,[2,20–22] although representations most commonly show a slight upward tilt. The curvature of the surface of the fossa is greater in the frontal plane (length) than in the sagittal plane (width) with substantial variability in curvature.[23] The humerus is the distal segment of the GH joint. The humeral head has an articular surface that is invariably larger than that of the proximal segment, forming one-third to

one-half of a sphere.[5,13] As a general rule, the head faces medially, superiorly, and posteriorly with respect to the shaft of the humerus and the humeral condyles. An axis through the humeral head and longitudinal axis of the shaft of the humerus may form an angle of 130° to 150° in the frontal plane (Fig. 7–16a).[2,5] This is commonly known as the **angle of inclination** of the humerus. In the transverse plane the axis through the humeral head and an axis through the humeral condyles form an angle that varies far more than other parameters but may be given for illustration as 30° posteriorly (Fig. 7–16b).[2] This angle is known as the **angle of torsion.** The normal posterior position of the humeral head with respect to the humeral condyles may be termed **posterior torsion** or **retrotorsion** of the humerus.

Glenoid Labrum

When the arms hang dependently at the side, the two articular surfaces of the GH joint have little contact. The majority of the time the inferior surface of the humeral head rests only on a small inferior portion of the fossa[5,24,25] (see

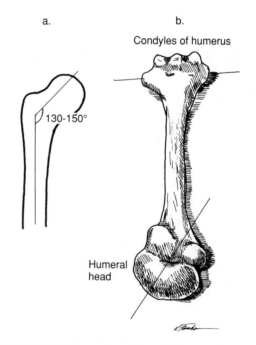

FIGURE 7–16. Humeral head is angled in two planes. (a) The head in the frontal plane is angled 130° to 150° with respect to the shaft. (b) The head in the transverse plane is commonly angled posteriorly with respect to an axis through the humeral condyles (retroversion).

Fig. 7–15). The total available articular surface of the glenoid fossa is somewhat enhanced by an accessory structure known as the **glenoid labrum.** This structure surrounds and is attached to the periphery of the glenoid fossa (Fig. 7–17), enhancing the depth or curvature of the fossa.[19] Although the labrum was traditionally thought to be synovium-lined fibrocartilage,[26] more recently it has been proposed that it is actually a redundant fold of dense fibrous connective tissue with little fibrocartilage other than at the attachment of the labrum to the periphery of the fossa.[27] The labrum superiorly is loosely attached, whereas the inferior portion is firmly attached and relatively immobile.[28]

Glenohumeral Capsule and Ligaments

The entire GH joint in the resting position (arm dependent at the side) is surrounded by a large, loose capsule that is taut superiorly and slack anteriorly and inferiorly (Fig. 7–18). The capsule is twice the size of the humeral head[29] and, when slack, allows more than 1 inch of distraction of the head from the glenoid fossa in the loose-packed position.[6] The relative laxity of the GH capsule is necessary for the large excursion of joint surfaces but provides little stability without the reinforcement of ligaments and muscles. When the humerus is abducted and laterally rotated on the glenoid, the capsule twists on itself and tightens, making abduction and lateral rotation the close-packed position for the GH joint.[30] The capsule is rein-

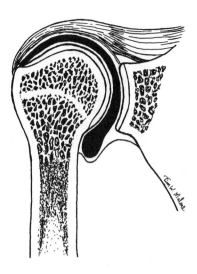

FIGURE 7–18. GH capsule. When the arm is at rest at the side, the large capsule is taut superiorly and lax inferiorly.

forced by the **superior, middle,** and **inferior glenohumeral** ligaments. However, a thin area of capsule between the superior and the middle GH ligaments (known as the **foramen of Weitbrecht**) is a particular point of weakness in the capsule. Although reinforced anteriorly by the subscapularis tendon, it is a common site of extrusion of the humeral head with anterior dislocation of the joint.

The ligaments that reinforce the GH joint capsule are the three GH ligaments and the coracohumeral ligament. The three GH ligaments (superior, middle, and inferior) vary considerably in size and extent and may change with age. Figure 7–19a shows the three ligaments as they would appear on the surface of the joint capsule. Recent work has shown the GH ligaments to be more complex than once thought. The superior glenohumeral ligament passes from the superior glenoid labrum and base of the coracoid process (deep to the **coracohumeral ligament**) to the upper neck of the humerus. Harryman and colleagues[31] described connections between the superior GH ligament, the superior capsule, and the coracohumeral ligament. These interconnected structures bridge the gap over the humeral head between the **supraspinatus** and **subscapularis** muscle tendons and may also be attached to the sheaths of these muscles. Harryman and colleagues termed these interrelated structures the **rotator interval capsule** (Fig. 7–19b). The inferior GH ligament has been described as having at least three portions and, thus, has

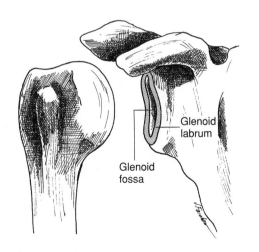

FIGURE 7–17. The glenoid labrum. As either a fibrocartilage structure or as a redundant capsular fold, the labrum deepens the glenoid fossa.

Glenoid labrum

Glenoid fossa

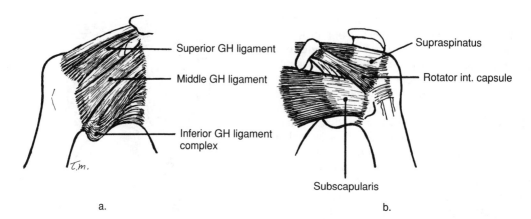

a.   b.

FIGURE 7–19. (a) The superior, middle, and inferior GH ligaments as they would appear on the surface of the joint capsule. (b) The superior capsule and superior GH ligament (deep to the supraspinatus tendon) and the coracohumeral ligament comprise the rotator interval capsule that bridges the gap between the supraspinatus and subscapularis tendons.

been termed the **inferior glenohumeral ligament complex.**[32] The three components of the complex (anterior and posterior bands and the axillary pouch in between) show position-dependent variability in function,[33] as well as variations in viscoelastic behavior.[19] Numerous studies of the restraints provided by the GH ligaments indicate different contributions to GH stability. There appears to be reasonable consensus, however, that the superior GH ligament (and its associated rotator interval capsule structures) contribute most to stability when the arm is at the side (0°), and the inferior GH ligament complex contributes most to stability when the GH joint is at 90° or more.[19,32-34] Most, if not all, of the GH ligaments tighten with lateral rotation of the humerus, consequently increasing their role in GH stabilization.

The coracohumeral ligament originates from the coracoid process and has two bands. The first inserts into the edge of the supraspinatus and onto the greater tubercle where it joins the superior GH ligament; the other band inserts into the subscapularis and lesser tubercle.[31,35] The two bands form a tunnel through which the tendon of the **long head of the biceps brachii** passes.[36] The interesting anatomic relations of the ligament would appear to position it to serve a more complex function than one would expect from a simple passive structure. As part of the rotator interval capsule, its stabilizing function would appear to be most important in preventing inferior translation of the humeral head in the dependent arm. However, there is some indication that it may also assist in preventing superior translation, especially when

the dynamic stabilizing force of the rotator cuff muscles is impaired.[35]

Bursae

Several bursae are associated with the shoulder complex in general and the GH joint specifically. Although all contribute to function, the most important are the **subacromial** and **subdeltoid** bursae (Fig. 7–20). These bursae separate the supraspinatus tendon and head of the humerus from the acromion, coracoid process, coracoacromial ligament, and deltoid muscle. The bursae may be separate but are commonly continuous with each other. Collectively the two are known as the subacromial bursa. The subacromial bursa permits smooth gliding be-

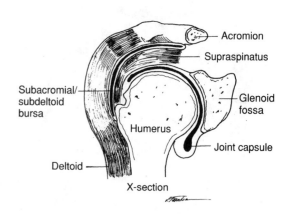

FIGURE 7–20. Subacromial and subdeltoid bursae permit smooth gliding of the supraspinatus muscle and the humeral head under the deltoid muscle and the acromion process.

tween the humerus and supraspinatus tendon and its surrounding structures. Interruption or failure of this gliding mechanism is a common cause of pain and limitation of GH motion, although it rarely occurs as a primary problem. The inferior wall of the subacromial bursa is also the superior portion of the supraspinatus tendon sheath. Subacromial bursitis is most commonly secondary to inflammation or degeneration of the supraspinatus tendon.[11]

Coracoacromial Arch

The **coracoacromial** (or **suprahumeral**) **arch** is formed by the coracoid process, the acromion, and the coracoacromial ligament that spans the two bony projections (Fig. 7–21). The coracoacromial arch forms an osteoligamentous vault that covers the humeral head and forms a space within which the subacromial bursa, the supraspinatus tendon, and a portion of the tendon of the long head of the biceps lie. The coracoacromial arch protects the structures beneath it from direct trauma from above. Such trauma is common and can occur through such simple daily tasks as carrying a heavy bag slung over the shoulder. The arch also prevents the head of the humerus from dislocating superiorly, because an unopposed upward translatory force on the humerus would cause the head of

the humerus to hit the coracoacromial arch. Paradoxically, the impact of the humeral head into the arch (while beneficially preventing dislocation) simultaneously can cause painful impingement of the structures lying in the suprahumeral space. When the suprahumeral space is narrowed, the likelihood of impingement of the supraspinatus tendon and subacromial bursa increases. Narrowing of the space can be caused by factors such as changes in the shape of the acromion inferiorly, changes in the slope of the acromion, acromial bone spurs, AC joint osteophytes or a large coracoacromial ligament.[35]

Glenohumeral Motions

GLENOHUMERAL OSTEOKINEMATICS

The GH joint is usually described as having 3° of freedom: flexion/extension, abduction/adduction, and medial/lateral rotation. The range of each of these motions occurring solely at the GH joint varies considerably. The joint is generally, though not universally, considered to have 120° of flexion and about 50° of extension.[37] The range of medial/lateral rotation of the humerus varies with position. With the arm at the side, medial and lateral rotation may be limited to as little as 50° of combined motion. Abducting the humerus to 90° frees the arc of rotation to 120°.[5] The restricted arc of medial/lateral rotation when the arm is at the side is due to the impact of the lesser tubercle on the anterior glenoid fossa with medial rotation and the impact of the greater tubercle on the acromion with lateral rotation. When the arm is abducted, these bony restrictions play little role, so the checks of motion become capsular and muscular.

The maximum range of abduction at the GH joint is the topic of much disagreement. There is consensus, however, that the range of abduction of the humerus in the frontal plane (whether done actively or passively) will be diminished if the humerus is maintained in neutral or medial rotation. When the humerus is medially rotated, the humerus will not abduct on the glenoid fossa beyond 60°; at neutral rotation, 90° of GH abduction can be obtained.[11,38] The restriction to abduction is caused by the impingement of the greater tubercle on the coracoacromial arch. When the humerus is laterally rotated 35° to 40°,[39,40] the greater tubercle will pass under or behind the arch so that abduction can continue unim-

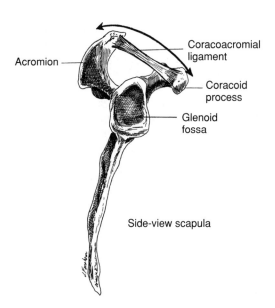

FIGURE 7–21. Coracoacromial arch. The arch is formed by the coracoid process anteriorly, the acromion posteriorly, and the coracoacromial ligament superiorly.

Coracoacromial ligament

Acromion

Coracoid process

Glenoid fossa

Side-view scapula

peded. There is apparently not the same need for rotation of the humerus for flexion to achieve its full range. Given the forward movement of the humerus in flexion, the greater tubercle slides behind or under the acromion process regardless of rotation.

The ROMs for abduction of the GH joint (presuming impact of the greater tubercle is avoided) are reported to be anywhere from 90°[2,5] to 120°,[11,38] with varying citations in between.[26,41] Inman and coworkers[42] found active abduction to be limited to 90° when the scapula did not participate in the motion, but claimed 120° of motion was available passively. Adding to the confusion, some studies examined the range of abduction in the traditional frontal plane, whereas others have investigated elevation in the so-called **plane of the scapula**. The plane of the scapula lies through the resting scapula and lies, therefore, 30° to 40° anterior to the frontal plane. When the humerus elevates in the plane of the scapula (referred to as abduction in the plane of the scapula, or more simply as **scaption**[43]), there is presumably less restriction to motion because the capsule is less twisted than when the humerus is brought further back into the frontal plane. Browne and colleagues,[39] however, found maximum elevation not in the plane of the scapula, but 23° anterior to that plane. Although it has been proposed that scaption does not require concomitant lateral rotation to achieve maximal range, this premise has also been disputed.[39,40] The range for scaption does not appear to differ from those cited for abduction in the frontal plane. Soslowski and colleagues[40] found five of nine cadaver shoulders to have a maximum of 120° of GH joint scaption, whereas three had 90° and one had less.

GLENOHUMERAL ARTHROKINEMATICS

The glenoid fossa and humeral head are incongruent surfaces; the convex humeral head is a substantially larger surface and may have a different radius of curvature than the shallow concave fossa. Given this incongruence, rotations of the joint around its three axes do not occur as pure spins, but have changing centers of rotation and shifting contact patterns within the joint. There is a somewhat surprising lack of consensus on the extent and direction of movement of the humeral head on the fossa.[19] However, there is agreement that elevation of the humerus requires that the humeral head glide inferiorly (caudally) in a direction opposite to movement of the shaft of the humerus. For example, abduction of the humerus would cause a superior (cephalad) rolling of the humeral head on the fossa. The large humeral head would soon run out of glenoid surface and the head of the humerus would impact on the overhanging coracoacromial arch (Fig. 7–22a). However, if the head of the humerus glides inferiorly while it rolls up the fossa, full ROM can be achieved (Fig. 7–22b). Although inferior glide of the humeral head is necessary to minimize upward roll of the humeral head, it would appear that the center of rotation of the head still moves superiorly on the glenoid even though the magnitude of reported shift differs.[19,40,44] Additionally, the humeral head may glide anteriorly or posteriorly and medially or laterally on the fossa. Howell and colleagues[45] found that the cocking phase of pitching a ball resulted in a posterior glide of the humeral head on the fossa, and the acceleration phase of the throw was accompanied by an anterior glide of the head on the fossa. Although some investigators found a similar posterior migration of the humeral head with maximum elevation,[19,40] Wuelker and colleagues[44] found the opposite. Most investigators seem to agree that many variables determine the pattern of movement within the fossa, including articular geometry, capsuloligamentous influences, positional influences, and muscle dynamics.

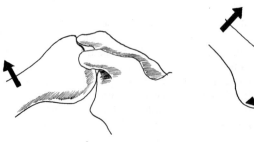 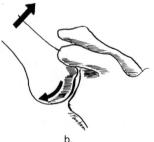

a.   b.

FIGURE 7–22. (a) Abduction of the humerus as a pure rolling of the large humeral head on the small glenoid fossa would cause impaction of the head into the acromion. (b) Abduction of the humerus occurring as a combination of rolling and sliding prevents impaction and allows a full ROM.

Static Stabilization of the Dependent Arm

Given the incongruence of the GH articular surfaces, the bony surfaces alone cannot maintain joint contact in the dependent position (arm hanging at the side). As the humeral head rests on the fossa, gravity acts on the humerus parallel to the shaft in a downward direction (negative translatory force). This would appear to require a vertical upward pull to restore equilibrium. Such a vertical force could only be supplied by muscles such as the anterior deltoid or the long heads of the biceps brachii and triceps brachii. Basmajian and Bazant[20] and Mac-Conaill and Basmajian[30] have shown that all muscles of the shoulder complex are electrically silent in the relaxed, unloaded limb and even when the limb is tugged vigorously downward. The mechanism of joint stabilization, therefore, must be passive. As can be seen in Figure 7–23, gravity (G) acting on the humerus is a pure translatory force but lies at a distance from the eccentrically located center of rotation of the humeral head.[5] Given the axis and the line of pull, gravity creates an adduction moment (counterclockwise torque in Fig. 7–23) on the humerus. Gravity must be offset by a force that can apply a torque of equal magnitude in the direction of abduction. Such a force can be applied by the structures of the rotator interval capsule (superior capsule, superior glenohumeral ligament, and coracohumeral ligament) that are taut when the arm is at the side.[31,33,34] Given the attachment of rotator in-terval capsule structures on the greater tubercle, the moment arm (MA) of this passive force is nearly twice that of the more centrally located force of gravity. The action line of the rotator interval capsule is upward (offsetting the downward translatory component of gravity) and into the glenoid fossa (compressing joint surfaces).

When the passive force of the rotator interval capsule is inadequate for static stabilization, as it may be in the heavily loaded arm, activity of the supraspinatus is recruited.[20] This is not surprising when one recalls that the supraspinatus tendon has attachments to the rotator interval capsule.[35] In fact, the role of the supraspinatus may be more critical than its electromyographic (EMG) activity indicates. Although *not* active when the unloaded arm hangs at the side, paralysis or dysfunction in the supraspinatus may lead to gradual inferior subluxation of the GH joint. Without the reinforcing passive tension of the intact supraspinatus muscle, the sustained load on the structures of the rotator interval capsule apparently causes these structures to gradually stretch and results in a loss of joint stability. Although the subscapularis does not show activity in the loaded dependent arm, resting tension in this muscle may also, through its connections to the rotator interval cuff, provide some support to those structures. Inferior GH subluxation is commonly encountered in patients with diminished rotator cuff function due to stroke.

Dynamic Stabilization of the Glenohumeral Joint

THE DELTOID AND GLENOHUMERAL STABILIZATION

It is generally accepted that the **deltoid** muscle is a prime mover (along with the supraspinatus) for GH abduction. The anterior deltoid is also considered the prime mover in GH flexion. Both abduction and flexion are elevation activities with many biomechanical similarities. Although the segments of the deltoid that participate will vary with role and function,[46,47] examination of the resultant action lines of the deltoid muscle in abduction can be used to highlight the stabilization needs of the GH joint in elevation activities. Figure 7–24 shows the action line of the deltoid muscle with the arm at the side (the action line of the three segments of the deltoid acting together coincide

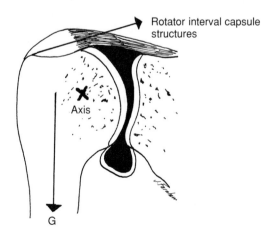

Rotator interval capsule structures

Axis

G

FIGURE 7–23. Mechanism for stabilization of the dependent arm. When the arm is relaxed at the side, the dislocation effect of gravity (G) is counteracted by the passive tension in the structures of the rotator interval capsule.

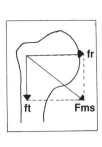

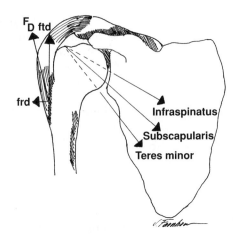

FIGURE 7–24. Force couple of the deltoid muscle (F_D) and the muscles of the musculotendinous cuff. The infaspinatus, subscapularis, and teres minor muscles together (Fms) have a negative translatory component (ft, inset) that nearly offsets the positive translatory component (ftd) of the deltoid force.

with the fibers of the middle deltoid). When the muscle action line (F_D) is resolved into its translatory (f_{td}) and rotatory (f_{rd}) components, the translatory component is by far the larger. That is, the majority of the force of contraction of the deltoid causes the humeral head to translate superiorly; only a small proportion of force causes rotation (abduction) of the humerus. The component forces of the deltoid provides an example in which a translatory force applied in the direction of the joint is *not* a stabilizing influence. The articular surface of the humerus is not in line with the shaft of the humerus; therefore, a force parallel to the bone creates a dislocating rather than a stabilizing (compressive) effect. The superior (caudal) translatory force of the deltoid, if unopposed, would cause the humeral head to impact the coracoacromial arch before much abduction had occurred. Once the inferiorly directed force of the coracoacromial arch is introduced by humeral head contact, rotation of the humeral head could, theoretically, continue against the leverage provided by the arch. However, but pain from impinged structures would prevent much motion. The inferior translatory pull of gravity cannot offset f_{td}, because the resultant force of the deltoid must exceed that of gravity before any rotation can occur. Another force or set of forces must be introduced. This is a major function of the muscles of the rotator, or musculotendinous, cuff.

THE ROTATOR CUFF AND GLENOHUMERAL STABILIZATION

The supraspinatus, **infraspinatus, teres minor,** and subscapularis muscles compose the **rotator** or **musculotendinous cuff.** These mus-

cles are considered to be part of a "cuff" because the inserting tendons of each muscle of the cuff blend with and reinforce the GH capsule. More importantly, all have action lines that significantly contribute to the dynamic stabilization of the GH joint. The action lines of the infraspinatus, teres minor, and subscapularis are shown in Figure 7–24. When the force of any one (or all three taken together) is resolved into its components (inset), it can be seen that the rotatory force (fr) not only tends to cause at least some rotation of the humerus, but f_r also compresses the head into the glenoid fossa. Now we have an example of a rotatory component creating joint stabilization! This is due, once again, to the fact that the articular surface of the humerus lies nearly perpendicular to the shaft.

Although the muscles of the rotator cuff are important GH joint compressors, equally (or perhaps more) critical to the stabilizing function of cuff muscles is the inferior (caudal) translatory pull (f_t) of the muscles. The sum of the three negative translatory components of the rotator cuff nearly offsets the superior translatory force of the deltoid muscle. Sharkey and Marder[48] showed that abduction without the infraspinatus, teres minor, and subscapularis muscles resulted in substantial superiorly directed shifts in humeral position in cadaver models.

In addition to their stabilizing role, the teres minor and infraspinatus muscles contribute to abduction by providing the lateral rotation necessary to prevent the greater tubercle from impacting the acromion. Although the weak adduction force of the teres minor muscle and the medial rotatory force of the subscapularis would appear to contradict their role in elevation of the arm, Otis and colleagues[49] found the effectiveness of these muscles in their contradictory functions to be diminished during abduction of the arm. That is, the infraspinatus and subscapularis added to the abduction torque, whereas the teres minor added to the lateral rotatory torque. The medial and lateral rotatory forces also help center the humeral head, with increased anterior and posterior displacements evident when rotator cuff forces are reduced.[50] Saha[23] referred to these muscles as "steerers." A steering muscle causes a changeover of surfaces within the joint, usually by gliding, and directs the articular surfaces to the appropriate points of contact. He noted that muscles serve both as vertical steerers and, later in the elevation range, as horizontal steerers. He particularly credits the subscapularis with being able to posteriorly steer the humeral head, thus offsetting anterior dislocating forces.

The action of the deltoid along with the combined actions of the infraspinatus, teres minor, and subscapularis form a **force couple.** In a force couple, the divergent pulls of the forces create a pure rotation. In this case, the divergent pulls create an *almost* perfect spinning of the humeral head around a fixed axis of rotation.

THE SUPRASPINATUS AND GLENOHUMERAL STABILIZATION

Although the supraspinatus muscle is also part of the rotator cuff, the action line of the supraspinatus muscle has a superior (cephalad) translatory component, rather than the inferior (caudal) component found in the other muscles of the cuff. Given its line of pull, the supraspinatus is of no use in offsetting the upward dislocating action of the deltoid.[51] The supraspinatus still is effective as a stabilizer of the GH joint because, like the other cuff muscles, its rotatory component generates a strong compressive force. Unlike the other cuff muscles, the rotatory component of the supraspinatus has a large enough MA that it is capable by itself of producing a full or nearly full range of GH joint abduction and, with the assistance of gravity, stabilizing the joint.[30] Gravity acts as a stabilizing synergist to the supraspinatus by offsetting the small upward translatory pull of the muscle (Fig. 7–25). Gravity and the supraspinatus, using Saha's terminology,[23] act as vertical steerers; the resultant of the two forces causes an inferior gliding of the humeral

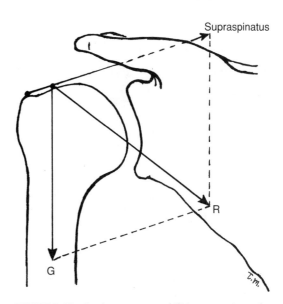

FIGURE 7–25. Gravity acts as a stabilizing synergist to the supraspinatus muscle. Activity of the supraspinatus and gravity (G) produce a resultant force (R) that abducts the humerus and causes the downward sliding of articular surfaces necessary for a full ROM.

head during abduction of the shaft, allowing full articulation of the surfaces and preventing abnormal superior displacement.

THE LONG HEAD OF THE BICEPS AND GLENOHUMERAL STABILIZATION

The long head of the biceps runs superiorly from the anterior shaft of the humerus through the bicipital groove between the greater and lesser tubercles to attach to the supraglenoid tubercle and superior labrum. It enters the GH joint capsule through an opening between the supraspinatus and subscapularis muscles where it penetrates the capsule but not the synovium (Fig. 7–26). Within the bicipital groove, the biceps tendon is enveloped by a tendon sheath and tethered there by the **transverse humeral ligament** that runs between the greater and lesser tubercles. The long head of the biceps, because of its position at the superior capsule and its connections to structures of the rotator interval capsule,[35] is sometimes considered to be part of the reinforcing cuff of the GH joint. The biceps muscle is capable of contributing to the force of flexion and can, if the humerus is laterally rotated, contribute to the force of abduction and anterior stabilization.[42] Although elbow and shoulder position may influence its function, the long head appears to contribute to GH stabilization by cen-

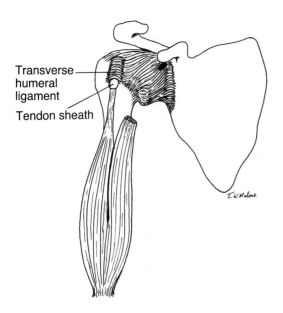

Transverse
humeral
ligament

Tendon sheath

FIGURE 7–26. The long head of the biceps brachii passes through a fibro-osseous tunnel formed by the bicipital groove and the transverse humeral ligament. It is protected within the tunnel by a tendon sheath.

tering the head in the fossa, and by reducing vertical (superior and inferior) and anterior translations.[52–55] Pagnani and colleagues hypothesize that the long head may produce its effect by tightening the relatively loose superior labrum and transmitting increased tension to the superior and middle GH ligaments.[55] This concept follows from their observation that lesions of the anterosuperior labrum did not affect stability of the GH joint unless the attachment of the long head of the biceps was also disrupted.[56] The overall contribution of the long head to GH stabilization is supported by the observation that the tendon hypertrophies with rotator cuff tears.[55,57]

COSTS OF DYNAMIC STABILIZATION

Given what we know about the GH joint thus far, we can summarize that dynamic stabilization at any point in the range is a function of (1) the force of the prime mover(s), (2) the force of gravity, (3) the force of the compressors and steerers, (4) articular surface geometry, and (5) passive capsuloligamentous forces. Inman and colleagues[42] appropriately add (6) the force of friction and (7) the joint reaction force because any shear force within the GH joint creates some friction across its joint surfaces and because all compressive forces that snug the

head into the glenoid fossa must be opposed by an equal force from the glenoid fossa in the opposite direction (joint reaction force). When all stabilization factors are intact, the head of the humerus rotates into flexion or abduction around a relatively fixed axis with minimal superior gliding. Over time, however, even normal stresses resulting from the complex dynamic stabilization process may lead to degenerative changes or dysfunction at the GH joint. Any disruption in the synergistic action of the dynamic stabilization factors may accelerate degenerative changes in or around the joint.

As the humerus rotates around a relatively fixed axis during elevation, some superior gliding may occur. Even a small amount of gliding may be responsible for changes that occur in the pressure within the subacromial bursa as the humerus elevates. These pressures are related to both arm position and load, with greater pressures in the bursa evidenced as the arms are loaded and maintained in an elevated position.[58] The swelling pressure of the subacromial bursa, especially with a concomitant supraspinatus contraction as the arm elevates, may narrow the suprahumeral space and decrease blood supply to the "critical zone" of the supraspinatus tendon where small anastomosing vessels are responsible for tendon nutrition.[11] Such restriction to blood supply may be responsible for an increasing incidence of supraspinatus tendon tears from minor trauma with increasing age.[59] Supraspinatus tendon tears, however, do not seem to be attributable to the aging process alone, but are considered multifactorial. The supraspinatus is either passively tensed or actively contracting when the arm is at the side (depending on load); it also participates in elevation throughout the ROM. Consequently, the tendon is under tension most of one's waking hours and is vulnerable to tensile overload and chronic overuse.[8] Impingement of the stressed supraspinatus tendon can occur when the suprahumeral space is reduced by osteoligamentous factors (see Coracohumeral Arch), when there is increased upward migration of the humeral head with less favorable GH mechanics, or when occupational factors demand heavy lifting or sustained overhead arm postures. Although the supraspinatus tendon is the most vulnerable of the cuff muscles, the overuse and potential impingement issues also apply to the other cuff muscles as well. Symptomatic and asymptomatic rotator cuff tears are seen in almost all people over the age of 70, with the supraspinatus likely to show lesions before the other tendons of the cuff.[60] Rotator cuff lesions typically produce pain between 60° and 120° of combined GH elevation and scapular upward rotation. This range constitutes what is known as the **painful arc.**

Degenerative changes in the AC joint may result in pain in the same area of the shoulder as pain from supraspinatus or rotator cuff lesions. Pain due to AC degeneration is more typically found when the arm is raised beyond the painful arc.[61] The long head of the biceps similarly can produce pain in anterosuperior shoulder. Because the long head of the biceps, like the supraspinatus tendon, is poorly vascularized,[61] it is subject to some of the same degenerative changes and the same trauma seen in the tendons of the rotator cuff. Whether the biceps is actively contributing to elevation of the arm, to joint stabilization or is passive, the tendon of the biceps must slide within the bicipital groove and under the transverse humeral ligament as the humerus moves around any of its three axes. If the bicipital tendon sheath is worn or inflamed or if the tendon is hypertrophied (as seen with rotator cuff tears), the gliding mechanism may be interrupted and pain produced. A tear in the transverse humeral ligament may result in the tendon of the long head popping in and out of the bicipital groove with rotation of the humerus, a potentially wearing and painful microtrauma.

Mechanical deviations in GH stabilization factors may result in degenerative changes in other structures of the joint besides the rotator cuff (e.g., the glenoid labrum) and to subluxation of the joint. Dislocation of the GH joint can also occur. Capsuloligamentous and muscle reinforcement to the GH is weakest inferiorly, but it is most common for the GH joint to dislocate anteriorly. Although the subscapularis and the glenohumeral ligaments reinforce the capsule anteriorly, a force applied to an abducted, laterally rotated arm can force the humeral head through the foramen of Weitbrecht. A predisposition to actual dislocation most typically exists when the individual structural variations are in the direction of (1) anterior tilt of the glenoid fossa; (2) excessive retrotorsion of the humeral head; or (3) weakened horizontal steerers (rotator cuff).[23]

Integrated Function of the Shoulder Complex

The shoulder complex acts in a coordinated fashion to provide the smoothest and greatest ROM possible to the upper limb. Motion available to the GH joint alone would not account for the full range of elevation (abduction or flexion) available to the humerus. The remainder of the range is contributed by the scapulothoracic joint through its SC and AC linkages. Combined scapulohumeral motion (1) distributes the motion between two joints (GH and ST), permitting a large ROM with less compromise of stability than would occur if the same range occurred at one joint; (2) maintains the glenoid fossa in an optimal position to receive the head of the humerus, increasing joint congruency while decreasing shear forces; and (3) permits muscles acting on the humerus to maintain a good length-tension relation while minimizing or preventing active insufficiency of the GH muscles.

Scapulothoracic and Glenohumeral Contributions

The scapulothoracic joint contributes to both flexion and abduction (elevation) of the humerus by upwardly rotating the glenoid fossa 60° from its resting position. If the humerus were fixed to the fossa, this alone would result in 60° of elevation of the humerus. The humerus is not fixed, of course, but can move independently on the glenoid fossa. The GH joint contributes 120° of flexion and anywhere from 90° to 120° of abduction (depending on individual structural variations and on one's philosophy of available GH abduction). The combination of scapular and humeral movement results in what is commonly held to be a maximum range of elevation to 180° (Fig. 7–27) and in an *overall* ratio of 2° of GH to 1° of scapulothoracic motion.

During the initial 60° of flexion or the initial 30° of abduction of the humerus, an inconsistent amount and type of scapular motion takes place relative to GH motion. During this period the scapula seeks a position of stability in relation to the humerus (setting phase).[42,47] In this early phase, motion occurs primarily at the GH joint, although stressing the arm may increase the scapular contribution.[41,62] With increasing range, the scapula increases its contribution, approaching a 1:1 ratio with GH movement. In

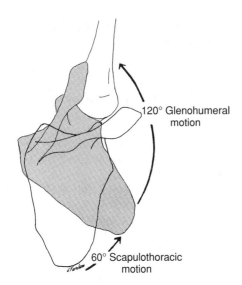

120° Glenohumeral
motion

60° Scapulothoracic
motion

FIGURE 7–27. Elevation of the arm through a full ROM normally requires 60° of scapulothoracic motion and 120° of GH motion. These motions occur concomitantly, not sequentially.

the latter part of the range, the GH joint again increases its contribution.[23,26,41] Although Poppen and Walker[22] found the GH to scapulothoracic ratio to be 5:4 between 24° and maximum elevation in the plane of the scapula, they note that the absolute angles achieved at each joint yield an overall ratio of 2° of GH motion for each 1° of ST motion. The combination of concomitant GH and ST motion is most commonly referred to as **scapulohumeral rhythm.** However, the rhythm varies among individuals and may vary with external constraints.[63] Högfors and colleagues[64] used in vivo imaging and bony implantation of tantalum balls in three subjects. Although generally confirming the findings of Poppen and Walker, they concluded that individual differences resulted in qualitative similarities but quantitative differences. Because there does not appear to be a specific scapulohumeral rhythm that should serve as a standard and because scapulohumeral rhythm is irrelevant when pathologies are encountered, the utility of the term seems limited.

Sternoclavicular and Acromioclavicular Contributions

Scapulohumeral motion involves motion of the SC and AC joints, as well as the ST and GH joints. Because the ST joint is part of a closed chain, movement of the scapula occurs only with motion at both the AC and SC joints. The

60° arc of upward rotation through which the scapula moves during elevation of the arm can be attributed primarily to SC and secondarily to AC motion produced by the force couple of the **trapezius** and **serratus anterior** muscles. These two muscles are the *only* muscles capable of upwardly rotating the scapula.

Phase One

The upper portion of the trapezius muscle elevates the clavicle; the lower portion of the trapezius muscle combines with the upper and lower portions of the serratus anterior muscle (Fig. 7–28) to produce an upward rotatory force on the scapula. The middle trapezius may also contribute to upward rotation. Although upward rotation of the scapula would appear to occur at the AC joint, the coracoclavicular ligament prevents this AC movement because the ligament binds the coracoid process of the scapula to the clavicle (see discussion of coracoclavicular ligament of the AC joint). The upward rotatory force on the scapula from the contracting muscles, therefore, must produce movement at the next available joint: the SC joint. The pull of the trapezius and serratus anterior muscles on the scapula (and the direct pull of the upper trapezius on the lateral clavicle) force the clavicle to elevate. Clavicular elevation carries the scapula through 30° of upward rotation as the scapula rides on the lateral end of the rising clavicle while main-

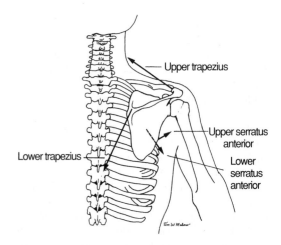

FIGURE 7–28. The action lines of the upper trapezius, lower trapezius, upper serratus anterior, and lower serratus anterior combine to produce almost pure upward rotation of the scapula.

taining a relatively fixed scapuloclavicular angle (Fig. 7–29a). Elevation of the clavicle is checked when the costoclavicular ligament becomes taut. Because the ST upward rotation and clavicular elevation occur *concurrently* with GH motion, the GH joint can be expected under normal conditions to simultaneously flex or abduct about 60° (using an overall 2:1 ratio with the understanding that individual differences exist). Given 30° of ST upward rotation and 60° of GH flexion or abduction, the arm will be elevated approximately 90° to 100° from the side of the body.[42,47] During the initial 30° of ST motion, the AC joint maintains a relatively fixed relation between the scapula and clavicle, although allowing 10° of medial rotation and some anterior tipping of the scapula to maintain the scapula against the changing contour of the rib cage.[46]

Phase Two

As the lower trapezius and the serratus anterior continue to generate an upward rotatory force on the scapula, upward rotation at the AC joint is still restrained by the coracoclavicular ligament while the SC joint is now constrained by tension in the costoclavicular ligament (which checked further clavicular elevation). With no

other available motion to dissipate the upward rotatory force being created by the trapezius and serratus muscles, tension in the coracoclavicular ligament (especially the conoid portion[7]) builds as the coracoid process of the scapula gets pulled downward. The tensed conoid ligament draws its posteroinferior clavicular attachment forward and down as the coracoid process drops, causing the clavicle to posteriorly rotate.[46] Posterior rotation of the clavicle around its longitudinal axis will flip the lateral end of the crank-shaped clavicle up (Fig. 7–29 inset) without causing further elevation at the SC joint and while still maintaining a relatively fixed scapuloclavicular angle. The magnitude of posterior rotation of the clavicle may be anywhere from 30°[2] to 55°.[7] The scapula that is attached to the lateral end of the rotating clavicle, however, will be carried through an additional 30° of upward rotation (Fig. 7–29b). As the scapula finds its final position on the rib cage, the AC joint absorbs varying amounts of anterior/posterior tipping and medial/lateral rotation. The magnitudes of AC motion can be expected to differ between flexion, scaption, and abduction of the arm, as well as to differ with variations in scapular resting position, rib cage configuration, and muscle dynamics.

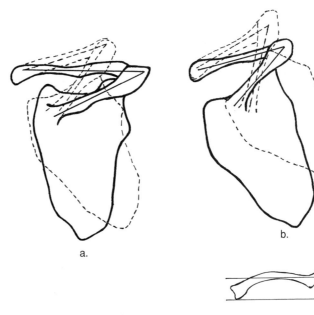

a.

b.

inset

FIGURE 7–29. (a) The first 30° of scapular upward rotation is produced by elevation of the clavicle. (b) The second 30° of scapular upward rotation occurs when posterior rotation of the clavicle flips the lateral end of the clavicle up (inset), carrying the scapula up with it.

If 180° is accepted as the maximal range of flexion and abduction of the humerus, raising the arm *to the horizontal* involves 60° of GH motion and 30° of ST motion, with the scapular contribution produced by clavicular elevation at the SC joint. Raising the arm *from the horizontal to vertical position* involves an additional 60° of GH movement (with lateral rotation needed for scaption and abduction) and 30° of ST movement produced by clavicular rotation and AC motion (Fig. 7–30). For the clavicle to rotate about its longitudinal axis, it would appear to require mobility of both the SC and the AC joints. However, internal fixation of the AC joint does not significantly impair range of elevation, whereas attempted internal fixation of the SC joint most often results in extrusion of the fixating hardware.[3,7] These observations would lead one to conclude that the SC joint is of primary importance both for the first 30° of ST upward rotation and for the second 30° of ST upward rotation, with the AC joint playing a supporting role.

The sequence of phase one and phase two scapulohumeral motions occurs regardless of the plane in which the arm is elevated. That is, although the range may vary somewhat, the component events are similar whether the motion is performed as flexion, abduction, or scaption. One difference already noted is that abduction of the arm in the frontal plane requires concomitant lateral rotation of the humerus to permit full GH range. There is also another difference between performance of sagittal plane and frontal plane elevation. Although the scapula must upwardly rotate in both instances, flexion requires simultaneous protraction of the scapula. Protraction of the scapula brings the glenoid fossa forward, keeping the fossa in line with the shaft of the humerus. If this did not occur, the head of the humerus would be unprotected posteriorly; posterior dislocations could occur with relatively little force. In abduction of the arm in the frontal plane, the scapula tends to remain in neutral protraction-retraction or is slightly retracted.

Structural Dysfunction

Completion of the range of elevation of the arm depends on the ability of GH, ST, SC, and AC joints each to make the needed contribution. Disruption of movement in any of the participating joints will result in a loss of ROM. Once restrictions to function are introduced, the concept of scapulohumeral rhythm is no longer relevant; that is, a reduction in GH joint range will *not* result in a proportional decrease in scapulothoracic range. The ratio of movement is no longer pertinent because the body will automatically recruit any and all remaining motion at other joints. In fact, though not necessarily predictable, restriction to motion at any one joint in the shoulder complex commonly results in the development of some hypermobility (and reduced stability) in remaining articulations.

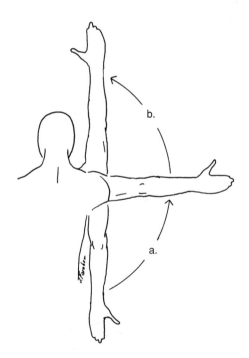

FIGURE 7–30. (a) Bringing the arm from the side to the horizontal requires concomitant GH motion and SC elevation. (b) Arm horizontal to overhead position requires concomitant GH motion and SC-AC rotation.

EXAMPLE 1: If motion at the GH joint is restricted by pain or disease, the total range available to the humerus will be reduced. Whatever portion of the motion remains at the GH joint will still be accompanied by the full 60° of ST motion. For example, restriction of the humerus in a position of medial rotation will limit GH joint abduction to approximately 60°. The 60° of available GH range in the medially rotated humerus will combine with 60° of unimpeded ST motion to give a total available range of 120° as the arm is raised from the side.

EXAMPLE 2: Hypothetical fusion of the SC joint would eliminate ST movement. Because both clavicular elevation and rotation occur through the SC joint, SC fusion would eliminate both components of scapular upward rotation. The arm would elevate only at the GH joint, with the amount of available motion at that joint influenced by whether the motion is performed actively or passively (see the discussion of deltoid function in the next section). It should be noted, however, that fixation of the very stable SC joint rarely occurs. In such an unusual instance, however, one would expect over time to develop hypermobility and increased instability of the AC joint.

Muscles of Elevation

Perry describes elevation and depression as the two primary patterns of shoulder complex function.[65] Elevation activities are described as those requiring muscles to overcome or control the weight of the limb and its load, and usually involve components of GH flexion or abduction, and scapular upward rotation. The completion of normal elevation depends not only on freedom of movement and integrity of the joints involved but also on the appropriate strength and function of the muscles producing and controlling movement. A closer look at the activity of these muscles should enhance an understanding of normal function, as well as contribute to an understanding of the deficits seen in pathologic situations.

Deltoid Muscle

The deltoid is at resting length (optimal length-tension) when the arm is at the side. When at resting length, the deltoid's angle of pull will result in a predominance of superior translatory pull on the humerus with an active contraction (see Fig. 7–24). With an appropriate synergistic downward pull from the infraspinatus, teres minor, and subscapularis, the rotatory components of the anterior and middle deltoid are effective primary movers for flexion and abduction, respectively. The anterior deltoid can assist with abduction after 15° of GH motion.[49] When the humerus is in the plane of the scapula, the anterior and middle deltoid are optimally aligned to produce elevation of the humerus.[22] The action line of the posterior deltoid has too small an MA (and too small a rotatory component) to contribute effectively to abduction; it serves primarily as a joint compressor[24,46] and in functions such as horizontal abduction.

As the humerus elevates, the translatory component of the deltoid diminishes its superior dislocating influence and shifts its line of pull increasingly toward the glenoid fossa. At the same time, the rotatory component of the deltoid must counteract the increasing torque of gravity as the arm moves toward horizontal. Analysis by EMG shows gradually increasing activity in the deltoid, peaking at 90° of humeral abduction and plateauing for the remainder of the motion (Saha[23] found a peak at 120° with a drop off to moderate activity at 180°). The peak activity in flexion does not occur until the end of the range and there is less total activity.[23,42] Although the MA of the deltoid gets larger as the humerus elevates[25] and the torque of gravity diminishes once the arm is above the horizontal, the high activity level of the deltoid continues. The deltoid's shortening fibers are approaching active insufficiency. As a result of the loss of tension due to extreme shortening, a greater number of motor units must be recruited to maintain even equivalent force output. The multipennate structure and considerable cross section of the deltoid help compensate for the relatively small MA, low mechanical advantage, and less-than-optimal length/tension.

Maintenance of appropriate length/tension of the deltoid is strongly dependent on simultaneous scapular movement. When the scapula is restricted, the deltoid becomes actively insufficient and can only achieve and barely maintain 90° of GH abduction (whether the supraspinatus is available for assistance or not).[5,38,42] The synergy that occurs between the scapular upward rotators and the deltoid is further discussed in the section on trapezius and serratus anterior function. As already noted, deltoid activity also depends on an intact rotator cuff. With complete derangement of the cuff, a contraction of the deltoid results in a shrug of the shoulder rather than in abduction of the humerus. Stimulation of the axillary nerve (innervating the deltoid and teres minor alone) produces approximately 40° of abduction.[66] Partial tears in or partial paralysis of the cuff will weaken the rotation produced by the deltoid.[18]

Supraspinatus Muscle

The supraspinatus muscle is considered an abductor of the humerus. Like the deltoid muscle, however, it functions in both flexion and abduction of the humerus. Its role, according to MacConaill and Basmajian,[30] is quantitative rather than specialized. The pattern of activity of the supraspinatus is essentially the same as that found in the deltoid.[42] The MA of the supraspinatus is fairly constant throughout the ROM and is larger than that of the deltoid for the first 60° of shoulder abduction.[24] When the deltoid is paralyzed, the supraspinatus alone can bring the arm through most if not all of the GH range, but the motion will be weaker. With a suprascapular nerve block that paralyzes the supraspinatus and the infraspinatus, the strength of elevation in the plane of the scapula is reduced by 35% at 0° and by 60% to 80% at 150°.[67] The secondary functions of the supraspinatus are to compress the GH joint, to act as a vertical steerer for the humeral head, and to assist in maintaining the stability of the dependent arm. With isolated and complete paralysis of the supraspinatus muscle, some loss of abduction force is evident, but most of its functions can be performed by remaining musculature. Isolated paralysis of the supraspinatus is unusual, however, because its innervation is the same as the infraspinatus and related to that of the teres minor. Most commonly, lesions of the rotator cuff muscles occur together, producing a more extensive deficit than seen with paralysis of the supraspinatus alone.

Infraspinatus, Teres Minor, and Subscapularis Muscles

When Inman and coworkers[42] assessed the combined actions of the infraspinatus, teres minor, and subscapularis muscles, electromyographic activity indicated a nearly linear rise in action potentials from 0° to 115° elevation. Activity dropped slightly between 115° and 180°. Total activity in flexion was slightly greater than that in abduction. In abduction an early peak in activity of these muscles appeared at 70° of elevation. Steindler[5] hypothesized that the early peak was a response to the need for depression (downward sliding) of the humeral head, whereas the latter peak at 115° was a result of increased activity of these muscles in producing lateral rotation of the humerus. The medial rotatory function of the subscapularis acts to steer the head of the humerus horizontally, while continuing to work with the other cuff muscles to compress and stabilize the joint.[23]

Upper and Lower Trapezius and Serratus Anterior Muscles

The upper trapezius and upper serratus anterior muscles form one segment of a force couple that drives the scapula in elevation of the arm. These two muscle segments, along with the levator scapula muscle, also support the shoulder girdle against the downward pull of gravity. Although support of the scapula in the pendant limb in many individuals is passive, loading the limb will produce activity in these muscles.[30,42] The second segment of the force couple is formed by the lower trapezius and lower serratus anterior muscles. When activity of the upper and lower trapezius and serratus anterior muscles was monitored by EMG during humeral elevation, the curves were similar and complementary. Activity in the trapezius rises linearly to 180° in abduction, with more undulating activity in flexion. The serratus anterior shows a linear increase in action potentials to 180° in flexion, with undulating activity in abduction.[42] Saha found the upper and lower trapezius activity peaked and plateaued before the end of the range, with some decrease in activity at maximal elevation.[23] The middle trapezius is also active during elevation (especially abduction) and may contribute to upward rotation of the scapula.

In abduction of the arm, the force of the trapezius seems more critical to the production of upward rotation of the scapula than the force of the serratus anterior. When the trapezius is intact and the serratus anterior is paralyzed, abduction of the arm can occur through its full range although it is *weakened*. When the trapezius is paralyzed (even though the serratus anterior may be intact), abduction of the arm is both weakened and *limited in range* to 75°.[5] This is only slightly better than the range that can be obtained when neither of the upward rotators of the scapula are present.[66] The remaining range occurs exclusively at the GH joint. Without the trapezius (with or without the serratus anterior), the scapula rests in a downwardly rotated position due to the unopposed effect of gravity on the scapula. When abduction of the arm is attempted, the middle and posterior fibers of the activated deltoid (originating on the acromion and spine of the scapula) increase the downward rotatory pull on the scapula (Fig. 7–31). Although the deltoid can still achieve the 90° of GH motion attributed to it when the scapula has been immobilized, the 90° occurs on a downwardly rotated scapula; the net effect is that the arm will rise from the side only about 60° to 75° (Fig. 7–32).[68]

Although the trapezius seems to be the more critical of the two upward rotators in abduction of the arm, the reverse set of circumstances occurs with flexion of the arm. In flexion the anterior orientation of the scapula is important in that this can be produced only by the serratus anterior. If the serratus anterior is intact, trapezius paralysis results in loss of *force* of shoulder flexion but there is no range deficit. If the serratus anterior is paralyzed (even in the presence of a functioning trapezius), flexion will be both *diminished in strength* and *limited in range* to 130° or 140° of flexion. When the scapular retraction component of the trapezius is unopposed by the serratus anterior, the trapezius is unable to upwardly rotate the scapula more than 20° of its potential 60°.[5]

Although the serratus anterior and trapezius are the prime movers for scapulothoracic upward rotation, these muscles serve an equally important function as stabilizing synergists for the deltoid acting at the GH joint. All muscles pull on both proximal and distal attachments equally. When both ends are free to move, the

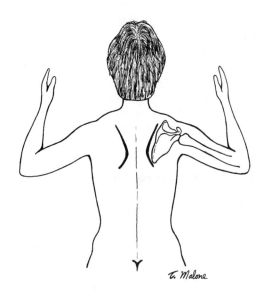

FIGURE 7–32. With paralysis of the trapezi, attempted abduction of the arms causes the deltoids to have a downward rotatory effect on the scapulae. Although 90° of GH joint motion can be achieved, the position of the scapulae results in the arms only being raised from the side 60° or less.

lighter end will usually move first. In most instances, the lighter of the two segments of the joint is the distal segment. Rather uniquely, the lighter segment of the GH joint is the proximal scapular segment. If the deltoid acted on its lighter proximal segment rather than the heavier humerus (with its appended forearm and hand), the scapula would rotate downward before the humerus would elevate. The deltoid muscle would become actively insufficient before much humeral elevation was produced. The trapezius and serratus anterior muscles, as upward scapular rotators, prevent the undesired downward rotatory movement of the scapula during deltoid contraction. The trapezius and serratus anterior maintain optimal length-tension in the deltoid and permit the deltoid to carry its heavier distal lever through full ROM. Thus, the role of the scapular force couple of the trapezius and the serratus anterior is both agonistic to scapular movement and synergistic to GH movement. The trapezius and serratus anterior produce desired scapular upward rotation, while preventing undesired movement by the deltoid as it elevates the GH joint.

Rhomboid Muscles

The **rhomboid major** and **minor** muscles are active in elevation of the humerus, especially

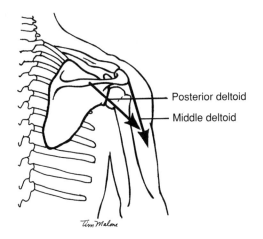

FIGURE 7–31. Without the trapezius, the scapula rests in a downwardly rotated position due to the unopposed effect of gravity on the scapula. When abduction of the arm is attempted, the middle and posterior fibers of the activated deltoid increase the downward rotatory pull on the scapula.

in abduction. These muscles serve a critical function as stabilizing synergists to the muscles that rotate the scapula. They contract eccentrically to control the change in position of the scapula produced by the trapezius and the serratus anterior. Paralysis of these muscles causes disruption of the normal scapulohumeral rhythm and may result in diminished ROM.[5]

Muscles of Depression

Depression is the second of the two primary patterns of shoulder complex function.[65] It involves the *forceful* downward movement of the arm in relation to the trunk. If the arm is fixed by weight bearing or by holding on to an object (e.g., a chinning bar), depression is then the forceful movement of the trunk upward in relation to the arm. In depression activities, the scapula tends to rotate downward and adduct during the humeral motion, but there is not a consistent ratio of one segment to the other.

Latissimus Dorsi and Pectoral Muscles

When the upper extremity is free to move in space, the **latissimus dorsi** muscle serves an important function in adduction and medial rotation of the humerus, as well as in extension of the humerus. When the latissimus pulls on its attachment to the scapula and on its humeral attachment, it can also adduct and depress the shoulder girdle. When the hand is fixed in weight bearing, the latissimus dorsi muscle will pull its caudal attachment on the pelvis toward its cephalad attachment on the scapula and humerus. This results in

lifting the body up as in a seated pushup. When the hands are bearing weight on the handles of a pair of crutches, a contraction of the latissimus will unweight the feet as the trunk rises beneath the fixed scapula; this will allow the legs to swing forward through the crutches.

Some studies have found the latissimus dorsi muscle to be active in abduction and flexion of the arm.[23,24] Its activity may contribute to joint stability because it causes compression of the GH joint when the arm is above the horizontal.

The clavicular portion of the **pectoralis major** can assist the deltoid in flexion of the GH joint but the sternal and abdominal portions are primary depressors of the shoulder complex. The combined action of the pectoralis major's sternal and abdominal portions parallels that of the latissimus dorsi, although the pectoralis is located anterior rather than posterior to the GH joint as is the latissimus. In activities involving weight-bearing on the hands, both the pectoralis major and the latissimus can depress the shoulder complex, while anterior/posterior movement of the humerus and protraction/retraction of the scapula are neutralized. The depressor function of these muscles is further assisted by the **pectoralis minor** muscle, which acts directly on the scapula to depress and rotate it downward.

Teres Major and Rhomboid Muscles

The **teres major** muscle, like the latissimus dorsi, adducts, medially rotates, and extends the humerus. The teres major is active primarily during resisted activities, but may also be active during unresisted extension and adduction activities behind the back.[69]

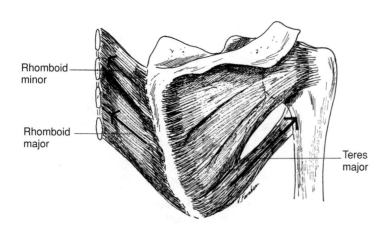

Rhomboid minor

Rhomboid major

Teres major

FIGURE 7–33. Scapular synergy of the teres major and rhomboid muscles. The rhomboid major and rhomboid minor offset the unwanted scapular upward rotation force produced by teres major activity.

Function of the teres major muscle is strongly dependent on activity of the rhomboid muscles. The teres major muscle originates on the scapula and attaches to the humerus. Consequently, the segment it attaches to proximally is lighter than the segment it attaches to distally. The proximal scapula must be stabilized to permit the teres major to act effectively as an extensor and adductor of the humerus. Without stabilization, the teres major would upwardly rotate the lighter scapula rather than move the heavier humerus. The rhomboid muscles, as downward rotators of the scapula, offset the undesired upward rotatory force of the teres major (Fig. 7–33). By fixing the scapula as the teres major contracts, the rhomboids allow the teres major to move the heavier humerus.

Summary

In this chapter, we laid the foundation for understanding more distal upper extremity joint function by exploring the intricate dynamic stabilization of the shoulder complex. The more distal joints of the upper extremity depend on the dual mobility/stability roles of the shoulder complex. Whereas function in the hand, for instance, can continue on a limited basis with loss of shoulder mobility, loss of shoulder stability can render the remaining function in the hand unusable. We will next explore the elbow as the intermediary between the shoulder and the hand.

REFERENCES

1. Dempster, W: Mechanics of shoulder movement. Arch Phys Med Rehabil 45:49, 1965.
2. Kapandji, I: The Physiology of the Joints ,Vol. 1, ed 5. Churchill Livingstone, Edinburgh and London, 1982.
3. Flatow, E: The biomechanics of the acromioclavicular, sternoclavicular and scapulothoracic joints. Inst Course Lect 42:237–245, 1993.
4. Ludewig, P, et al: Three-dimensional scapular orientation and muscle activity at selected positions of humeral elevation. J Orthop Sports Phys Ther 24:57–65, 1996.
5. Steindler, A: Kinesiology of the Human Body. Charles C. Thomas, Springfield, IL, 1955.
6. Williams, P (ed.): Gray's Anatomy, ed 38. Churchill Livingstone, New York, 1995.
7. Pronk, G, et al: Interaction between the joints of the shoulder mechanism: The function of the costoclavicular, conoid and trapezoid ligaments. Proc Inst Mech Eng 207[H]:219–229, 1993.
8. Pratt, N: Anatomy and biomechanics of the shoulder. J Hand Ther 7:65–76, 1994.
9. Sarrafian, S: Gross and functional anatomy of the shoulder. Clin Orthop 173:11–18, 1983.
10. Depalma, A: Degenerative Changes in Sternoclavicular and Acromioclavicular Joints in Various Decades. Charles C. Thomas, Springfield, IL, 1957.
11. Cailliet, R: Shoulder Pain, ed 2. FA Davis, Philadelphia, 1991.
12. Sadr, B, and Swann, M: Spontaneous dislocation of the sterno-clavicular joint. Acta Orthop Scand 50:269–274, 1979.
13. Morris, J: Joints of the shoulder girdle. Aust J Physiother 24:63–66, 1978.
14. Petersson, C: Degeneration of the acromio-clavicular joint. Acta Orthop Scand 54:434, 1983.
15. Post, M: Current concepts in the diagnosis and management of acromioclavicular dislocations. Clin Orthop 200:234–247, 1985.
16. MacDonald, P, et al: Comprehensive functional analysis of shoulders following complete acromioclavicular separation. Am J Sports Med 16:475–480, 1988.
17. Bargen, J, et al: Biomechanics and comparison of two operative methods of treatment of complete acromioclavicular separation. Clin Orthop 130:267–272, 1978.
18. Fenlin, J: Total glenohumeral joint replacement. Orthop Clin North Am 6:565, 1975.
19. Bigliani, L, et al: Glenohumeral stability. Clin Orthop 330:13–30, 1996.
20. Basmajian, J, and Bazant, F: Factors preventing downward dislocation of the adducted shoulder. J Bone Joint Surg 41:1182, 1959.
21. Saha, A: Dynamic stability of the glenohumeral joint. Acta Orthop Scand 42: 490, 1971.
22. Poppen, N, and Walker, P: Normal and abnormal motion of the shoulder. J Bone Joint Surg [Am] 58:195, 1976.
23. Saha, A: Theory of Shoulder Mechanism: Descriptive and Applied. Charles C. Thomas, Springfield, IL, 1961.
24. Poppen, N, and Walker, P: Forces at the glenohumeral joint in abduction. Clin Orthop 135:165, 1978.
25. Walker, P, and Poppen, N: Biomechanics of the shoulder joint during abduction on the plane of the scapula. Bull Hop Joint Dis Orthop Inst 38:107, 1977.
26. Freedman, L, and Monroe, R: Abduction of the arm in the scapular plane: Scapular and glenohumeral movements. J Bone Surg [Am] 48:150, 1966.
27. Moseley, H, and Overgaarde, K: The anterior capsule mechanism in recurrent dislocation of the shoulder. Morphological and clinical studies with special references to the glenoid labrum and glenohumeral ligaments. J Bone Joint Surg [Br] 44:913, 1962.
28. Cooper, D, et al: Anatomy, histology and vascularity of the glenoid labrum: An anatomical study. J Bone Joint Surg 74A:46–52, 1992.
29. Rothman, R, et al: Anatomic considerations in the glenohumeral joint. Orthop Clin North Am 6:341, 1975.
30. MacConaill, M, and Basmajian, J: Muscles and Movement: A Basis for Human Kinesiology. Williams & Wilkins, Baltimore, 1969.
31. Harryman, DT, et al: The role of the rotator interval capsule in passive motion and stability of the shoulder. J Bone Joint Surg 74-A(1):53–66, 1992.
32. O'Brien, SJ, et al: The anatomy and histology of the inferior glenohumeral ligament complex of the shoulder. Am J Sports Med 18:449–456, 1990.
33. Warner, JJP, et al: Static capsuloligamentous restraints to superior-inferior translation of the glenohumeral joint. Am J Sports Med 20:675–685, 1992.
34. O'Connell, PW, et al: The contribution of the glenohumeral ligaments to anterior stability of the shoulder joint. Am J Sports Med 18:579–584, 1990.

35. Soslowsky, L, et al: Biomechanics of the rotator cuff. Orthop Clin North Am 28:17–30, 1997.

36. Ferrari, DA: Capsular ligaments of the shoulder. Am J Sports Med 18:20–24, 1990.

37. Norkin, C, and White, D: Measurement of Joint Motion: A Guide to Goniometry, ed 2. FA Davis, Philadelphia, 1995.

38. Lucas, D: Biomechanics of the shoulder joint. Arch Surg 107:425, 1973.

39. Browne, A, et al: Glenohumeral elevation studied in three dimensions. J Bone Joint Surg 72B:843–845, 1990.

40. Soslowsky, L, et al: Quantitation of in situ contact areas at the glenohumeral joint: A biomechanical study. J Orthop Res 10:524–534, 1992.

41. Doody, S, and Waterland, J: Shoulder movements during abduction in the scapular plane. Arch Phys Med Rehabil 51: 595, 1970.

42. Inman, B, et al: Observations of function of the shoulder joint. J Bone Joint Surg [Br] 26:1, 1944.

43. McMahon, P, et al: Comparative electromyographic analysis of shoulder muscles during planar motions: Anterior glenohumeral instability versus normal. J Shoulder Elbow Surg 5:11–123, 1996.

44. Wuelker, N, et al: Translation of the glenohumeral joint with simulated active elevation. Clin Orthop 309:193–200, 1994.

45. Howell, S, et al: Normal and abnormal mechanics of the glenohumeral joint in the horizontal plane. J Bone Joint Surg [Am] 70:227–232, 1988.

46. DeDuca, C, and Forrest, W: Force analysis of individual muscles acting simultaneously on the shoulder joint during isometric abduction. J Biomech 6:385, 1973.

47. Dvir, Z, and Berme, N: The shoulder complex in elevation of the arm: A mechanism approach. J Biomech 1:219, 1978.

48. Sharkey, N, and Marder, R: The rotator cuff opposes superior translation of the humeral head. Am J Sports Med 23:270–275, 1995.

49. Otis, J, et al: Changes in moment arms of the rotator cuff and deltoid muscles with abduction and rotation. J Bone Joint Surg 76-A:1994.

50. Wuelker, N, et al: Dynamic glenohumeral joint stability. J Shoulder Elbow Surg 7:43–52, 1998.

51. Wuelker, N, et al: Function of the supraspinatus muscle. Acta Orthop Scand 65:442–446, 1994.

52. Itoi, E, et al: Stabilising function of the biceps in stable and unstable shoulders. J Bone Joint Surg 75-B:546–550, 1993.

53. Itoi, E, et al: Biomechanical investigation of the glenohumeral joint. J Shoulder Elbow Surg 5:407–424, 1996.

54. Malicky, D, et al: Anterior glenohumeral stabilization factors: Progressive effects in a biomechanical model. J Orthop Res 14:22–288, 1996.

55. Pagnani, M, et al: Role of the long head of the biceps brachii in glenohumeral stability: A biomechanical study in cadavera. J Shoulder Elbow Surg 5:255–262, 1996.

56. Pagnani, M, et al: Effect of lesions of the superior portion of the glenoid labrum on glenohumeral translation. J Bone Joint Surg 77[A]:1003–1010, 1995.

57. Sakurai, G, et al: Morophologic changes in long head of biceps brachii in rotator cuff dysfunction. J Orthop Sci 3:137–142, 1998.

58. Sigholm, G, et al: Pressure recording in the subacromial bursa. J Orthop Res 6:123–128, 1988.

59. Ozaki, J, et al: Tears of the rotator cuff of the shoulder associated with pathological changes in the acromion. J Bone Joint Surg [Am] 70:1224–1230, 1988.

60. Gschwend, N, et al: Rotator cuff tear—relationship between clinical and anatomopathological findings. Arch Orthop Trauma Surg 107:7–15, 1988.

61. Kessel, L, and Watson, M: The painful arc syndrome. J Bone Joint Surg 59:1166–1172, 1977.

62. Saha, A: The classic: Mechanism of shoulder movements and a plea for the recognition of "zero position" of the glenohumeral joint. Clin Orthop 173:3–9, 1983.

63. McQuade, K, and Smidt, G: Dynamic scapulohumeral rhythm: the effects of external resistance during elevation of the arm in the scapular plane. J Ortho Sports Phys Ther 27:125–133, 1998.

64. Hogfors, C, et al: Biomechanical model of the human shoulder joint—II. the shoulder rhythm. J Biomech 24:699–709, 1991.

65. Perry, J: Normal upper extremity kinesiology. Phys Ther 58:265, 1978.

66. Celli, L, et al: Some new aspects of the functional anatomy of the shoulder. Ital J Orthop Traumat 11:83, 1985.

67. Colachis, SC, and Strohm, BR: Effects of suprascapular and axillary nerve block on muscle force in the upper extremity. Arch Phys Med Rehabil 52:22–29, 1971.

68. Smith, L, et al: Brunnstrom's Clinical Kinesiology, ed 5. FA Davis, Philadelphia, 1996.

69. Basmajian, J, and DeLuca, C: Muscles Alive, ed 5. Williams & Wilkins, Baltimore, 1985.

Study Questions

1. *Identify the intra-articular motions of the SC for evaluation/depressions and protraction/retraction.*

2. *What are the roles of the costoclavicular and interclavicular ligaments at the SC joint?*

3. *Discuss the relevance of the sternoclavicular disk to SC joint congruency and joint motion.*

4. *Identify the scapular movements that take place at the AC joint.*

5. *Discuss the relevance of the coracoclavicular ligament and the AC joint disk to the AC joint function.*

6. *Discuss the configuration of the humerus and the glenoid fossa as they relate to GH joint stability. What role do the glenoid labrum and joint capsule play in joint stability?*

7. *What is the most frequent direction of GH dislocation? Why is this true?*

8. *Compare the relative stability and tendency toward degenerative changes in the GH, AC, and SC joints.*

9. *What are the advantages of the coracohumeral arch? What are the disadvantages?*

10. *What intra-articular motions must occur at the GH joint for full abduction to occur? What is the normal range? What range will be available to the joint if the humerus is not able to laterally rotate?*

11. *What muscle is the prime mover in shoulder GH flexion and abduction? What synergy is necessary for normal function of this muscle? Why?*

12. *Why is the supraspinatus able to abduct the shoulder without additional muscular synergy?*

13. What accounts for the static stabilization of the GH joint when the arm is at the side? What happens if you excessively load the hanging (dependent) limb?

14. Identify five factors that play a role in the dynamic stabilization of the GH joint in either flexion or abduction of that joint (both flexion and abduction are elevation functions).

15. What is the total ROM available to the humerus in elevation? How is this full range achieved?

16. How does the shape of the clavicle contribute to elevation of the arm?

17. What muscles are necessary to produce the normal scapular and humeral movements in elevation of the arm?

18. If the scapulothoracic joint were fused in neutral position, what range of elevation would still be available to the upper extremity actively?

19. What is the most common traumatic problem at the AC joint? What deficits is a person with this disability likely to encounter?

20. What are the consequences of a rupture of the coracoclavicular ligaments?

21. If the GH joint were immobilized by osteoarthritis, what range of elevation would be available to the upper extremity?

22. If isolated paralysis of the supraspinatus were to occur, what would be the likely functional deficit?

23. If the muscles of the rotator cuff were paralyzed, what would be the effect when abduction of the arm was attempted?

24. When there is paralysis of the trapezius and the serratus anterior, what is the functional deficit when abduction of the arm is attempted?

25. If the deltoid alone were paralyzed, what would happen with attempted abduction of the arm? With attempted flexion of the arm?

26. What is the role of the rhomboids in elevation of the arm?

27. What differences would you see in attempted abduction if the trapezius alone were paralyzed compared with paralysis of both the trapezius and the serratus anterior?

28. What muscular synergy does the teres major require to perform its function?

29. Describe why electromyographic activity of the deltoid in normal abduction shows a gradual rise in activity to between 90° and 120°, with a plateau thereafter.

30. Which of the joints of the shoulder complex is most likely to undergo degenerative changes over time? Which is least likely?

CHAPTER 8
THE ELBOW COMPLEX

OBJECTIVES

Following the study of this chapter, the reader should be able to:

Describe

1. All of the articulating surfaces associated with each of the following joints: humeroulnar, humeroradial, and the proximal and distal radioulnar.
2. The ligaments associated with all the joints of the elbow complex.
3. The muscles associated with all of the joints of the elbow complex.

Identify

1. Axes of motion for supination and pronation and flexion and extension.
2. The degrees of freedom associated with each of the joints of the elbow complex.
3. Structures limiting the range of motion in flexion and extension.
4. Structures that create the carrying angle.
5. Structures limiting motion in supination and pronation.

Compare

1. The translatory and rotatory component of the brachioradialis and brachialis at all points in the range of motion.

2. The moment arms of the flexors at any point in the range of motion.
3. Muscle activity of the extensors in a closed kinematic chain with activity in an open kinematic chain.
4. The role of the pronator teres with the role of the pronator quadratus.
5. The role of the biceps with that of the brachialis.
6. The resistance of the elbow joint to longitudinal tensile forces with its resistance to compressive forces.
7. The features of a classic tennis elbow with the features of cubital tunnel syndrome.
8. The role and structure of the annular ligament with the role and structure of the articular disk.
9. The role of the medial collateral ligament with the role of the lateral collateral ligament at 90° of flexion and in full extension.
10. The etiology of avascular necrosis of the capitulum.

Introduction

The joints and muscles of the elbow complex are designed to serve the hand. They provide mobility for the hand in space by apparent shortening and lengthening of the upper extremity. This function allows the hand to be brought close to the face for eating or placed at a distance from the body equal to the length of the upper extremity. Rotation at the elbow complex provides additional mobility for the hand. In conjunction with providing mobility for the hand, the elbow complex structures also provide stability for skilled or forceful movements of the hand when performing activities using tools or implements. Many of the 15 muscles that cross the elbow complex[1] also act either at the wrist or shoulder, and therefore the wrist and shoulder are linked with the elbow in enhancing function of the hand.

The elbow complex consists of the elbow joint (humeroulnar and humeroradial articulations) and the proximal and distal radioulnar joints. The apparent shortening and lengthening of the upper extremity occur at the elbow joint, which is formed by the distal end of the humerus and the proximal ends of the radius and ulna. The elbow joint is considered to be a compound joint that functions as a hinge joint and therefore as a uniaxial diarthrodial joint with 1° of freedom of motion. Flexion and extension occur in the sagittal plane around a coronal axis. Two major ligaments and five muscles are directly associated with the elbow joint. Three of the muscles are flexors that cross the anterior aspect of the joint. The other two muscles are extensors that cross the posterior aspect of the joint.

The proximal and distal radioulnar joints are linked and function as one joint. Therefore, the two joints acting together to produce rotation of the forearm have 1° of freedom of motion. These joints are diarthrodial uniaxial joints of the pivot (trochoid) type. Rotation (supination and pronation) occurs in the transverse plane around a longitudinal axis. Six ligaments and four muscles are associated with these joints. Two muscles are for supination and two are for pronation. The elbow joint and the proximal radioulnar joint are enclosed in a single joint capsule, but constitute distinct articulations.

Structure: Elbow Joint (Humeroulnar and Humeroradial Articulations)

Articulating Surfaces on the Humerus

The articulating surfaces on the humerus are the hourglass-shaped **trochlea** and the spherically shaped **capitulum** (Fig. 8–1). These structures, which are covered with articular cartilage, are located between the two epicondyles on the distal end of the humerus. The trochlea, which forms part of the humeroulnar articulation, lies on the anterior medial aspect of the distal humerus. The **trochlear groove** spirals obliquely around the trochlea and divides the trochlea into a medial and lateral portion. The medial portion of the trochlea projects distally more than the lateral portion and the entire trochlea is set at an angle and slightly anterior to the shaft of the humerus. Individual varia-

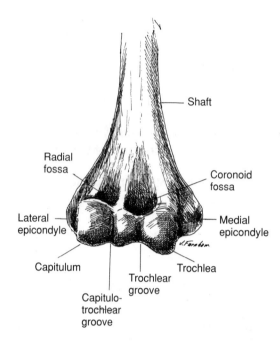

FIGURE 8–1. Articulating surfaces on the anterior aspect of the right distal humerus.

tions in the obliquity of the trochlear groove affect the direction of movement of the forearm during flexion and extension. The trochlea has an asymmetrical sellar (or saddle-shaped) surface that is concave transversely and convex anteroposteriorly.[2] An indentation located just above the trochlea is called the **coronoid fossa.** The capitulum, which is part of the humeroradial articulation, is located on the anterior lateral surface of the distal humerus. The capitulum, like the trochlea, lies anterior to the shaft of the humerus. A groove, called the **capitulotrochlear groove,** separates the capitulum from the trochlea. An indentation located just above the capitulum is called the **radial fossa.** Posteriorly, the distal humerus is indented by a deep fossa called the **olecranon fossa** (Fig. 8–2).

Articulating Surfaces on the Radius and Ulna

The articulating surfaces of the ulna and radius correspond to the humeral articulating surfaces (Fig. 8–3). The ulnar articulating surface of the humeroulnar joint is a semicircular-shaped concave surface called the **trochlear notch.** The proximal portion of the notch is divided into two unequal parts by the **trochlear**

ridge. The ridge corresponds to the **trochlear groove** on the humerus. The radial articulating surface of the humeroradial joint is composed of the proximal end of the radius (**head of the radius**). The head has a slightly cup-shaped concave surface that is surrounded by a rim. The concavity of the radial head corresponds to the convex surface of the capitulum and the radial head's convex rim fits into the capitulotrochlear groove (see Fig. 8–1).

Articulation

Articulation between the ulna and humerus at the humeroulnar joint occurs primarily as a sliding motion of the trochlear notch of the ulna on the trochlea. In extension, sliding continues until the olecranon process enters the olecranon fossa (Fig. 8–4a). In flexion, the trochlear ridge of the ulna slides along the trochlear groove until the coronoid process reaches the floor of the coronoid fossa in full flexion[3] (Fig. 8–4b). Eckstein and coworkers[4] studied the distribution of subchondral mineralization and the size and position of contact areas on the trochlear notch to determine load

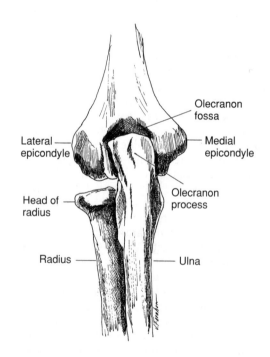

FIGURE 8–2. Posterior aspect of a left elbow joint in the extended position. The olecranon fossa is shown partially obscured by the olecranon process of the ulna. In the fully extended position, there is no contact between the radial head and the capitulum.

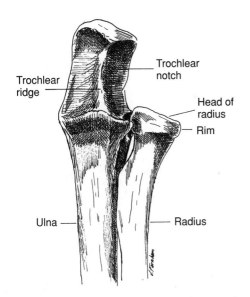

FIGURE 8–3. An anterior view of the articulating surfaces on the radius and ulna. Drawing depicts a left forearm.

distribution at the humeroulnar joint. Based on the results of their study, they concluded that at 90° of elbow flexion a physiologic incongruity is present between the articulating surfaces on the trochlea and the trochlear notch.[4] The notch is somewhat deeper than is necessary to accommodate the trochlea. The incongruity was found to decrease as the load on the joint increased. In all 16 specimens examined by these authors, more load was accepted by the olecranon and coronoid surfaces than by the central aspects of the trochlear notch. The same authors conducted two additional studies. In the first study, Eckstein and colleagues[5] determined that at loads of 25 N (simulating resisted elbow extension) with the elbow positioned at 30°, 60°, 90°, and 120° of flexion no articulating surface contact occurred

between the trochlea and the depths of the trochlear notch in all six specimens studied. At a load of 500 N the articulating surface contact areas expanded from the sides toward the depths of the notch. In the second study, the authors[6] found that the density of the subchondral bone under the articulating surfaces of the sides of the trochlear notch was far greater than the densities found in the depth of the notch. The lack of density in the depth of the notch tended to confirm their previous findings of a "concave incongruity" at the humeroulnar joint. The authors postulated that the regular change of articulating surface contact areas inherent in the incongruent joint promotes the movement of synovial fluid and thus of nutrients. However, in later studies the authors[7] found that the pattern of cartilage thickness in 14 notches studied differed significantly from the subchondral mineralization zone. Jacobs and Eckstein, in a study using finite element simulation, concluded that the density of subchondral bone could not be regarded as a direct measure of the adjacent articular pressure in incongruent joints with deep sockets. Apparently, in these joints, tensile stresses appear to play a dominant role in subchondral bone remodeling.[8]

Articulation between the radial head and the capitulum at the humeroradial joint involves sliding of the shallow concave radial head over the relatively large convex surface of the capitulum. In full extension, no contact occurs between the articulating surfaces (Fig. 8–5a). In flexion, the rim of the radial head slides in the capitulotrochlear groove and enters the radial fossa as the end of the flexion range is reached[9] (Fig. 8–5b). Schenck and associates found significant differences in the mechanical properties of the articular cartilage and in the articular cartilage thickness both within and between

FIGURE 8–4. Schematic representation of motions of the ulna on the humerus at the humeroulnar joint. (a) In extension, the olecranon process enters the olecranon fossa. (b) In flexion, the coronoid process reaches the coronoid fossa.

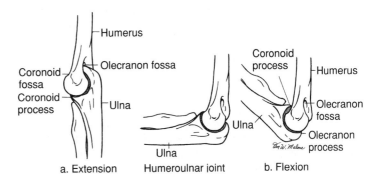

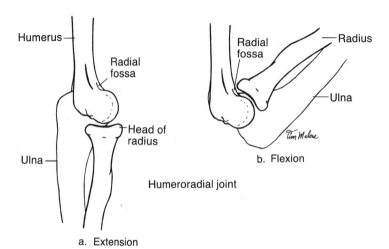

a. Extension

Humeroradial joint

b. Flexion

FIGURE 8–5. Schematic representation of motions of the radius at the humeroradial joint. (a) In full extension, there is no contact between the capitulum and the radial head. (b) During flexion, the rim of the radius slides in the capitulotrochlear groove and in full flexion reaches the radial fossa on the humerus.

the capitulum and the radial head.[10] For example, these authors found that the central section of the radial head was significantly stiffer than the lateral aspect of the capitulum. They hypothesized that the difference in stiffness was related to the prevalence of pathology involving the capitulum in individuals engaged in throwing sports.

Joint Capsule

The humeroulnar and humeroradial joints and the superior radioulnar joint are enclosed in a single joint capsule. Anteriorly, the proximal attachment of the capsule is just above the coronoid and radial fossae, and distally it is inserted into the ulna on the margin of the coronoid process and into the annular ligament. Laterally, the capsule's attachment to the radius blends with the fibers of the lateral collateral ligament. Medially, the capsule blends with fibers of the medial collateral ligament. Posteriorly, the capsule is attached to the humerus along the upper edge of the olecranon fossa. The capsule is fairly large, loose, and weak anteriorly and posteriorly, but ligaments reinforce its sides. Fat pads are located between the capsule and the synovial membrane adjacent to the olecranon, coronoid, and radial fossae.[2,11]

Ligaments

Most hinge joints in the body have collateral ligaments, and the elbow is no exception. Collateral ligaments are located on the medial and lateral sides of hinge joints to provide me-

dial/lateral stability to the joint and to keep joint surfaces in apposition. The two main ligaments associated with the elbow joints are the **medial (ulnar)** and **lateral (radial) collateral** ligaments.

MEDIAL (ULNAR) COLLATERAL LIGAMENT

The medial or ulnar collateral ligament (**MCL**) is described as consisting of two (anterior and posterior)[12–14] or three parts (anterior, oblique (transverse), and posterior.[15–17] Callaway and coworkers[18] in a study of 28 cadaveric elbows found that the MCL was composed of anterior, posterior, and occasionally transverse bundles (Fig. 8–6a). Fuss argues that the so-called oblique or transverse portion is actually Cooper's ligament and should not be considered part of the MCL because it does not span the joint.[12] Regan and coworkers also describe the MCL as consisting of two parts superficially, but these authors found no distinction between the two parts when they observed the ligament from its inferior or deep capsular surface. Instead they found a series of fibers that are inserted sequentially along the radial fossa of the ulna from anterior to posterior coexistent with the capsular insertion.[13] Although the composition of the MCL remains controversial, most authors are in agreement that the anterior part of the ligament is the most functionally significant.

The anterior part of the MCL extends from the anterior aspect, tip, and medial edge of the medial epicondyle of the humerus to attach on the ulnar coronoid process. Mechanoreceptors (Golgi organs, Ruffini terminals, Pacini corpuscles, and free nerve endings) are densely dis-

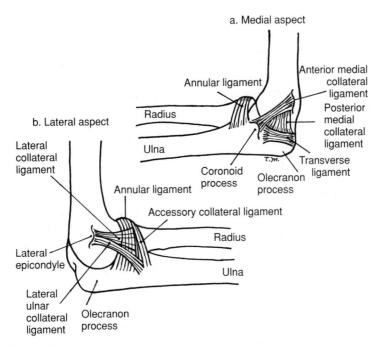

a. Medial aspect

Annular ligament

Anterior medial collateral ligament

Radius

Posterior medial collateral ligament

b. Lateral aspect

Lateral collateral ligament

Ulna

Coronoid process

Olecranon process

τ.m.

Transverse ligament

Annular ligament

Accessory collateral ligament

Radius

Lateral epicondyle

Ulna

Lateral ulnar collateral ligament

Olecranon process

FIGURE 8–6. (a) Three parts of the medial (ulnar) collateral ligament are shown on the medial aspect of the right elbow. The musculature and joint capsule have been removed to show the ligament's attachments. The anterior portion of the ligament arises from the medial epicondyle of the humerus and attaches on the ulnar coronoid process. The fibers of the transverse portion arise from the olecranon process and attach to the ulnar coronoid process. The posterior portion of the ligament arises from the medial epicondyle and attaches to the ulnar coronoid and olecranon processes. (b) The lateral (radial) collateral ligament is shown on the lateral aspect of the right elbow. The musculature and the joint capsule have been removed to show the ligament's attachments. The lateral collateral ligament arises from the lateral epicondyle of the humerus and attaches to the annular ligament and the olecranon process. The lateral ulnar collateral portion of the lateral collateral ligament arises as a narrow band from the lateral epicondyle to insert on the ulna.[13, 22] Proximally between the annular ligament and the lateral epicondyle the lateral ulnar collateral ligament cannot be separated from the lateral collateral ligament.[22] The accessory collateral ligament arises from the annular ligament and inserts into the ulna.

tributed near the ligament's humeral and ulnar attachments.[19] The collagen fiber bundles in the anterior part of the ligament are more closely packed than the fibers in the posterior part of the ligament. Fuss has identified three anatomic and functionally distinct fiber components in the anterior portion of the ligament: (1) fibers that arise from the anterior surface of the medial condyle that are taut in full extension; (2) fibers that arise from below the tip of the medial epicondyle that are taut from 90° of flexion to full flexion; and (3) fibers that arise from the inferior edge of the medial epicondyle that are always taut throughout the full range of motion (ROM) and limit the extremes of extension. The third group of fibers Fuss designated as a "guiding bundle."[12] This bundle of fibers is the only part of the anterior ligament that is taut in the range of motion from 0° to 90° and according to Fuss aid in guiding joint movement. The anterior portion of the MCL is

considered to be the primary stabilizer of the elbow to valgus stress in the range of elbow flexion from 20° to 120° of flexion.[20,21] Callaway and colleagues[18] describe the composition of the anterior portion of the MCL as having an anterior and a posterior band that tighten in reciprocal fashion as the elbow flexes and extends. The anterior band of the anterior portion was found by these authors to be the primary restraint to valgus at 30°, 60°, and 90° of flexion and the coprimary restraint to valgus at 120° of flexion. The posterior band of the anterior MCL was found to be a coprimary restraint to valgus at 120° of flexion and a secondary restraint at 30° and 90° of flexion.[18]

The posterior part of the MCL is not as distinct as the anterior medial collateral and sometimes its fibers blend with the fibers of the medial portion of the joint capsule. The fibers of the posterior portion of the MCL extend from the posterior aspect of the medial epicondyle of the humerus to attach to the ulnar coronoid and olecranon processes. Mechanoreceptors are densely distributed near the humeral and ulnar attachments.[19] The posterior MCL limits elbow extension[12] but plays a less significant role than the anterior medial collateral in providing valgus stability for the elbow.[20,21] The oblique (transverse) fibers of the medial collateral extend between the olecranon and ulnar coronoid processes. This portion of the ligament assists in providing valgus stability and helps to keep the joint surfaces in approximation. A summary of the function of the MCL is presented in Table 8–1.

LATERAL (RADIAL) COLLATERAL LIGAMENT

The lateral (radial) collateral ligament (**LCL**) is a fan-shaped, poorly demarcated structure that extends from the inferior lateral epicondyle of the humerus and attaches to the annular ligament (ligament encircling the head of the radius) and to the olecranon process (Fig. 8–6b). Mechanoreceptors are densely distributed near the humeral and ulnar attachments.[19] According to Regan and colleagues, the ligamentous complex also consists of various capsular thickenings extending from the lateral humeral epicondyle to the olecranon process, as well as

a short narrow band of ligamentous tissue that extends from the annular ligament to insert on the ulna.[13] The ligamentous tissue extending from the lateral epicondyle to the lateral aspect of the ulnar is sometimes referred to as the **lateral ulnar collateral ligament (LUCL)** and is considered by some authors to be part of the lateral collateral ligamentous complex.[13,15,22] In a study of 10 specimens, Olson and associates could not separate the LCL from the LUCL.[22] The LCL provides reinforcement for the humeroradial articulation, offers some protection against varus stress in some positions of the elbow, and assists in providing resistance to distraction of the joint surfaces.[23] Some fibers of the LCL remain taut throughout the flexion ROM with either a varus or valgus moment applied.[13] The LCL is considered to be weaker but more elastic than the MCL and apparently plays a lesser role than the MCL in providing reinforcement for the elbow joint. However, Olsen and coworkers concluded that the LCL is an important stabilizer of the humeroradial joint in forced varus and prevents posterior translation of the radial head.[22]

The LUCL maintains tension throughout the total ROM in flexion when a varus stress is applied. The ligament's fibers are taut at more

Table 8–1. **Summary: Medical Collateral Ligament Function**

Fibers	Joint Position/ROM	Function	Authors
Anterior portion MCL (fibers arising from anterior surface of medial epicondyle)	Full extension	Limits extension	Fuss[12]
Anterior portion MCL (fibers arising from below tip of medial epicondyle.)	90° to full flexion	Fibers are taut	Fuss[12]
Anterior portion MCL (fibers arising from the inferior edge of the medial epicondyle)	0° to full flexion	Fibers are taut— guides joint motion	Fuss[12]
Anterior portion MCL	0° to full flexion	Resists valgus stress and limits extension	Regan et al[13]
Anterior portion MCL	20–120° flexion	Primary stabilizer to valgus stress	Soberg, Ovelson, and Nielsen[20] Hotchkiss and Weiland[21]
Anterior band anterior portion MCL	30°, 60°, and 90° flexion	Primary stabilizer to valgus stress	Callaway et al[18]
Posterior band of anterior portion MCL	120° flexion	Coprimary restraint to valgus	Callaway et al[18]
Posterior portion of MCL	55°, 85°, and 95° flexion to full flexion	Less significant role than anterior portion. Limits flexion.	Regan et al[13]

Table 8–2. **Summary: Lateral Collateral and Lateral Ulnar Collateral Ligaments**

Fibers	Joint Position/ROM	Function	Author
LCL (posterior fibers)	0–90°		Regan et al[13]
LCL (middle fibers)	0° to full flexion	Fibers taut with either a varus or valgus moment applied	Regan et al[13]
LCL		Fibers taut in forced varus	Olsen et al[22]
LUCL	0° to full flexion	Fibers taut when varus stress applied	Regan et al[13]

than 110° of flexion when either a varus or valgus stress is applied or when no load is applied. It would appear that the LUCL has the potential for assisting the LCL in resisting varus stress at the elbow and assisting in providing lateral support. A summary of the function of the LCL is presented in Table 8–2.

Muscles

Nine muscles cross the anterior aspect of the elbow joint but only three of these muscles (the **brachialis, biceps brachii,** and the **brachioradialis**) have primary functions at the elbow joint. The remaining six muscles (**pronator teres, flexor carpi radialis, flexor carpi ulnaris, flexor digitorum superficialis,** and the **palmaris longus**), which arise by a common tendon from the medial epicondyle of the humerus, are considered to be weak flexors of the elbow, but have primary functions at other joints including the radioulnar, wrist, hand, and fingers.

The major flexors of the elbow are the brachialis, the biceps brachii, and the brachioradialis. The brachialis muscle arises from the anterior surface of the lower portion of the humeral shaft and attaches by a thick broad tendon to the ulnar tuberosity and coronoid process. The biceps brachii arises from two heads, a short and long head. The short head arises as a thick flat tendon from the coracoid process of the scapula and the long head arises as a long, narrow tendon from the scapula's supraglenoid tubercle. The muscle fibers arising from the two tendons unite in the middle of the upper arm to form the prominent muscle bulk of the upper arm. Muscle fibers from both heads insert by way of the strong flattened tendon on the rough posterior area of the tuberosity of the radius. Other fibers of the biceps brachii insert into the bicipital aponeurosis that extends medially to blend with the fascia that lies over the forearm flexors.[2,24] The bra-

chioradialis muscle arises from the lateral supracondylar ridge of the humerus and inserts into the distal end of the radius just proximal to the radial styloid process.

The two extensors of the elbow are the triceps and the anconeus. The triceps has three heads, a long, medial, and lateral. The long head crosses both the glenohumeral joint at the shoulder as well as the elbow joint. The long head arises from the infraglenoid tubercle of the scapula by a flattened tendon that blends with the glenohumeral joint capsule. The medial and lateral heads cross only the elbow joint. The medial head covers an extensive area as it arises from the entire posterior surface of the humerus. In contrast, the lateral head arises from only a narrow ridge on the posterior humeral surface. The three heads insert via a common tendon into the olecranon process. The anconeus is a small triangular muscle that originates from the lateral epicondyle of the humerus and inserts into both the olecranon process and the adjacent posterior surface of the ulna.[24]

Function: Elbow Joint (Humeroulnar and Humeroradial Articulations)

Axis of Motion

The axis for flexion and extension is relatively fixed and passes through the center of the trochlea and capitulum bisecting the longitudinal axis of the shaft of the humerus[3,25–27] (Fig. 8–7). When the upper extremity is in the anatomic position, the long axis of the humerus and the long axis of the forearm form an acute angle medially when they meet at the elbow. The angulation is due to the configuration of the articulating surfaces and results in a normal valgus angulation of the forearm in relation to the humerus (Fig. 8–8). This angle is

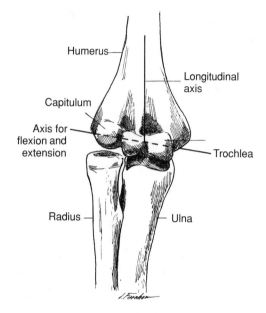

FIGURE 8–7. The axis of motion for flexion and extension. The axis of motion is centered in the middle of the trochlea on a line that intersects the longitudinal (anatomic) axis of the humerus.

called the **carrying angle** and is slightly greater in women than men. The average angle in men is about 5°, whereas in women it is about 10° to 15°.[28] An increase in the carrying angle is considered to be abnormal, especially

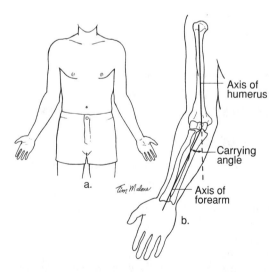

FIGURE 8–8. The carrying angle of the elbow. (a) The forearm lies slightly lateral to the humerus when the elbow is fully extended in the anatomic position. (b) The long axis of the humerus and the long axis of the forearm form the carrying angle.

if it occurs unilaterally. When the angle is increased beyond the average, it is called **cubitus valgus.**

Normally, the carrying angle disappears when the forearm is pronated and the elbow is in full extension and when the forearm is flexed against the humerus in full elbow flexion.[9] The configuration of the trochlear groove determines the pathway of the forearm during flexion and extension. In the most common configuration of the groove, the ulna is guided progressively medially from extension to flexion so that in full flexion, the forearm comes to rest in the same plane as the humerus[9] (Fig. 8–9a). In extension, the forearm moves laterally until it reaches a position slightly lateral to the axis of the humerus in full extension. Variations in the direction of the groove will alter the pathway of the forearm so that when the elbow is passively flexed, the forearm will come to rest either medial[9,27] (Fig. 8–9b) or lateral (Fig. 8–9c) to the humerus[9] in full flexion. Different methods of measuring the carrying angle have led to conflicting conclusions regarding the carrying angle.[26] For example, London,[3] who used the axis of the forearm and a perpendicular to the axis of rotation of the elbow joint rather than the axes of the humerus and forearm to measure the carrying angle, concluded that the carrying angle did not change during the range of elbow flexion/extension.

Range of Motion

A number of factors determine the amount of motion that is available at the elbow joint. These factors include the type of motion (active or passive), the position of the forearm (relative pronation-supination), and the position of the shoulder. The range of active flexion at the elbow is usually less than the range of passive motion, because the bulk of the contracting flexors on the anterior surface of the humerus interferes with the approximation of the forearm with the humerus. The active ROM for elbow flexion with the forearm supinated is typically considered to be from about 135° to 145°, whereas the range for passive flexion is between 150° and 160°.[9] The position of the forearm also affects the flexion ROM. When the forearm is in either pronation or midway between supination and pronation, the ROM is less than it is when the forearm is supinated. The position of the shoulder may affect the ROM available to the elbow. Two joint muscles,

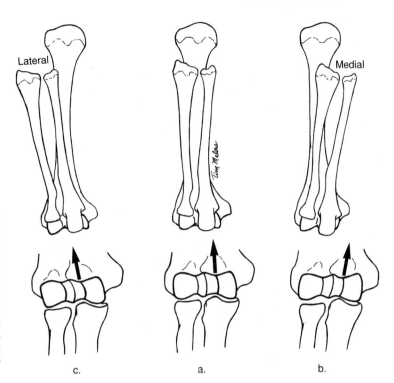

FIGURE 8–9. Position of the forearm in passive flexion. (a) In the most common configuration of the trochlear groove, the ulna is guided progressively medially from extension to flexion so that in full flexion the forearm comes to rest in the same plane as the humerus. (b) The forearm comes to rest slightly medially to the humerus in passive flexion. (c) The forearm comes to rest slightly laterally in the least common configuration of the trochlear groove.

c.

a.

b.

such as the biceps brachii and the triceps, that cross both the shoulder and elbow joints may become actively or passively insufficient when a full ROM is attempted at both joints. Passive tension in the triceps may limit elbow flexion when the shoulder is simultaneously moved into full flexion. Concomitantly, the biceps brachii, if active, may lose tension as it attempts to shorten over both joints. Passive tension created in the long head of the biceps by shoulder hyperextension may limit full elbow extension. If the elbow extension is being produced by the triceps, the long head may become actively insufficient.

Other factors that limit the ROM and help to provide stability for the elbow are the configuration of the joint surfaces, the ligaments, and joint capsule. The elbow has inherent articular stability at the extremes of extension and flexion.[11,20] In full extension the humeroulnar joint is in a close-packed position. In this position, bony contact of the olecranon process in the olecranon fossa limits the end of the extension range and the configuration of the joint structures helps to provide valgus and varus stability. The bony components, MCL, and anterior joint capsule contribute equally to resist valgus stress in full extension.[23] The bony components provide one-half of the resistance to

varus stress in full extension, and the lateral collateral and joint capsule provide the other half of the resistance.[23] Resistance to joint distraction in the extended position is entirely provided by soft-tissue structures. The anterior portion of the joint capsule provides the majority of the resistance to anterior displacement of the distal humerus out of the olecranon fossa, whereas the MCL and LCL contribute only slightly.[21,23]

Approximation of the coronoid process with the coronoid fossa and of the rim of the radial head in the radial fossa limits extremes of flexion. In 90° of flexion the anterior part of the MCL provides the primary resistance to both distraction and valgus stress. If the anterior portion of the MCL becomes lax through overstretching, medial instability will result when the elbow is in flexed positions. Also, the carrying angle will increase. The majority of the resistance to varus stress when the elbow is flexed to 90° is provided by the osseous structures of the joint and only a slight amount by the LCL and the joint capsule. The anterior joint capsule contributes only slightly to varus/valgus stability and provides little resistance to distraction when the elbow is flexed.[21,23] Co-contractions of the flexor and extensor muscles of the elbow, wrist, and hand help to provide stability for the elbow during forceful motions of the wrist and fingers and in activities in which the arms are used to support the body weight. During pulling activities such as when one grasps and attempts to pull a fixed rod toward the body, the elbow joints are compressed by the contractions of muscles that cross the elbow and act on the wrist and hand.[29]

Muscle Action

Flexors

The role that the three flexor muscles play in motion at the elbow is determined by a number of factors, including the location of muscles, position of the elbow and adjacent joints, position of the forearm, the magnitude of the applied load, the type of muscle contraction, and the speed of motion. The brachialis is inserted close to the joint axis and therefore is considered to be a mobility muscle. The brachialis has a large strength potential (large physiologic cross-sectional area) and a large work capacity (volume).[1] The moment arm (MA) of the brachialis is greatest at slightly more than 100° of elbow flexion,[2,30] and, therefore, its ability to produce torque is greatest at that particular elbow position. The brachialis is inserted on the ulna and, therefore, is unaffected by changes in the forearm position brought about by rotation of the radius. As a one-joint muscle, the brachialis is not affected by the position of the shoulder. Studies of muscle activity at the elbow have been performed using electromyography (EMG). This technique is used to monitor the electrical activity that is produced by the firing of motor units. Using EMG, it is possible to determine the relative proportion of motor units that are firing in a particular muscle during a specific muscle contraction. According to EMG studies, the brachialis muscle works in flexion of the elbow in all positions of the forearm, with and without resistance. It also is active in all types of contractions (isometric, concentric, and eccentric) during slow and fast motions.[31]

The biceps brachii is also considered to be a mobility muscle because of its insertion close to the joint axis. The long head of the biceps has the largest volume among the flexors, but the muscle has a relatively small physiologic cross-sectional area.[1] The MA of the biceps is largest between 80° and 100° of elbow flexion and, therefore, the biceps is capable of pro-

ducing its greatest torque in this range.[30] The MA of the biceps is rather small when the elbow is in full extension and most of the muscle force is translatory (joint compression). Therefore, when the elbow is fully extended the biceps is less effective as an elbow flexor than when the elbow is flexed to 90°. When the elbow is flexed beyond 100°, the translatory component of the muscle force is directed away from the elbow joint and, therefore, acts as a distracting or dislocating force as shown in Figure 1–57 in Chapter 1. The biceps is active during unresisted elbow flexion with the forearm supinated and when the forearm is midway between supination and pronation in both concentric and eccentric contractions, but it tends *not* to be active when the forearm is pronated. When the magnitude of the resistance increases much beyond limb weight, the biceps is active in all positions of the forearm.[31] The biceps with both heads crossing two joints may become actively insufficient when full flexion of the elbow is attempted with the shoulder in full flexion especially when the forearm is supinated.

The brachioradialis is inserted at a distance from the joint axis and therefore during muscle contraction, the largest component of muscle force goes toward compression of the joint surfaces and hence toward stability (see Fig. 1–58). Like the biceps, the brachioradialis has a relatively small physiologic cross-sectional area.[1] The peak MA for the brachioradialis occurs between 100° and 120° of elbow flexion.[30] The brachioradialis shows no electrical activity during eccentric flexor activity when the motion is performed slowly with the forearm supinated. Activation of the brachioradialis during concentric contractions is greater than during eccentric contractions particularly when the range of elbow flexion is between 0° and 60°.[32] However, the brachioradialis shows no activity during slow, unresisted, concentric elbow flexion. When the speed of the motion is increased, the brachioradialis shows moderate activity if a load is applied and the forearm is in either a position midway between supination and pronation or in full pronation.[31] The brachioradialis does not cross the shoulder and therefore is unaffected by the position of the shoulder.

The pronator teres as well as the palmaris longus, flexor digitorum superficialis, flexor carpi radialis, and flexor carpi ulnaris are weak elbow flexors.[2]

Extensors

The effectiveness of the triceps as a whole is affected by changes in the position of the elbow but not by changes in position of the forearm because the triceps attaches to the ulna and not the radius. The long head of the triceps crosses two joints; therefore, activity of the long head is affected by changing shoulder joint positions. The long head becomes actively insufficient when full elbow extension is attempted with the shoulder in hyperextension. In this instance the muscle is shortened over both the elbow and shoulder simultaneously.

The medial and lateral heads of the triceps are not affected by the position of the shoulder. The medial head is active in unresisted active elbow extension.[31] All three heads are active when heavy resistance is given to extension or when quick extension of the elbow is attempted in the gravity-assisted position. The maximum isometric torque that the triceps can generate is at an elbow position of 90° of elbow flexion.[33,34] However, the total amount of extensor torque generated at 90° varies with the position of the shoulder and the body.[35] The triceps is active eccentrically to control elbow flexion as the body is lowered to the ground in a push-up (Fig. 8–10a). The triceps is active concentrically to extend the elbow when the triceps acts in a closed kinematic chain such as in a push-up (Fig. 8–10b). The triceps may be active during activities requiring stabilization

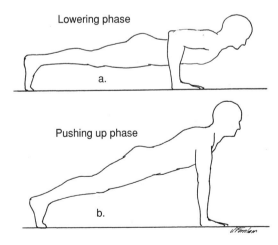

FIGURE 8–10. Action of the triceps in a push-up. (a) The triceps muscle works eccentrically in reverse action to control elbow flexion during the lowering phase of a push-up. (b) The triceps works concentrically in reverse action to produce the elbow extension that raises the body in a push-up.

of the elbow. For example, it acts as a synergist to prevent flexion of the elbow when the biceps is acting as a supinator. The other extensor of the elbow, the anconeus, assists in elbow extension and apparently also acts as a stabilizer during supination and pronation.

Synergistic actions of elbow flexor and extensor muscles have been investigated during isometric contractions in response to a variety of stresses including varus, valgus, flexion, and extension.[36] Some muscle pairs like the brachialis and brachioradialis and the anconeus and medial head of the triceps brachii are coactivated in a similar manner for all stresses. However, the synergistic patterns of other muscles at the elbow complex are complex and vary with the direction of the stress. For example, the brachialis and the long head of the biceps work synergistically during isometric contractions only from 0° to 45° of flexion.

In addition to the fact that synergies are affected by the direction and variety of stress, synergistic activity also appears to be affected by the type of muscle contraction being used (isometric, concentric, eccentric).[32] Nakazawa and associates using EMG found that activation patterns in the biceps brachii and the brachioradialis varied with the type of muscle contraction during elbow flexion against a load.[32] The synergistic actions of the muscles of the elbow and their relation to elbow and wrist function are still being investigated. Dounskaia and coworkers in an EMG study of arm cycling suggested that a hierarchical organization of control for elbow-wrist coordination was operative in this activity. Muscles of the elbow were responsible for movement of the entire linkage and the wrist muscles were responsible for making the corrections to the movement that were necessary to complete the task.[37]

Structure: Superior and Inferior Radioulnar Joints

Superior Radioulnar Joint

The articulating surfaces of the proximal radioulnar joint include the **ulnar radial notch,** the **annular ligament,** the capitulum of the humerus, and the head of the radius. The radial notch is located on the lateral aspect of the proximal ulna directly below the trochlear notch (Fig. 8–11a). The surface of the radial notch is concave and covered with articular car-

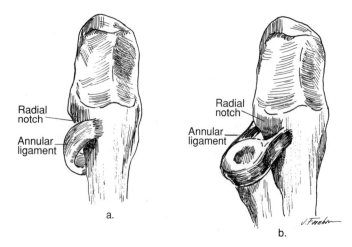

Radial notch

Annular ligament

Radial notch

Annular ligament

a.

b.

FIGURE 8–11. The annular ligament. (a) Attachments of the annular ligament. (b) The head of the radius has been pulled away from its normal position adjacent to the radial notch to show how the ligament partially surrounds the radial head.

tilage. A circular ligament called the annular ligament is attached to the anterior and posterior edges of the notch. The ligament is lined with articular cartilage, which is continuous with the cartilage lining of the radial notch. The annular ligament encircles the rim of the radial head, which is also covered with articular cartilage (Fig. 8–11b). Mechanoreceptors are evenly distributed throughout the ligament.[19] The capitulum and the proximal surface of the head of the radius are actually part of the elbow and have already been discussed under the elbow joint.

Inferior Radioulnar Joint

The articulating surfaces of the distal radioulnar joint include the **ulnar notch** of the radius, the **articular disk,** and the **head of the ulna** (Fig. 8–12). The ulnar notch of the radius is located at the distal end of the radius along the interosseous border. The radius of curvature of the concave ulnar notch is 4 to 7 mm larger than that of the ulnar head. The articular disk is sometimes referred to as either the **triangular fibrocartilage (TFC)** because of its triangular shape or as a part of **the triangular fibrocartilage complex (TFCC)** due to its extensive fibrous connections.

The disk has been described as resembling a shelf that has its medial border embedded in a wedge of vascular connective tissue containing fine ligamentous bands joining the disk to the ulna and articular capsule.[38] The base of the articular disk is attached to the distal edge of the ulnar notch of the radius. The apex of the articular disk has two attachments. One attachment is to the fovea on the ulnar head. The other attachment is to the base of the ulnar styloid

process.[39,40] Medially the articular disk is continuous with the fibers of the ulnar collateral ligament, which arises from the sides of the styloid process.[40] The margins of the articular disk are thickened and are either formed by or are integral parts of the dorsal and palmar capsular radioulnar ligaments (Fig. 8–13). The ligaments are firmly attached to the radius; the ulnar attachments are somewhat less firmly attached. The thickness of the dorsal and palmar margins and of the apex of the disk is approximately 3 to 6 mm[40,41] in contrast to the central area of the articular disk, which may only be 0.5 to 3 mm in thickness and is often so thin that it is transparent.[40] The central area may be perforated and the number of perforations in-

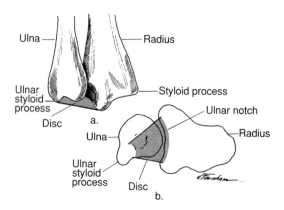

Ulna

Radius

Ulnar styloid process

Styloid process

Disc

a.

Ulnar notch

Ulna

Radius

Ulnar styloid process

Disc

b.

FIGURE 8–12. The inferior radioulnar joint of a left forearm. (a) An anterior view of the inferior radioulnar joint shows the disk in its normal position in a supinated left forearm. (b) An inferior view of the disk shows how the disk covers the inferior aspect of the distal ulna and separates the ulna from the articulation at the wrist.

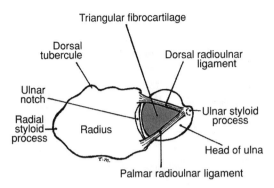

Triangular fibrocartilage
Dorsal tubercle
Dorsal radioulnar ligament
Ulnar notch
Radial styloid process
Radius
Ulnar styloid process
Head of ulna
Palmar radioulnar ligament

FIGURE 8–13. The illustration includes the distal aspects of a left radius and ulnar as well as the articular disk and articulating surfaces of the distal radioulnar joint. The articular disk is shown with radioulnar ligaments bordering the sides of the disk.

creases with age from 7% in the third decade to 53.1% for individuals who are in the sixth decade and above.[40] Chidgey and colleagues in a study of 12 fresh cadaver wrists found that the articular disks had a high collagen content with sparsely but equally distributed elastin fibers. The same authors found that 80% of the central portion of the articular disk was avascular compared to the peripheral area, which was only 15% to 20% avascular. The radioulnar ligaments were well vascularized.[42] Ohmori and Azuma found free nerve endings in the ulnar side of the articular disk particularly around the periphery. The authors suggest that in view of their findings the disk may be a source of wrist pain.[43]

The articular disk has two articulating surfaces: the proximal (superior) surface and the distal (inferior) surface. The proximal surface of the disk articulates with the ulnar head at the distal radioulnar joint while the distal surface articulates with the carpal bones as part of the radiocarpal joint.[2] Both the proximal and distal surfaces of the articular disk are concave. The superior surface of the articular disk is deepened to accommodate the convexity of the ulnar head; the distal surface is adapted to accommodate the carpal bones.[40] The peripheral parts of both the ulnar and carpal disk surfaces are covered by synovium coming from their respective joint capsules.[40]

The ulnar head is convex and is covered with articular cartilage beneath the disk.[44,45] The head has two articular surfaces, the pole and the seat, which articulate with the articular disk and the ulnar notch of the radius, respectively. The convex pole is U shaped and faces the disk.

The convex seat faces the ulnar notch of the radius.[39]

Radioulnar Articulation

The proximal and distal radioulnar joints are mechanically linked; therefore, motion at one joint is always accompanied by motion at the other joint. The distal radioulnar joint is also considered to be functionally linked to the wrist in that compressive loads are transmitted through the distal radioulnar joint from the hand to the radius and ulna. The radius carries approximately 80% of the compressive load from the hand and the ulna 20% of that load.[45]

Pronation of the forearm occurs as a result of the radius crossing over the ulna at the superior radioulnar joint. During pronation and supination, the rim of the head of the radius spins within the osteoligamentous enclosure formed by the radial notch and the annular ligament. At the same time the surface of the head spins on the capitulum of the humerus. At the distal radioulnar joint, the concave surface of the ulnar notch of the radius slides around the ulnar head, while the disk follows the radius by twisting at its apex and sweeping along beneath the ulnar head. Joint surface contact is optimal only with the forearm in a neutral position between supination and pronation. In maximal pronation and supination the articulating surfaces have only minimal contact.[46] In full supination the seat of the ulnar head rests on the palmar aspect of the ulnar notch, whereas in full pronation it rests against the dorsal lip of the ulnar notch[39,47] (Fig. 8–14).

Ligaments

The three ligaments associated with the proximal radioulnar joint are the annular and quadrate ligaments and the oblique cord (Fig. 8–15). The **annular ligament** is a strong band that forms four-fifths of a ring that encircles the radial head (see Fig. 8–11). The inner surface of the ligament is covered with cartilage and serves as a joint surface. The proximal border of the annular ligament blends with the joint capsule, and the lateral aspect is reinforced by fibers from the lateral collateral ligament.[2] The **quadrate ligament** extends from the inferior edge of the ulna's radial notch to insert in the neck of the radius. The quadrate ligament reinforces the inferior aspect of the joint capsule and helps to maintain

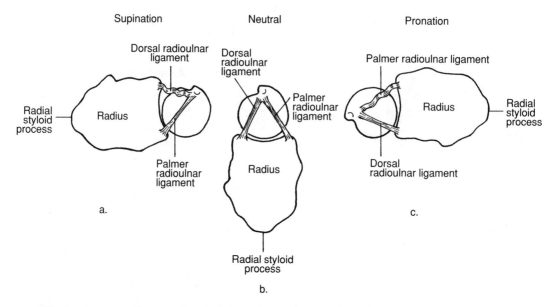

FIGURE 8–14. Articulating surfaces and dorsal and palmar radioulnar ligaments at the distal radioulnar joint. (a) The head of the ulna is shown in contact with the palmar aspect of the ulnar notch in full supination. The palmar radioulnar ligament is taut and the dorsal ligament is lax. (b) In the neutral position, the articulating surface of the head of the ulna has maximum contact with the radial articulating surface. (c) In full pronation the head of the ulna has contact only with the dorsal lip of the ulnar notch. The dorsal radioulnar ligament is taut and the palmar ligament is lax.

the radial head in apposition to the radial notch.[11] The quadrate ligament also limits the spin of the radial head in supination and pronation. The **oblique cord** is a flat fascial band on the ventral forearm that extends from an attachment just inferior to the radial notch on the ulna to insert just below the bicipital tuberosity on the radius. The fibers of the oblique cord are at right angles to the fibers of the interosseous membrane.[2] The functional significance of the oblique cord is not clear, but it may assist in preventing separation of the radius and ulna.

The dorsal and palmar radioulnar ligaments, as well as the interosseous membrane, which stabilizes both proximal and distal joints, reinforce the distal radioulnar joint. The dorsal and palmar ligaments are formed by longitudinally oriented collagen fiber bundles originating from the dorsal and palmar aspects of the ulnar notch of the radius.[46] The two ligaments extend along the margins of the articular disk to insert on the ulnar fovea and base of ulnar styloid process[39] (see Fig. 8–14). The palmar radioulnar ligament is at least 2 mm longer than the dorsal radioulnar ligament.[48] According to Linscheid, the dorsal radioulnar ligament averages 18 mm in length, whereas the palmar averages 22 mm.[39]

The interosseous membrane is described simply as a broad collaginous sheet that runs between the radius and ulna.[2] However, Skahen and associates consider the interosseous membrane to be a complex structure consisting of a central band, a variable number of accessory bands (1 to 5), a proximal interosseous band, and membranous portions.[49] The fibers of the central band run distally and medially from the radius to the ulna. Maximum strain in the fibers of the central band occurs when the forearm is in a neutral position (midway between supination and pronation). The fibers in the central band are relaxed in both supinated and pronated positions.[2,49] The interosseous membrane provides stability for both the superior and inferior radioulnar joints. When under tension, the membrane not only binds the joints together, but also provides for the transmission of forces from the hand and distal end of the radius to the ulna. A tract extends from the interosseus membrane and inserts in the distal radioulnar joint capsule between the tendon sheaths of the extensor digiti minimi and the extensor carpi ulnaris muscles. The tract's deep fibers insert directly into the articular disk (triangular fibrocartilage). The tract of the interosseus membrane is taut in pronation and loose in supination.[50] The articular disk also provides stability for the inferior radioul-

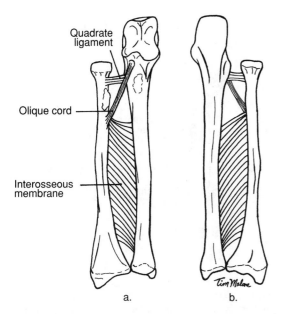

FIGURE 8–15. Ligamentous structures that provide stability for the proximal and distal radioulnar joints. The head of the radius has been slightly separated from the ulna and the annular ligament has been removed to show the quadrate ligament. (a) The anterior aspect of the radius and ulna are shown with the right forearm in a supinated position. The quadrate ligament is shown extending from the inferior edge of the radial notch on the ulna to attach on the neck of the radius. The oblique cord is shown extending from below the radial notch to attach just below the bicipital tuberosity. (b) A posterior view of the right radius and ulna in the supinated position. The interosseous membrane is shown extending between the radius and ulna for a considerable portion of their length.

nar joint by binding the distal radius and ulna together. The distal radioulnar joint capsule, which is a separate entity from the triangular fibrocartilage, can be a source of limitation of motion when it is invaded by scar tissue following wrist injuries.[51]

Muscles

The muscles associated with the radioulnar joints are the **pronator teres, pronator quadratus, biceps brachii,** and the **supinator.** The pronator teres has two heads, a humeral head and an ulnar head. The humeral head comes from the common flexor tendon on the medial epicondyle of the humerus. The smaller ulnar head arises from the medial aspect of the coronoid process of the ulna. The muscle attaches distally to the surface of the lateral side of the radius at its greatest convexity. The pronator quadratus is located at the distal end of the

forearm. It arises by two heads (superficial and deep) from the ulna and crosses the interosseous membrane anteriorly to insert on the radius. The fibers of the superficial head pass transversely to insert on the radius while the fibers of the deep head extend obliquely to insert on the radius.[52] The biceps brachii has been discussed previously. The supinator is a short and broad muscle that arises from the lateral epicondyle of the humerus, radial collateral ligament, annular ligament, and the lateral aspect of the ulna. The muscle crosses the posterior aspect of the interosseous membrane to insert into the radius just medial and inferior to the bicipital tuberosity.

Function: Radioulnar Joints

Axis of Motion

The axis of motion for pronation and supination is a longitudinal axis extending from the center of the radial head to the center of the ulnar head.[9,53] In supination the radius and ulna lie parallel to one another, whereas in pronation, the radius crosses over the ulna (Fig. 8–16). There is very little motion of the ulna

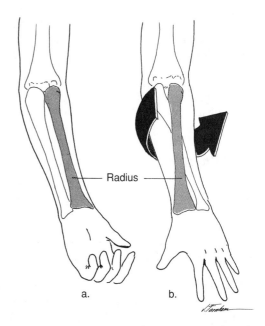

FIGURE 8–16. Supination and pronation. (a) The radius and ulna are parallel to each other in the supinated position of the forearm. (b) In the pronated position, the radius crosses over the ulna. Drawing shows a left upper extremity.

during pronation and supination. Motion of the proximal ulna is negligible. Motion of the distal ulna is of less magnitude than that of the radius and opposite in direction to motion of the radius.[45] The ulnar head moves distally and dorsally in pronation and proximally and medially in supination. Therefore, at the distal radioulnar joint, the ulnar head glides in the ulnar notch of the radius from the dorsal lip of the ulnar notch in pronation to a position on the palmar aspect of the ulnar notch in full supination.[39]

Range of Motion

A total ROM of 150° has been ascribed to the radioulnar joints.[2,44,54] The ROM of pronation and supination is assessed with the elbow in 90° of flexion. This position stabilizes the humerus so that radioulnar joint rotation may be distinguished from rotation that is occurring at the shoulder joint. When the elbow is fully extended, active supination and pronation occur in conjunction with shoulder rotation. Limitation of pronation when the elbow is extended may be caused by passive tension in the biceps brachii. Pronation in all positions is limited by bony approximation of the radius and ulna and by tension in the dorsal radioulnar ligament and the posterior fibers of the medial collateral ligament of the elbow.[21] Supination is limited by passive tension in the palmar radioulnar ligament and the oblique cord. The quadrate ligament limits spin of the radial head in both pronation and supination, and the annular ligament helps to maintain stability of the proximal radioulnar joint by holding the radius in close approximation to the radial notch.

Muscle Action

The pronators produce pronation by exerting a pull on the radius, which causes its shaft and distal end to turn over the ulna (Fig. 8–17). The pronator teres is a two-joint muscle that has a slight role in elbow flexion although its major action is at the radioulnar joints. As a two-joint muscle, the pronator teres may become actively insufficient when a full range of pronation is attempted simultaneously with the full range of shoulder flexion. The pronator teres contributes some of its force toward stabilization of the proximal radioulnar joint. The translatory component of the force produced by the

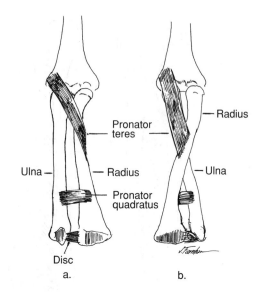

FIGURE 8–17. Pronation of the forearm. The pronator teres and pronator quadratus produce pronation by pulling the radius over the ulna. Drawing shows a left forearm (a) in the supinated position and (b) in the pronated position.

pronator teres helps to maintain contact of the radial head with the capitulum. The pronator quadratus, a one-joint muscle, is unaffected by changing positions at the elbow. The pronator quadratus is active in unresisted and resisted pronation and in slow or fast pronation. The deep head of the pronator quadratus also acts to maintain compression of the distal radioulnar joint.[29,52]

The supinators, like the pronators, act by pulling the shaft and distal end of the radius over the ulna (Fig. 8–18). The supinator muscle acts alone during unresisted slow supination in all positions of the elbow or forearm. The supinator also can act alone during unresisted fast supination when the elbow is extended. However, activity of the biceps is always evident when supination is performed against resistance and during fast supination when the elbow is flexed to 90°. Activity of the biceps is most evident when using a screwdriver to drive a screw into the wood. The anconeus muscle is active in supination and pronation. An elbow stabilization role has been suggested to explain this activity.

The strength of the flexors versus the extensors as determined by isometric testing of these muscle groups at 90° of elbow flexion shows that the elbow flexors are stronger than the elbow extensors and that the supinators are stronger than the pronators.[55]

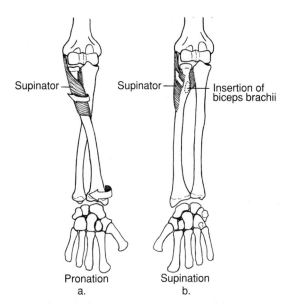

Supinator — Supinator — Insertion of biceps brachii

Pronation
a.

Supination
b.

FIGURE 8–18. Supination of the right forearm. (a) In the pronated position the supinator muscle wraps around the proximal radius. A contraction of the supinator or the biceps or both pulls the radius over the ulna. (b) The supinator muscle and the insertion site of the biceps are shown in the supinated position.

Stability

Muscular support of the distal radioulnar joint is attributed to the pronator teres,[39] the pronator quadratus,[48,52,54,56,57] and the extensor carpi ulnaris tendon.[39,48,58] According to Linscheid, the ulnar head of the pronator teres binds the ulna to the radius while the humeral head depresses the ulna during pronation.[39] The superficial head of the pronator quadratus is the prime mover for forearm pronation; the deep head provides dynamic stabilization for the distal radioulnar joint. Activity in the extensor carpi ulnaris muscle exerts a slight depressive force on the dorsal aspect of the ulnar head as the tendon is stretched over the head during supination. Tension in the tendon helps to maintain the position of the ulnar head during both supination and pronation.[58]

The dorsal and palmar radioulnar ligaments, the interosseous membrane and tract, and the articular disk provide ligamentous support of the distal radioulnar joint. The dorsal radioulnar ligament becomes taut in pronation, whereas the palmar radioulnar ligament becomes taut in supination[39,46,48,54,56,59] (see Fig. 8–14). According to Schiend, the radioulnar ligaments have limited cross sectional areas and low structural stiffness, but they are able to pre-

vent separation of the radius from the ulna during loading and allow for force transmission from the radius to the ulna through the distal radioulnar joint.[58] However, these ligaments do not augment longitudinal stability. They allow approximately 5 mm of play between the radius and ulna before providing resistance to further distraction.[39] The radioulnar ligaments, the articular disk, and the pronator quadratus maintain the ulna within the ulnar notch and prevent the ulna from subluxating or dislocating. Yet these ligaments allow a high degree of mobility. The interosseous membrane provides stability for the distal joint by binding the radius and ulna together. Also, according to Skahen and coworkers, the interosseous membrane in combination with the triangular fibrocartilaginous complex provide important longitudinal stabilization.[60] The interosseous membrane also transfers loads from the wrist to the forearm.[61] Markolf and associates studied radioulnar load sharing at the wrist and elbow with the elbow in varus, valgus, and neutral positions.[62] When the elbow was in varus (no contact between the radial head and capitulum), force was transmitted from the distal radius through the interosseous membrane to the proximal ulna. When the elbow was in valgus (contact between the radial head and the capitulum), the force was transmitted through the radius. When the forearm was in the neutral position, the mean force in the distal end of the ulna averaged 7% of the applied load, whereas the force in the proximal ulna averaged 93% of the load applied to the wrist.[62] The tract associated with the interosseous membrane is taut in pronation and loose in supination. During pronation the tract protects the ulnar head in a sling. It also provides stability for the joint by reinforcing the dorsal aspect of the joint capsule.[50]

The articular disk acts as a cushion in allowing compression force transmission from the carpals to the ulna and acts as a stabilizer of the ulnar side of the carpals.[47] Also the disk assists in the transmission of compressive forces from the radius to the ulna.[61–63] Adams and associates[59] used a distractive force to study the relationship between strains in the disk and forearm position. The distractive force was designed to simulate the effects of the separation of articulating surfaces that accompanies a power grip. These authors found that strain distribution in the disk was dependent on the forearm position.[59] Changes in disk configuration occurred consistently during forearm motion

Table 8–3. **Ligamentous and Muscular Contributions to Stability at the Proximal and Distal Radioulnar Joints**

Joint	Ligamentous	Muscular
Proximal radioulnar joint	Annular and quadrate ligaments[11] Oblique cord[21] (limits supination) Interosseous membrane	Passive tension in the biceps brachii in the full extended elbow position Pronator teres (helps maintain contact of radial head and capitulum)
Distal radioulnar joint	Interosseous membrane[49,50] Dorsal radioulnar ligament (limits pronation)[39,46,56] Palmar radioulnar ligament (limits supination)[39,46,56] Triangular fibrocartilage[39,40,47,59] Joint capsule	Pronator quadratus[39,52,57] Anconeus Extensor carpi ulnaris[39,48,58] Pronator teres

and resulted in non-uniform strain in the articular disk. Tension across the entire disk decreased in supination, whereas tension increased in the radial portion of the disk in pronation.[59] During the midrange portion of the pronation/supination motion the disk provided minimal resistance to forearm movement because the articular disk attachment to the ulnar head is near the axis of rotation of the distal radioulnar joint. The authors concluded that the articular disk regularly bears both compressive and tensile strains.[59] According to Mikic, compressive forces are transmitted through the central portion of the disk and some of the load is converted to tensile loading within the peripheral margins.[40] A summary of ligamentous and muscular support for the distal radioulnar joint is presented in Table 8–3.

Mobility and Stability: Elbow Complex

Functional Activities

The joints and muscles of the elbow complex are used in almost all activities of daily living such as dressing, eating, carrying, and lifting. They are also used in tasks such as splitting firewood, hammering nails, and playing tennis. Most of the activities of daily living require a combination of motion at both the elbow and radioulnar joints. A total of about 100° of elbow flexion and 100° of supination/pronation is sufficient to accomplish simple tasks such as eating, brushing one's hair, brushing one's teeth, and dressing. The range of elbow flexion required is from about 30° of flexion to 130° of flexion. Fifty degrees of pronation and 55° of supination are necessary to allow the hand to function normally in these activities. For example, about 40° of pronation and 20° of supination are required to use a telephone.[64] Therefore, mobility of the complex is necessary for normal functioning in most areas of activity.

The design of the radioulnar joints enhances the mobility of the hand. In primitive species the ulna was a major weight-bearing structure and was connected directly to the carpals through a dense immobile syndesmosis.[54] The complete separation of the ulna from the carpals by the articular disk and the formation of a true diarthrodial joint lined with articular cartilage are features that permit pronation and supination to occur in every position of the hand to the forearm. Pronation and supination of the forearm, when the elbow is flexed at 90°, rotates the hands so that the palm faces either superiorly or inferiorly. The mobility afforded the hand is achieved at the expense of stability because the movable forearm is unable to provide a stable base for attachment of the wrist and hand muscles. Therefore, many of the muscles that act on the wrist and hand are attached on the distal end of the humerus rather than on the forearm. The flexors of the wrist and fingers include the flexor carpi radialis, flexor carpi ulnaris, palmaris longus, flexor digitorum superficialis, and flexor digitorum profundus.

All of these muscles, except the flexor digitorum profundus, originate on the medial epicondyle of the humerus. The flexor digitorum profundus originates on the proximal ulna. The extensors of the wrist and fingers, which originate in the region of the lateral epicondyle of the humerus, include the extensor carpi radialis longus, extensor carpi radialis brevis, extensor carpi ulnaris, and extensor digitorum.

Relationship to the Hand and Wrist

The location of the hand and wrist muscles at the elbow and the fact that these muscles cross the elbow create close structural and functional relationships between the elbow and wrist/hand complexes. The elbow complex affects and is affected by the wrist and hand muscles; therefore, these muscles need to be considered in any discourse on the elbow complex. Anatomically, the hand and wrist muscles help to reinforce the elbow joint capsule and contribute to stability of the elbow complex. In a study of 11 cadaveric specimens, Davidson and coworkers[65] found that the humeral head of the flexor carpi ulnaris muscle is the only muscle that lies directly over the anterior portion of the medial collateral ligament at elbow flexion positions between 90° and 120°. Because the medial elbow is subjected to the largest valgus stress during the cocking and acceleration phases of throwing, which occur between 80° and 120° of elbow flexion, the flexor carpis ulnaris muscle has the potential to provide significant reinforcement for the MCL during throwing activities.[65] During muscular contractions, the wrist muscles may contribute to the torque production of the elbow muscles although their primary action is at the wrist and hand. However, the muscles may have a more important functional role by producing compression of the articulating surfaces at the elbow. The importance of compression or stabilization of the elbow can be seen in the work of Amis and associates,[29] who investigated the effect of tensile loads on the forearm during a pulling activity. They found that both the humeroradial and humeroulnar articulations are subjected to compressive forces during pulling activities and that the MCL was heavily loaded. Andersson found that during a pulling task, the flexors, at an elbow position of 90° of flexion, exerted a flexor force of 6000 N.[66]

Relationship to the Head, Neck, and Shoulder

Head and neck positions can affect the elbow flexor torque production in healthy young adults.[67] Clinically, it has been observed that restrictions of motion in the neck and shoulder also may affect function of the elbow. Limitations of shoulder joint internal rotation may cause a subject to excessively pronate the arm during throwing or racquet swinging activities. A lack of shoulder external rotation may cause a person to compensate for the lost motion by supinating the forearm.[68]

Effects of Immobilization and Injury

Like other joints in the body, the joints and muscles of the elbow complex may be subject to the effects of immobilization and injury. Immobilization may cause decreases in muscle strength.[69] If the flexors happen to be weakened more than the extensors, the flexors may not be able to counteract the pull of the extensors and the elbow joint may hyperextend during extension. Also the flexor muscles' contributions to joint compression would be decreased, and therefore joint stability would be diminished. Prolonged immobilization of the elbow in 90° of flexion results in adaptive shortening of the elbow flexors and lengthening of the elbow extensors. Consequently the elbow ROM in extension is limited.

Injuries to the elbow are fairly frequent and these injuries usually disrupt normal function. Therefore, an understanding of the mechanisms of these injuries and their relation to elbow joint structures is necessary for determining the effects of the injuries on joint function.

Compression Injury

Resistance to longitudinal compression forces at the elbow is provided for mainly by the contact of bony components; therefore, excessive compression forces at the elbow often result in bony failure. Falling on the hand when the elbow is in a close-packed position may result in the transmission of forces through the bones of the forearm to the elbow (Fig. 8–19a). If the forces are transmitted through the radius as may happen with a concomitant valgus stress, a fracture of the radial head may result from impact of the radial head on the capitulum (Fig. 8–19b). If the force from the fall is transmitted to the ulna, a fracture of either the coronoid or olecranon processes may occur from impact of the ulna on the humerus (see Fig. 8–19b). If neither the radius nor the ulna absorbs the excessive force through a fracture,

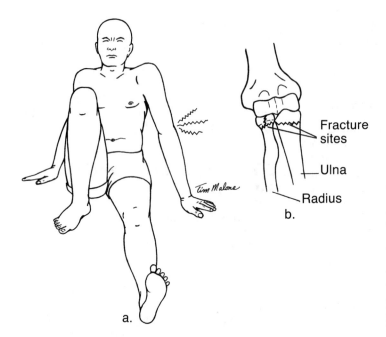

a.

b.

FIGURE 8–19. A fall on the hand with the elbow in a close-packed position may involve transmission of forces through the bones of the forearm to the elbow. (a) Transmission of forces from the hand to the elbow may occur through either or both the radius and ulna. (b) Impact of the radial head on the capitulum may cause either a fracture of the radial head or neck or both. A fracture of the coronoid or olecranon process (or both) may result from forces transmitted through the ulna.

then the force may be transmitted to the humerus and may result in a fracture of the supracondylar area.

Distraction Injury

Ligaments and muscles provide for resistance of the joints of the elbow complex to longitudinal traction. A distraction force of sufficient magnitude exerted on the radius may cause the radius to slip out of the annular ligament. Small children are particularly susceptible to this type of injury because the radial head is not fully developed. Lifting a small child up into the air by one or both hands or yanking a child by the hand is the usual causative mechanism and therefore the injury is referred to as **nursemaid's elbow** (Fig. 8–20). However, the distractive pull will rarely cause problems if the child is expecting the pull and has contracted the compressive elbow flexors. When the pull is unexpected, the muscles are not ready to provide the appropriate stabilization.

Varus/Valgus Injury

The MCL and LCL, articular configuration, and the joint capsule provide resistance to medial and lateral stresses at the elbow. If either one of the ligaments is overstretched, one aspect of the joint will be subjected to abnormal tensile stresses and the other to abnormal compres-

sive forces. The MCL is subjected to tensile stress during the backswing or "cock up" portion of throwing a ball (Fig. 8–21). If the stress on the MCL is repetitive, such as in baseball pitching, the ligament may become lax and unable to reinforce the medial aspect of the joint. In a study of 40 uninjured professional baseball

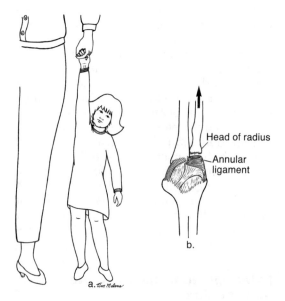

FIGURE 8–20. Nursemaid's elbow. (a) A pull on the hand creates tensile forces at the elbow. (b) The radial head is shown being pulled out of the annular ligament.

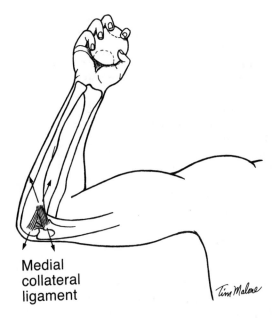

Medial collateral ligament

Tim Malone

FIGURE 8–21. Stretching of the medial collateral ligament during throwing.

pitchers, Ellenbacher and colleagues found increased elbow laxity in players' pitching arms.[70] The resulting medial instability may cause an increase in the normal carrying angle and excessive compression of the radial head on the capitulum. If the abnormal compression forces on the articular cartilage are prolonged, these forces may interfere with the blood supply of the cartilage and result in avascular necrosis. Repetitive microtrauma from valgus stress can cause epiphyseal plate fractures of the proximal radius.[71] In a magnetic resonance study of throwing injuries, full-thickness tears of the MCL were found in the elbows of 34 of 63 subjects tested and undersurface tears were found in 5 subjects. In addition 30 loose bodies were detected in the elbows of 14 subjects and cartilaginous damage was present in 21 elbows.[72]

Overuse and Other Injuries

The current interest in racquetball, Little League softball, paddle tennis, squash, and tennis predisposes participants to the possibility of elbow injuries. The use of a racquet greatly increases the length of the forearm lever (resistance arm) and subjects the elbow complex structures to great stresses. The classic tennis elbow (epicondylitis of the lateral epicondyle) is caused by repeated forceful contractions of the wrist exten-

sors, primarily the extensor carpi radialis brevis. The tensile stress created at the origin of the extensor carpi radialis brevis may cause microscopic tears that lead to inflammation of the lateral epicondyle.[73,74] Repeated tensile stress on the inelastic tendon may result in microscopic tears at the musculotendinous junction and result in tendinitis. Repetitive microtrauma injury can lead to mucinoid degeneration of the extensor origin and subsequent failure of the tendon.[75] Medial tendinitis or medial epicondylitis may be caused by forceful repetitive contractions of the pronator teres, flexor carpi radialis, and occasionally by the flexor carpi ulnaris. These muscles are involved in the tennis serve when the combined motion of elbow extension, pronation, and wrist flexion is used. High-speed video analysis shows that the elbow moves from 116° to 20° of flexion during serving. Ball impact occurs at an average of 35° of flexion. The forearm is in about 70° pronation at full impact.[76] One method of treatment for tennis elbow uses a brace or a band or cuff that is placed around the proximal forearm. Theoretically, the band is supposed to diminish the potential force that the forearm muscles generate by preventing full muscle expansion during a contraction.[77]

In certain phases of baseball pitching, muscle contractions also may cause high compression forces at the elbow. For example, during the acceleration and deceleration phases of baseball pitching, the compression forces at the elbow can attain 90% of body weight. EMG shows that the triceps, anconeus, wrist flexors and pronators as well as the biceps are all active in an attempt to prevent elbow distraction during pitching. Activity in the same muscles during peak valgus stress may assist the medial collateral ligament in stabilization of the elbow.[78] However, stretching of the MCL resulting in ligamentous sprain, medial epicondylitis, and flexor/pronator muscle strain are common injuries in baseball pitchers as well as in swimmers, golfers, and tennis players among others.[79] In a study of windmill softball pitchers, Barrentine and coworkers found that the compression forces that act at the elbow to resist elbow distraction equaled 67% to 79% of the values that had been calculated for overhand pitching.[80]

Other injuries to the elbow complex that may occur as a result of muscular contraction include nerve compression and bony fracture or dislocation. Repetitive forceful contraction of the flexor carpi ulnaris may compress the ulnar nerve as it passes through the cubital tunnel between the medial epicondyle of the humerus and the olecranon process of the ulna (Fig. 8–22). The resulting injury, called **cubital tunnel syndrome,** results in impaired motion of the thumb and fourth and fifth digits.[81] Sudden forceful contractions of the biceps brachii when the forearm is supinated and flexed at 90° may cause a rupture of the biceps tendon, or fracture or dislocation of the radius.

The interrelationship between the elbow complex and the wrist and hand complex makes normal functioning of the elbow of vital importance. If elbow function is impaired, function of the hand also may be impaired. For example, if the elbow cannot be flexed, it is impossible for the hand to bring food to the mouth. The fact that many important vascular and neural structures that supply the hand are closely associated with the elbow makes it important to prevent excessive stress and to protect the elbow from injury. Supracondylar humeral fractures, which are common in the skeletally immature individual, may injure either the radial or median nerves or the brachial artery.[71] If the radial nerve is injured at the level of the epicondyle, the wrist extensors, supinator, thumb, and finger extensors will be affected. If the median nerve is injured at the level of the elbow, the pronators, flexor carpi radialis, finger flexors, thenar muscles, and lumbricales will be affected. In the following chapter the reader will learn the specific functions of the hand muscles and will be better able to appreciate the significance of injury to some of the muscles.

Summary

Some of the interrelationships between the structure and function of elbow, shoulder, wrist, and hand have been introduced in this chapter. Muscles that have their primary actions at the wrist and hand also cross the elbow and contribute to its stability and function, whereas the stability and ROM at the shoulder and elbow help to enhance the function of the wrist and hand. Compensations at the elbow complex often are necessary when the ROM is limited at the shoulder or wrist. New relationships for the joints and muscles of the upper extremity will be introduced in the detailed study of the wrist and hand that follows in the next chapter.

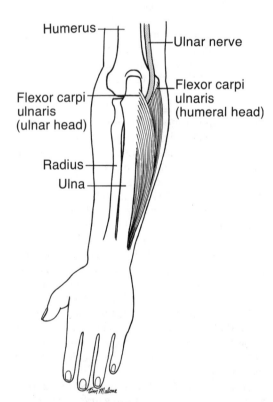

FIGURE 8–22. Location of the ulnar nerve as it passes through the cubital tunnel. A contraction of the flexor carpi ulnaris muscle can cause compression of the ulnar nerve between the two heads of the muscle, which are located on either side of the ulnar nerve at the elbow.

Humerus

Ulnar nerve

Flexor carpi ulnaris (ulnar head)

Flexor carpi ulnaris (humeral head)

Radius

Ulna

REFERENCES

1. An, KN et al: Muscles across the elbow joint: A biomechanical analysis. J Biomech 14:659–669, 1981.
2. Williams, PL, et al (eds): Gray's Anatomy, ed 38. Churchill Livingstone, New York, 1995.
3. London, JT: Kinematics of the elbow. J Bone Joint Surg 63A:529–535, 1981.
4. Eckstein, F, et al: Stress distribution in the trochlear notch. J Bone Joint Surg (Br)76:647, 1994.
5. Eckstein, F, et al: Morphomechanics of the humero-ulnar joint: I Joint space width and contact area as a function of load and angle. Anat Rec 243:318, 1995.
6. Eckstein, F, et al: Morphomechanics of the humero-ulnar joint: II Concave incongruity determines the distribution of load and subchondral mineralization. Anat Rec 243:327, 1995.
7. Milz, S, et al: Thickness distribution of the subchondral mineralization zone of the trochlear notch and its correlation with the cartilage thickness: An expression of functional adaptation to mechanical stress acting on the humeroulnar joint. Anat Rec 248:189, 1997.
8. Jacobs, CR, and Eckstein, F: Computer simulation of subchondral bone adaptation to mechanical loading in an incongruous joint. Anat Rec 249:317, 1997.
9. Kapandji, IA: The Physiology of the Joints, Vol I. E&S Livingstone, Edinburgh and London, 1970.

10. Schenck, RC et al: A biomechanical analysis of articular cartilage of the elbow and a potential relationship to osteochondritis dessicans. Clin Orthop Rel Res 299:305, 1994.

11. Palastanga, N, et al: Anatomy and Human Movement: Structure and Function. Heinemann Medical Books, Oxford, 1989.

12. Fuss, F: The ulnar collateral ligament of the human elbow joint. Anatomy, function and biomechanics. J Anat 175:203, 1991.

13. Regan, WD, et al: Biomechanical study of ligaments around the elbow joint. Clin Orthop 271:170, 1991.

14. Bowling, RW, and Rockar, PA: The elbow complex. In Malone, TR, et al (eds): Orthopedic and Sports Physical Therapy, ed. 3. Mosby-Yearbook, St Louis. 1997, p 382.

15. Sobel, J, and Nirschl, RP. Elbow Injuries. In Zachazewski, JE, et al (eds): Athletic Injuries and Rehabilitation. WB Saunders, Philadelphia. 1996, p 544.

16. Richardson, JK, and Iglarsh, ZA: Clinical Orthopaedic Physical Therapy. WB Saunders, Philadelphia, 1994, p 222.

17. Reid, DC, and Kushner, S. The elbow. In Donatelli, R, and Wooden, MJ (eds): Orthopaedic Physical Therapy, ed 2. Churchill Livingstone, New York, 1994.

18. Callaway, GH, et al: Biomechanical evaluation of the medial collateral ligament of the elbow. J Bone Joint Surg 79:123, 1997.

19. Petrie, S, et al: Mechanoreceptors in the human elbow ligaments. J Hand Surg 23:512, 1998.

20. Sojberg, JO, et al: Experimental elbow instability after transection of the medial collateral ligament. Clin Orthop Rel Res 218:186–190, 1987.

21. Hotchkiss, RN, and Weiland, AJ: Valgus stability of the elbow. J Orthop Res 5:372–377, 1987.

22. Olsen, BS, et al: Lateral collateral ligament of the elbow joint: Anatomy and kinematics. J Shoulder Elbow Surg 5:103, 1996.

23. Morrey, BF, and An, KN: Articular and ligamentous contributions to the stability of the elbow joint. Am J Sports Med 11:315–318, 1983.

24. Netter, F: The Ciba Collection of Medical Illustrations, Vol 8. Musculoskeletal System Part 1. Ciba-Geigy, Summit, NJ, 1987.

25. Youm, Y, et al: Biomechanical analysis of forearm pronation-supination and elbow flexion-extension. J Biomech 12:245, 1979.

26. Deland, JT, et al: Biomechanical basis for elbow hinge-distractor design. Clin Orthop Rel Res 215:303–312, 1987.

27. Morrey, BF, and Chao, YS: Passive motion of the elbow joint. J Bone Joint Surg 58A:501–508, 1976.

28. Hoppenfeld, S: Physical Examination of the Spine and Extremities. Appleton-Century-Crofts, New York, 1976.

29. Amis, AA, et al: Elbow joint force predictions for some strenuous isometric actions. J Biomech 13:765–775, 1980.

30. Murray, WM, et al: Variation of muscle moment arms with elbow and forearm position. J Biomech 28:513, 1995.

31. Basmajian, JV: Muscles Alive, ed 4. Williams & Wilkins, Baltimore, 1978.

32. Nakazawa, K, et al: Differences in activation patterns in elbow flexor muscles during isometric, concentric and eccentric contractions. Eur J Applied Physiol 66:214, 1993.

33. Provins, KA, and Salter, N: Maximum torque exerted about the elbow joint. J Appl Physiol 7:393–398, 1955.

34. Currier, DP: Maximal isometric tension of elbow extensors at varied positions. Phys Ther 52:1043–1049, 1972.

35. Bohannon, RW: Shoulder position influences elbow extension force in healthy individuals. JOSPT 12:111–114, 1990.

36. Buchanan, TS, et al: Characteristics of synergistic relations during isometric contractions of human elbow muscles. J Neurophysiol 56:1225–1241, 1986.

37. Dounskaia, NV, et al: Hierarchal control of different elbow/wrist coordination patterns. Exp Brain Res 121:239, 1998.

38. Mohiuddin, A, and Zanjua, MZ: Form and function of radioulnar joint articular disc. The Hand 14:61–66, 1982.

39. Linscheid, RL: Biomechanics of the distal radioulnar joint. Clin Orthop 275:46, 1992.

40. Mikic, Z: Detailed anatomy of the articular disc of the distal radioulnar joint. Clin Orthop Rel Res 245:123, 1989.

41. Chiou, HJ, et al: Triangular fibrocartilage of wrist: Presentation on high resolution ultrasonography. J Ultrasound Med 17:41, 1998.

42. Chidgey, LK, et al: Histologic anatomy of the triangular fibrocartilage. J Hand Surg 16A:1084, 1991.

43. Ohmori, M, and Azuma, H: Morphology and distribution of nerve endings in the human triangular fibrocartilage complex. J Hand Surg (Br) 23:522, 1998.

44. Palmer, AK: The distal radioulnar joint. Orthop Clin North Am 15:321–335, 1984.

45. Palmer, AK, and Werner, FW: Biomechanics of the distal radioulnar joint. Orthop Clin North Am 15:27–35, 1984.

46. Ekenstam, F: Anatomy of the distal radioulnar joint. Clin Orthop 275:14, 1992.

47. Schiend, F, et al: The distal radioulnar ligaments: A biomechanical study. J Hand Surg 16A:1116, 1991.

48. Van Der Heijden, ED, and Hillen, B: A two-dimensional kinematic analysis of the distal radioulnar joint. J Hand Surg (Br) 21:824, 1996.

49. Skahen, JR 3rd, et al: The interosseous membrane of the forearm: Anatomy and function. J Hand Surg (Am) 22:981, 1997.

50. Gabl, M, et al: The interosseous membrane and its influence on the distal radioulnar joint. An investigation of the distal tract. J Hand Surg (Br) 23:179, 1998.

51. Kleinman, WB, and Graham, JJ. The distal radioulnar joint capsule: Clinical anatomy and role in post traumatic limitation of forearm rotation. J Hand Surg (Am) 23:588, 1998.

52. Johnson, RK, and Shrewsbury, MM: The pronator quadratus in motions and in stabilization of the radius and ulna at the distal radioulnar joint. J Hand Surg (Am) 1:205, 1976.

53. Hollister, AM, et al: The relationship of the interosseous membrane to the axis of rotation of the forearm. Clin Orthop 298:272, 1994.

54. Drobner, WS, and Hausman, MR: The distal radioulnar joint. Hand Clin 8:631, 1992.

55. Askew, LJ, et al: Isometric elbow strength in normal individuals. Clin Orthop Rel Res 222:261–266, 1987.

56. Kihara, H, et al. The stabilizing mechanisms of the distal radioulnar joint during pronation and supination. J Hand Surg (Am) 20:930, 1995.

57. Stuart, PR: Pronator quadratus revisited. J Hand Surg 21:741, 1996.

58. Kauer, JM: The distal radioulnar joint. Clin Orthop Rel Res 275:37 1991.

59. Adams, BD, and Holley, KA: Strains in the articular disk of the triangular fibrocartilage complex: A biomechanical study. J Hand Surg 18A:919, 1993.

60. Skahen, JR 3rd, et al: Reconstruction of the interosseous membrane of the forearm in cadavers. J Hand Surg (Am) 22:786, 1997.

61. Birkbeck, DP, et al: The interosseous membrane affects load distribution in the forearm. J Hand Surg (Am) 6:975, 1997.

62. Markolf, KL, et al: Radioulnar load-sharing in the forearm: A study in cadavera. J Bone Joint Surg (Am) 80:879, 1998.

63. Bade, H, et al: Morphology of the articular surfaces of the distal radioulnar joint. Anat Rec 246:410, 1996.

64. Morrey, BF, et al: A biomechanical study of normal functional elbow motion. J Bone Joint Surg 63A: 872–876, 1981.

65. Davidson, PA, et al: Functional anatomy of the flexor pronator muscle group in relation to the medial collateral ligament of the elbow. Am J Sports Med 23:245, 1995.

66. Andersson, GBJ, and Schultz, AB: Transmission of moments across the elbow joint and the lumbar spine. J Biomech 12:747–755, 1979.

67. Deutsch, H, et al: Effect of head-neck position on elbow flexor muscle torque production. Phys Ther 67: 517–521, 1987.

68. Dilorenzo, CE, et al: The importance of shoulder and cervical dysfunction in the etiology and treatment of athletic elbow injuries. J Orthop Sports Phys Ther 11:402–409, 1990.

69. Vaughan, VC: Effects of upper limb immobilization on isometric muscle strength, movement time, and triphasic electromyographic characteristics. Phys Ther 69:119–129, 1989.

70. Ellenbacher, TS, et al: Medial elbow joint laxity in professional baseball pitchers. A bilateral comparison using stress radiography. Am J Sports Med 26:420, 1998.

71. Ireland, ML, and Andrews, JR: Shoulder and elbow injuries in the young athlete. Clin Sports Med 7:473–494, 1988.

72. Sugimoto, H, et al: Throwing injury of the elbow: Assessment with gradient three-dimensional Fourier transform gradient-echo and short term inversion recovery images. J Magn Reson Imaging 8:487, 1998

73. Priest, JD, et al: The elbow and tennis. Part 1: An analysis of players with and without pain. Phys Sports Med 8:4, 1980.

74. La Freniere, JG: "Tennis elbow" evaluation, treatment and prevention. Phys Ther 59:6, 1979.

75. Field, LD, and Savoie, FH: Common elbow injuries in sport. Sports Med 26:193, 1998.

76. Kibler, WB: Clinical biomechanics of the elbow in tennis: Implications for evaluation and diagnosis. Med Sci Sports Exerc 26:1203, 1994.

77. Nirschi, RP, and Sobel, J: Conservative treatment of tennis elbow. Phys Sports Med 9:6, 1981.

78. Werner, SL, et al: Biomechanics of the elbow during baseball pitching. J Ortho Sports Phys Ther 17:274, 1993.

79. Andrews, JR, and Whiteside, JA: Common elbow problems in the athlete. J Orthop Sports Phys Ther 17:289, 1993.

80. Barrentine, SW, et al: Biomechanics of windmill softball pitching with implications about injury mechanisms at the shoulder and elbow. J Orthop Sports Phys Ther 28:405, 1998.

81. Craven, PR, and Green, DP: Cubital tunnel syndrome. J Bone Joint Surg 62(A):986, 1980.

Study Questions

1. Name and locate all of the articulating surfaces of the joints of the elbow complex. Describe the method of articulation at each joint including axes of motion and degrees of freedom.

2. Explain the stabilizing function of the brachioradialis by diagramming the translatory and rotatory components at different joint angles.

3. Explain why active elbow flexion is more limited than passive flexion. Which structures limit extension?

4. Describe the "carrying angle" and explain why it is present.

5. Which structures limit supination and pronation?

6. If slow pronation of the forearm is attempted without resistance, which muscle will be used?

7. What does the term "concave incongruity" mean? Where is it found?

8. How does the structure and function of the annular ligament differ from that of the medial collateral ligament?

9. Describe the activity of the biceps brachii during a chin-up.

10. What is the mechanism of injury in tennis elbow?

11. Which position of the elbow is most stable? Why?

12. Compare the biceps brachii with the brachialis on the basis of structure and function.

13. Describe the mechanism of injury involved in cubital tunnel syndrome.

CHAPTER 9

THE WRIST AND HAND COMPLEX

OBJECTIVES

Following the study of this chapter, the reader should be able to:

Define

1. The terminology unique to the wrist and hand complexes.

Describe

1. The articular surfaces of the joints of the wrist and hand complexes.
2. The ligaments of the joints of the wrist and hand, including the functional significance of each.
3. Accessory joint structures found in the wrist and hand complexes, including the function of each.
4. Types of movements and ranges of motion of the radiocarpal joint, the midcarpal joint, and the total wrist complex.
5. The sequence of joint activity occurring from full wrist flexion to extension, including the role of the scaphoid; the sequence of joint activity in radial and ulnar deviation from neutral.
6. The role of the wrist musculature in producing wrist motion.
7. Motions and ranges available to joints of the hand complex.
8. The gliding mechanisms of the extrinsic finger flexors.
9. The structure of the extensor mechanism, including the muscles and ligaments that compose it.
10. How metacarpophalangeal extension occurs, including the muscles that produce and control it.
11. How flexion and extension of the proximal interphalangeal joint occur, including the muscular and ligamentous forces that produce and control these motions.
12. How flexion and extension of the distal interphalangeal joint occur, including the muscular and ligamentous forces that produce and control these motions.

13. The role of the wrist in optimizing length-tension in the extrinsic hand muscles.
14. The muscles that most commonly participate in release of objects from the hand.
15. The functional position of the wrist and hand.

Differentiate Between

1. The role of the interossei and lumbrical muscles at the metacarpophalangeal and interphalangeal joints.
2. The muscles used in cylindrical grip and those active in spherical grip, hook grip, and lateral prehension.
3. The muscles that are active in pad-to-pad, tip-to-tip, and pad-to-side prehension.

Compare

1. The activity of muscles of the thumb (in opposition of the thumb to the index finger) with the activity of those active in opposition to the little finger.
2. The characteristics of power grip with those of precision handling.
3. The most easily disrupted form of precision handling with the form of precision handling that may be used by someone without any active hand musculature; what are the prerequisites for each?

Introduction

The human hand may well surpass all body parts except the brain as a topic of universal interest. The human hand has been characterized as a symbol of power,[1] as an extension of intellect,[2] and as the seat of the will.[3] The symbiotic relation of the mind and hand is exemplified by sociologists' claim that the brain is responsible for the design of civilization, but the hand is responsible for its formation. The hand cannot function without the brain to control it; likewise the encapsulated brain needs the hand as a primary tool of expression. The entire upper limb is subservient to the hand. Any loss of function in the upper limb, regardless of the segment, ultimately translates into diminished function of its most distal joints. It is the significance of this potential loss that has led to detailed study of the finely balanced intricacies of the normal upper limb and hand.

The Wrist Complex

The wrist (**carpus**) consists of two compound joints: the **radiocarpal** and the **midcarpal joints,** referred to collectively as the **wrist complex.** Each joint proximal to the wrist complex serves to broaden the placement of the hand in space and to increase the degrees of freedom available to the hand. The shoulder serves as a dynamic base of support; the elbow allows the hand to approach or extend away from the body; and the forearm adjusts the approach of the hand to an object. The carpus, unlike the more proximal joints, serves placement of the hand in space to only a minor degree. The major contribution of the wrist complex seems to be to control length-tension relationships in the multiarticular hand muscles and to allow fine adjustment of grip. The wrist muscles appear to be designed for balance and control rather than for maximizing torque production.[4] The adjustments in length-tension of the extrinsic hand muscles that occur at the wrist cannot be replaced by compensatory movements of the shoulder, elbow, or forearm. The wrist has been called the most complex joint of the body from both an anatomic and physiologic perspective.[5] The intricacy and variability of the interarticular and intra-articular relations within the wrist complex are such that the wrist has received a large amount of attention with consensus on relatively few points. One point on which there appears to be consensus is that the structure and biomechanics of the wrist, as well as the hand, vary tremendously from person to person and that even subtle variations can produce differences in how a given function occurs. The intent of this chapter, therefore, is less to provide details on what is "normal" and more to describe the wrist complex (and hand) in such a way that general structure is clear and a conceptual framework is developed within which normal function and pathology can be understood.

The wrist complex as a whole is considered

to be biaxial, with motions of flexion/extension (volar flexion/dorsiflexion) around a coronal axis, and radial deviation/ulnar deviation (abduction/adduction) around an anteroposterior axis. Some will argue that some degree of pronation/supination may also be found, especially at the radiocarpal joint.[6] The ranges of motion (ROMs) of the entire complex are variable and reflect the differences in carpal kinematics due to such factors as ligamentous laxity, shape of articular surfaces and constraining effects of muscles.[7] Normal ranges are cited as 78° to 85° of flexion, 60° to 85° of extension, 15° to 21° of radial deviation, and 38° to 45° of ulnar deviation.[8–10] The ranges are contributed in various proportions by the compound radiocarpal and midcarpal joints. Gilford and colleagues[11] proposed that the two-joint, rather than single-joint, system of the wrist complex: (1) permitted large ROMs with less exposed articular surface and tighter joint capsules, (2) had less tendency for structural pinch at extremes of ranges, and (3) allowed for flatter multijoint surfaces that are more capable of withstanding imposed pressures.

Structural Components of the Wrist Complex

Radiocarpal Joint Structure

The radiocarpal joint is formed by the radius and radioulnar disk (as part of the **triangular fibrocartilage complex [TFCC]**) proximally and by the scaphoid, lunate, and triquetrum distally (Fig. 9–1). The proximal radiocarpal joint surface has a single continuous biconcave curvature that is long and shallow side to side (frontal plane) and shorter and sharper anteroposteriorly (sagittal plane). The proximal joint surface is composed of (1) the lateral radial facet that articulates with the scaphoid; (2) the medial radial facet that articulates with the lunate; and (3) the **TFCC** that articulates predominantly with the triquetrum although it also has some contact with the lunate in the neutral wrist (Fig. 9–2). The scaphoid and lateral facet of the radius account on average for slightly more than half the radiocarpal surface contact; the TFCC accounts for only about 10%.[12–14]

The TFCC consists of the radioulnar disk, a connective tissue wedge, and the various fibrous attachments[15] (see Fig. 9–2). The TFCC structural components are difficult to differentiate one from another.[16] Mohiuddin and Janjua[17] and Benjamin and colleagues,[18] however,

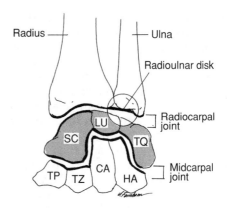

FIGURE 9–1. Wrist complex. The radiocarpal joint is composed of the radius and the radioulnar disk, with the scaphoid (SC), lunate (LU), and the triquetrum (TQ). The midcarpal joint is composed of the scaphoid, lunate, and triquetrum with the trapezium (TP), the trapezoid (TZ), the capitate (CA), and the hamate (HA).

provide descriptions that represent a reasonable consensus. The articular disk is a fibrocartilaginous continuation of the articular cartilage of the distal radius. The disk is connected medially via two dense fibrous connective tissue laminae. The upper lamina attaches to the ulnar head and ulnar styloid; the lower lamina has connections to the sheath of the extensor carpi ulnaris and to the triquetrum, hamate, and the base of the fifth metacarpal via fibers from the ulnar collateral ligament. The so-called meniscus homolog is a region of irregular connective tissue that lies within and is part of the lower lamina. The medial connective tissue structures may facilitate ROM because connective tissue is more compressible than fibrocartilage.[17] Overall, the TFCC should be considered to function at the wrist as an extension of the distal radius, just as it does at the

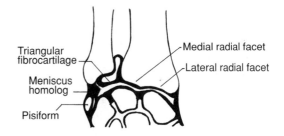

FIGURE 9–2. The proximal surface of the radiocarpal joint is formed by the medial and lateral facets of the distal radius and by the triangular fibrocartilage or radioulnar disk. The radioulnar disk and meniscus homologue are together part of the triangular fibrocartilage complex.

distal radioulnar joint. Effectively, the ulna does not participate as part of the radiocarpal joint other than as an attachment site for segments of the TFCC. As a whole, the compound proximal radiocarpal joint surface is oblique, angled slightly volarly and ulnarly. The angulation is due primarily to the articular margins of the radius, which extend farther on the dorsal and radial sides of the bone.

The scaphoid, lunate, and triquetrum compose the proximal carpal row. The proximal carpal row is the distal surface of the radiocarpal joint. These bones are connected by numerous interosseous ligaments that, like the carpals themselves, are covered with cartilage proximally.[19] The proximal carpal row and ligaments together appear to present a single biconvex joint surface that, unlike a rigid segment, can change shape somewhat to accommodate to the demands of space between the forearm and hand.[20] The pisiform, anatomically part of the proximal row, does not participate in the radiocarpal articulation. The pisiform functions entirely as a sesamoid bone, presumably to increase the moment arm (MA) of the flexor carpi ulnaris that attaches to it. The curvature of the distal radiocarpal joint surface is sharper than the proximal surface in both directions, making the joint somewhat incongruent. The concept of articular incongruence is supported by the finding that the overall contact between the proximal and distal radiocarpal surfaces is typically only about 20% of available surface, with never more than 40% of available surface in contact at any one time.[13] Joint incongruence and the angulation of the proximal joint surface result in a greater range of flexion than extension,[21] and in greater ulnar deviation than radial deviation for the radiocarpal joint.[19] The total range of flexion/extension is greater than the total range of radial/ulnar deviation. Incongruence and ligamentous laxity may account for as much as 45° of combined passive pronation/supination at the radiocarpal and midcarpal joints together,[6] although this motion is rarely considered to be an additional degree of freedom available to the wrist complex.

The radiocarpal joint is enclosed by a strong but somewhat loose capsule and is reinforced by capsular and intracapsular ligaments. Most ligaments that cross the radiocarpal joint also contribute to stability at the midcarpal joint, so all the ligaments will be presented together after introduction of the midcarpal joint. Similarly, the muscles of the radiocarpal joint also

function at the midcarpal joint. In fact, the radiocarpal joint is not crossed by any muscles that act on the radiocarpal joint alone. The flexor carpi ulnaris (FCU) is the only muscle that crosses the radiocarpal joint and attaches to any of the bones of the proximal carpal row. Although the FCU tendon ends on the pisiform, the pisiform is only loosely connected to the triquetrum below.[22] Consequently, forces applied to the pisiform by the FCU are translated not to the triquetrum on which it sits, but to the hamate and fifth metacarpal via pisiform ligaments. Motions occurring at the radiocarpal joint are a result of forces applied by the abundant passive ligamentous structures and by muscles that are attached to the distal carpal row and metacarpals. Consequently, movements of the radiocarpal and midcarpal joints must be examined together.

Midcarpal Joint Structure

The midcarpal joint is the articulation between the scaphoid, lunate, and triquetrum proximally and the distal carpal row composed of the trapezium, trapezoid, capitate, and hamate (see Fig. 9–1). The midcarpal joint is a functional rather than anatomic unit. It does not form a single uninterrupted articular surface, nor does it have its own capsule as does the radiocarpal joint. However, it is anatomically separate from the radiocarpal joint and has a capsule and synovial lining that is continuous with each intercarpal articulation and may be continuous with some of the carpometacarpal articulations[19] (Fig. 9–3). The midcarpal joint surfaces are complex with an overall reciprocally concave-convex configuration. The complexity of surfaces and ligamentous connections, however, simplify its movements. Functionally, the carpals of the distal row (with their attached metacarpals) move as an almost fixed unit. The capitate and hamate are most strongly bound together with, at most, a small amount of play between them.[23-25] The union of the distal carpals also results in nearly equal distribution of loads across the scaphoid-trapezium-trapezoid, the scaphoid-capitate, the lunate-capitate and the triquetrum-hamate articulations.[13,26] Together the bones of the distal carpal row contribute 2° of freedom to the wrist complex, with varying amounts of radial/ulnar deviation and flexion/extension credited to the joint. The excursions permitted by the articular surfaces of the midcarpal joint generally favor the range of

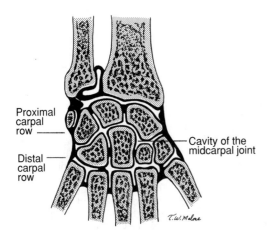

Proximal
carpal
row

Distal
carpal
row

Cavity of the
midcarpal joint

T.W.Malone

FIGURE 9–3. The midcarpal joint formed by the articulation of the bones of the proximal and distal carpal rows is anatomically separated from the radiocarpal joint by interosseous ligaments.

extension over flexion and radial deviation over ulnar deviation—the opposite of what was found for the radiocarpal joint.[19,21,27] The functional union of the distal carpals with each other and with their contiguous metacarpals not only serve the wrist complex, but also are the foundation for the transverse and longitudinal arches of the hand.[24]

Ligaments of the Wrist Complex

The tremendous individual differences that exist in the structure of the carpus can, perhaps, best be appreciated when one reviews the ligaments of the wrist. There are substantive differences in names, anatomic descriptions, and ascribed functions from investigator to investigator. We will identify those ligaments for which there is consensus as to their existence and criticality to function. Although there may not be universal agreement as to the structure and function of individual ligaments, there is consensus that the ligamentous structure of the carpus is responsible not only for articular stability, but also for guiding and checking motion between and among the carpals. When we examine the function of the wrist complex, we shall see that the variability of ligaments will, among other factors, translate into substantial and widely acknowledged differences among individuals on movement of the joints of the wrist complex.

The ligaments of the wrist complex are designated as either extrinsic or intrinsic ligaments.[28] The extrinsic ligaments are those that connect

the carpals to the radius or ulnar proximally or to the metacarpals distally; the intrinsic ligaments are those that interconnect the carpals themselves and are also known as intercarpal or interosseous ligaments. Nowalk and Logan[28] found the intrinsic ligaments to be stronger and less stiff than the extrinsic ligaments. They conclude that the intrinsic ligaments lie within the synovial lining and, therefore, must rely on synovial fluid for nutrition rather than contiguous vascularized tissues as do the extrinsic ligaments. The extrinsic ligaments, therefore, are more likely to fail but also have better potential for healing and help protect the slower to heal intrinsic ligaments by accepting forces first.[28]

VOLAR CARPAL LIGAMENTS

On the volar surface of the wrist complex, the numerous intrinsic and extrinsic ligaments are variously described by either composite or separate names, depending on the investigator. The composite ligament known as the **volar radiocarpal ligament** has been described most commonly as having three distinct bands: the **radioscaphoid, radiotriquetral,** and **radiocapitate**[9,19,29,30] (Fig. 9–4b). Nowalk and Logan[28] identified the radiocapitate as an extrinsic ligament, whereas Blevens and colleagues[30] identified it as part of their "palmar intracapsular radiocarpal ligaments." The composite **ulnocarpal** ligament arises from the TFCC and has been described as having bands attaching to the lunate (**ulnolunate**) and to the capitate either directly (**ulnocapitate**) or indirectly (via the **ulnotriquetral** and **capitotriquetral ligaments**)[31] (see Fig. 9–4b). Weak **radial** and **ulnar collateral ligaments** have also classically been described as part of the ligamentous complex.[19] More recently, however, it has been proposed that the ulnar collateral is really part of the ill-defined tissues of the TFCC,[16,18] whereas the radial collateral may be considered an extension of the volar radiocarpal ligament and capsule.[16]

Two volar intrinsic ligaments have received particular attention and acknowledgment of their importance to wrist function. The first of these, the **scapholunate interosseous ligament,** is generally, though not universally,[32] credited with being a key factor in maintaining scaphoid stability and, therefore, stability of much of the wrist.[30,33,34] Injury to this ligament, as we shall see when we discuss wrist pathology, appears to contribute largely to scaphoid instability and, therefore, to one of the most common

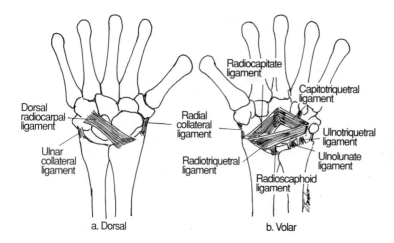

FIGURE 9–4. (a) Dorsal ligaments of the wrist complex. (b) Volar ligaments of the wrist complex, including the volar radiocarpal ligament (radiocapitate, radiotriquetral, and radioscaphoid) and the ulnocarpal ligament (ulnolunate, ulnotriquetral, and capitotriquetral).

wrist problems. As an intrinsic ligament, however, the scapholunate interosseous is largely avascular and, therefore, more susceptible to degenerative change and less amenable to surgical repair.[35] The second key intrinsic ligament is the **lunotriquetral interosseous ligament.** This ligament is credited with maintaining stability between the lunate and triquetrum. Injury to this ligament appears to be largely responsible for lunate instability, another problematic wrist pathology.

DORSAL CARPAL LIGAMENTS

Dorsally, the major wrist ligament is the **dorsal radiocarpal ligament** (Fig. 9–4a). This ligament, as is true of the volar radiocarpal, varies somewhat in description but is obliquely oriented. Essentially, the ligament as a whole converges on the triquetrum from the distal radius, with possible attachments along the way to the lunate and lunotriquetral interosseous ligament.[31,36] Garcia-Elias and colleagues suggest that the obliquity of the volar and dorsal radiocarpal ligaments help offset the sliding of the proximal "carpal condyle" on the inclined radius.[37] A second dorsal ligament is the **dorsal intercarpal ligament** that courses horizontally from the triquetrum to the lunate, scaphoid, and trapezium.[16,36] The two dorsal ligaments together form a horizontal V that contributes to radiocarpal stability.[36]

Function of the Wrist Complex

Movements of the Radiocarpal and Midcarpal Joints

Motions at the radiocarpal and midcarpal joints are caused by a rather unique combination of active muscular and passive ligamentous and joint reaction forces. Although there are abundant passive forces on the proximal carpal row, no muscular forces are applied directly to the articular bones of the proximal row, given that the flexor carpi ulnaris applies its force via the pisiform to the more distal bones. The proximal carpals, therefore, are effectively a mechanical link between the radius and the distal carpals and metacarpals to which the muscular forces are actually applied. Gilford and associates[11] suggested that the proximal carpal row is an **intercalated segment,** a relatively unattached middle segment of a three-segment linkage. When compressive forces are applied across an intercalated segment, the middle segment tends to collapse and move in the opposite direction from the segments above and below. For example, application of compressive muscular extensor forces across the biarticular wrist complex would cause an unstable proximal carpal row to collapse into flexion while the distal carpal row extended. An intercalated segment requires some type of stabilizing mechanism to normalize combined midcarpal/radiocarpal motion and prevent collapse of the middle segment (the proximal carpal row). The stabilization mechanism appears to involve the scaphoid and its functional and anatomic connections both to the adjacent lunate and to the distal carpal row. Garcia-Elias and colleagues[37] support the hypothesis that the stability of the proximal carpal row depends on the interaction of two opposite tendencies when the carpals are axially loaded (compression across a neutral wrist); the scaphoid tends to flex while the lunate and triquetrum tend to extend. These counterrotations within the proximal row are prevented by the ligamentous structure (including the key scapholunate interosseous and lunotriquetral interosseous ligaments). Linking the scaphoid to the lunate and triquetrum, according to Garcia-Elias and colleagues,[37] will cause the proximal carpals to "collapse synchronously" into flexion and pronation, while the distal carpals move into extension and supination. They proposed that the counterrotation between rows and the resulting ligamentous tension increases coaptation of midcarpal articular surfaces and adds to stability.

Although the proposed carpal stability mechanism of Garcia-Elias and colleagues appears to hold as a conceptual framework, findings of other investigators differ in detail if not in substance. Recent advances in technology, including computer modeling, suggest that intercarpal motion is far more complex and individualistic than was once thought. There is general agreement that the three bones of the proximal carpal row do not move as a unit, but that motions of the three carpals vary both in magnitude and in direction with axial loading, with radiocarpal flexion/extension, and with radial/ulnar deviation.[5,37–39] In fact, Short and colleagues[34] found that carpal motions differed not only with individual osteoligamentous configuration and position, but with direction of motion; that is, relations in the carpus differed when the wrist reached neutral position depending on whether the position was reached from full flexion, full extension, or deviation.

FLEXION/EXTENSION OF THE WRIST

During flexion/extension, the scaphoid seems to show the greatest motion of the three proximal carpals while the lunate moves least.[5,25] Some investigators found that flexion and extension of the radiocarpal joint occurs almost exclusively as flexion and extension, respectively, of the proximal carpal row,[34,40] whereas others found simultaneous but lesser amounts of radial/ulnar deviation and pronation/supination of two or all three proximal carpal bones during radiocarpal flexion/extension.[5,19] Motion of the more tightly bound distal carpals and their attached metacarpals during midcarpal flexion/extension appears to be a fairly simple corresponding flexion and extension, with movement of the distal segments proportional to movement of the hand.[38]

Given the apparent variability of findings, a conceptual framework for flexion/extension of the wrist is in order. The following sequence of events proposed by Conwell[31,41] gives an explanation of the relative motions of the various segments and of their interdependence. It can easily be appreciated, however, that the conceptual framework is oversimplified and ignores some of the simultaneous interactions that occur among the key carpal bones. The motion begins with the wrist in full flexion. Active extension is initiated at the distal carpal row and the attached metacarpals by the wrist extensor muscles attached to those bones. The distal carpals (capitate, hamate, trapezium, and trapezoid) glide on the relatively fixed proximal bones (scaphoid, lunate, and triquetrum). Although the surface configurations of the midcarpal joint are complex, the distal carpal row effectively glides in the same direction as motion of the hand. When the wrist complex reaches neutral (long axis of the third metacarpal in line with the long axis of the forearm), the ligaments spanning the capitate and scaphoid draw the capitate and scaphoid together into a close-packed position. Continued extensor force now moves the combined unit of the distal carpal row and the scaphoid on the relatively fixed lunate and triquetrum. At approximately 45° of hyperextension of the wrist complex, the scapholunate interosseous ligament brings the scaphoid and lunate into close-packed position. This unites all the carpals and causes them to function as a single unit. Wrist complex extension is completed as the proximal articular surface of the carpals move as a solid unit on the radius and radioulnar disk. All ligaments become taut as full extension is reached and the entire wrist complex is close-packed.

Wrist motion from full extension to full flexion occurs in the reverse sequence. In this conceptual framework, the scaphoid (through mediation of the wrist ligaments) participates at different times in scaphoid-capitate, scaphoid-lunate, or radioscaphoid motion (Fig. 9–5). Crumpling of the proximal carpal row (intercalated segment) is prevented and full ROM is achieved. Interestingly, computer modeling and cadaver study of radiocarpal intra-articular contact patterns showed that radiocarpal extension is accompanied by increased contact dorsally. One would expect extension of the hand to be accompanied by sliding of the convex proximal carpal surface volarly in a direction opposite to hand motion. If this contact

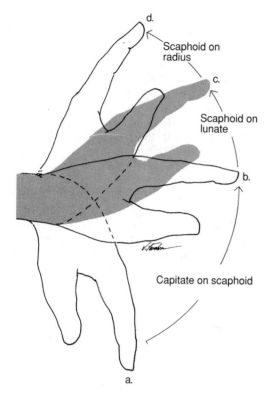

d.

Scaphoid on
radius

c.

Scaphoid on
lunate

b.

Capitate on scaphoid

a.

FIGURE 9–5. Wrist complex extension. From a to b movement occurs entirely at the midcarpal joint. From b to c the scaphoid locks onto the distal carpal row to move on the stable lunate and triquetrum. From c to d all the carpals lock and motion occurs entirely at the radiocarpal joint.

pattern exists in vivo, it likely reflects the complexity of radiocarpal motion and may contradict assumptions about movement between convex and concave surfaces.

RADIAL/ULNAR DEVIATION OF THE WRIST

Radial and ulnar deviation of the wrist seems to be an even more complex, but perhaps less varied, motion than flexion/extension. Radial deviation produces not only deviation of the proximal and distal carpals radially, but simultaneous flexion of the proximal carpals and extension of the distal carpals (with accompanying pronation/supination components varying among investigators).[5,12,20,40,44] The opposite motions of the proximal and distal carpals occur with ulnar deviation. During radial/ulnar deviation the distal carpals, once again, move as a relatively fixed unit, although the magnitude of motion between the bones of the proximal carpal row may differ.[5,25] Garcia-Elias and colleagues[7] found that the magnitude of scaphoid flexion during radial deviation (and

extension during ulnar deviation) related to ligamentous laxity. Volunteer subjects with ligamentous laxity showed more scaphoid flexion/extension and less radial/ulnar deviation than others. Ligamentous laxity was more common among women than men. The investigators proposed that ligamentous laxity led to less binding of the scaphoid to the distal carpal row and, therefore, more out-of-plane motion for the scaphoid.

In full radial deviation, both the radiocarpal and midcarpal joints are in close-packed position.[27,43,45,46] The ranges of wrist complex radial and ulnar deviation are greatest when the wrist is in neutral flexion/extension. When the wrist is extended and is in close-packed position, the carpals are all locked and very little radial or ulnar deviation is possible. In wrist flexion the joints are loose-packed and the bones splayed. Further movement of the proximal row cannot occur and, as in extreme extension, little radial or ulnar deviation is possible in the fully flexed position.[47]

What appears to be a redundancy in function at the midcarpal and radiocarpal joints ensures maintenance of the minimum ROM required for activities of daily living. Brumfield and Champoux[48] found that a series of hand activities necessary for independence required a functional wrist motion of 10° of flexion and 35° of extension. Ryu and colleagues[10] included a wide range of hand functions in their test battery and determined that all could be completed with minimum wrist motions of 60° extension, 54° flexion, 40° ulnar deviation, and 17° radial deviation. There is consensus that wrist extension and ulnar deviation are most important for wrist activities. Wrist extension and ulnar deviation was also found to be the position of maximum scapholunate contact.[13] Given the key role of the scaphoid in stability of the carpus, this would imply maximum stability in the wrist position where maximum hand grip occurs.

Muscles of the Wrist Complex

The primary role of the muscles of the wrist complex is to provide a stable base for the hand, while permitting positional adjustments that allow for optimal length-tension in the long finger muscles. Hazelton and associates[2] investigated the peak force that could be exerted at the interphalangeal (IP) joints of the fingers during different wrist positions. The study found the greatest IP flexor force occurs with ulnar deviation of the wrist (neutral flexion/extension), whereas the least force occurred with wrist flexion (neutral deviation). The muscles of the wrist, however, are not structured merely to optimize the force of finger flexion. If optimizing finger flexor force outweighed other concerns, one might expect the wrist extensors to be stronger than the wrist flexors. Rather, the work capacity (ability of a muscle to generate force per unit of cross-section) of the wrist flexors is more than twice that of the extensors. Again contrary to expectation in optimizing finger flexor force, the work capacity of the radial deviators slightly exceeds that of the ulnar deviators.[49] The function of the wrist muscles cannot be understood by looking at any one factor or function, but should be assessed by electromyography (EMG) in various patterns of use against the resistance of gravity and external loads. Although an introduction to muscles of the wrist is in order, discussion of the synergies between hand and wrist musculature must be discussed in the context of hand function.

VOLAR WRIST MUSCULATURE

Six muscles have tendons crossing the volar aspect of the wrist and, therefore, are capable of creating a wrist flexion movement. These are the **palmaris longus (PL)**, the **flexor carpi radialis (FCR)**, the **flexor carpi ulnaris (FCU)**, the **flexor digitorum superficialis (FDS)**, the **flexor digitorum profundus (FDP)**, and the **flexor pollicis longus (FPL)**. The first three of these muscles are primary wrist muscles. The last three are flexors of the digits with secondary actions at the wrist. All pass under the proximal flexor retinaculum of the wrist, except the PL and FCU.

The positions of the FCR and FCU tendons at the wrist indicate that the tendons can, respectively, radially deviate and ulnarly deviate the wrist as well as flex. However, the FCR does not appear to be effective as a radial deviator of the wrist in an isolated contraction. Its distal attachment on the bases of the second and third metacarpals places it in line with the long axis of the hand. Along with the PL, the FCR functions as a wrist flexor with little concomitant deviation.[9] The FCR is active during radial deviation, however. The FCR either augments the strong radial deviating force of the extensor carpi radialis longus or offsets the extension also produced by the extensor carpi radialis

longus. The PL is a wrist flexor without producing either radial or ulnar deviation. The muscle and tendon are absent unilaterally or bilaterally in approximately 14% of people without any apparent strength or functional deficit.[50] Given its apparent redundancy with other muscles, the PL tendon (when present) is commonly used for surgical reconstruction of other structures.

The FCU attaches to the pisiform, a sesamoid bone that increases the FCU MA for flexion. Through the pisiform's ligaments,[22] the FCU acts on the hamate and fifth metacarpal, effectively producing flexion and ulnar deviation of the wrist complex. The FCU tendon crosses the wrist farther from the axis for wrist radial/ulnar deviation than does the FCR, so it is more effective in its ulnar deviation function than the FCR is in its radial deviation function.

The FDS, FDP, and the FPL are predominantly flexors of the digits. As multijoint muscles, their capacity to produce an effective wrist flexion force depends on a synergistic stabilizer to prevent full excursion of the more distal joints they cross. If these muscles attempt to act over both the wrist and the more distal joints, they will become actively insufficient. The FDS and FDP show varied activity in wrist radial/ulnar deviation as one might anticipate from the central location of the tendons. The FDS seems to function more consistently as a wrist flexor than does the profundus.[51] This is logical considering the FDP is a longer, deeper muscle, crosses more joints and is, therefore, more likely to become actively insufficient. The effect of the FPL on the wrist has received relatively little attention. The position of the tendon suggests the ability to contribute to both flexion and radial deviation of the wrist if its more distal joints are stabilized.

DORSAL WRIST MUSCULATURE

The dorsum of the wrist complex is crossed by the tendons of nine muscles. Three of the nine muscles are primary wrist muscles; the **extensor carpi radialis longus and brevis (ECRL, ECRB)** and the **extensor carpi ulnaris (ECU)**. The other six are finger and thumb muscles that may act secondarily on the wrist; these are the **extensor digitorum communis (EDC)**, the **extensor indicis proprius (EIP)**, the **extensor digiti minimi (EDM)**, the **extensor pollicis longus (EPL)**, the **extensor pollicis brevis (EPB)**, and the **abductor pollicis longus (APL)**. The EDC and the EIP are also known, more simply, as the extensor digitorum and the extensor indicis, respectively. The tendons of all nine muscles pass under the extensor retinaculum that is divided into six distinct tunnels by septa. The septa help stabilize the tendons on the dorsum of the hand and allow the muscles to be effective stabilizers of the wrist.[16]

The ECRL and ECRB together make up the predominant part of the wrist extensor mass.[52] The ECRB is somewhat smaller than the ECRL, but has a more central location and generally shows more activity during wrist extension activities.[9,53] One study found the ECRB to be active during all grasp-and-release hand activities, except those performed in supination.[54] The ECRL has a smaller moment arm for wrist flexion than does the ECRB.[4] The ECRL shows increased activity when either radial deviation or support against ulnar deviation is required, or when forceful finger flexion motions are performed.[42,53] The ongoing activity of the ECRB makes it vulnerable to overuse and is more likely than the quieter ECRL to be inflamed in lateral epicondylitis.

The ECU extends and ulnarly deviates the wrist. It is active not only in wrist extension, but frequently in wrist flexion as well.[53] Backdahl and Carlsoo[51] hypothesized that the ECU activity in wrist flexion adds an additional component of stability to the structurally less stable position of wrist flexion. This is not needed on the radial side of the wrist that has more developed ligamentous and skeletal control. The connection of the ECU tendon sheath to the TFCC also appears to help tether the ECU and prevent loss of excursion efficiency with bowstringing. Tang and colleagues[55] found a 30% increase in excursion of the ECU after release of the TFCC from the distal ulna. The effectiveness of the ECU as a wrist extensor is also affected by forearm position. When the forearm is pronated, the crossing of the radius over the ulna causes a reduction in the MA of the ECU, making it less effective as a wrist extensor.[52,54]

The EDM and the EIP insert into the tendons of the EDC and, therefore, have a common function with the EDC.[56] The EIP and EDM are capable of extending the wrist, but wrist extension is credited more to the EDC. The EDC is a finger extensor muscle but functions also as a wrist extensor (without radial or ulnar deviation). There appears to be some reciprocal synergy of the EDC with the ECRB in providing wrist extension because less ECRB activity is seen when the EDC is active.[53]

The three extrinsic thumb muscles cross the wrist. The APL and the EPB are both capable of radially deviating the wrist and may serve a minor role in that function. However, radial deviation of the wrist may detract from their prime action on the thumb. A synergistic contraction of the ECU may be required to offset the unwanted wrist motion when the APL and EPB act on the thumb. When muscles producing ulnar deviators are absent, the thumb extrinsics may produce a significant radial deviation deformity at the wrist. Little evidence has been found to indicate that the more centrally located EPL has any notable effect on the wrist.

Wrist Joint Pathology

The wrist accounts for 6% of all fractures and dislocations in the body, with the bones of the proximal row the most common site of debilitating injury.[28] The scaphoid is the most frequently fractured of the carpal bones. Maximum strain of the scaphoid was found at neutral radial/ulnar deviation and wrist extension,[57] the position of a fall on the outstretched hand. The scaphoid is also involved in the most common carpal instability problem known as **scapholunate instability** or **radial perilunate instability.** When injury to one or more ligaments attached to the scaphoid unlinks the lunate from the stabilizing influence of the scaphoid, the lunate (and the attached triquetrum) are left to act as an unconstrained intercalated segment. When ligamentous constraint on the scaphoid is reduced or removed, the scaphoid tends to follow its natural tendency to collapse into flexion on the volarly inclined radius (potentially including some out-of-plane motion as well). The flexed scaphoid slides dorsally on the radius and subluxes. Released from scaphoid stabilization, the lunate and triquetrum follow their natural tendency to extend, and the muscular forces applied to the distal carpals cause them to flex on the extended lunate and triquetrum (Fig. 9–6a). The flexed distal carpals glide dorsally on the lunate and triquetrum, accentuating the extension of the lunate and triquetrum. This zigzag pattern of the three segments (the scaphoid, the lunate and triquetrum, and the distal carpal row) is known as **dorsal intercalated segmental instability,** more commonly referred to as **DISI.**[12,20] The scaphoid subluxation may be dynamic, occurring only with compressive loading of the wrist with muscle

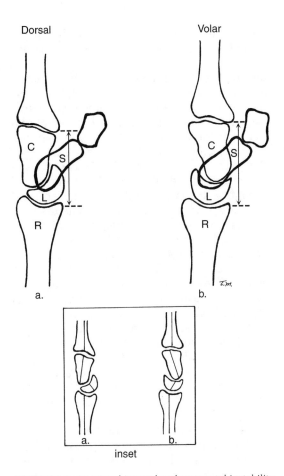

Dorsal   Volar

a.   b.

inset

a.   b.

FIGURE 9–6. (a) Dorsal intercalated segmental instability (DISI). The lunate, released from the flexed scaphoid, extends on the radius. The capitate moves in the opposite direction (flexion) on top of the lunate. (b) Volar intercalated segmental instability (VISI). The lunate and scaphoid flex on the radius while the trapezium (not shown) extends. The capitate follows the trapezium into extension.

forces, or may become fixed or static. With subluxation of the scaphoid, the contact pressures at the radioscaphoid articulation increase because the contact occurs over a smaller area.[13,30] DISI, therefore, may result over time in degenerative changes at the radioscaphoid joint and then, ultimately, at the other intercarpal joints.[29] With sufficient ligamentous laxity, the capitate may sublux dorsally off the extended lunate and migrate into the gap between the flexed scaphoid and extended lunate. At this point, the deformity has been termed **scapholunate advanced collapse** or **SLAC.**[30] Although it is arguable whether the load on the radiolunate joint increases or decreases with DISI,[13,21,34] there is agreement that the radiolunate articulation is less likely to

show degenerative changes than the radioscaphoid. This has been attributed to a more spherical configuration of the radiolunate facets that better center applied loads across the articular surfaces.[30]

The other common form of carpal instability occurs when the ligamentous union of the lunate and triquetrum is disrupted through injury.[20] The lunate and triquetrum together normally tend to move toward extension and offset the tendency of the scaphoid to flex. When the lunate is no longer linked with the triquetrum, the lunate and scaphoid together fall into flexion, and the triquetrum and distal carpal row extend (Fig. 9–6b). This **ulnar perilunate instability** is known as **volar intercalated segmental instability** or **VISI.** VISI and DISI illustrate the importance of proximal carpal row stabilization to wrist function and of maintenance of the scaphoid as the bridge between the distal carpal row and the two other bones of the proximal carpal row.

Now that we have examined the wrist complex, let's look at the hand complex that the wrist serves.

The Hand Complex

The hand consists of five digits, or four fingers and a thumb. Each digit has a **carpometacarpal (CMC)** joint and a **metacarpophalangeal (MCP)** joint. The fingers each have two **interphalangeal (IP)** joints, and the thumb has only one. There are 19 bones and 19 joints distal to the carpals that make up the hand complex. Although the joints of the fingers and the joints of the thumb have structural similarities, function differs significantly enough that the joints of the fingers shall be examined separately from those of the thumb. In examining the joints of the fingers, however, one should be cautious about generalizations that we will make. Ranney[58] pointed out that each digit of the hand is unique and that models proposed for, and conclusions drawn, about one finger may not be accurate for all.

Structure of the Fingers

CMC Joints of the Fingers

The CMC joints of the fingers are composed of the articulations between the distal carpal row and the bases of the second through fifth metacarpals (Fig. 9–7). The distal carpal row, of course, also is part of the midcarpal joint. One

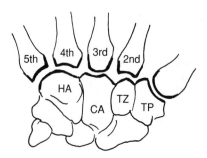

FIGURE 9–7. Carpometacarpal joints of the fingers. The articulations between the second through fifth metacarpals and distal carpal row (TP, trapezium; TZ, trapezoid; CA, capitate; HA, hamate).

attribute of the distal carpals that affects CMC and hand function but not wrist function is the volar concavity, or **carpal arch,** formed by the trapezoid, trapezium, capitate, and hamate. The concavity of the palm of the hand persists even when the hand is fully opened. The carpal arch is created not only by the curved shape of the carpals but also by the ligaments that maintain the concavity (Fig. 9–8). The ligaments that maintain the arch are the **transverse carpal ligament** (TCL) and the transversely oriented intercarpal ligaments. The TCL is the portion of the **flexor retinaculum** that attaches to the pisiform and hook of the hamate medially, and the scaphoid and trapezium laterally; the more proximal portion of the flexor retinaculum is continuous with the fascia overlying the forearm muscles. The TCL and intercarpal ligaments that link the four distal carpals maintain the relatively fixed concavity that will contribute to the arches of the

palm. These structures also form the **carpal tunnel.** The carpal tunnel contains the median nerve, the extrinsic finger and thumb flexors, and the flexor carpi radialis tendon (held in a separate compartment medially). When the median nerve becomes compressed within the tunnel, a neuropathy known as **carpal tunnel syndrome** may develop. Cobb and colleagues[59] propose that the proximal edge of the TCL is the most common site for wrist flexion-induced median nerve compression. The tunnel is narrowest, however, at the level of the hook of the hamate where median nerve compression is unlikely to be affected by changes in wrist position.[59] When the TCL is cut to release median nerve compression, the carpal arch may widen somewhat, but was found to maintain its dorso-volar stiffness as long as the stronger transverse intercarpal ligaments were intact.[60] A number of intrinsic hand muscles attach to the TCL and bones of the distal carpal row. These may also contribute to maintaining the carpal arch.

The proximal portion of the four metacarpals of the fingers articulate with the distal carpals to form the second through fifth CMC joints. The second metacarpal articulates primarily with the trapezoid and secondarily with the trapezium and capitate. The third metacarpal articulates primarily with the capitate, and the fourth metacarpal articulates with the capitate and hamate. Lastly, the fifth metacarpal articulates with the hamate. Each of the metacarpals also articulates at its base with the contiguous metacarpal or metacarpals, with the exception of the second metacarpal that articulates at its base with the third but not the first metacarpal. All finger CMCs are supported by strong transverse and weaker longitudinal ligaments volarly and dorsally. The **deep transverse metacarpal ligament** spans the heads of the second through fourth metacarpals volarly. The deep transverse metacarpal ligament tethers together the metacarpal heads and effectively prevents the attached metacarpals from any more than minimal abduction at the CMC joints. Although the transverse metacarpal ligament contributes directly to CMC stability, it also is structurally part of the MCP joints of the fingers and will be discussed again in that context. The ligamentous structure is primarily responsible for controlling the total ROM available at each CMC joint, although some differences in articulations also exist.

The range of CMC motion of the fingers is observable at the metacarpal heads and in-

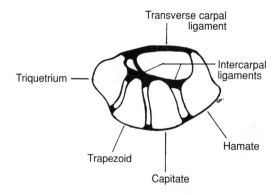

FIGURE 9–8. The transverse (fixed) carpal arch with the transverse carpal ligament and intercarpal ligaments that assist in maintaining the concavity.

creases from the radial to the ulnar side of the hand. The second through fourth CMC joints are plane synovial joints with 1° of freedom: flexion/extension. Although structured to permit flexion/extension, the second and third CMCs are essentially immobile and may be considered to have "zero degrees of freedom."[27,58] The fourth CMC joint has perceptible flexion/extension, whereas the fifth CMC joint is a saddle joint with 2° of freedom, including flexion/extension, some abduction/adduction, and a limited amount of opposability.[9,58,61] The immobile second and third metacarpals provide a fixed and stable axis about which the very mobile first metacarpal (thumb) and the fourth and fifth metacarpals can move.[23,58,62] The motion of the fourth and fifth metacarpals facilitates the ability of the ring and little fingers to oppose the thumb. The adjustable positions of the first, fourth, and fifth metacarpal heads around the fixed second and third form a **mobile transverse arch** at the level of the metacarpal heads that augments the fixed arch of the distal carpal row. The deep transverse metacarpal ligament contributes to stability of the mobile arch during grip functions.[63] The function of the finger CMC joints and their segments overall is to contribute (with the thumb) to the **palmar arches.** The palmar arches allow the palm and the digits to conform optimally to the shape of the object being held. This maximizes the amount of surface contact, enhancing stability as well as increasing sensory feedback. Including the fingers and the thumb, the palmar arches can easily be visualized as occurring transversely across the palm and longitudinally down the palm (Fig. 9–9).

Muscles that cross the CMC joints will contribute to palmar cupping by acting on the mobile segments of the palmar arches. Hollowing of the palm accompanies finger flexion, and relative flattening of the palm accompanies finger extension. The fifth CMC is crossed and acted on by the **opponens digiti minimi (ODM)**. This oblique muscle is attached proximally to the hamate and TCL and distally to the ulnar side of the fifth metacarpal. It is optimally positioned, therefore, to flex and rotate the fifth metacarpal about its long axis. No other muscles cross or act on the finger CMC joints alone. However, increased arching occurs with activity of the FCU and with intrinsic hand muscles that insert on the TCL.[8,64] The radial wrist muscles (FCR, ECRL, and ECRB) cross the second and third CMC joints to insert on the bases

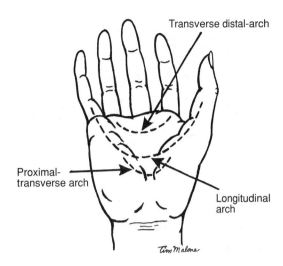

FIGURE 9–9. The palmar arches that assist with grasp. The proximal transverse arch is fixed while the distal transverse and longitudinal arches are mobile.

of those metacarpals, but produce little or no motion at these fixed articulations. The stability of the second and third CMCs can be viewed as a functional adaptation that enhances the efficiency of the FCR, ECRL, and ECRB. If the second and third CMC joints were mobile, the radial flexor and extensors would act first on the CMC joints and, consequently, would be less effective at the midcarpal and radiocarpal joints given the loss in length-tension.

MCP Joints of the Fingers

Each of the four MCP joints of the fingers is composed of the convex metacarpal head proximally and the concave base of the first phalanx distally (Fig. 9–10). The MCP joint is condyloid with 2° of freedom: flexion/extension and abduction/adduction. The large metacarpal head has 180° of articular surface in the sagittal plane, with the predominant portion lying volarly. This is apposed to approximately 20° of articular surface on the phalanx. In the frontal plane the articular surfaces are more congruent. The joint is surrounded by a capsule that is generally considered to be lax in extension and, in conjunction with the poorly mated surfaces, allows some passive axial rotation of the proximal phalanx in that position.[58] The presence of a volar and two collateral ligaments contributes to joint stability, but the joint must still be considered incongruent given the differential in its articular surfaces. When joints are this incongruent, it is common to find an accessory joint structure to

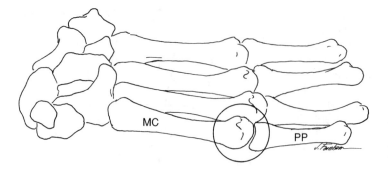

FIGURE 9–10. Metacarpophalangeal joints of the fingers. A view of the volar surface of the hand shows the articulation between the large head of the metacarpal (MC) and the smaller base of the proximal phalanx (PP).

enhance stability. At the MCP joint, this function is served by the volar plate.

THE VOLAR PLATE

The **volar plate** (volar ligament) at the MCP joint is a unique structure that increases joint congruence. The volar plate is composed of fibrocartilage and is firmly (but not rigidly) attached to the base of the proximal phalanx. The plate becomes membranous proximally to blend with the capsule. Through its capsular connection, the plate attaches to the metacarpal head just proximal to the articular surface (Fig. 9–11a). The volar plate can also be visualized as a fibrocartilage impregnation of the volar portion of the capsule that overlies the metacarpal head. The four volar plates of the MCP joints of the fingers also blend with and are interconnected superficially by the deep transverse metacarpal ligament that, as we saw earlier, tethers together the heads of the metacarpals of the four fingers. The volar plate at each finger MCP joint is part of a multilayered structure. From deep to superficial, we have (1) the volar plate that is in contact with the metacarpal head; (2) the MCP joint capsule that blends with the volar aspect of the plate; (3) the superficial longitudinal fibers of the capsule that are reinforced superficially (volarly) by the perpendicular fibers of the deep transverse ligament; and (4) the deep transverse metacarpal ligament that has grooves on its volar surface for the long flexor tendons of the fingers. The deep transverse metacarpal ligament also has fibers on its dorsal surface at each MCP joint that pass to the dorsal expansion of the extensor tendons (Fig. 9–12). The connections of each volar plate to the collateral ligaments of the MCP joint (via the capsule) and the extensor expansion (via the deep transverse metacarpal ligament) help stabilize the volar plates on the four metacarpal heads.[19,58,63] The inner surface of the volar plate is effectively a continuation of the articular surface of the base of the proximal phalanx. In extension, the plate adds to the amount of surface in contact with the large metacarpal head. Its fibrocartilage composition is consistent with its ability both to resist tensile stresses in restrict-

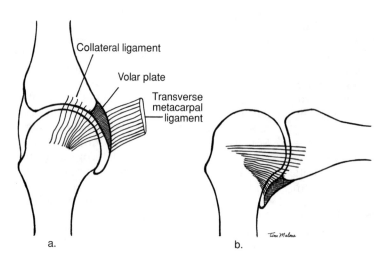

a.   b.

FIGURE 9–11. (a) The volar plate at the MCP joint attaches to the base of the proximal phalanx and to the joint capsule beneath the metacarpal head. It blends with the capsule and the deep transverse metacarpal ligament volarly (not shown: the A1 annular pulley that lies superficial to the transverse metacarpal ligament). (b) In MCP joint flexion, the flexible attachments of the plate allow it to slide proximally on the metacarpal head without impeding motion.

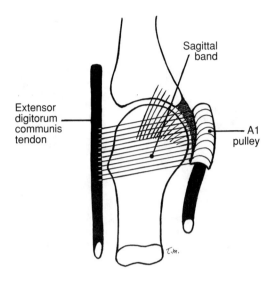

FIGURE 9–12. The connections of the sagittal bands to each side of the volar plate, the collateral ligaments of the MCP joint (via the capsule), and the extensor expansion help stabilize the EDC tendons over the MCP joint dorsally and the volar plates on the four metacarpal heads volarly.

ing MCP hyperextension and compressive forces needed to protect the volar articular surface of the metacarpal head from objects held in the palm.[65] The flexible attachment of the plate to the phalanx permits the plate to glide proximally down the volar surface of the metacarpal head in flexion without restricting motion, while also preventing pinching of the long flexor tendons in the MCP joint (Fig. 9–11b).

THE COLLATERAL LIGAMENTS

The collateral ligaments of the MCP joint are generally considered to be slack in extension, permitting a full range of abduction/adduction. Tension in the collateral ligaments at full MCP flexion (the close-packed position for the MCP joint) is considered to account for the minimal amount of abduction/adduction that can be obtained at the MCP joint in full flexion. Shultz and associates[66] concluded that the collateral ligaments provided stability throughout the MCP ROM with parts of the fibers taut at various points in the range. They proposed that the bicondylar shape of the volar surface of the metacarpal head provided a bony block to abduction/adduction at about 70° of MCP flexion, rather than collateral ligamentous tension.

Fisher and associates[67] did a series of dissections of fingers seeking an explanation for the relatively small incidence of osteoarthritis in MCP joints as compared to the fairly common changes seen in the distal interphalangeal (DIP) joints and, to a lesser extent, in the proximal interphalangeal (PIP) joints. They found fibrocartilage that projected into the MCP, PIP, and DIP joints from the inner surface of the extensor hood, from the volar plates, and from the collateral ligaments. The fibrocartilage projections were most impressive in the MCP joints and may, like the volar plate itself, increase the surface area on the small base of the phalange for contact with the large metacarpal (and phalangeal) heads.

RANGE OF MOTION

The total ROM available at the MCP joint varies with each finger. Flexion/extension increases radially to ulnarly, with the index finger having approximately 90° of MCP flexion and the little finger approximately 110°. Hyperextension is fairly consistent between fingers but varies widely among individuals. The range of passive hyperextension has been used as a measure of generalized body flexibility.[68] The range of abduction/adduction is maximal in MCP extension; the index and little finger have more frontal plane mobility than the middle and ring fingers. As previously mentioned, abduction/adduction is most restricted in MCP flexion.

IP Joints of the Fingers

Each of the **proximal interphalangeal (PIP)** and **distal interphalangeal (DIP)** joints of the fingers are composed of the head of a phalanx and the base of the phalanx distal to it. Each IP joint is a true synovial hinge joint with 1° of freedom (flexion/extension), a joint capsule, a volar plate, and two collateral ligaments (Fig. 9–13).

The base of each middle and distal phalanx has two shallow concave facets with a central ridge. The distal phalanx sits on the pulley-shaped head of the phalanx proximal to it. The joint structure is similar to that of the MCP joint in that the proximal articular surface is larger than the distal articular surface. Unlike

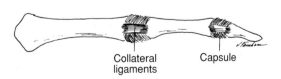

Collateral ligaments   Capsule

FIGURE 9–13. Capsule and collateral ligaments of the proximal and distal interphalangeal joints.

the MCP joints, there is little posterior articular surface at the PIP or DIP and, therefore, little hyperextension. The DIP joint may have some passive hyperextension, but the proximal joint has essentially none. Volar plates reinforce each of the joint capsules and enhance stability. The plates at the IP joints are structurally and functionally identical to those at the MCP joint, except that the plates are not connected by a deep transverse ligament. Fisher and associates[67] found fibrocartilage projections from the extensor mechanism, the volar plate, and the collateral ligaments attached to the bases of the phalanges at both the PIPs and the DIPs, with the structures more obvious at the PIPs. The collateral ligaments of the IP joints are not fully understood but some portions remain taut and provide support throughout PIP and DIP motion.[69,70] Injuries to the collateral ligaments of the PIP joint are common, particularly in sports and workplace injuries, with the radial or lateral collateral twice as likely to be injured than the ulnar or medial collateral.[71] Dzwierzynski and colleagues[71] found the lateral collateral of the index finger to be the strongest of the PIP collaterals, whereas the fifth PIP joint had the weakest. When one considers that the thumb is most likely to oppose the lateral side of the index (creating a varus stress at the PIP joint) and least likely to do so at the fifth, the relative strengths of the lateral collateral ligaments meet functional expectations.

The total range of flexion/extension available to the index finger is greater at the PIP joint (100° to 110°) than it is at the DIP joint (80°). The ranges for PIP and DIP flexion at each finger increase ulnarly, with the fifth PIP and DIP joints achieving 135° and 90°, respectively. The increasing flexion/extension ROM from the radial to the ulnar side of the hand is consistent at the CMC, MCP, and PIP joints and, to a less significant degree at the DIP joints. The pattern that results from simultaneous flexion at all joints is shown in Figure 9–14a. The additional range allocated to the more ulnarly located fingers angles them toward the scaphoid and facilitates opposition of the fingers with the thumb. The greater available range ulnarly also produces a grip that is tighter, or has greater closure, on the ulnar side of the hand. Many objects are constructed so that the shape is narrower at the ring and little fingers and widens toward the long and index fingers to fit the ROM pattern (Fig. 9–14b).

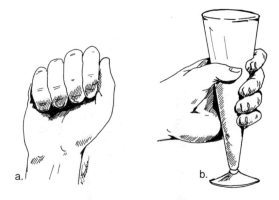

FIGURE 9–14. (a) Pattern of increasing flexion from the radial to the ulnar side of the hand. (b) The ring and little fingers have more flexion ROM so can accommodate a narrower shape for more contact.

Finger Musculature

Extrinsic Finger Flexors

There are two muscles originating outside the hand that contribute to finger flexion. These are the **flexor digitorum superficialis (FDS)** and the **flexor digitorum profundus (FDP)**. The FDS can flex the MCP joint and the PIP joint. The profundus can flex the MCP, PIP, and the DIP joints and is considered to be the more active of the two muscles. With gentle pinch or grasp, the FDP alone will be active. However, when hand closure is attempted by a person with long-standing paralysis of the intrinsic hand musculature, the DIP and PIP joints flex well before the MCP joint. The result is that the fingertips catch at or just below the metacarpal heads.[72] Grasp is ineffective because the fingers are already flexed as an object approaches the palm. Although the intrinsic finger muscles (lumbricals and interossei) are not active in gently closing the hand, their passive viscoelastic constraints at the MCP and IP joints must be necessary for normal function.

The FDS functions alone in finger flexion only when flexion of the DIP joint is not required. When simultaneous PIP and DIP flexion are called for, the FDS acts as a reserve muscle. It joins the FDP by increasing its activity as increased flexor force is needed or when finger flexion with wrist flexion is desired.[51,56,73,74] Although the FDS is commonly considered to be stronger at PIP flexion because it crosses few joints, it reverses its position with the FDP at the PIP joint. The FDS is superficial to the FDP at the MCP joint. Because the FDS is farther from the MCP joint axis, the FDS has a greater moment arm for MCP flexion. Just proximal to the PIP, however, the deeper FDP tendon emerges through the split in the FDS tendon (**Camper's chiasma**) so the that FDS tendon can attach to the base of the middle phalanx. Consequently, at the PIP joint, the FDP is farther from the PIP joint axis than the FDS.[58] Although the MA may not be optimal at the PIP joint, the FDS is important for balance at that joint. When the FDS is absent, forceful pinch (thumb to fingertip) activity of the FDP may create PIP *extension* along with DIP flexion, rather than flexion at both joints.[75] This phenomenon can be observed in many normal hands because the FDS of the little finger is commonly absent or may have anomalous distal attachments.[75,76]

Both the FDS and FDP are dependent on wrist position for optimal length-tension. If there is not a counterbalancing extensor force at the wrist, the volarly located forces of the FDS and FDP muscles will cause wrist flexion to occur. If these muscles are permitted to shorten over the wrist, there will be a concomitant loss of tension at the more distal joints. In fact, it is almost impossible to fully flex the fingers actively if the FDS and FDP are also permitted to simultaneously flex the wrist. The counterbalancing wrist extensor force is usually supplied by an active wrist extensor such as the ECRB or, in some instances, the EDC.

The greater available range of MCP and IP flexion in the ring and little fingers than in the index or long fingers may result in some relative loss of tension in the ulnar FDS and FDP muscles during active finger flexion. Because the long flexors of the ring and little fingers must shorten over a greater range, the muscles are more likely to become actively insufficient. This is not a problem if strong grip is not required (e.g., holding a glass). Then the object may be tapered ulnarly to accommodate the greater ROM. Conversely, if the object to be held by the fingers is heavy or requires strong grip, the object may be shaped so that it is wider ulnarly than radially, a so-called pistol grip (Fig. 9–15). This limits the MCP/IP flexion in the ring and little fingers and minimizes loss of FDS/FDP tension. The so-called pistol grip of most tools is an example of modifying an object to optimize hand function.

MECHANISMS OF FINGER FLEXION

Optimal function of the FDS and FDP depends not only on the wrist musculature but also on

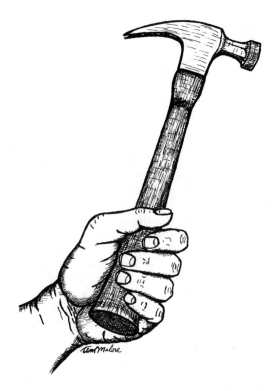

FIGURE 9–15. In pistol-grip, the object has a larger circumference ulnarly to prevent full flexion of the ring and little fingers. Restricting ROM maintains better length-tension for stronger grip in these two fingers when using heavy objects or using objects forcefully.

intact flexor gliding mechanisms. The gliding mechanisms consist of retinaculae, ligaments, bursae, and digital tendon sheaths. The fibrous structures tether the long flexor tendons to the hand; the bursae and sheaths facilitate friction-free excursion of the tendons. The retinaculae and ligaments prevent bowstringing of the tendons that would result in loss of excursion and work efficiency in the contracting muscles. The tendons must be anchored without interfering with their pull or creating frictional forces that would cause degeneration of the tendons over time.

As the tendons of the FDS and FDP cross the wrist to enter the hand, they first pass beneath the proximal flexor retinaculum and through the carpal tunnel. Friction between the tendons themselves and friction of the tendons on the overlying TCL are prevented by the radial and ulnar bursae that envelop the flexor tendons at this level. All eight tendons of the profundus and superficialis are invested in a common bursa known as the **ulnar bursa.** The bursa is compartmentalized to prevent friction of tendon on tendon. The FPL that accompanies the FDS and FDP through the carpal tunnel is encased in its own **radial bursa.** The radial and ulnar bursae contain a synovial-like fluid that minimize frictional forces. The pattern of bursae and tendon sheaths may vary among individuals. The most common representation shows the ulnar bursa to be continuous with the digital tendon sheath for the little finger. However, Phillips and colleagues[77] found continuity between the ulnar bursa and tendon sheath of the little finger in only 30% of 60 specimens. The ulnar bursa is typically not continuous with the digital tendon sheaths for the index, middle, and ring fingers. Rather, for these fingers, the ulnar bursa ends just distal to the proximal palmar crease, and the digital tendon sheaths begin at the middle or distal palmer creases.[9] The radial bursa encases the flexor pollicis longus and is continuous with its digital tendon sheath (Fig. 9–16). The extent and communication of the digital tendon sheaths is functionally relevant because infection within a sheath will travel its full length, producing painful tenosynovitis. If a sheath is continuous with the ulnar or radial bursa, the infection will spread into the palm (or visa versa).[50] The tendon sheaths for each finger

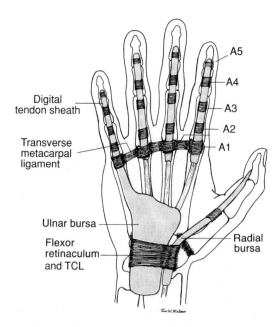

FIGURE 9–16. The flexor mechanisms of the fingers and thumb include the flexor retinaculum and transverse carpal ligament (TCL) at the wrist, the annular pulleys (A1-A5), the radial and ulnar bursae, and the digital tendon sheaths.

Digital tendon sheath

Transverse metacarpal ligament

Ulnar bursa

Flexor retinaculum and TCL

Radial bursa

A5
A4
A3
A2
A1

end proximal to the insertion of the FDP on the base of the distal phalanx. Consequently, common puncture wounds or injuries to the pad of the fingers are unlikely to introduce infection into the digital tendon sheaths.

The FDS and FDP tendons of each finger pass through as many as five fibro-osseous tunnels formed by what are known as **annular pulleys** (or **vaginal ligaments**), as well as under three cruciate ligaments[19,78] (see Fig. 9–16). The first two annular pulleys lie closely together, with one (designated the A1 pulley) at the head of the metacarpal and a second larger one (A2) along the volar midshaft of the proximal phalanx. The floor of the first pulley is formed by the flexor groove in the deep transverse metacarpal ligament, whereas all the other annular pulleys attach directly to bone. The third annular pulley (A3) lies at the distal most part of the proximal phalanx, and the fourth (A4) lies centrally on middle phalanx. A fifth pulley (A5) may lie at the base of the distal phalanx. The base of the pulleys on the bone is longer than the roof superficially, and the roof has a slight concavity volarly. This structure allows the pulleys to approximate at extremes of flexion, forming nearly one continuous tunnel.[19] The curvature also allows the fibro-osseous tunnel to contour to the slight bowstringing of the tendon during flexion, distributing pressure throughout the tunnel rather than just at the edges.[78] Three cruciate (crisscrossing) ligaments also tether long flexor tendons. One is located between the A2 and A3 pulleys and is designated as C1; the next cruciate (C2) lies between the A3 and A4 pulleys; and the last cruciate (C3) lies between the A4 and A5 pulleys. The A4, A5, and C3 structures contain only the FDP tendon because the FDS inserts on the middle phalanx proximal to these structures. The annular pulleys and cruciate ligaments vary among individuals in both number and extent.[78] An additional annular pulley found proximal to the A1 is also described by some and has been named the palmar aponeurosis (PA) pulley.[79]

Friction of the FDS and FDP tendons on the annular pulleys and cruciate ligaments is minimized by the digital tendon sheaths that envelop the tendons from the point at which the tendons pass into the most proximal annular pulley (PA or A1) to the point at which the tendon of the FDP passes through the most distal cruciate or pulley (C3 or A5). The synovial-like fluid contained in each of the digital tendon sheaths permits gliding of the tendons beneath their ligamentous constraints and between each other. This is particularly important over the proximal phalanx where the FDS tendon splits to either side of the FDP tendon and rejoins *beneath* the FDP tendon to insert on the middle phalanx. The FDP tendon, consequently, must pass through Camper's chiasma. Once the FDP tendon is distal to the last annular pulley, the tendon sheath ends because lubrication of the tendon is no longer needed. Vascular supply to the gliding mechanism is critical to maintaining synovial fluid and tendon nutrition. Direct vascularization of each tendon occurs through vessels that reach the tendon via the **vincula tendinum.** These are folds of the synovial membrane (usually four in number) that carry blood vessels to the body of the tendon and to the tendinous insertions of the two flexors of each finger.[19] The tendons also receive some of their nutrition directly from the synovial fluid within the sheath and, through that mechanism, can withstand at least partial loss of direct vascularization.[80]

The function of the annular pulleys is to keep the flexor tendons close to the bone, allowing only a minimum amount of bowstringing and migration volarly from the joint axes.[81] This sacrifices the increase in MA that might occur with substantial bowstringing of the tendons, but enhances both tendon excursion efficiency and work efficiency of the long flexors.[75,82] Any interruption in either the annular pulleys or the digital tendon sheaths can result in substantial impairment of FDS and FDP functioning or in structural deformity. Of the potential six annular pulleys (PA, A1 through 5), integrity of pulleys A2, A3, or A4 is variously credited with being most critical to maintaining FDS/FDP efficiency.[82,83] The gliding mechanism of the fingers is critical not only to proper application of active finger flexion forces but also to the ability of the tendons to undergo passive excursion in finger extension. **Trigger finger** is one example of the disability that can be created when repetitive trauma to a flexor tendon results in the formation of nodules on the tendon and thickening of the annular pulley. Finger flexion may be prevented completely or the finger may be unable to re-extend.[8]

Extrinsic Finger Extensors

The extrinsic finger extensors are the EDC, the EIP, and the EDM. As each of these muscles passes from the forearm to the hand, it passes beneath the extensor retinaculum that maintains proximity to the joints and improves excursion efficiency. As the tendons pass deep to the retinaculum, each tendon is encased within its own tendon sheath to prevent friction between tendons and friction on the retinaculum. The septa of the retinaculum through which the tendons pass are attached to the dorsal carpal ligaments and help maintain stability of the extensor tendons on the dorsum, as well as allowing those muscles to contribute to wrist extension.[16] There are no commonly shared bursae dorsally. The tendon sheaths are also not as variable or as extensive as the sheaths associated with the flexor tendons and there are no annular pulleys. At approximately the MCP joint, the EDC tendon merges with a broad aponeurosis known as the **extensor expansion** or the **extensor hood.** Distal to the hood, the EDC tendon continues as three bands: the **central tendon** that inserts on the base of the middle phalanx and two **lateral bands** that rejoin as the **terminal tendon** to insert into the base of the distal phalanx (Fig. 9–17). The EIP and EDM insert into the EDC tendons of the index and little fingers, respectively, at or just proximal to the extensor hood. Given the attachments of the EIP and EDM to the EDC structure, these muscles appear to add independence of action to the index and ring fingers, rather than additional strength or actions. The tendons of the EDC, EIP, and EDM also show a good deal of variability. Most of the time, the index finger has one EDC tendon leading to the extensor hood and one EIP tendon inserting on to its ulnar side.[84–86] At the lit-

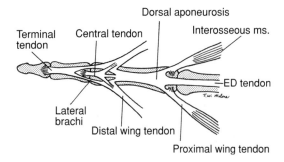

FIGURE 9–17. Dorsal view of the extensor mechanism including the tendon of the extensor digitorum (ED), the dorsal aponeurosis, the proximal and distal wing tendons of the interossei, and the central tendon, lateral bands, and terminal tendon.

tle finger, the EDM tendon may merge with the extensor hood, with no EDC tendon at all in as many as 30% of specimens.[87] The middle and ring fingers do not have their own auxiliary extensor muscles, but frequently have two or even three EDC tendons leading to the hood.[86] The EDC tendons of one finger may also be connected to the tendon(s) of an adjacent finger by **junctura tendinae.** These fibrous connections (frequently visible along with the extensor tendons on the dorsum of the hand) cause active extension of one finger to be accompanied by passive extension of the adjacent finger—with the patterns of interdependence varying with the connections. Generally, the EDC, EIP, EDM, and junctura tendinae connections result in the index finger having the most independent extension, with extension of the little, middle, and ring fingers in declining order of independence.[58]

The EDC, EIP, and EDM are the only muscles capable of extending the MCP joints of the fingers. They are also wrist extensors by continued action. Active tension on the extensor hood from one or more of these muscles will extend the MCP even though there are no direct attachments to the proximal phalanx.[88] Although tension on the hood can produce MCP extension, the central tendon and terminal tendon distal to the extensor expansion cannot be tightened sufficiently by the extrinsic extensor muscles alone to produce extension at either the PIP or DIP joints. Rather, an isolated contraction of one of the extrinsic extensors will result in MCP hyperextension with IP flexion.[72,89,90] The flexion is produced by passive tension in the FDS and FDP when the MCP joint is extended. Active IP extension requires contributions from two intrinsic muscle groups (the interossei and lumbricals) that attach to the extensor hood, central tendon, or the lateral bands. These intrinsic muscles, along with the extrinsic extensors, the extensor hood, the central tendon, the lateral bands, terminal tendon, and oblique retinacular ligament, together comprise the **extensor mechanism.** Because the EIP and EDM share innervation, insertion, and function with the EDC in its role as part of the extensor mechanism, discussion of the EDC from this point on should be assumed to include contributions from the EIP or the EDM muscles. For the sake of clarity and brevity, all three muscles will not be named each time.

We will now examine in more detail the ex-

tensor mechanism and the contributions made by the extrinsic extensors and intrinsic musculature.

THE EXTENSOR MECHANISM

The structure of the extensor mechanism of each finger (see Fig. 9–17) is made up of the EDC tendon, its connective tissue expansions and connections (including the central tendon, lateral bands, central tendon, and oblique retinacular ligaments), and fibers from the **dorsal interosseous (DI), volar interosseous (VI), and lumbrical** muscles of each finger. More detailed information about the component parts will be presented after the extensor expansion structure is described.

The foundation of the extensor expansion is formed by the tendons of the EDC (with EIP and EDM). Additionally, the extensor hood has sagittal bands that connect the volar surface of the hood to the volar plates and transverse metacarpal ligament. The sagittal bands help stabilize the hood at the MCP joint and help prevent bowstringing of the extensor mechanism with MCP extension.[58] The dorsal and volar interossei attach proximally to the sides of the metacarpals. Distally, some muscle fibers go deep to insert directly into the proximal phalanx, whereas others join with and become part of the hood that wraps around the proximal phalanx. The interossei also contribute fibers to the central tendon and both lateral bands (Fig. 9–18). The lumbricals attach proximally to the FDS tendons and distally to the radial lateral band. The lateral bands are interconnected dorsally by a triangular band of superficial fibers known as the **triangular,** or **transverse retinacular, ligament.** With the

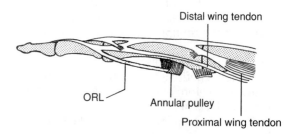

FIGURE 9–18. Each of the oblique retinacular ligaments (ORL) arises from the annular pulley on the proximal phalanx and passes distally to a lateral band of the extensor mechanism. The ORL lies volar to the axis of the PIP joint and dorsal to the axis of the DIP axis through its attachment to the lateral band.

addition of the oblique retinacular ligaments, the structure of the extensor mechanism for each finger is complete. The **oblique retinacular ligaments** (**ORL**s) arise from both sides of the proximal phalanx and from the sides of the A2 annular pulley volarly. The ORLs continue distally as slender bands to insert on the lateral bands distal to the PIP joint (see Fig. 9–18).[91,92] Function of the extensor mechanism can now be presented by looking in more detail at the active and passive elements that compose it and by referencing the relation of relevant segments to each joint individually.

Extensor Mechanism Influence on MCP Joint Function. At each MCP joint, the EDC tendon passes *dorsal* to the MCP joint axis. An active contraction of the muscle creates tension on the hood, pulls the hood proximally over the MCP joint, and extends the proximal phalanx. The other active forces that are part of the extensor mechanism are the dorsal interosseous, volar interosseous, and lumbrical muscles. Each of these muscles passes *volar* to the MCP joint axis and, therefore, creates a flexor force at the joint. When the EDC, interossei, and lumbricals all contract simultaneously, the MCP joint will extend (as will the IP joints) because the torque produced by the EDC at the MCP exceeds the MCP flexor torque of the intrinsic muscles. If the intrinsics are inactive, the EDC (as already noted) will hyperextend the MCP and cause passive flexion of the IP joints. This position of the finger, known as **clawing,** is the classic zigzag pattern seen with an unstable intercalated segment as the unstable proximal phalanx extends on the metacarpal below while the middle and distal phalanx flex over it. Normally the collapse is prevented by active tension in the lumbricals or interossei that cross the MCP joint anteriorly.[58] When these muscle are not present as in an ulnar nerve injury, the EDC is unopposed and the finger claws, also known as an **intrinsic minus** position because it is attributed to the absence of the finger intrinsic muscles (Fig. 9–19).

Extensor Mechanism Influence on IP Joint Function. The PIP and DIP joints are joined by both active and passive forces in such a way that DIP extension and PIP extension are interdependent: when the PIP is actively extended, the DIP will also extend. Similarly, active DIP extension will create PIP extension. The interdependence can be understood by examining structural relationships in the extensor mecha-

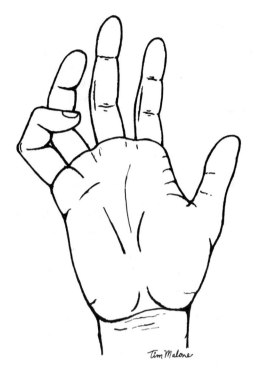

Tim Malone

FIGURE 9–19. In the ulnar nerve-deficient hand (claw hand), the ring and little fingers are hyperextended at the MCP from unopposed EDC tension and flexed at the IP joints from passive long flexor tension. The little finger may also be abducted (Wartenberg's sign) from the unopposed pull of the EDM.

nism. Each PIP joint is crossed dorsally by the central tendon and lateral bands of the extensor mechanism. The EDC, the interossei, and lumbrical muscles all have attachments to the hood, central tendon, or lateral bands at or proximal to the PIP joint. Consequently, the EDC, interossei, and lumbricals are each capable of producing at least some tension in the central tendon, the lateral bands, and (via the lateral bands) the terminal tendon that will simultaneously create some extensor force at both the PIP and DIP joints. An EDC contraction alone will not produce IP extension. An active contraction of a DI, VI, or lumbrical muscle *is* capable of extending the IP joints. However, if one or more of the intrinsic muscles contracts without a contraction of the EDC, the MCP will simultaneously flex because each passes volar to the MCP joint axis. Although it may appear that the intrinsics are independently extending the IP joints, a second source of passive tension in the extensor mechanism may be assisting the active intrinsic muscles. Stack[93] proposed that the interossei and lumbricals would not be able to generate sufficient tension to cause IP extension if the EDC tendon was completely slack or severed. *Two* sources of tension in the extensor expansion appear to be necessary to fully extend the IP joints. Source 1 is normally provided by an active contraction of one or more of the intrinsic finger muscles. Source 2 may be provided either by (2a) an *active contraction* of the EDC (with active MCP extension) or by (2b) *passive stretch* (created by MCP flexion resulting from a contraction of the intrinsic muscles). When the intrinsic musculature is paralyzed, the EDC may be able to extend the IP joints, but *only* if the MCP joint is maintained in flexion by some external force. The ability to use the EDC to extend the IPs with passively maintained MCP flexion is known as **Bunnell's sign.**[94] With the stretch imposed on the extensor mechanism by passive MCP flexion (source 1), additional tension is provided by an active contraction of the EDC (source 2). These two sources may be sufficient to produce full or nearly full PIP and DIP extension.[89] The passive MCP flexion can be provided either by a splinting device or by surgical fixation of the MCP joints in a semiflexed position.

Tension in the lateral bands distal to the PIP joint and some of the linkage between the PIP and DIP may be contributed by passive action of the oblique retinacular ligaments. The ORLs pass just volar to the PIP joint axis and attach distally to the lateral bands. Tension will increase in the ORLs as the PIP is extended (actively or passively) *if* the lateral bands and their terminal tendon are already tensed by DIP flexion. Consequently, PIP extension, through passive tension in the ORLs, may contribute to DIP extension. The lengths of the ORLs are such, however, that the contribution to DIP extension may be significant only during the first half of the DIP extension range (90° to 45° flexion) when the ORLs are most stretched.[91,93] Overall, the structure of the extensor expansion and its contributing active and passive elements contribute to linking PIP and DIP extension.[8,9,72,90]

Flexion of the DIP joint produces flexion of the PIP joint by a similar combination of active and passive forces that link extension of these two joints. When the DIP joint is flexed by the FDP, a simultaneous flexor force is applied over both joints it crosses. However, the active force might not be sufficient to produce PIP flexion if extensor restraining forces were not released at the same time. When the DIP begins flexing, the terminal tendon and its lateral bands are stretched over the dorsal aspect of the DIP joint. The stretch in the lateral bands pulls the extensor hood (from which the lateral bands arise) distally. The distal migration in the extensor hood causes the central tendon of the extensor expansion to relax, facilitating flexion of the PIP. The combination of active (FDP) and passive forces (release of the central tendon) still might not be sufficient to flex the PIP joint if the lateral bands remained taut on the dorsal aspect of the PIP joint. The bands, however, are permitted to migrate volarly by the elasticity of the interconnecting triangular ligament. Through the combination of active and passive mechanisms, both active and passive DIP flexion ordinarily result in simultaneous PIP flexion.

The normal coupling of DIP and PIP flexion can be overridden by some individuals. That is, some people can actively flex a DIP while maintaining the PIP in extension. This "trick" is due to the influence of the ORLs and requires some PIP hyperextension of the finger. When the PIP can be sufficiently hyperextended, the ORLs (ordinarily lying just volar to the PIP joint axis) pass *dorsal* to the PIP joint axis. Now, tension in the ORLs produced with active DIP flexion will accentuate PIP *extension* because the ORLs have been placed dorsal to the PIP joint and function as passive joint extensors. The trick of active DIP flexion and PIP extension serves no functional purpose and can be accomplished only by those individuals and in those fingers where PIP hyperextension is available.

The functional coupling of PIP/DIP joint action can be demonstrated by one other PIP/DIP relation. When the PIP is fully flexed actively by the FDS or flexed passively by some outside force, the DIP cannot be actively extended. When the PIP joint is flexed, the dorsally located central tendon is increasingly stretched. The tensed central tendon pulls the extensor hood (from which the central tendon arises) distally. This distal movement of the hood releases some of the tension in the lateral bands. The lateral bands are further released as the bands separate slightly and migrate volarly around the flexing PIP joint. Relaxation of the lateral bands relaxes the terminal tendon on the distal phalanx. As 90° of PIP flexion is reached, loss of tension in the terminal tendon completely eliminates any extensor force at the DIP joint, including any potential contribution from the ORLs that have also been released by PIP flexion.[95] Although the DIP joint can be actively flexed by the FDP when the PIP is already flexed, it cannot be actively re-extended as long as the PIP joint remains flexed.

The coupled actions of the PIP and DIP joints are summarized as follows:

- Active extension of the PIP joint will normally be accompanied by extension of the DIP joint.
- Active or passive flexion of the DIP joint will normally be accompanied by flexion of the PIP.
- Full flexion of the PIP joint (active or passive) will prevent the DIP joint from being actively extended.

Intrinsic Finger Musculature

DORSAL AND VOLAR INTEROSSEI

The dorsal interossei (DI) and volar interossei (VI) are sets of muscles arising from between the metacarpals and attaching to the bases of the proximal phalanges or to the extensor expansion. There are four DI muscles (one to each finger) and three to four VI muscles. Many (but not all) anatomy texts describe the thumb as having the first VI. Mardel and Underwood[96] suggest that the discrepancy may be in whether the muscle is considered a separate volar interosseous or as part of the flexor pollicis brevis. Although we will consider the thumb as having the first VI, we will consider at this time only the action of the VI and DI at the fingers. Because the DI and VI are alike in location and in some of their actions, they are characterized by their ability to produce MCP abduction and adduction, respectively. More recently, additional detail on the attachments of these muscles has increased our understanding of their contribution to hand function. We will now look at how the attachments of the interossei affect their role as MCP flexors or stabilizers and as IP extensors.

The interossei muscle fibers join the extensor expansions in two locations. Some fibers attach *proximally* to the proximal phalanx and to the extensor hood via what are termed **proximal wing tendons;** some fibers attach more *distally* to the lateral bands and central tendon via **distal wing tendons** (see Figs. 9–17 and 9–18). Although individual variations in muscle attachments exist, studies have found some consistency in the point of attachment of the different interossei.[92,93,97] The first DI muscle has the most consistent attachment of its group, inserting entirely into the bony base of the proximal phalanx and the extensor hood via proximal wing tendons, with no distal wing tendons present. The three DI of the middle and ring fingers have both proximal wing tendons *and* distal wing tendons attaching them to the lateral bands and central tendon. The proximal and distal wing tendons of the DI usually arise from separate bellies; the belly from which the distal wing tendon arises resembles a volar interosseous muscle. The little finger does not have a DI. The abductor digiti minimi (ADM) muscle is, in effect, a DI and typically has only a proximal wing tendon.[58] The three VI consistently appear to have distal wing tendons only, with no proximal attachments.

Given the proximal and distal wing tendons of the DI, VI, and ADM, these muscles can be characterized not only as abductors or adductors of the MCP, but also as proximal or distal interossei according to the pattern of attachment. Proximal interossei will have their predominant effect at the MCP joint alone, whereas the distal interossei will produce their predominant action at the IP joints, with some effect by continued action at the MCP joint.

All of the DI and VI muscles (regardless of their designation as proximal or distal) pass *dorsal* to the transverse metacarpal ligament (see Fig. 9–18) but just volar to the axis for MCP joint flexion/extension. All the interossei, therefore, are potentially flexors of the MCP joint. The ability of the interossei to flex the MCP joint, however, will vary somewhat with MCP joint position and with the presence of proximal versus distal wing tendons.

Role of the Interossei at the MCP Joint in MCP Extension. When the MCP joint is in extension, the MA (and rotatory component) of all the interossei for MCP flexion is so small that little flexion torque is produced (see Fig. 9–18). Given that the action lines pass almost directly through the coronal axis, the interossei are very effective stabilizers (joint compressors) of the MCP when the MCP is in extension. This stabilizing function is credited with helping to prevent collapse of the unstable proximal segment into a clawed position.[58,72] The stabilizing force of the interossei appears to be provided by *passive* viscoelastic tension in the muscle. There is typically no EMG activity recorded in the interossei when the hand is at rest, when there is isolated EDC activity, or when there is combined EDC-FDP activity. Yet, when these activities are performed in a hand with long-standing ulnar nerve paralysis (therefore, no interossei), an exaggerated MCP joint hyperextension (clawing) results. Clawing does not occur in the ulnar nerve-deficient hand when the hand is at rest until the viscoelastic tension in the interossei has been lost through atrophy. Once such atrophy occurs, the predominance of EDC tension even in relaxation is evidenced by the MCP posture assumed by each finger of the hand at rest. In a low ulnar nerve injury, the index and middle finger retain a lumbrical as well as the extrinsic flexors. The loss of the interossei is reflected by a resting MCP posture of neutral flexion/extension rather than slight flexion as one would expect. The ring and little finger will be missing both interossei and lumbricals. Despite the presence of the FDS and FDP, the resting posture of the ring and little fingers over time is one of MCP hyperextension or clawing.[8,9,49,72] The little finger may also assume an MCP abducted position with loss of the intrinsics. Abduction of the little finger (**Wartenberg's sign**) in an ulnar nerve-deficient hand may derive from the unbalanced pull of the EDM among those individuals having a direct connection of the EDM to the abductor tubercle—the only one of the extensor tendons that has an insertion on the proximal phalanx in any substantial number of people.[87]

When the MCP is extended, the interossei (and ADM) lie at a relatively large distance from the AP axis for MCP joint abduction/adduction. Consequently, in the MCP extended position, the interossei (and ADM) are effective abductors or adductors of the MCP without the loss of tension that would occur if the muscles were simultaneously producing MCP flexion. The interossei with proximal wing tendons are better as MCP joint abductors/adductors because proximal wing tendons act directly on the proximal phalanx. Interossei with distal wing tendons are less effective at the MCP joint because they must act on the MCP joint by continued action. In our conceptual framework, all the DI (MCP abductors) have proximal wing tendons and the VI (MCP adductors) have only distal wing tendons. Therefore, MCP abduction is stronger than MCP adduction. The DI muscles also have twice the muscle mass of the VI muscles. In a progressive ulnar nerve paralysis, the relatively ineffective MCP adduction component of the VI is the first to show weakness.

Role of the Interossei at the MCP Joint in

MCP Flexion. When the MCP joint is in flexion, the action lines of the interossei lie more volar to the MCP joint axis than they do in MCP extension. In fact, in full MCP flexion, the action lines of the interossei are nearly perpendicular to the moving segment (proximal phalanx) (Fig. 9–20). Consequently, the ability of the interossei muscles to create an MCP flexion torque increases as the joint moves from full extension to full flexion. At the same time, the collateral ligaments of the MCP joint become increasingly taut. The increasing tension in the collateral ligaments helps prevent the loss of tension in the interossei that would occur with simultaneous MCP flexion and abduction/adduction. In full MCP flexion, abduction and adduction are completely restricted by tight collateral ligaments, by the shape of the condyles of the metacarpal head, and by active insufficiency of the fully shortened interossei muscles. Even in full MCP flexion, the MA of the interossei for flexion is restricted by the location of the interossei tendons behind the transverse metacarpal ligament. The ligament limits the amount of volar excursion that can occur. However, even with a relatively small MA for MCP flexion (in the MCP flexed position), the interossei are considered powerful MCP flexor muscles[98] that contribute to grip when strong pinch or grip is required.[74]

Role of the Interossei at the IP Joint in IP Extension. The ability of the interossei to produce IP joint extension is governed by the distal wing tendons of the DI and VI muscles. To create sufficient tension in the extensor mechanism to extend the IP joints, the muscles must attach to the central tendon or lateral bands. All the interossei (volar and dorsal) typically

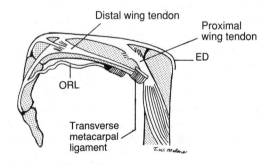

FIGURE 9–20. Full flexion of the PIP joint releases tension in the lateral bands and the ORL. Consequently, the terminal tendon is relaxed and the DIP cannot be actively extended.

have distal wing tendons except the first DI (index finger) and the ADM (little finger). In other words, all "interossei" have distal attachments except the two outside abductors.

When the MCP joint is extended, the action lines of the distal wing tendons are ineffective in producing MCP flexion but capable of extending the IP joints. Because the distal wing tendons attach directly to the central tendon and lateral bands, the IP extension produced by the distal wing tendons is stronger than their MCP abduction/adduction action (which is performed by continued action). When the MCP joint is in flexion, the action lines of the distal wing tendons migrate volarly at the MCP but are restricted in their volar excursion by the transverse metacarpal ligament. The transverse metacarpal ligament prevents the distal wing tendons from becoming slack through volar migration and has a pulley effect on the distal tendons. The pulley effect of the transverse metacarpal ligament appears to enhance the function of the distal wing tendons, because IP extension by the distal wing tendons

of the interossei appears to be more effective in MCP flexion than in MCP extension.

The index and little fingers each have only one interosseous muscle with a distal wing tendon (second VI and fourth VI, respectively). The middle and ring finger each have two distal wing tendons (second and third DI for the middle finger, and fourth VI and DI for the ring finger). The index and little fingers, therefore, are weaker in IP extension than are the middle and ring fingers.[97]

Overall, in approaching or holding the position of MCP flexion and IP extension, both proximal and distal wing tendons of the interossei contribute to the MCP flexion torque. The proximal components are effective MCP flexors, and the distal components are maximally effective as both MCP flexors and IP extensors. The most consistent activity of all the interossei apparently occurs when the MCPs are being flexed and the IP joints are simultaneously extended.[72,99] If the interossei are shortened, this position may not be able to be reversed passively. A summary of actions of the interossei is presented in Table 9–1.

Table 9–1. **Summary of Interossei Muscle Action**

Muscle	Attachments	Action	
		MCP Extended	**MCP Flexed**
FIRST FINGER			
DI	Proximal only	MCP abduction	MCP flexion
VI	Distal only	IP extension and MCP adduction*	IP extension and MCP flexion*
SECOND FINGER			
DI	Proximal and distal	MCP abduction and IP extension	MCP flexion and IP extension
DI	Proximal and distal	MCP abduction and IP extension	MCP flexion and IP extension
THIRD FINGER			
DI	Proximal and distal	MCP abduction and IP extension	MCP flexion and IP extension
VI	Distal only	IP extension and MCP adduction*	IP extension and MCP flexion*
FOURTH FINGER			
DI	Proximal only	MCP abduction	MCP flexion
VI	Distal only	IP extension and MCP adduction*	IP extension and MCP flexion*

*Occurs indirectly by continued action.
DI, dorsal interossei; VI, volar interossei; MCP, metacarpophalangeal; IP, interphalangeal.

LUMBRICAL MUSCLES

The lumbricals are the only muscles in the body that attach at both ends to tendons of other muscles. Each muscle arises from a tendon of the FDP in the palm, passes volar to the transverse metacarpal ligament, and attaches to the lateral band of the extensor mechanism on the radial side (Fig. 9–21a). Like the interossei, the lumbricals cross the MCP joint volarly and the IP joints dorsally. Differences in function in the two muscle groups can be attributed to the more distal insertion of the lumbricals on the lateral band, to their profundus tendon origin, and to their great contractile range.

The insertion of the lumbricals on the distal lateral bands makes them consistently effective IP extensors, regardless of MCP position. In MCP extension, the transverse metacarpal ligament prevents the lumbrical muscle from migrating dorsally and losing tension as the IP joints extend. Studies have found the lumbricals to be more frequently active as IP extensors in the MCP extended position than are the interossei.[72,100] When the lumbrical contracts, it pulls not only on its distal attachment (the lateral band) but also on its proximal attachment (the FDP tendon). Because the proximal attachment of the lumbrical muscle is on a somewhat movable tendon, shortening of the lumbrical muscle not only pulls the lateral bands proximally to extend the IP joints but also pulls the FDP tendon distally in the palm. The distal migration of the FDP tendon releases much of the passive flexor force of the inactive FDP at the MCP and IP joints (Fig. 9–21b). Ranney and Wells[94] confirmed this, finding that the IP joints did not extend until the tension within the lumbrical equaled the tension within the FDP, which permitted the lumbrical to pull the FDP tendon distally. That is, the lumbricals might be considered to be both agonists and synergists for IP extension. Tension in the lumbricals on the lateral bands produces IP extension, while the lumbrical simultaneously releases antagonistic tension in the FDP tendon.[101] The distal wing tendons of the interossei can also extend the IP joints. However, they are less effective as IP extensors in the absence of the lumbricals, because the interossei do not have the same ability to release the passive resistance of the FDP tendon to IP extension. It should also be emphasized that tension in the FDP and extensor mechanism is critical to lumbrical function. If passive tension were not present in the inactive FDP, an active lumbrical contraction would pull the FDP tendon so far distally that the muscle would become actively insufficient and there would be no effective pull of the lumbrical on the extensor expansion. Similarly, tension (active or passive) in the EDC tendon and extensor expansion are necessary before the second source of tension, the lumbrical, can be effective in fully extending both IP joints.[93]

The lumbricals have a greater MA for MCP flexion than the interossei because the lumbricals lie volar to the interossei. Functionally, however, this component of lumbrical action is weaker in the lumbricals than in the interossei.[72,97,98,100,102] This relative weakness may be attributed to the small cross section of the lumbricals compared with the interossei. However, it may also have to do with the moving attachment of the lumbrical on the FDP tendon. A contraction of a lumbrical causes the associated FDP tendon to migrate distally and carries the lumbrical along with it. The distal migration of the FDP tendon and lumbrical has the effect both of releasing passive tension in the inactive FDP that might contribute to MCP flexion, and of minimizing the active force of the lumbrical at the MCP joint. Although the lum-

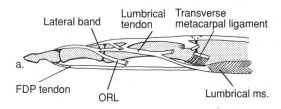

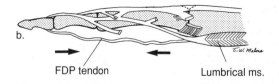

FIGURE 9–21. (a) The lumbrical muscle arises from the tendon of the flexor digitorum profundis (FDP). The lumbrical lies volar to the transverse metacarpal ligament and passes dorsally to attach to the lateral band of the extensor mechanism. (b) An active contraction of the lumbrical pulls on both the FDP tendon and the lateral band. The pull on the FDP tendon will move the tendon distally, releasing the passive tension of the tendon at the PIP and DIP.

bricals do not contribute much to MCP flexion, MCP flexion does not appear to weaken their effectiveness as IP extensors. The unusually large contractile range of the lumbrical muscles seems to prevent them from becoming actively insufficient when shortening both at the MCP and at the IP joints. The lumbricals may also assist the FDP indirectly with hand closure. When the FDP muscle contracts, the FDP tendon moves proximally as does its associated lumbrical. This creates a passive pull of the lumbrical on the lateral band during hand closure that may assist the FDP in flexing the MCP joint *before* the IPs, avoiding the problem of catching the fingertips in the palm as is seen in the intrinsic minus hand.[98]

In summary, the function of the lumbricals is simpler than that of the interossei. The lumbricals are strong extensors of the IP joints, regardless of MCP joint position; they are also relatively weak MCP flexors regardless of MCP joint position. The ability of the lumbricals to extend the IPs appears to depend only on intact tension in the extensor mechanism and in the FDP tendons. When the lumbricals and interossei contract together without any extrinsic finger muscles, these muscles produce MCP flexion and IP extension, the so-called **intrinsic plus** position of the hand.

Structure of the Thumb

CMC Joint of the Thumb

The CMC joint of the thumb is the articulation between the trapezium and the base of the first metacarpal. Unlike the CMC joints of the fingers, it is a saddle joint with 2° of freedom: flexion/extension and abduction/adduction (Fig. 9–22). The joint also permits some axial rotation, which occurs concurrently with the other motions. The net effect at this joint is a circumduction motion commonly termed **opposition.** Opposition permits the tip of the thumb to oppose the tips of the fingers.

FIRST CMC JOINT STRUCTURE

Zancolli and associates[103] proposed that the first CMC joint surfaces consist not only of the traditionally described saddle-shaped surfaces but also of a spherical portion located near the anterior radial tubercle of the trapezium. The saddle-shaped portion of the trapezium is concave in the sagittal plane (abduction/adduction) and convex in the frontal plane (flexion/extension). The spherical portion is convex in all directions. The base of the first metacarpal has a reciprocal shape to that of the trapezium (see Fig. 9–22). Flexion/extension and abduction/adduction occur on the saddle-shaped surfaces, whereas the axial rotation of the metacarpal that accompanies opposition occurs on the spherical surfaces.[103] Flexion/extension of the joint occurs around a somewhat oblique anteroposterior axis, whereas abduction/adduction occurs around an oblique coronal axis. The obliquity of the motions occurs because of the inclination of the trapezium. As a consequence, flexion/extension occurs nearly parallel to the palm, with abduction/adduction occurring nearly perpendicular to the palm. Cooney and associates[104] measured the first CMC joint ROM as an average of 53° of flexion/extension, 42° of abduction/adduction, and 17° of rotation.

The capsule of the CMC joint is relatively lax but is reinforced by radial, ulnar, volar, and dorsal ligaments. There is also an **intermetacarpal ligament** that helps tether the bases of the first and second metacarpals, preventing extremes of radial and dorsal displacement of the base of the first metacarpal.[103,105] Although some investigators hold that the axial rotation seen in the metacarpal during opposition is a function of incongruence and joint laxity,[9,106] Zancolli and associates[103] theorize that it is a result of the congruence of the

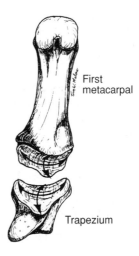

First metacarpal

Trapezium

FIGURE 9–22. The saddle-shaped portion of the trapezium is concave in the sagittal plane (abduction/adduction) and convex in the frontal plane (flexion/extension). The spherical portion found near the anterior radial tubercle is convex in all directions. The base of the first metacarpal has a reciprocal shape to that of the trapezium.

spherical surfaces and resultant tensions encountered in the supporting ligaments. It would seem, however, that some incongruence must exist at the joint. Osteoarthritic changes with aging are common at the first CMC and may be attributable to the high loads imposed on this joint by pinch and grasp across incongruent surfaces. Ateshian and colleagues[107] found gender differences in the fit of the trapezium with the metacarpal, with the trapezium of women showing more incongruence than that of men in a group of older individuals. This matches an increased incidence of osteoarthritis of the first CMC among older women, but it does not address whether the incongruence of the trapezium is a cause or effect of degenerative changes. The first CMC is close-packed both in extremes of abduction and adduction, with maximal motion available in neutral position.[61]

FIRST CMC JOINT FUNCTION

It is the unique range and direction of motion at the first CMC that produces opposition of the thumb. Opposition is, sequentially: abduction, flexion, and adduction of the first metacarpal, with simultaneous rotation. These movements change the orientation of the metacarpal, bring the thumb out of the palm, and position the thumb for contact with the fingers. The functional significance of the CMC joint of the thumb and of the movement of opposition can be appreciated when one realizes that use of the thumb against a finger occurs in almost all forms of **prehension** (grasp and handling activities). When the first CMC joint is fused in extension and adduction, opposition cannot occur. The importance of opposition is such that fusion of the first CMC may be followed over time by an adaptation of the trapezioscaphoid joint, which develops a more saddle-shaped configuration that can restore some of the lost opposition.[64] This amazing shift in joint function is an excellent example of the body's ability to replace essential functions whenever possible.

MCP and IP Joints of the Thumb

The MCP joint of the thumb is the articulation between the head of the first metacarpal and the base of its proximal phalanx. It is considered to be a condyloid joint with 2° of freedom: flexion/extension and abduction/adduction.[58] There is an insignificant amount of passive rotation.[64] The metacarpal head is not covered

with cartilage dorsally or laterally, and more closely resembles the head of the proximal phalanx, minus its central groove. The joint capsule, the reinforcing volar plate, and the collateral ligaments are similar to those of the other MCP joints. The main functional contribution of the first MCP joint is to provide additional flexion range to the thumb in opposition and to allow the thumb to grasp and contour to objects. Despite the structural similarities between the MCP joints, the first MCP joint is far more restricted in motion than those of the fingers. Although the available range varies among individuals, the first MCP joint rarely has more than half the flexion available at the fingers and little if any hyperextension. Abduction/adduction and rotation are extremely limited. This limitation to motion is probably attributable to the major structural difference between the MCP joints of the thumb and fingers. The first MCP joint is reinforced extracapsularly on its volar surface by two sesamoid bones (Fig. 9–23). These are maintained in position by fibers from the collaterals and by an intersesamoid ligament. Goldberg and Nathan[108] propose that the sesamoids are the result of friction and pressure on the tendons in which they are embedded. They support this by noting that the sesamoids of the first MCP do not appear until around 12 years of age and that sesamoids in some investigations have also been found in as many as 70% of fifth MCP joints and 50% of second MCPs.

The IP joint of the thumb is the articulation between the head of the proximal phalanx and

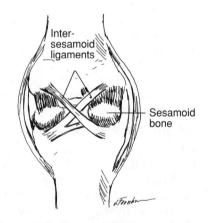

FIGURE 9–23. Metacarpophalangeal joint of the thumb. Unlike the MCP joints of the fingers, this joint is reinforced volarly by two sesamoid bones and the intersesamoid ligaments that secure them to the joint.

the base of the distal phalanx. It is structurally and functionally identical to the IP joints of the fingers.

Thumb Musculature

The muscles of the thumb have been compared to guy wires supporting a flagpole, where there must be a continuous effective pull in every direction to maintain stability. The metacarpal, proximal, and distal phalanx form an articulated shaft that sits on the trapezium. Like the flagpole, tension from the muscular guy wires must be provided in every direction for stability to be maintained. Because the stability comes from the muscles more than from articular constraints (at least at the CMC joint), the majority of muscles that attach to the thumb tend to be active during most thumb motions. There is also substantial individual variability in motor strategies among normal subjects.[109] Consequently, exploration of muscle function in the thumb (and, to a somewhat lesser extent, function through the hand) is largely an issue not of when a muscle functions but when the preponderance of muscle activity might be expected with shifting tasks. The role of the extrinsic and intrinsic thumb muscles will be presented as generalizations, as will the final section of this chapter on hand prehension.

Extrinsic Thumb Muscles

There are four extrinsic muscles, one located volarly and three dorsoradially. The FPL inserts on the distal phalanx and is the correlate of the FDS. The FPL tendon at the wrist is invested by the radial bursa that is continuous with its digital tendon sheath. It is the only muscle capable of flexing the distal phalanx of the thumb. Its tendon sits between the sesamoid bones and would appear to derive some protection from those bones. The EPB and APL run a common course from the dorsal forearm, crossing the wrist on its radial aspect to their insertion. The short extensor (EPB) inserts on the proximal phalanx; the long abductor (APL) inserts on the base of the metacarpal. Both muscles radially deviate the wrist slightly and abduct the CMC joint. The EPB also extends the MCP joint. Both the APL and EPB tendons pass through a common compartment in the extensor retinaculum of the wrist, close to the radial styloid process. Entrapment and inflammation of these tendons at this point is not uncom-

mon, producing a tenosynovitis of one or both of these tendons known as **De Quervain disease.**[8] The EPL originates with the APL and EPB but courses around the dorsal radial (**Lister's**) tubercle before turning toward the thumb and inserting on the distal phalanx. At the level of the proximal phalanx, the EPL tendon is joined by expansions from the abductor pollicis brevis, the first VI muscle, and the adductor pollicis.[19] There is no further elaboration of the extensor expansion on the thumb, but we see the same balance of MCP abductors and adductors contributing to extensor tension and to stabilization of the long extensor tendon. The thenar muscles that attach to the EPL tendon can extend the IP joint to neutral, but cannot complete the range into hyperextension in those individuals with that additional range.

The EPL can complete the full range of extension at the IP joint, as well as applying an extensor force at the MCP joint. The EPL also extends and adducts the CMC joint of the thumb. Unlike in the fingers, there is a separate extensor tendon for each joint of the thumb. The APL attaches to the base of the metacarpal, the EPB to the base of the proximal phalanx, and the EPL to the base of the distal phalanx.

As is true for other extrinsic hand muscles, wrist positioning is an essential factor in providing optimal length-tension for the extrinsic muscles of the thumb. The FPL is ineffective as an IP flexor in wrist flexion. The EPL cannot complete IP extension when the wrist, CMC, and MCP are simultaneously extended. The APL and EPB require the synergy of an ulnar deviator of the wrist to prevent the muscles from creating wrist radial deviation, thus affecting their ability to generate tension over the joints of the thumb.

Intrinsic Thumb Muscles

There are five **thenar,** or intrinsic thumb, muscles that primarily take their origin from the carpal bones and the flexor retinaculum. The **opponens pollicis (OP)** is the only intrinsic thumb muscle to have its distal attachment on the first metacarpal. Its action line is nearly perpendicular to the long axis of the metacarpal and is applied to the lateral side of the bone. The OP, therefore, is very effective in positioning the metacarpal in an abducted, flexed, and rotated posture. **The abductor pollicis brevis**

(APB), flexor pollicis brevis (FPB), adductor pollicis (ADP), and first VI all insert on the proximal phalanx. The FPB has two heads of insertion. Its larger lateral head attaches distally with the APB and also applies some abductor force. The FPB crosses the sesamoid bones at the MCP, which increases its MA for flexion. The medial head of the FPB attaches distally with the ADP and assists in thumb adduction. The first VI muscle arises from the first metacarpal and attaches to the ulnar sesamoid bone and then on to the proximal phalanx.

Although not generally considered a thenar muscle, the first DI may also contribute to thumb function. The first DI is a bipennate muscle arising from both the first and second metacarpals and from the intercarpal ligament that joins the metacarpal bases. Brand and Hollister[98] propose that it is a CMC joint distractor, rather than a typical joint compressor, because it pulls the first metacarpal distally toward the first DI's insertion on the base of the index proximal phalanx. They also argue that thumb attachment of the first DI has little or no ability to move the thumb, but that it is important in offsetting the compressive and dorsoradially directed forces that the flexor/adductor muscles create across the CMC joint in lateral pinch and power grip. When these forces were created in lab specimens without tension in the first DI, the CMC subluxed.[98] Belanger and Noel[110] suggest that the first DI can assist with thumb adduction.

The thenar muscles are active in most grasping activities, regardless of the precise position of the thumb as it participates. The OP works together most frequently with the APB and the FPB, although the intensity of the relation varies. When the thumb is gently brought into contact with any of the other fingers, activity of the OP predominates in the thumb and APB activity exceeds that of the FPB. When opposition to the index finger or middle finger is performed firmly, activity of the FPB exceeds that of the OP. With firm opposition to the ring and little fingers, however, the relation changes; OP activity increases with firm opposition to the ring finger, equaling activity of the FPB with firm opposition to the little finger.[42] The change in balance of muscle activity with firm opposition and with increasingly ulnar opposition can be accounted for by the increased need for abduction and metacarpal rotation. Increased pressure in opposition additionally appears to bring in activity of the adductor pol-

licis. The ADP stabilizes the thumb against the opposed finger. In firm opposition to the index and middle fingers, ADP activity exceeds the very minimal activity of the APB. With more ulnarly located position, the increased need for abduction results in simultaneous activity of the abductor and adductor.[42] Activity of the extrinsic thumb musculature in grasp appears to be partially a function of helping to position the MCP and IP joints. The main function of the extrinsics, however, is in returning the thumb to extension from its position in the palm. Although release of an object is essentially an extrinsic function, some OP and abductor brevis activity have been identified.[42] This muscular activity would assist in maintaining the thumb in abduction and in maintaining metacarpal rotation, which facilitates the next move of the thumb back into opposition.

The joint structure and musculature of the wrist complex, the fingers and the thumb have now each been examined. Some instances of specific muscle activity have been presented to clarify the potential function of the muscle. A summary of wrist and hand function, however, can best be presented through the assessment of purposeful hand activity. Because the entire upper limb is geared toward execution of movement of the hand, it is appropriate to complete the description of the upper limb by looking at an overview of the wrist and hand in prehension activities.

Prehension

Prehension activities of the hand involve the grasping or taking hold of an object between any two surfaces in the hand; the thumb participates in most but not all prehension tasks. The number of ways that objects of varying sizes and shapes may be grasped is nearly infinite, with strategies also varying among individuals. However, a broad classification system for grasp has evolved that will permit observations about the coordinated muscular function generally required to produce or maintain a position.

Prehension can be categorized as either **power grip** or **precision handling.** Each of these two categories has subgroups that further define the grasp. Power grip is generally a forceful act resulting in flexion at all finger joints. When the thumb is used, it acts as a stabilizer to the object held between the fingers and, most commonly, the palm. Precision handling, in contrast, is the skillful placement of an object between fingers, or finger and thumb.[111] The palm is not involved. Landsmeer[112] has suggested that power grip and precision handling can be differentiated on the basis of the dynamic and static phases involved. Power grip is the result of a sequence of opening the hand, positioning the fingers, approaching the fingers to the object, and maintaining a static phase that actually constitutes the grip. This is contrasted to precision handling, which shares the first three steps of the sequence but does not contain a static phase at all. In precision handling the fingers and thumb grasp the object with the intention of manipulating it within the hand; in power grip the object is grasped so that the object can be moved through space by the more proximal joints.

When assessing muscular function during each type of grasp, synergy of the hand muscles results in almost constant activity of all intrinsic and extrinsic muscles. The task becomes more one of identifying when muscles are *not* working or when the balance of activity between muscles might change. It should also be emphasized that the muscular activity documented by EMG studies is specific to the activity as performed in a given study. Even in studies using similar forms of prehension, variables such as size of object, firmness of grip, timing, and instructions to the subject can cause substantial changes in reported muscle activity. However, as indications of general muscular activity patterns, the studies are useful in the development of a conceptual framework within which hand function can be understood.

Power Grip

The fingers in power grip usually function in concert to clamp onto and hold an object into the palm. The fingers assume a position of sustained flexion that varies in degree with the size, shape, and weight of the object. The palm is likely to contour to the object as the palmar arches form around it. The thumb may serve as an additional surface to the finger-palm vise by adducting against the object, or it may be removed from the object. When the thumb is involved, it generally is adducted to clamp the object to the palm. This is in contrast to precision handling where the thumb is more likely to assume a position of abduction.[113] Three varieties of power grip studied by Long and associates[73] exemplify the similarities and differences seen in power grip. They examined hook grip (Fig. 9–24a), spherical grip (Fig. 9–24b) and cylindrical grip (Fig. 9–24c). A fourth variety, lateral prehension, will also be considered with power grip.

Cylindrical Grip

Cylindrical grip (see Fig. 9–24c) almost exclusively uses flexors to carry the fingers around and maintain grasp on an object. The function in the fingers is performed largely by the FDP, especially in the dynamic closing action. In the static phase the FDS assists when the intensity of the grip requires greater force. Although power grip traditionally has been thought of as an extrinsic activity, recent studies have indicated considerable interosseous muscle activity. The interossei are considered to be functioning as MCP flexors and abductors/adductors. In strong grip the magnitude of force of the interossei in metacarpal flexion has been found to nearly equal that of the extrinsic flex-

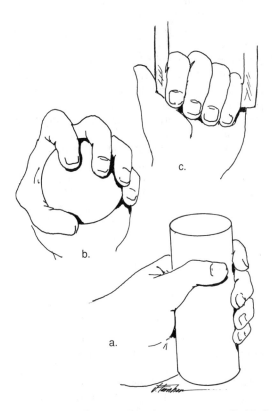

FIGURE 9–24. Three varieties of power grip: (a) cylindrical, (b) spherical, and (c) hook.

ors.[102,111,114] Because the IP joints are being flexed, the MCP flexion task most likely falls to the proximal (dorsal) interossei. The interossei may also position the MCP joint in abduction or adduction to ulnarly deviate the MCP joint and align the distal phalanges of the thumb and fingers. The combination of MCP flexion and ulnar deviation (adduction for the index finger and abduction for the middle, ring and little fingers) points the fingers toward the thumb but also tends to produce ulnar subluxation forces on the MCP joints and on the tendons of the long flexors at the MCP. The subluxing forces are ordinarily counteracted by the radial collateral ligaments and by the annular pulleys that anchor the long tendons in place. These structures are assisted, especially in isometric functions, by the active or passive tension in the EDC. The EDC contraction increases joint compression and enhances joint stability during power grip.[111] Although the location of the lumbricals indicates a possible contribution to MCP flexion in power grip, their lack of EMG activity, regardless of strength grip, is consistent with their role as IP extensors.[73]

Thumb position in cylindrical grip is the most variable of the digits. The thumb usually comes around the object, then flexes and adducts to close the vise. The FPL and the thenar muscles are all active. The activity of the thenar muscles will vary with the width of the web space, with the CMC rotation required, and with increased pressure or resistance. A distinguishing characteristic of power grip over precision handling is the magnitude of activity of the adductor pollicis. The EPL may be variably active as an MCP stabilizer or as an adductor.

Muscles of the hypothenar eminence usually are active in cylindrical grip. The ADM functions as a proximal interosseous muscle to flex and abduct (ulnarly deviate) the fifth MCP joint. The opponens digiti minimi (ODM) and the flexor digiti minimi (FDM) are more variable but frequently reflect the amount of abduction and rotation of the first metacarpal. In fact, increased activity of the OP automatically results in increased activity of the ODM and FDM.

Cylindrical grip is typically performed with the wrist in neutral flexion/extension and slight ulnar deviation. Ulnar deviation also puts the thumb in line with the long axis of the forearm; this alignment better positions the object in the hand to be turned by pronation/supination of the forearm[113] as, for example, in turning a door knob. Ulnar deviation of the wrist is the posi-tion that optimizes force of the long finger flexors. The least flexion force is generated at these joints in wrist flexion.[2] The heavier an object is, the more likely it is that the wrist will ulnarly deviate. Additionally, a strong contraction of the flexor carpi ulnaris at the wrist will increase tension on the flexor retinaculum. This provides a more stable base for the active hypothenar muscles that originate from that ligament. It is interesting to note that regardless of wrist position, the percent of total IP flexor force allocated to each finger is relatively constant. The ring and little fingers can generate only 70% of the flexor force of the index and middle fingers.[2] The ring and little fingers seem to serve as weaker but more mobile assists to the more stable and stronger index and middle fingers. The contribution of the ring and little finger to grip can be improved if full flexion of (and concomitant loss of tension over) the joints in those fingers is prevented by an object that is wider ulnarly than radially (the pistol-grip shape).

Spherical Grip

Spherical grip (see Fig. 9–24b) is similar in most respects to cylindrical grip. The extrinsic finger and thumb flexors and the thenar muscles follow similar patterns of activity and variability. The main distinction can be made by the greater spread of the fingers to encompass the object. This evokes more interosseous activity than is seen in other forms of power grip.[73] The MCP joints do not deviate in the same direction (e.g., ulnarly) but tend to abduct. The phalanges are no longer parallel to each other as they commonly are in cylindrical grip. The MCP abductors must be joined by the adductors to stabilize the joints that are in the loose-packed position of semiflexion. Although flexor activity predominates in the digits as it does in all forms of power grip, the extensors do have a role. The extensors not only provide a balancing force for the flexors but are also essential for smooth and controlled opening of the hand and release of the object. Opening the hand during object approach and object release are primarily an extensor function, calling in the lumbricals, the EDC, and thumb extrinsics.

Hook Grip

Hook grip (see Fig. 9–24a) is actually a specialized form of prehension. It is included in power grip because it has more characteristics of power grip than of precision handling. It is a function primarily of the fingers. It may include the palm but never includes the thumb. It can be sustained for prolonged periods of time as anyone who has carried a briefcase or books at his side or hung onto a commuter strap on a bus or train can attest. The major muscular activity is provided by the FDP and FDS. The load may be sustained completely by one muscle or the other, or by both muscles in concert. This depends on the position of the load relative to the phalanges. If the load is carried more distally so that DIP flexion is mandatory, the FDP must participate. If the load is carried more in the middle of the fingers, the FDS may be sufficient. Some interosseous muscle activity has been demonstrated on EMG, but its purpose is not fully understood. It may help prevent clawing at the MCP joints, although the activity is not evident in every finger.[73] In hook grip the thumb is held in moderate to full extension by thumb extrinsics.

Lateral Prehension

Lateral prehension is a rather unique form of grasp. Contact occurs between two adjacent fingers. The MCP and IP joints are usually maintained in extension as the contiguous MCP joints simultaneously abduct and adduct. This is the only form of prehension in which the extensor musculature plays a part in the maintenance of the posture; the EDC and the lumbricals are active to extend the phalanges. MCP abduction and adduction are performed by the interossei. Lateral prehension is included here as a form of power grip because it involves the static holding of an object that is then moved by the more proximal joints of the upper extremity. Although not a "powerful" grip, neither is lateral prehension used to manipulate objects in the hand. It is generally typified by the holding of a cigarette.

Precision Handling

The positions and muscular requirements of precision handling are somewhat more variable than those of power grip, require much finer motor control, and are more dependent on intact sensation. The thumb is one jaw of what has been termed a two-jaw chuck; the thumb is generally abducted and rotated from the palm. The second and opposing jaw is formed by either the distal tip, the pad, or the

side of a finger. When two fingers oppose the thumb, it is called a three-jaw chuck. The three varieties of precision handling that exemplify this mode are **tip-to-tip prehension** (Fig. 9–25a), **pad-to-pad prehension** (Fig. 925b), and **pad-to-side prehension** (Fig. 9–25c). Each tends to be a dynamic function with relatively little static holding.

Pad-to-Pad Prehension

Pad-to-pad prehension involves opposition of the pad, or pulp, of the thumb to the pad, or pulp, of the finger. It is in the pad of the distal phalanx of each digit that the greatest concentration of tactile corpuscles are found; 80% of precision handling uses this mode of prehension.[1] The finger used in two-jaw chuck is usually the index; in three-jaw chuck the middle finger is added. The MCP and PIP joints of the fingers are partially flexed, with the degree of flexion being dependent on the size of the object being held. The DIP joint may be fully

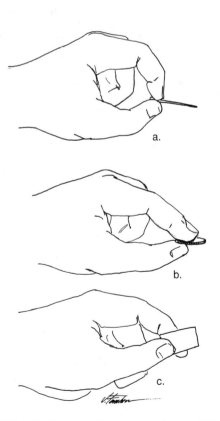

FIGURE 9–25. Three varieties of precision handling: (a) tip-to-tip prehension, (b) pad-to-pad prehension, and (c) pad-to-side prehension.

extended or in slight flexion. When the DIP joint is extended, the FDS alone performs the function without assistance of the FDP. The DIP extension is caused by the pull of the FDS down on the middle phalanx against the pressure of the thumb on the distal phalanx. When partial DIP flexion is required by the task, the FDP must be activated. Interosseous activity is present both in supplementing MCP flexor force and in providing the MCP abduction or adduction required in object manipulation. In dynamic manipulation the VI and DI muscles tend to work reciprocally, rather than in the synergistic co-contraction pattern observed during power grip. In a static but firm pad-to-pad pinch, the interossei may again co-contract.[73]

The thumb in pad-to-pad prehension is held in CMC flexion, abduction, and rotation. The first MCP and IP joints are partially flexed to fully extended. The thenar muscle control is provided by the OP, FPB, and APB, each of which is innervated by the median nerve. The ADP activity (ulnar nerve) increases with increased pressure of pinch. In ulnar nerve paralysis, loss of ADP function (as well as function of the first DI and first VI) renders the thumb less stable.

Fine adjustments in the angulation of the DIP joint of the finger and the IP joint of the thumb provide the control for the points of contact on the pads of the digits. In full finger DIP and thumb IP extension, contact occurs on the more proximal portion of the distal phalanx. As flexion of the finger DIP and thumb IP joint increases, the contact moves distally toward the nails. The flexion, when required, is provided by the FDP for the finger and by the FPL for the thumb. DIP flexion in the finger is accompanied by a proportional flexion in the PIP joint.

As is found in power grip, the extensor musculature is used for opening the hand to grasp, for release, and for stabilization when necessary. In the thumb, the EPL may be used to maintain the IP joint in extension, when contact is light and on the proximal pad. Synergistic wrist activity must also occur to balance the forces created by the FDS and FDP. The wrist is more typically held in neutral radial/ulnar deviation and slight extension.[113]

Tip-to-Tip Prehension

Although the muscular activity found in tip-to-tip prehension is nearly identical to that of pad-to-pad prehension,[73] there is a significant difference. In tip-to-tip prehension the IP joints of the finger and thumb must have the range and available force to create nearly full joint flexion. The MCP joint of the finger must also be ulnarly deviated (with fingertip pointed radially) to present the tip of the finger to the thumb. In the first finger, the ulnar deviation occurs as MCP adduction. In the remaining fingers, MCP abduction produces ulnar deviation. If the flexion range for the distal phalanx in either the finger or the thumb is not available, or if the active force for IP flexion and MCP ulnar deviation (abduction or adduction) cannot be provided, tip-to-tip prehension cannot be performed. As the most precise form of grasp, it is also the most easily disturbed. Tip-to-tip prehension has all the same muscular requirements as pad-to-pad in both fingers and thumb. Additionally, however, tip-to-tip prehension requires activity of the FDP, the FPL, and the interossei; although these muscles may assist in pad-to-pad prehension, they are not required.

Pad-to-Side Prehension

Pad-to-side prehension is also know as **key grip** because a key is held between the pad of the thumb and side of the index finger. Pad-to-side prehension differs from the other forms of precision handling only in that the thumb is more adducted and less rotated. The activity level of the FPB increases and that of the OP decreases, as compared with tip-to-tip prehension. Activity of the adductor pollicis also increases over that seen in either tip-to-tip or pad-to-pad prehension.[11] Slight flexion of the distal phalanx of the thumb is required. If the pad-to-side prehension is being used for something like turning a key, the wrist will again assume neutral flexion/extension and drop into slight ulnar deviation to put the key in line with the forearm so that pronation or supination can be used to turn the key.

Pad-to-side prehension is the least precise of the forms of precision handling; it can actually be performed by a person with paralysis of all hand muscles. If the hand muscles are paralyzed as they would be in a person with a spinal cord injury above the C7 level, active wrist extensors (assuming they are present) can create pad-to-side prehension. The force needed to flex the MCP and IP joints of the fingers and thumb is provided by the passive tension created in the extrinsic tendons as the tendons are stretched over the extending wrist. The grip may be released by allowing gravity to flex the wrist. As the wrist flexes, the extrinsic flexors become slack, and the EDC (EIP, EDM) and EPL become stretched. The passive tension in the extensors in a dropped wrist is adequate to partially extend both MCP and IP joints. The phenomenon of using wrist extension to close the fingers and wrist flexion to open them is known as **tenodesis.** The same tenodesis action can achieve a cylindrical grip if the proper balance of tension exists in the extrinsic flexors. The flexors must be loose enough to permit the partially flexed fingers of the "open" hand to surround the object in wrist flexion while still being tight enough to hold onto the object when the wrist is extended. Active control of a wrist extensor muscle is the minimal requirement for functional use of tenodesis in a person without more distal hand musculature. Tenodesis was described in Chapter 2 when we first discussed passive insufficiency. As was noted then, tenodesis can and does also occur in the fully intact hand although the presence of balancing muscles permits us to override it.

Functional Position of the Wrist and Hand

Although it is difficult to isolate any one joint or function as being singularly important among all those examined, grasp would have to take precedence. There can be little doubt that the hand cannot function either as a manipulator or as a sensory organ unless an object can enter the palmar surface and unless moderate finger flexion and thumb opposition are available to allow sustained contact. Application of either an active muscular or passive tendinous flexor force to the digits requires the wrist to be stabilized in moderate extension and ulnar deviation. Delineation of the so-called functional position of the wrist and hand takes into account these needs and is the position from which optimal function is most likely to occur. It is *not necessarily* the position in which a hand should be immobilized. Position for immobilization depends on the disability.

The functional position is (1) wrist complex in slight extension (20°) and slight ulnar deviation (10°) and (2) fingers moderately flexed at the MCP joint (45°), slightly flexed at the PIP joint (30°), and slightly flexed at the DIP joint.[1]

The wrist position optimizes the power of the finger flexors so that hand closure can be accomplished with the least possible effort. It is also the position in which all wrist muscles are under equal tension. With similar considerations for the position of the joints of the digits, the functional position provides the best opportunity for the disabled hand to interact with the brain that controls it.

Summary

Despite the many articulations that make up the hand and wrist complex, the bony and ligamentous components of these joints have less potential for problems than the musculotendinous structures that cross and act on other joints. The motor control of and sensory feedback from the wrist and hand alone occupy more space topographically on the primary motor and sensory cortices of the brain than does the entire lower extremity. As we proceed to examine the joints of the lower extremity, analogy to the corresponding joints of the upper extremity can and should be made. However, the primary weight-bearing function of the lower extremities does not require the complexity and delicate balance of muscular control that can so profoundly affect functional performance in the hand.

REFERENCES

1. Harty, M: The hand of man. Phys Ther 51:777, 1974.
2. Hazelton, F, et al: The influence of wrist position on the force produced by the finger flexors. Biomechanics 8:301, 1975.
3. Simpson, D: The functioning hand, the human advantage. J R Coll Surg Edinb 21:329, 1976.
4. Lieber, R, and Friden, J: Musculoskeletal balance of the human wrist elucidated using intraoperative laser diffraction. J Electromyogr Kinesiol 8(2):93–100, 1998.
5. Kobayashi, M, et al: Intercarpal kinematics during wrist motion. Hand Clinics 13:143–149, 1997.
6. Ritt, M, et al: Rotational stability of the carpus relative to the forearm. J Hand Surg 20A:305–311, 1995.
7. Garcia-Elias, M, et al: Influence of joint laxity on scaphoid kinematics. J Hand Surg 20B:379–382, 1995.
8. Cailliet, R: Hand Pain and Impairment, ed 4. FA Davis, Philadelphia, 1994.
9. Kapandji, I: The Physiology of the Joints, Vol. 1, ed 5. Churchill Livingstone, Edinburgh and London, 1982.
10. Ryu, J, et al: Functional ranges of motion of the wrist joint. J Hand Surg 16A:409–419, 1991.
11. Gilford, V, et al: The mechanism of the wrist joint. Guy's Hosp Rep 92:52, 1943.
12. Linscheid, R: Kinematic considerations of the wrist. Clin Orthop 202:27–39, 1986.

13. Patterson, R, and Viegas, S: Biomechanics of the wrist. J Hand Ther 8:97–105, 1995.
14. Schuind, F, et al: Force and pressure transmission through the normal wrist. A theoretical two-dimensional study in the posteroanterior plane. J Biomech 28:57–601, 1995.
15. Palmer, AK, and Werner, FW: Biomechanics of the distal radioulnar joint. Clin Orthop 187:26–35, 1984.
16. Mizuseki, T, and Ikuta, Y: The dorsal carpal ligaments: Their anatomy and function. J Hand Surg 14B:91–98, 1989.
17. Mohuiddin, A, and Janjua, M: Form and function of the radioulnar disc. Hand 14:61–66, 1982.
18. Benjamin, M, et al: Histological studies on the triangular fibrocartilage complex of the wrist. J Anat 172:59–67, 1990.
19. Williams, P (ed): Gray's Anatomy, ed. 38. Churchill Livingstone, New York, 1995.
20. Taleisnik, J: Current concepts review: Carpal instability. J Bone Joint Surg 70A:1262–1268, 1988.
21. Viegas, S, and Patterson, R: Load mechanics of the wrist. Hand Clin 13:109–128, 1997.
22. Pevny, T, et al: Ligamentous and tendinous support of the pisiform, anatomy and biomechanical study. J Hand Surg 20A:299–304, 1995.
23. Ritt, M, et al: The gross and histologic anatomy of the ligaments of the capitohamate joint. J Hand Surg 21A:1022–1028, 1996.
24. Ritt, M, et al: The capitohamate ligaments. J Hand Surg 21B:451–454, 1996.
25. Li, G, et al: Carpal kinematics of lunotriquetral dissociations. Biomed Sci Instrum 27:273–281, 1991.
26. Viegas, S, et al: Load mechanics of the midcarpal joint. J Hand Surg 18A:14–18, 1993.
27. Youm, Y, et al: Kinematics of the wrist. I: An experimental study of radial-ulnar deviation and flexion-extension. J Bone Joint Surg 6A:423, 1978.
28. Nowalk, M, and Logan, S: Distinguishing biomechanical properties of intrinsic and extrinsic human wrist ligaments. J Biomech Engr 113:85–93, 1991.
29. Mayfield, J: Wrist ligamentous anatomy and pathogenesis of carpal instability. Orthop Clin North Am 15:209–216, 1984.
30. Blevens, A, et al: Radiocarpal articular contact characteristics with scaphoid instability. J Hand Surg 14A:781–790, 1989.
31. Mayfield, J, et al: The ligaments of the human wrist and their functional significance. Anat Rec 186:417, 1976.
32. Boabighi, A, et al: The distal ligamentous complex of the scaphoid and the scapho-lunate ligament. An anatomic, histological and biomechanical study. J Hand Surg 18B:65–69, 1993.
33. Kauer, J: The interdependence of the carpal articulation chains. Acta Ant 88:481, 1976.
34. Short, W, et al: A dynamic biomechanical study of scapholunate ligament sectioning. J Hand Surg 20A:986–999, 1995.
35. Berger, R: The gross and histologic anatomy of the scapholunate interosseous ligament. J Hand Surg 21A:170–178, 1996.
36. Viegas, S, et al: The dorsal ligaments of the wrist: anatomy, mechanical properties, and function. J Hand Surg 24A:456–468, 1999.
37. Garcia-Elias, M: Kinetic analysis of carpal stability during grip. Hand Clin 13:151–158, 1997.
38. Savelberg, H, et al: Carpal bone kinematics and ligament lengthening studied for the full range of joint movement. J Biomech 26:1389–1402, 1993.
39. Kobayahsi, M, et al: Axial loading induces rotation of the proximal carpal row bones around unique screw-displacement axes. J Biomech 30:1165–1167, 1997.
40. Short, W, et al: Analysis of the kinematics of the scaphoid and lunate in the intact wrist joint. Hand Clin 13:93–108, 1997.
41. Conwell, H: Injuries to the Wrist. CIBA Pharmaceutical, Summit, NJ, 1970.
42. MacConaill, M, and Basmajian, J: Muscles and Movement: A Basis for Human Kinesiology. Williams & Wilkins, Baltimore, 1969.
43. Wright, R: A detailed study of movement of the wrist joint. J Anat 70:137, 1935.
44. Kauer, J: The mechanism of the carpal joint. Clin Orthop 202:16–26, 1986.
45. Sarrafian, S: Functional characteristics of the foot and plantar aponeurosis under tibiotalar loading. Foot Ankle 8:4–18, 1987.
46. Fisk, G: Carpal instability and the fractured scaphoid. Ann R Coll Surg (Engl) 46:63, 1970.
47. MacConaill, M: The mechanical anatomy of the carpus and its bearing on some surgical problems. J Anat 75:166, 1941.
48. Brumfield, RH, and Champoux, JA: A biomechanical study of normal functional wrist motion. Clin Orthop 187:23, 1984.
49. Steindler, A: Kinesiology of the Human Body. Charles C. Thomas, Springfield, IL, 1955.
50. Moore, K, and Dalley, AI: Clinically Oriented Anatomy, ed 4. Lippincott Williams & Wilkins, Philadelphia, 1999.
51. Backdahl, M, and Carlsoo, S: Distribution of activity in muscles acting on the wrist. Acta Morph Neer Scand 4:136, 1961.
52. Ketchum, L, et al: The determination of moments for extension of the wrist generated by muscles of the forearm. J Hand Surg 3:105, 1978.
53. Radonjic, F, and Long, C: Kinesiology of the wrist. Am J Phys Med 50:57, 1971.
54. Perry, J: Normal upper extremity kinesiology. Phys Ther 58:265, 1978.
55. Tang, J, et al: The triangular fibrocartilage complex: An important component of the pulley for the ulnar wrist flexor. J Hand Surg 23A:986–991, 1998.
56. Boivin, J, et al: Electromyographic kinesiology of the hand: Muscles driving the index finger. Arch Phys Med Rehabil 50:17, 1969.
57. Romdhane, L, et al: Experimental investigation of the scaphoid strain during wrist motion. J Biomech 23:1277–1284, 1990.
58. Ranney, D: The hand as a concept: digital differences and their importance. Clin Anat 8:281–287, 1995.
59. Cobb, T, et al: Anatomy of the flexor retinaculum. J Hand Surg 18A:91–99, 1993.
60. Garcia-Elias, M, et al: Stability of the transverse carpal arch: An experimental study. J Hand Surg 14A:277–282, 1989.
61. Batmanabane, M, and Malathi, S: Movements at the carpometacarpal and metacarpophalangeal joints of the hand and their effect on the dimensions of the articular ends of the metacarpal bones. Anat Rec 213:1002–1010, 1985.
62. Joseph, R, et al: Chronic sprains of the carpometacarpal joints. J Hand Surg 6:172–180, 1981.
63. Al-Qattan, M, and Robertson, G: An anatomical study of the deep transverse metacarpal ligament. J Anat 12:443–446, 1993.

64. Kaplan, E: The participation of the metacarpopha-langeal joint of the thumb in the act of opposition. Bull Hosp Joint Dis 27:39, 1966.

65. Benjamin, M, et al: Capsular tissues of the proximal interphalangeal joint: Normal composition and effects of Dupuytren's disease and rheumatoid arthritis. J Hand Surg 18B:370–376, 1993.

66. Shultz, R, et al: Metacarpophalangeal joint motion and the role of the collateral ligaments. Intern Orthop (SICOT) 11:149–155, 1987.

67. Fisher, D, et al: Descriptive anatomy of fibrocartilaginous menisci in the finger joints of the hand. J Orthop Res 3:484–491, 1985.

68. Cailliet, R: Scoliosis: Diagnosis and Management. FA Davis, Philadelphia, 1975.

69. Minamikwa, Y, et al: Stability and constraint of the proximal interphalangeal joint. J Hand Surg 18A:198–204, 1993.

70. Rhee, R, et al: A biomechanical study of the collateral ligaments of the proximal interphalangeal joint. J Hand Surg 17A:157–163, 1992.

71. Dzwierzynski, W, et al: Biomechanics of the intact and surgically repaired proximal interphalangeal joint collateral ligaments. J Hand Surg 21A:679–683, 1996.

72. Long, C: Intrinsic-extrinsic muscle control of the fingers. J Bone Joint Surg 50A:973, 1968.

73. Long, C, et al: Intrinsic-extrinsic muscle control of the hand in power grip and precision handling. J Bone Joint Surg 52A:853, 1970.

74. Brook, N, et al: A biomechanical model of index finger dynamics. Med Eng Phys 17:54–63, 1993.

75. Hamman, J, et al: A biomechanical study of the flexor digitorum superficialis: Effects of digital pulley excision and loss of the flexor digitorum profundus. J Hand Surg 22A:328–335, 1997.

76. Baker, D, et al: The little finger superficialis. Clinical investigation of its anatomic and functional shortcomings. J Hand Surg 6:374–378, 1981.

77. Phillips, C, et al: The flexor synovial sheath anatomy of the little finger: A macroscopic study. J Hand Surg 20A:636–641, 1995.

78. Lin, G, et al: Functional anatomy of the human digital flexor pulley system. J Hand Surg 14A:949–956, 1989.

79. Phillips, C, and Mass, D: Mechanical analysis of the palmar aponeurosis pulley in human cadavers. J Hand Surg 21A:240–244, 1996.

80. Hunter, J, et al: Rehabilitation of the Hand: Surgery and Therapy, Vol. I, ed 4. CV Mosby, St. Louis, 1995.

81. Mester, S, et al: Biomechanics of the human flexor tendon sheath investigated by tenography. J Hand Surg 20B:500–504, 1995.

82. Rispler, D, et al: Efficiency of the flexor tendon pulley system in human cadaver hands. J Hand Surg 21A:444–450, 1996.

83. Manske, P, and Lesker, P: Palmar aponeurosis pulley. J Hand Surg 8:259–263, 1983.

84. Gonzalez, M, et al: Anatomy of the extensor tendons to the index finger. J Hand Surg 21A:988–991, 1996.

85. von Schroeder, H, and Botte, M: Anatomy of the extensor tendons of the fingers: Variations and multiplicity. J Hand Surg 20A:27–34, 1995.

86. El-Badawi, M, et al: Extensor tendons of the fingers: Arrangement and variations. II. Clin Anat 8:391–398, 1995.

87. Gonzalez, M, et al: The extensor tendons to the little finger: An anatomic study. J Hand Surg 20A:844–847, 1995.

88. Van Sint Jan, S et al: The insertion of the extensor digitorum tendon on the proximal phalanx. J Hand Surg 21A:69–76, 1996.

89. von Schroeder, H, and Botte, M: The functional significance of the long extensors and juncturae tendinum in finger extension. J Hand Surg 18A:641–647, 1993.

90. Brand, P: Paralytic claw hand. J Bone Joint Surg 40B:618, 1958.

91. El-Gammel, T, et al: Anatomy of the oblique retinacular ligament of the index finger. J Hand Surg 18A:717–721, 1993.

92. Salisbury, C: The interosseous muscles of the hand. J Anat 71:395, 1936.

93. Stack, H: Muscle function in the fingers. J Bone Joint Surg 44B:899, 1962.

94. Ranney, D, and Wells, R: Lumbrical muscle function as revealed by a new and physiological approach. Anat Rec 222:110–114, 1988.

95. Landsmeer, J: The anatomy of the dorsal aponeurosis of the human fingers and its functional significance. Anat Rec 104:31, 1949.

96. Mardel, S, and Underwood, M: Adductor pollicis. The missing interosseous. Surg Radiol Anat 13:49–52, 1991.

97. Eyler, D, and Markee, J: The anatomy and function of the intrinsic musculature of the fingers. J Bone Joint Surg 36A:1, 1954.

98. Brand, P, and Hollister, A: Clinical Mechanics of the Hand, ed. 2. Mosby Year Book, St. Louis, 1993.

99. Close, J, and Kidd, C: The functions of the muscles of the thumb, the index and the long fingers. J Bone Joint Surg 51A:1601, 1969.

100. Backhouse, K, and Catton, W: An experimental study of the functions of the lumbrical muscles in the human hand. J Anat 88:133, 1954.

101. Leijnse, H, and Kalker, J: A two-dimensional kinematic model of the lumbrical in the human finger. J Biomech 28:237–249, 1995.

102. Ketchum, L, et al: A clinical study of the forces generated by the intrinsic muscles of the index finger and extrinsic flexor and extensor muscles of the hand. J Hand Surg 3:571, 1978.

103. Zancolli, E, et al: Biomechanics of the trapeziometacarpal joint. Clin Orthop 220:14–26, 1987.

104. Cooney, W, et al: The kinesiology of the thumb trapeziometacarpal joint. J Bone Joint Surg 63A:1371–1380, 1981.

105. Pagalidis, T, et al: Ligamentous stability of the base of the thumb. Hand 13:29–35, 1981.

106. Kauer, J: Functional anatomy of the carpometacarpal joint of the thumb. Clin Orthop 220:7–13, 1987.

107. Ateshian, G, et al: Curvature characteristics and congruence of the thumb carpometacarpal joint: Differences between female and male joints. J Biomech 25:591–607, 1992.

108. Goldberg, I, and Nathan, H: Anatomy and pathology of the sesamoid bones. Int Orthop (SICOT) 11:141–147, 1987.

109. Johanson, M, et al: Phasic relationships of the intrinsic and extrinsic thumb musculature. Clin Orthop 322:120–130, 1996.

110. Belanger, A, and Noel, G: Force-generating capacity of thumb adductor muscles in the parallel and perpendicular plane of adduction. J Orthop Sports Phys Ther 21:139–146, 1995.

111. Chao, E, et al: Three-dimensional force analysis of the

finger joints in selected isometric hand functions. J Biomech 9:387, 1976.

112. Landsmeer, J: Power grip and precision handling. Ann Rheum Dis 22:164, 1962.

113. Bejjani, F, and Landsmeer, J. In Nordin, M and Frankel, V (eds): Basic Biomechanics of the Musculoskeletal System. Lea & Febiger, Philadelphia, 1989.

114. Kozin, S, et al: The contribution of the intrinsic muscles to grip and pinch strength. J Hand Surg 24A: 64–72, 1999.

Study Questions

1. Name the bones of the wrist complex; describe the articulations that occur between these bones and the functional joints that are formed.

2. Describe the components and role of the triangular fibrocartilage complex in wrist function.

3. What is the total ROM normally available at the wrist complex? How are the motions distributed between the radiocarpal and midcarpal joints of the complex?

4. Describe the sequence of carpal motion occurring from full wrist flexion to full extension, emphasizing the role of the scaphoid.

5. What effect does release of the scapholunate stabilizers or of the lunotriquetral stabilizers have on wrist position?

6. Identify the muscles that can extend the wrist; include the joints crossed, actions produced, and activity levels of each.

7. Describe the transverse carpal ligament, its attachments, and its role in wrist and hand function.

8. What is the function of the CMC joints of the fingers? How do the variations in ROM among the four CMC joints of the fingers contribute to function?

9. What role does the transverse metacarpal ligament play at the CMC joint? What role at the MCP joint?

10. Describe the locations and functions of the volar fibrocartilage plates.

11. What MCP joint position is most prone to injury and why?

12. Compare the joint structure of the MCP joints with that of the IP joints of the fingers. Identify both similarities and differences.

13. Describe the mechanisms, joint motions, and muscles that are necessary for the fingers to gently close into the palm without friction or loss of length-tension.

14. How does the "pistol-grip" design of most tools (larger ulnarly) relate to the MCP ROM and muscular function of the four fingers?

15. When is the FDS active as the primary finger flexor? When does it back up the FDP?

16. What muscles are active in gentle closure of the normal hand? What role, if any, do the intrinsic muscles play in this activity?

17. What wrist position is assumed when one needs to optimize finger flexion strength? Which wrist position is least effective for grasp?

18. What are annular pulleys and cruciate ligaments in the digits? Where are they found, and what functions do they serve?

19. Identify the bursae of the hand. What are their functions and how are they most typically related to the digital tendon sheaths?

20. Describe the active and passive elements that make up the extensor mechanism.

21. What role do the EDC, EIP, and EDM play in active extension of the PIP and DIP joints of the hand?

22. Describe the proximal and distal wing tendons of the interossei, including on which fingers they are located. How do the two different attachments affect function at the MCP and IP joints?

23. Describe the attachments of the lumbricals to the extensor mechanism. How do these muscles contribute to IP extension? What is their role at the MCP joint?

24. Why is active DIP flexion normally accompanied by PIP flexion at the same time?

25. Explain why the DIP cannot be actively extended if the PIP is fully flexed.

26. Why will an isolated contraction of the EDC produce flexion of the PIP and DIP joints? What is this finger position called?

27. How are the extrinsic flexors and extensors stabilized at the MCP joints?

28. Why is finger extension weaker in the index and little fingers?

29. Why does MCP adduction weaken more quickly than abduction in a progressive ulnar nerve problem?

30. Which are stronger flexors of the MCP joint, the lumbricals or the interossei?

31. Compare and contrast the MCP joint structure of the thumb with the MCP joint structure of the fingers.

32. What does the motion of thumb opposition require in terms of joint function and musculature?

33. What are the primary muscles of release in the wrist and hand?

34. In general, what is the difference between power grip and precision handling at the wrist, in the fingers and in the thumb? What do these two forms of prehension have in common?

35. Cylindrical grip is generally referred to as an extrinsic hand function. Why is this true?

36. What requirement does spherical grip have that differentiates it from cylindrical?

37. Which form of prehension requires only intrinsic musculature?

38. Which forms of prehension do not require the thumb?

39. What roles do interossei play in precision handling?

40. What requirements does tip-to-tip prehension have that are not necessary for pad-to-pad?

41. What is the finest (most precise) form of prehension that can be accomplished by someone without intact hand musculature, assuming availability of an active wrist extensor?

42. What is the functional position of the wrist and hand? Why is this the optimal resting position when there is no specific hand problem?

43. Why is an ulnar nerve injury called "claw hand"? What deficiency causes the clawing and in which fingers does it occur?

CHAPTER 10
THE HIP COMPLEX

· ·

· ·

OBJECTIVES
Following the study of this chapter, the reader should be able to:

Describe
1. The articulating surfaces of the pelvis and femur.
2. The structure and function of the trabecular systems of the pelvis and femur.
3. The structure and function of the ligaments of the hip joint.
4. The angle of inclination and angle of torsion.
5. The planes and axes of the following pelvic motions and the accompanying motions at the lumbar spine and hip joints: pelvic rotation and anterior, posterior, and lateral tilting of the pelvis.
6. The muscle activity that produces tilting and rotation of the pelvis.
7. Motions of the femur on the pelvis including planes and axes of motion.
8. The structure and function of all the muscles associated with the hip joints.
9. The forces that act on the head of the femur.
10. The position of greatest stability at the hip.
11. The position of greatest articular contact.

Explain
1. How sagittal and frontal plane equilibrium are maintained in erect bilateral stance.
2. How frontal plane equilibrium is achieved in unilateral stance.
3. Three ways to reduce forces acting on the femoral head.
4. How the function of the two-joint muscles at the hip are affected by changes in the position of the knee and hip.
5. The functional and structural relationship among the hip, knee, pelvis, and lumbar spine.

Compare

1. The forces acting on the femoral head in erect bilateral stance with the forces acting on the head in erect unilateral stance.
2. Coxa valga with coxa vara on the basis of hip joint stability and mobility.
3. Anteversion with retroversion on the basis of hip stability and mobility.
4. The motions that occur at the hip, pelvis, and lumbar spine during forward trunk bending with the motions that occur during anterior and posterior tilting of the pelvis in the erect standing position.
5. The structure and function of the following muscles: flexors and extensors, abductors and adductors, lateral and medial rotators.
6. The forces across the hip joint produced by using a cane on the same side as hip pain and using a cane on the side opposite hip pain.

Introduction

The hip joint, or **coxofemoral joint,** is the articulation of the acetabulum of the pelvis and the head of the femur. These two segments form a diarthrodial ball-and-socket joint with 3° of freedom: flexion/extension in the sagittal plane, abduction/adduction in the frontal plane, and medial/lateral rotation in the transverse plane. Although it is tempting to draw an analogy between the hip joint and the shoulder complex, the functional and structural adaptations of each to their respective roles has been so extensive that such comparisons are more of general interest than of functional relevance. The role of the shoulder complex is to provide a stable base on which a wide range of mobility for the hand can be superimposed. Shoulder complex structure gives precedence to open chain function. The primary function of the hip joint is to support the weight of the head, arms, and trunk (HAT) both in static erect posture and in dynamic postures such as ambulation, running, and stair climbing. The hip joint, like the other joints of the lower extremity that we will examine, is primarily structured to serve its weight-bearing functions. Although we examine hip joint structure and function as if the joint were designed to move the foot through space in an open chain, hip joint structure is more influenced by the demands placed on it when the limb is bearing weight. As we shall see later in this chapter, weight-bearing function of the hip joint and its related closed chain responses are basic to understanding the hip joint and the interactions that occur between the hip joint and the other joints of the spine and lower extremities.

Structure of the Hip Joint

Proximal Articular Surface

The cuplike concave socket of the hip joint is called the **acetabulum** and is located on the lateral aspect of the pelvic bone (**innominate** or **os coxa**). Three bones form the pelvis: the ilium, the ischium, and the pubis. Each of the three bones contributes to the structure of the acetabulum (Fig. 10–1). The pubis forms one-fifth of the acetabulum, the ischium two-fifths, and the ilium the remainder. Until full ossification of the pelvis occurs between 20 and 25 years of age, the separate segments of the acetabulum may remain visible.[1] The acetabulum appears to be a hemisphere, but only its upper

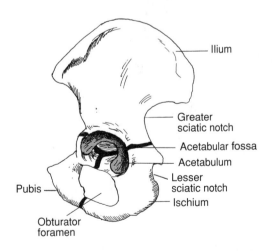

FIGURE 10–1. The acetabulum is formed by the union of the three bones of the pelvis, with only the upper horseshoe-shaped area being articular.

margin has a true circular contour,[2] and the roundness of the acetabulum as a whole decreases with age.[3] In actuality, only a horse-shoe-shaped portion of the periphery of the acetabulum (the **lunate surface**) is covered with hyaline cartilage and articulates with the head of the femur (see Fig. 10–1). The inferior aspect of the lunate surface (the base of the horseshoe) is interrupted by a deep notch called the **acetabular notch.** The acetabular notch is spanned by a fibrous band, the **transverse acetabular ligament,** that connects the two ends of the horseshoe. The transverse acetabular ligament also spans the acetabular notch to create a fibro-osseous tunnel beneath the ligament through which blood vessels may pass into the central or deepest portion of the acetabulum, called the **acetabular fossa.** The acetabular fossa is nonarticular; the femoral head does not contact this surface (Fig. 10–2). The acetabular fossa contains fibroelastic fat covered with synovial membrane.

Center Edge Angle of the Acetabulum

Although the acetabulum is oriented on each innominate to face laterally, it is also directed somewhat inferiorly and anteriorly. The magnitude of inferior orientation can be assessed using a line connecting the lateral rim of the acetabulum and the center of the femoral head. This line forms an angle with the vertical known as the **center edge (CE) angle** or the **angle of Wiberg** (see Fig. 10–2) and is the amount of inferior tilt of the acetabulum. Using computed tomography, Adna and associates[4] found CE angles in adults to average 38° in men and 35° in women (with ranges in both sexes to be about 22° to 42°). These values are in reasonable agreement with those ascertained by Brinckmann and associates[5] using roentgenograms, although the average values for men and women were the same in their larger sample. The similarity of the CE angle between men and women is somewhat surprising given the increased diameter and more vertical orientation of the sides of the female pelvis.[6] A smaller CE angle (or more vertical orientation) of the acetabulum may result in diminished coverage of the head of the femur and an increased risk of superior dislocation of the head of the femur. Because evidence indicates that the CE angle increases with age,[7] the implication is that children have less coverage over the head of the femur and therefore decreased joint stability as compared to adults. In fact, congenital dislocation is more common at the hip joint than at any other joint in the body.[6] This may be caused by deficiencies in the superior acetabulum (a diminished CE angle).

Acetabular Anteversion

The acetabulum not only faces somewhat inferiorly but also anteriorly. The magnitude of anterior orientation of the acetabulum may be referred to as the **angle of acetabular anteversion.** Adna and associates[4] found the average value to be 18.5° for men and 21.5° for women, although Kapandji[8] cites larger values of 30° to 40°. Pathologic increases in the angle of acetabular anteversion are associated with decreased joint stability and increased tendency for anterior dislocation of the head of the femur.

Acetabular Labrum

Given the need for stability at the hip joint, it is not surprising to find an accessory joint structure. The entire periphery of the acetabulum is rimmed by a ring of wedge-shaped fibrocartilage called the **acetabular labrum** (see labrum cross-section in Fig. 10–2). The acetabular labrum not only deepens the socket but in-

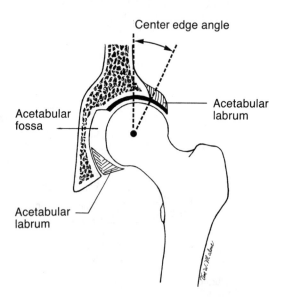

Center edge angle

Acetabular labrum

Acetabular fossa

Acetabular labrum

FIGURE 10–2. The center edge angle of the acetabulum is formed between a vertical line through the center of the femoral head and a line connecting the center of the femoral head and the bony edge of the acetabulum. The acetabular labrum deepens the acetabulum.

creases the concavity of the acetabulum through its triangular shape and grasps the head of the femur to maintain contact with the acetabulum. The transverse acetabular ligament is considered to be part of the acetabular labrum although, unlike the labrum, it contains no cartilage cells.[6]

Distal Articular Surface

The head of the femur is a fairly rounded hyaline cartilage-covered surface that may be slightly larger than a true hemisphere or as much as two-thirds of a sphere depending on body type.[8] The head of the femur is considered to be circular, unlike the more irregularly shaped acetabulum.[3] The radius of curvature of the femoral head is smaller in women than in men when compared to the dimensions of the pelvis.[5] Just inferior to the most medial point on the femoral head is a small roughened pit called the **fovea** or **fovea capitis** (Fig. 10–3). The fovea is not covered with articular cartilage and is the point at which the ligament of the head of the femur is attached.

The femoral head is attached to the femoral neck; the femoral neck is attached to the shaft of the femur between the greater trochanter and the lesser trochanter (see Fig. 10–3). Although the femoral neck is more distinct than the neck of the humerus, it is generally only about 5 cm long.[6] The femoral neck is angulated so that the femoral head most commonly

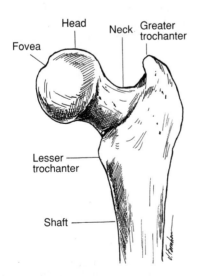

FIGURE 10–3. An anterior view of the proximal portion of the left femur shows the relationship between the head, neck, and femoral shaft.

faces medially, superiorly, and anteriorly. Although the angulation of the femoral head and neck is more consistent across the population than that of the humerus, there are still substantial individual differences and differences from side to side in the same individual.

Angulation of the Femur

There are two angulations made by the head and neck of the femur relative to the shaft. One angulation (**angle of inclination**) occurs in the frontal plane between an axis through the femoral head and neck and the longitudinal axis of the femoral shaft. The other angulation (**angle of torsion**) occurs in the transverse plane between an axis through the femoral head and neck and an axis through the distal femoral condyles. The origin and variability of these angulations can be understood in the context of the embryonic development of the lower limb. In the early stages of fetal development, both upper extremity and lower extremity limb buds project laterally from the body as if in full abduction. During the seventh and eighth weeks of gestational age and before full definition of the joints, adduction of the buds begins. At the end of the eighth week, the "fetal position" has been achieved, but the upper and lower limbs are no longer positioned similarly. Although the upper limb buds have torsioned somewhat laterally (bringing the ventral surface of the limb bud anteriorly), the lower limb buds have torsioned medially so that the ventral surface faces posteriorly.[9] The result for the lower limb is critical to understanding function. The knee flexes in the opposite direction from the elbow and the extensor (dorsal) surface of the limb is anteriorly rather than posteriorly located. The head and neck of the femur retain the original position of the limb bud; the shaft is inclined medially and medially torsioned with respect to the head and neck. The magnitude of medial inclination and torsion of the distal femur (with respect to the head and neck) is dependent on embryonic growth and, presumably, fetal positioning during the remaining months of uterine life. The development of the angulations of the femur appears to continue after birth and through the early years of development.

ANGLE OF INCLINATION OF THE FEMUR

The angle of inclination of the femur in early infancy is about 150° (referencing the medial

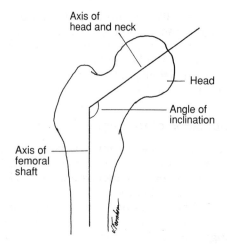

FIGURE 10–4. The axis of the femoral head and neck form an angle with the axis of the femoral shaft called the **angle of inclination**. This angle, measured medially, is approximately 125° in the adult.

angle formed by the axes of the head/neck and the shaft). The inclination decreases to an average of 125° in the normal adult (Fig. 10–4) and to about 120° in the normal elderly person.[10,11] The angle of inclination varies among individuals and between sexes. In women, the angle is somewhat smaller than it is in men, owing to the greater width of the female pelvis.[6] With a normal angle of inclination, the greater tro-chanter lies at the level of the center of the femoral head.[12] A pathologic increase in the medial angulation between the neck and shaft is called **coxa valga** (Fig. 10–5a), and a pathologic decrease is called **coxa vara** (Fig. 10–5b).

ANGLE OF TORSION OF THE FEMUR

The angle of torsion of the femur can best be viewed by looking down the length of the femur from top to bottom. An axis through the femoral head and neck will lie at an angle to an axis through the femoral condyles. This angulation reflects the twist in the bone that occurred during fetal development. However, rather than being seen as medial torsion of the femoral condyles (as occurs in the limb bud), the *normal* torsion in the femur is evident as anterior torsion (anterior twisting) of the head and neck of the femur (Fig. 10–6). The apparent reversal of perspective from distal to proximal occurs because the axis through the femoral condyles (which is also the knee joint axis) is normally aligned in the frontal plane (allowing the knee to flex and extend in the sagittal plane). If the axis through the femoral condyles lies in the frontal plane, then it appears that the head and neck of the femur are torsioned anteriorly on the femoral condyles, rather than the distal femoral condyles torsioned medially on the head and neck. The angle of torsion (which may also be known as the angle of anteversion) decreases with age. In the newborn, the angle of torsion is approximately 40°, decreasing substantially in the first 2 years.[13] Svenningsen and associates[7] found a decrease of approximately 1.5° per year until cessation of growth among children with both normal and exaggerated angles of anteversion. In the adult, the angle of torsion is normally 10° to 15°, but may vary from 7° to 30°.[6,8]

A pathologic increase in the angle of torsion is called **anteversion** (Fig. 10–7a), and a patho-

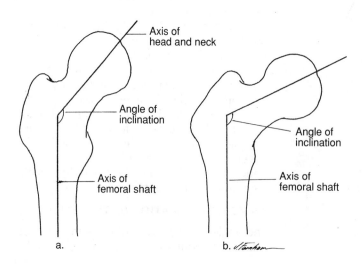

a.   b.

FIGURE 10–5. Abnormal angles of inclination. (a) A pathologic increase in the angle of inclination is called **coxa valga**. (b) A pathologic decrease in the angle is called **coxa vara**.

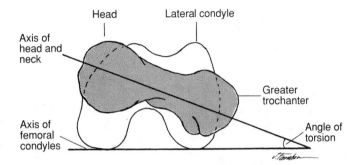

FIGURE 10–6. A line parallel to the posterior femoral condyles and a line through the head and neck of the femur normally make an angle with each other that averages 15° in the normal adult. The femoral head and neck are twisted anteriorly with respect to the femoral condyles.

logic decrease in the angle or reversal of torsion is known as **retroversion** (Fig. 10–7b).

Both normal and abnormal angles of inclination and torsion are *properties of the femur and exist independently of the hip joint.* However, abnormalities in the angulations of the femur can cause compensatory hip changes and can substantially alter hip joint stability, the weight-bearing biomechanics of the hip joint, and muscle biomechanics. Although some structural deviations such as femoral anteversion and coxa valga are commonly found together, each may occur independently of the other. Each structural deviation warrants careful consideration as to the impact on hip joint func-

tion *and* function of the joints both proximal and distal to the hip joint. As shall be evident when the knee and foot are discussed in subsequent chapters, femoral anteversion can create substantial dysfunction at both the knee and at the foot. The impact of abnormal angulations in the femur in hip joint function also will be discussed later in this chapter in the section on hip joint pathology.

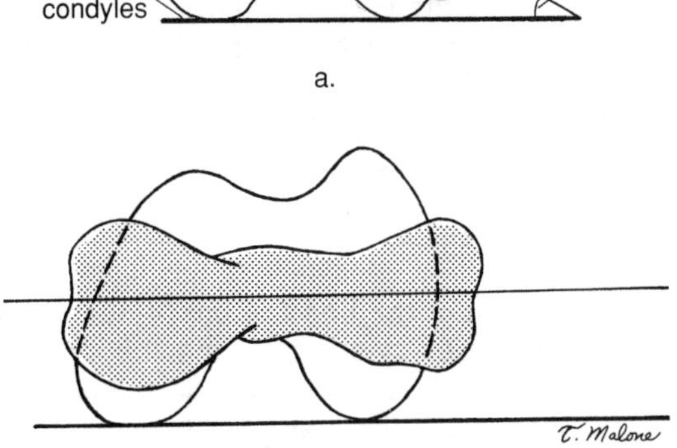

Articular Congruence of the Hip Joint

The hip joint is considered to be a congruent joint. Although this is relatively true, there is substantially more articular surface on the head of the femur than on the acetabulum. In the neutral or standing position, the articular surface of the femoral head remains exposed anteriorly and somewhat superiorly (Fig. 10–8a). Although the superiorly angled femoral head (angle of inclination) would appear to fit the inferiorly oriented acetabulum, this is not entirely the case. The acetabulum does not fully cover the head superiorly. The anterior torsion of the femoral head (angle of torsion) is poorly matched to the anterior orientation of the acetabulum, exposing a substantial amount of the femoral head's articular surface anteriorly. Structural deviations such as femoral anteversion, coxa valga, or a shallow acetabulum (decreased center edge angle) can result in increased articular exposure of the femoral head, less congruence, and reduced stability of the hip joint in the neutral (standing) position. Articular contact between the femur and the acetabulum can be increased in the normal hip joint by a combination of flexion, abduction, and slight lateral rotation[8] (Fig. 10–8b). This position (also known as the frog-leg position) corresponds to that assumed by the hip joint in a quadruped position and, according to Ka-

FIGURE 10–7. Abnormal angles of torsion in a right femur. (a) A pathologic increase in the angle of torsion is called **anteversion**. (b) A pathologic decrease in the normal angle of torsion is called **retroversion**.

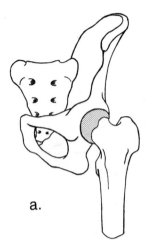
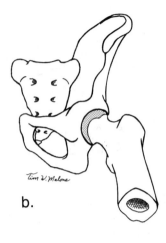

FIGURE 10–8. (a) In the neutral hip joint, articular cartilage from the head of the femur is exposed anteriorly and to a lesser extent superiorly. (b) Maximum articular contact of the head of the femur with the acetabulum is obtained when the femur is flexed, abducted, and laterally rotated slightly.

pandji,[8] is the true physiologic position of the hip joint. The position of combined flexion, abduction, and rotation is commonly used for immobilization of the hip joint when the goal is to improve articular contact and joint congruence in conditions such as congenital dislocation of the hip and in Legg-Calvé-Perthes disease.[14]

Articular contact within the hip joint is not based on joint position alone but is also affected by weight-bearing. We will examine the weight-bearing effects on the hip joint after examining the hip joint capsule and ligaments. An additional factor in articular congruence and coaptation of joint surfaces, however, is actually contributed by the nonarticular and non-weight-bearing portion of the acetabulum. The acetabular fossa may be important in setting up a partial vacuum in the joint so that atmospheric pressure contributes to stability by helping to maintain contact between the femoral head and the acetabulum. Wingstrand and colleagues[15] concluded that atmospheric pressure in hip flexion activities played a stronger role in stabilization than capsuloligamentous structures. It is also true that the head and acetabulum will remain together in an anesthetized patient even after the joint capsule has been opened. The pressure within the joint must be broken before the hip can be dislocated.[8]

Hip Joint Capsule and Ligaments

Hip Joint Capsule

The articular capsule of the hip is strong and dense. Unlike the relatively weak articular capsule of the shoulder, the hip joint capsule is a substantial contributor to joint stability. The capsule is attached proximally to the entire periphery of the acetabulum beyond the acetabular labrum.[6] The capsule covers the femoral head and neck like a sleeve and attaches to the base of the neck. The femoral neck is intracapsular, whereas the greater and lesser trochanters are both extracapsular. The synovial membrane lines the inside of the capsule. The capsule has two sets of fibers: The longitudinal fibers are more superficial and the circular fibers are deeper. The circular fibers form a collar around the femoral neck called the **zona orbicularis.** The capsule itself is thickened anterosuperiorly where the predominant stresses occur; it is relatively thin and loosely attached posteroinferiorly.[6] Anteriorly, there are longitudinal **retinacular fibers** deep in the capsule that travel along the neck toward the femoral head.[6] The retinacular fibers carry blood vessels that are the major source of nutrition to the femoral head and neck.[1] The retinacular blood vessels arise from a vascular ring located at the base of the neck and formed by the medial and lateral circumflex arteries (branches of the deep femoral artery).

Hip Joint Ligaments

The **ligament of the head of the femur** or **ligamentum teres** is an intra-articular but extrasynovial accessory joint structure. The ligament is a triangularly shaped band with its base on both sides of the peripheral edge of the acetabular notch. From there, the ligament passes under and blends with the transverse acetabular ligament to attach at its apex to the fovea of the femur (Fig. 10–9). The ligament of

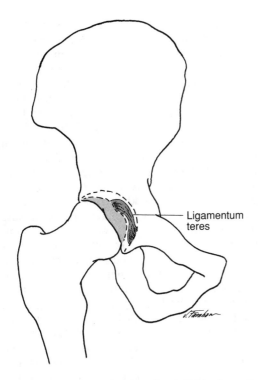

FIGURE 10–9. An anterior view of a right hip shows the centrally located ligamentum teres arising from the fovea on the femoral head. The joint capsule and other structures have been removed.

the head is encased in a flattened sleeve of synovial membrane so that it does not communicate with the synovial cavity of the joint. The material properties of the ligament of the head are similar to those of other ligaments,[16] and it is tensed in semiflexion and adduction.[6] However, it does not appear to play a significant role in joint stabilization regardless of joint position.[17] Rather, the ligament of the head appears to function primarily as a conduit for the secondary blood supply from the obturator artery and for the nerves that travel along the ligament to reach the head of the femur through the fovea. The importance of the secondary blood supply will vary across the life span, with a greater contribution to be made in childhood. While a child is still growing, the primary retinacular vessels cannot travel through the avascular cartilaginous epiphysis, but must travel across the surface where the vessels are more vulnerable to disruption. Crock[18] proposed that the femoral head was supplied predominantly by the blood vessels of the ligament of the head until bony maturation and epiphyseal closure. However, Tan and Wong[19]

found the ligament absent in 10% of their examined specimens. The vessels of the ligament of the head are commonly sclerosed in the elderly.[1] In the elderly, therefore, the secondary blood supply cannot be counted on to back up the primary retinacular supply when that supply is disrupted by such problems as femoral neck fracture.[19] The absence of a secondary blood supply to the head increases the risk of avascular necrosis of the femoral head with femoral neck trauma.

The hip joint capsule is typically considered to have three reinforcing capsular ligaments (two anteriorly and one posteriorly), although some investigators have further divided or otherwise renamed the ligaments.[8,17] For purposes of understanding hip joint function, the following three traditional descriptions would appear to suffice. The two anterior ligaments are the **iliofemoral ligament** and the **pubofemoral ligament.** The iliofemoral ligament is a fan-shaped ligament that resembles an inverted letter Y (Fig. 10–10). It often is referred to as the **Y ligament of Bigelow.** The apex of the ligament is attached to the anterior inferior

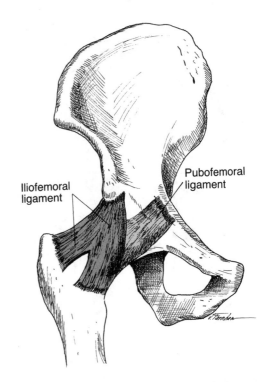

FIGURE 10–10. An anterior view of the right hip joint shows the two bands of the iliofemoral (Y) ligament and the more inferiorly located pubofemoral ligament.

iliac spine, and the two arms of the Y fan out to attach along the intertrochanteric line of the femur. The superior band of the iliofemoral ligament is the strongest and thickest of the hip joint ligaments.[8] The pubofemoral ligament (see Fig. 10–10) is also anteriorly located, arising from the anterior aspect of the pubic ramus and passing to the anterior surface of the intertrochanteric fossa. The bands of the iliofemoral and the pubofemoral ligaments form a Z on the anterior capsule similar to that of the glenohumeral ligaments. The **ischiofemoral ligament** is the posterior capsular ligament. The ischiofemoral ligament (Fig. 10–11) attaches to the posterior surface of the acetabular rim and the acetabulum labrum. Some of its fibers spiral around the femoral neck and blend with the fibers of the zona orbicularis. Other fibers are arranged horizontally and attach to the inner surface of the greater trochanter.

There is at the hip joint, as at other joints, some disagreement as to the roles of the joint ligaments. Fuss and Bacher[17] provide an excellent summary of the similarities and discrepancies to be found among of a number of investigators. It may be sufficient to conclude,

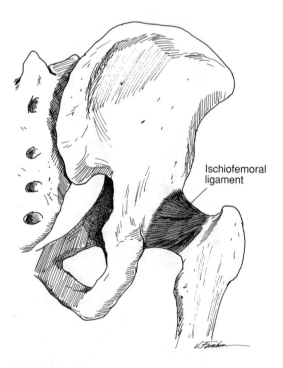

FIGURE 10–11. A posterior view of a right hip joint shows that the spiral fibers of this ligament are tightened during hyperextension and therefore limit hyperextension.

Ischiofemoral ligament

however, that each of the hip joint motions will be checked by at least one portion of one of the hip joint ligaments.[17] More functionally relevant is the consensus that the hip joint capsule and the majority of its ligaments are quite strong. The capsule and ligaments permit little or no joint distraction even under strong traction forces. The joint is also difficult to traumatically dislocate (unlike the glenohumeral joint). When hip joint dislocation does occur (as in a congenitally dislocated hip), the capsule and ligaments are strong enough to support the femoral head in weight-bearing. In such an instance, the stresses on the capsule imposed by the femoral head may lead to impregnation of the capsule with cartilage cells that contribute to a sliding surface for the head.[20] Under normal circumstances, the capsule and ligaments can and do support two-thirds of the body weight. In bilateral stance, the hip joint is typically in neutral position or slight extension. In this position, the capsule and ligaments are under some tension.[8] The normal line of gravity (LOG) in bilateral stance falls behind the hip joint axis, creating a gravitational extension moment. Further hip joint extension would create additional tension in the capsuloligamentous complex that is more than sufficient to offset the gravitation extension moment. As long as the LOG falls behind the hip joint axis, the capsuloligamentous structures are sufficient to support the superimposed body weight without active or passive assistance from the muscles crossing the hip.

Hip joint extension, with slight abduction and medial rotation, is the close-packed position for the hip joint.[6] It should be noted, however, that the close-packed and stable position for the hip joint is *not* the position of optimal articular contact. The hip joint is one of the few joints where the position of optimal articular contact (combined flexion, abduction, and lateral rotation) is not also the close-packed position. Under circumstances where the joint surfaces are *neither* maximally congruent *nor* close packed, the hip joint is at greatest risk for traumatic dislocation. A position of particular vulnerability occurs when the hip joint is flexed and adducted (as it is when sitting with the thighs crossed). In this position, a strong force up the femoral shaft toward the hip joint (as when the knee hits the dashboard in a car accident) may push the femoral head out of the acetabulum.[8,14]

The capsuloligamentous tension at the hip

joint is least when the hip is in moderate flexion, slight abduction and midrotation. In this position, the normal intra-articular pressure in minimized and the capacity of the synovial capsule to accommodate abnormal amounts of fluid is greatest.[15] This is the position assumed by the hip when there is pain arising from capsuloligamentous problems or from excessive intra-articular pressure arising from extra fluid (blood or synovial fluid) in the joint. Extra fluid in the joint may be a result of such conditions as synovitis of the hip joint or bleeding in the joint from tearing of blood vessels with femoral neck fracture. Wingstrand and colleagues[15] proposed that minimizing intra-articular pressure not only decreases pain in the joint but also prevents the excessive pressure from compressing the intra-articular blood vessels and interfering with the blood supply to the femoral head.

Weight-Bearing Structure of the Hip Joint

The internal architecture of the pelvis and femur reveal the remarkable adaptations that have occurred to accommodate the mechanical stresses and strains created by the transmission of forces between the femur and the pelvis. The trabeculae of bone line up along lines of stress and form systems to meet stress requirements. In Chapter 4, we followed the line of weight-bearing through the vertebrae of the spinal column to the sacral promontory and on through the sacroiliac joints. The weight-bearing lines of both the pelvis and the femur are evident by the arrangement of trabeculae (Fig. 10–12). Most of the weight-bearing stresses in the pelvis pass from the sacroiliac joints to the acetabulum, although trabeculae show evidence of some forces along the pubic ramus and additional forces running to the ischial tuberosities. The stresses along the pubic ramus most likely arise from the function of the pubic bones as compression struts against the medial femoral thrust.[6] The stress lines between the sacroiliac joints and the ischial tuberosities follow the weight-bearing forces in sitting.

The pelvic trabeculae that pass through the acetabulum of the pelvis form two major systems within the femur: the medial trabecular system and the lateral trabecular system. (See Fig. 10–12.) There are also two minor accessory systems of trabeculae. In bilateral static stance, the weight of the HAT is distributed between the left and right hip joints, with the force of at least half the superimposed body weight traveling down through the femoral head, while the ground reaction force (GRF) travels up the shaft. The distance between the superimposed body weight on the head and the GRF up the shaft create a bending (or shear) force at the femoral neck. The trabecular systems must resist this bending force.

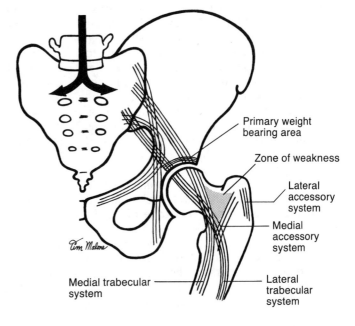

FIGURE 10–12. The trabeculae of the pelvis can be followed to the pubic ramus, the ischium, the dome of the acetabulum (primary weight-bearing areas), and the central area of the acetabulum. The trabeculae from the primary weight-bearing area are continuous with the medial trabecular system of the femur, whereas the trabeculae through the central acetabulum are continuous with the lateral trabecular system of the femur. With the addition of the medial accessory system and the lateral accessory system, an area of thin trabeculae (the zone of weakness) is evident.

Primary weight bearing area

Zone of weakness

Lateral accessory system

Medial accessory system

Medial trabecular system

Lateral trabecular system

The medial trabecular system arises from the medial cortex of the upper femoral shaft and radiates to the cortical bone of the superior aspect of the femoral head. The medial system of trabeculae is oriented along the vertical compressive forces passing through the hip joint.[8] The lateral trabecular system of the femur arises from the lateral cortex of the upper femoral shaft and, after crossing the medial system, terminates in the cortical bone on the inferior aspect of the head of the femur. The lateral trabecular system is oblique and may develop in response to shear stresses that are created by the weight of HAT pressing down on the femoral head while the GRF pushes up the femoral shaft.[8] The two accessory trabecular systems are confined primarily to the trochanteric area and neck of the femur[8] (Fig. 10–12). The medial accessory system arises from the medial aspect of the upper femoral shaft, crosses the lateral trabecular system, and fans out into the region of the greater trochanter. The lateral accessory trabecular system runs parallel to the greater trochanter.

The medial and lateral trabecular systems not only contribute to the structure of the head and neck of the femur, but also help resist the bending stresses that occur across the femoral neck and in the femoral shaft as the weight of HAT presses down on the femoral head.[8,21] The medial trabecular system, coinciding with cortical bone on the medial shaft of the femur, helps resist compression on the inside of the bending stresses of the shaft while the lateral system, coincident with the lateral cortical bone, helps resist tensile forces on the outside of the bending stresses on the shaft (Fig. 10–13). The lateral system is also is thought to help resist the compressive forces at the inferior femoral neck caused by bending stresses across the neck and accentuated by pull of the abductors on the greater trochanter[13] (Fig. 10–13, inset). The areas in which the various trabecular systems within both the pelvis and the femur cross each other at right angles are areas that offer the greatest resistance to stress and strain. There is an area in the femoral neck in which the trabeculae are relatively thin and do not cross each other. This **zone of weakness** has less reinforcement and thus more potential for injury. The zone of weakness of the femoral neck is particularly susceptible to the bending forces across the area and can fracture either when forces are excessive or when the tissues are no longer able to resist

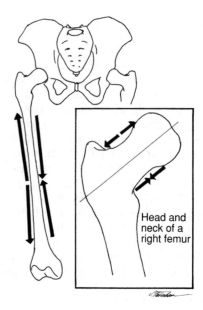

FIGURE 10–13. The weight-bearing line from the center of rotation of the femoral head causes a bending force on the shaft of the femur that results in compressive forces medially and tensile forces laterally. (Inset: The weight-bearing through the head of the femur and a contraction of the hip abductors can cause tensile stresses on the femoral neck superiorly and compressive stresses inferiorly.)

Head and neck of a right femur

normal forces. A more detailed description of the problems of hip fracture will be presented later in the chapter. Although questions have been raised recently about the validity of the classic theory of hip biomechanics first proposed by Pauwels,[22] Kummer[23] confirmed the validity of the theory using more recent technology to study the bony architecture and distribution of bone density.

The primary weight-bearing surface of the acetabulum, or **dome** of the acetabulum, is located on the superior portion of the lunate surface.[24,25] The dome can be found on a roetgenogram by drawing a line between the medial and lateral edges of the area of increased density. In the normal hip this line will be horizontal and will lie directly over the center of rotation of the femoral head.[25] This area is subject to the greatest prevalence of degenerative changes in the acetabulum.[24] Degenerative changes in the femoral head are most common around or immediately below the fovea, or around the peripheral edges of the head's articular surface. The primary weight-bearing area of the femoral head is its superior portion.[24] In contrast to the acetabulum, therefore, the primary weight-bearing area is *not* the area of greatest degenerative change. Athanasiou and colleagues[24] proposed that the variations in material properties, creep characteristics, and thickness may explain the differences in response of articular cartilage in the two primary weight-bearing areas. They further proposed that there is some persisting incongruence in the dome of the acetabulum in the moderately loaded hip (especially in young adults) that could result in incomplete compression of the dome cartilage and, therefore, inadequate fluid exchange to maintain cartilage nutrition. The superior femoral head receives compression not only from the dome in standing, but also from the posterior acetabulum in sitting and the anterior acetabulum in extension. The more frequent and complete compression of the cartilage of the superior femoral head, using this premise, accounts for better nutrition within the cartilage. It must be remembered, however, that avascular articular cartilage is dependent on both *compression* and *release* to move nutrients through the tissue; too little compression and excessive compression can both lead to compromise of the cartilage structure.

Function of the Hip Joint

Arthrokinematics

The hip joint motions are easiest to visualize as movement of the convex femoral head within the concavity of the acetabulum. The femoral head will glide within the acetabulum in a direction opposite to motion of the distal end of the femur. Flexion and extension occur from neutral position as an almost pure spin of the femoral head around a coronal axis through the head and neck of the femur. The head spins posteriorly in flexion and anteriorly in extension. However, flexion and extension from other positions must include both spinning and gliding of the articular surfaces, depending on the combination of motions. The motions of abduction and adduction and medial/lateral rotation must include both spinning and gliding of one surface on another, but again occur opposite to motion of the distal end of the femur when the femur is the moving segment. Whenever the hip joint is weight-bearing, the femur is relatively fixed and, in fact, motion of the hip joint is produced by movement of the pelvis on the femur. In this more common instance, the concave acetabulum moves in the same direction as the pelvis.

Osteokinematics

Motion of the Femur at the Hip Joint

The range of motion (ROM) available at the hip joint is, once again, most commonly described by movement of the femur and can best be visualized this way. As is true at most joints, ROM is influenced by whether the motion is performed actively or passively and whether passive tension in two-joint muscles is encountered or avoided. The following ranges of passive joint motion are typical of the hip joint.[26] Flexion of the hip is generally about 90° with the knee extended and 120° when the knee is flexed and passive tension in the two-joint hamstrings is released. Hip extension is considered to have a range of 10° to 30°. When hip extension is combined with knee flexion, passive tension in the two-joint rectus femoris may limit the movement. The femur can be abducted 45° to 50° and adducted 20° to 30°. Abduction can be limited by the two-joint gracilis muscle and adduction limited by the tensor fascia lata muscle and its associated iliotibial band. Medial and lateral rotation of the hip are usually measured with the hip joint in 90° of flexion, giving a typical range of 42° to 50°. Femoral anteversion is correlated with decreased range of lateral rotation and less strongly with increased range of medial rotation.[7] The limitation of lateral rotation ROM with femoral anteversion occurs because an anteverted femoral head is torsioned more anteriorly than normal. As lateral rotation of the femur turns the head out even more, the head is likely to encounter capsuloligamentous and muscular restrictions on the anterior aspect of the joint.

Normal gait on level ground requires at least the following hip joint ranges: 30° flexion, 10° hyperextension, 5° of both abduction and adduction, and 5° of both medial and lateral rotation.[27,28] Walking on uneven terrain or stairs will increase the need for joint range beyond that required for level ground, as will activities such as sitting in a chair or sitting cross-legged.

Motion of the Pelvis at the Hip Joint

When the proximal segment of a joint moves on the fixed distal segment, the motion across the joint is the same as if the distal segment were the moving part. However, the direction of movement of the lever reverses. For example, elbow flexion can be a rotation of the distal forearm upward or, conversely, a rotation of the proximal humerus downward. At the hip joint, this reversal of motion of the lever is further complicated by the horizontal orientation and shape of the pelvis. Unlike at other joints, there is also a new set of terms to identify joint motion when the pelvis (rather than femur) is the moving segment. The terms for pelvic motions are used with weight-bearing hip motion because these are the motions that are seen by the observer and, in fact, are key to what occurs at the joints above and below the pelvis. *The arthrokinematics and the available ROM at the hip joint remain unchanged, regardless of which segment is moving.*

ANTERIOR AND POSTERIOR PELVIC TILT

Anterior and posterior pelvic tilt are motions of the entire pelvis in the sagittal plane around a coronal axis. In the normally aligned pelvis, the anterior superior iliac spines of the pelvis lie on a horizontal line with the posterior superior iliac spines and on a vertical line with the symphysis pubis[29] (Fig. 10–14a). Anterior and posterior tilting of the pelvis on the fixed femur produce hip flexion and extension, respectively. Hip joint extension via posterior tilting of the pelvis brings the symphysis pubis up and the posterior aspect of the pelvis closer to the fe-

mur, rather than moving the femur posteriorly on the pelvis (Fig. 10–14b). Hip flexion through anterior tilting of the pelvis brings the anterior superior iliac spines anteriorly and inferiorly; the symphysis pubis moves down and closer to the femur rather than moving the femur toward the symphysis pubis (Fig. 10–14c). Anterior and posterior tilting can result in flexion and extension of both hip joints simultaneously or can occur at the stance hip joint alone if the opposite limb is non-weight-bearing.

LATERAL PELVIC TILT

Lateral pelvic tilt is a frontal plane motion of the entire pelvis around an anteroposterior axis. In the normally aligned pelvis, a line through the anterior superior iliac spines (ASISs) is horizontal. If a line through the ASISs is not horizontal, lateral tilt of the pelvis has occurred. Lateral tilt of the pelvis can occur in unilateral stance or in bilateral stance. Although both are functionally relevant, lateral tilt in unilateral stance contributes more to our understanding of hip joint structure and function and will be described first. In lateral tilt of the pelvis in unilateral stance, one hip joint is the pivot point or axis for motion of the *opposite* side of the pelvis as it elevates (hip hiking) or drops (pelvic drop). The

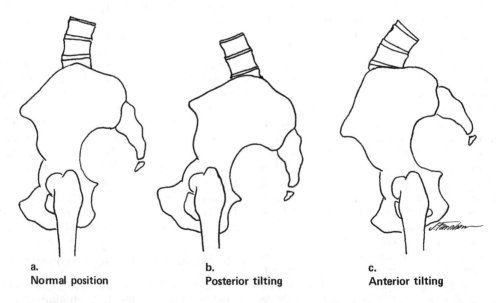

a.	b.	c.
Normal position	**Posterior tilting**	**Anterior tilting**

FIGURE 10–14. Representation of the tilting of the pelvis in the sagittal plane. (a) The pelvis is shown in its normal position in erect stance. The lumbar spine is in slight extension. (b) Posterior tilting of the pelvis moves the symphysis pubis superiorly and the lumbar spine flexes slightly. The hip joint extends. (c) In anterior tilting the symphysis pubis moves inferiorly and the lumbar spine is hyperextended (lordotic). The hip joint is flexed.

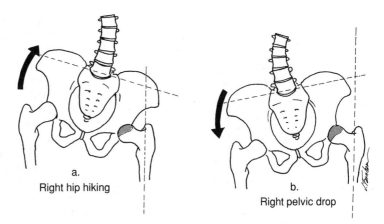

FIGURE 10–15. Lateral tilting of the pelvis around the left can occur either as hip hiking (elevation of the opposite side of the pelvis) or as pelvic drop (drop of the opposite side of the pelvis). (a) Hiking of the pelvis around the left hip joint results in left hip abduction. (b) Dropping of the pelvis around the left hip joint results in left hip joint adduction.

non-weight-bearing limb is in an open chain and has no obligatory position so will be ignored here. However, the non-weight-bearing leg typically hangs straight down as the pelvis moves. If one stands on the left limb and hikes the pelvis, the left hip joint is being abducted (Fig. 10–15a). The medial angle between the femur and a line through the ASISs increases just as it would if the pelvis were stationary and the femur abducted. If one stands on the left leg and drops the pelvis, the left hip joint will adduct (Fig. 10–15b). That is, the medial angle formed by the femur and a line through the ASISs will decrease just as it would if the pelvis were stationary and the femur adducted.

The relative hip joint motions in lateral pelvic tilt may be more difficult to visualize than those in anterior and posterior tilting because the eye tends to follow the iliac crest on the *same* side as the supporting hip joint rather than the opposite side. However, it should also be kept in mind that osteokinematic descrip-

tions reference the motion of the *end of the lever farthest from the joint axis.*

> **EXAMPLE 1:** An osteokinematic description of femoral motion references what is happening to the distal end of the femur, not to the proximally located greater trochanter that is close to the rotating head. Similarly, elbow flexion is viewed as the forearm approaching the humerus, not as the olecranon moving away from the humerus.

Visualizing the hip joint motions that occur when the pelvis moves on the femur is simpler if the neutral pelvis is visualized as a horizontal lever through the iliac crests (Fig. 10–16a). A hike of the pelvis will increase the angle between the two levers (Fig. 10–16b), producing hip joint abduction. A drop of the pelvis will decrease the angle between the two levers (Fig. 10–16c), producing hip joint adduction. The weight-bearing hip in unilateral stance will al-

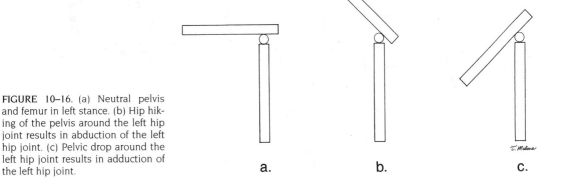

FIGURE 10–16. (a) Neutral pelvis and femur in left stance. (b) Hip hiking of the pelvis around the left hip joint results in abduction of the left hip joint. (c) Pelvic drop around the left hip joint results in adduction of the left hip joint.

a.   **b.**   **c.**

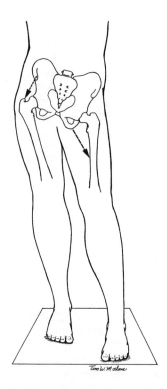

FIGURE 10–17. The pelvis and weight are shifted to the right, putting the right hip into a position of adduction and the left hip into abduction. To return to neutral position while continuing to bear weight on both feet, the right abductor and left adductor muscles work synergistically to shift the weight back to center.

the axis, the motion is defined by movement of the left side of the pelvis.

Lateral pelvic tilt can also occur in bilateral stance if the pelvis is shifted to one side. If both feet are weight-bearing, there is a closed chain between the two feet and the pelvis. Consequently, both hip joints will move. If the pelvis remains horizontal during the shift, the motion can not be named by referencing the pelvis. The hip joint motions can be identified, however. If the pelvis is tilted from horizontal, the side of the body and direction of tilt can be identified along with the resulting hip motions. If the pelvis is shifted to the right in bilateral stance (pelvis down on the left side), the right hip will be adducted and the left hip will be abducted (Fig. 10–17).

PELVIC ROTATION

Pelvic rotation is motion of the entire pelvis in the transverse plane around a vertical axis. Although rotation can occur around a vertical axis through the middle of the pelvis in bilateral stance, it most commonly and more importantly occurs in single-limb support around the axis of the supporting hip joint and will be initially defined in this way. Forward rotation of the pelvis occurs when the side of the pelvis opposite to the supporting hip joint moves anteriorly (Fig. 10–18a). Note again that the *opposite* side of the pelvis from the axis of rotation is referenced in identifying the motion. If the side of limb support is known, it should be redundant to specify *which* side of the pelvis is forwardly rotating. Forward rotation of the pelvis produces medial rotation of the supporting hip joint. The medial rotation of the hip joint that occurs during forward rotation of the pelvis can best be appreciated by

ways be the axis of rotation and the opposite side of the pelvis will always identify the movement. If a woman is standing on her right leg and hikes her pelvis, it should not be necessary to specify that the left side of the pelvis is the one that is rising. Because the right hip joint is

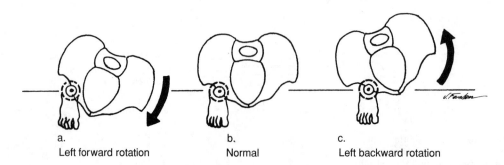

a.
Left forward rotation

b.
Normal

c.
Left backward rotation

FIGURE 10–18. A superior view of rotation of the pelvis in the transverse plane. (a) Forward rotation of the pelvis around the right hip joint results in medial rotation of the right hip joint. (b) Neutral position of the pelvis and the right hip joint. (c) Backward rotation of the pelvis around the right hip joint results in lateral rotation of the right hip joint.

doing the motion yourself. Standing on one leg and rotating the pelvis and trunk forward as much as possible will give a clear "feeling" of the relative medial rotation of the supporting limb. Backward rotation of the pelvis occurs when the side of the pelvis opposite the supporting hip moves posteriorly (Fig. 10–18c). Posterior rotation of the pelvis produces lateral rotation of the supporting hip joint. This again can be best appreciated by doing the motion.

As for lateral pelvic tilt, pelvic rotation can occur in bilateral stance. If both feet are bearing weight and the axis of motion occurs around a vertical axis through the center of the pelvis, the terms forward rotation and backward rotation must now be used by referencing a side (e.g., forward rotation on the right and backward rotation on the left).

Coordinated Motions of the Femur, Pelvis, and Lumbar Spine

When the pelvis moves on a relatively fixed femur, there are two possible outcomes to consider. Either the head and trunk will follow the motion of the pelvis (moving the head through space), or the head will continue to remain relatively upright and vertical despite the pelvic motions. These are open and closed chain responses, respectively. Each of these two situations produces very different reactions from the joints and segments proximal and distal to the hip joints and pelvis and must be examined separately.

Lumbar-Pelvic Motion

When the femur, pelvis, and spine move in a coordinated manner to produce a larger ROM than might be available to one segment alone, the hip joint is participating in an open chain and the term **lumbar-pelvic motion** can be used. Lumbar-pelvic motion can be considered analogous to scapulohumeral motion because the combination of motions at several joints serves to increase the range available to the distal segment. In the case of scapulohumeral motion, the joints are serving the hand. In the case of lumbar-pelvic motion, the joints may serve either end of the chain: the foot or the head.

EXAMPLE 2: If the goal is to bend forward to reach the floor, isolated flexion at the hip joints (anteriorly tilting the pelvis on the femurs) is generally insufficient to reach the ground. If the knees remain extended, the hips can only flex to 90°. The addition of flexion of the lumbar spine (and, perhaps, flexion of the thoracic spine) will incline the head and trunk forward sufficiently for the hands to reach the ground (Fig. 10–19). This is an example of an open chain response in the hips and trunk. It is *not* an example of how to pick up an object!

EXAMPLE 3: When a woman is side-lying, an attempt at maximal abduction of the top leg will bring the leg through as much as 90° of motion (Fig. 10–20). This is clearly not all from the hip joint that can only abduct to 45°, but includes lateral tilting of the pelvis (up on the abducting side) and lateral flexion of the lumbar spine toward the abducting hip joint.

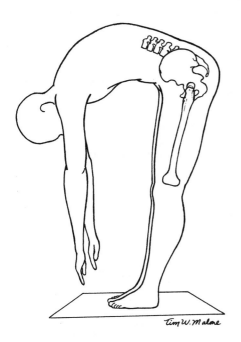

FIGURE 10–19. Lumbar-pelvic rhythm can increase the range of forward flexion of the body by combining hip flexion, anterior pelvic tilt, and flexion of the lumbar spine. This combination permits the hands to reach the ground.

The motions in these two examples are part of an open chain because *one* of the joints in the chain (just the pelvis in Example 2 or just the femur in Example 3) can move without, for the most part, necessitating motion of the other joints. However, open chain motions in stand-

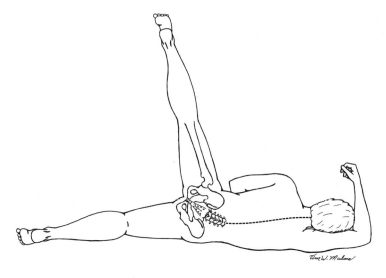

FIGURE 10–20. Lumbar-pelvic rhythm increases the range through which the foot can be moved by combining hip abduction, lateral pelvic tilt, and later flexion of the lumbar spine.

ing are not completely independent but typically require subtle adjustments or compensations by other joints to assure that the LOG remains within the base of support despite the rearrangement of segments. In Figure 10–19, the ankles have been plantarflexed slightly during the forward bend to move the pelvis posteriorly. This subtle shift in the pelvis will allow the LOG to remain within the base of support.

Closed Chain Hip Joint Function

Before we can examine closed chain hip joint function, we must first examine how the hip joint becomes part of the closed chain. For the hip joint to be part of a closed chain, we must identify the two ends and how each is "fixed." It is clear that the foot (one end of the chain) is frequently fixed by weight-bearing. However, the opposite end of the chain must also be fixed for a closed chain to exist. The other end of the functional closed chain in this instance is the head. Although the head is certainly free to move in space, the head most often remains upright and vertically oriented during upright activities. The drive to keep the head upright is due, in part, to the influence of the tonic labyrinthine and optical righting reflexes that are normally evident almost immediately at birth[30] and continue to operate throughout life. The drive to keep the head upright and over the sacrum will effectively *fix the head in relative space* even though this is not structurally the case; that is, the head is functionally rather than structurally fixed. When the head (one end of the chain) is held upright and over the base of support (the other end of the chain), all the seg-

ments between the head and the weight-bearing surface will be part of one closed chain. The premise of a closed chain is that movement at one joint will create movement in at least one other linkage in the chain. So, hip flexion (in our functional closed chain premise) cannot occur independently, but must be accompanied by motion in one or more joints above or below. Compensatory responses of the interposed segments will ensure that the head remains over the base of support and that the entire body does not become unstable. The closed chain response can be voluntarily overridden, however, because the head is not truly fixed.

EXAMPLE 4: A common example of open chain versus closed chain function is seen when the hip flexor musculature is tight and the hip joint is maintained in flexion as it is in both Figures 10–21a and 10–21b. A true open chain response would result in displacement of head and trunk forward over the flexed hips, with the LOG falling in front of the supporting feet. The person would be unstable and could not remain standing (see Fig. 10–21a). More commonly, sustained hip flexion in stance is accompanied by compensatory movements of the vertebral column that maintain the head in the upright position and keep the LOG well within the base of support (see Fig. 10–21b). Motion of one link in the chain is accompanied by motion at one or more others. Where hip flexion was accompanied by lumbar flexion to achieve more range (open chain), here we have hip flexion accompanied by lumbar extension to maintain the head over the sacrum.

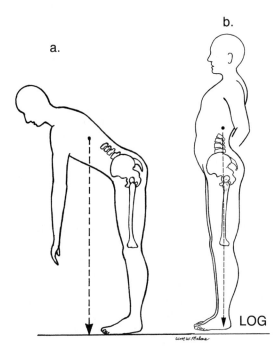

a.

b.

LOG

FIGURE 10–21. (a) In an open-chain response to tight hip flexors, the trunk will be inclined forward. The line of gravity (LOG) will fall outside the base of support if no other adjustments are made. (b) In a closed-chain response to tight hip flexors, the lumbar spine will extend to return the head to a position over the sacrum and maintain the LOG within the base of support.

EXAMPLE 5: If the pelvis is laterally tilted due to a short right leg (pelvis down on the right, right hip abduction), the trunk would fall to the right and the LOG would tend to fall to the right of the base of support. To keep the LOG within the center of the base, the lumbar spine will laterally flex to the left and away from the abducted hip joint. This is once again the opposite of what we saw in Example 4 of open chain function, where the lumbar spine laterally flexed to the *same* side as the abducted hip to increase the range available to the foot.

An important example of closed chain compensatory movements between the pelvis, hip, and lumbar spine can be seen during gait. When we walk, the pelvis will drop slightly (lateral pelvic tilt) around the supporting hip joint (hip joint adduction). If the head and trunk followed the pelvis, the body would lean away from the supporting extremity and the LOG would fall outside the supporting foot. Instead, the lumbar spine laterally flexes *toward* the side

of the supporting limb to prevent displacement of the head and trunk.

In any instance in which there is normal or abnormal pelvic motion during weight-bearing and the head must remain upright, compensatory motions of the lumbar spine will occur if available. This does not rule out the need for compensation at additional joints as well, but the lumbar spine tends to be the "first line of defense." As we examine the other joints of the lower extremity and move on to posture and gait, other compensatory motions will be encountered and discussed. Table 10–1 presents the compensatory motions of the lumbar spine that accompany given motions of the pelvis and hip joint in a functional closed chain.

Hip Joint Musculature

There have been numerous studies of the muscles of the hip joint. Most confirm underlying principles of muscle physiology seen at the other joints we have examined so far. That is, hip joint muscles work best in the middle of their contractile range or on a slight stretch (at optimal length-tension); two joint muscles generate greatest force when not required to shorten over both joints simultaneously; and tension generation is optimal with eccentric contractions, followed by isometric and then concentric contractions. The muscles of the hip joint, however, make their most important contributions to function during weight-bearing. In weight-bearing, the muscles are called on to move or support the HAT (two-thirds body weight) rather than the weight of one lower limb (one-sixth body weight). Given this task, the hip joint muscles are somewhat unique in their large areas of attachment, their length, and their large cross-section. These characteristics, in combination with the large ROM available at the hip joint, result in muscle function that is strongly influenced by hip joint position and availability of motion of the proximal and distal segments. For example, the adductor muscles may be hip flexors in the neutral hip joint, but will be hip extensors when the hip joint is already flexed.[31] Similarly, the pectineus and obturator externus muscles may switch from being lateral rotators of the hip joint to being medial rotators from a position of extreme medial rotation.[8] Such inversions of function are found in a few muscles at the shoulder (the clavicular portion of the pectoralis major, for example), but are fairly com-

Table 10–1. **Relationship of Pelvis, Hip Joint, and Lumbar Spine during Right Lower-Extremity Weight-Bearing and Upright Posture**

Pelvic Motion	Accompanying Hip Joint Motion	Compensatory Lumbar Spine Motion
Anterior pelvic tilt	Hip flexion	Lumbar extension
Posterior pelvic tilt	Hip extension	Lumbar flexion
Lateral pelvic tilt (pelvic drop)	Right hip adduction	Right lateral flexion
Lateral pelvic tilt (pelvic hike)	Right hip abduction	Left lateral flexion
Forward rotation	Right hip medial rotation	Rotation to the left
Backward rotation	Right hip lateral rotation	Rotation to the right

mon in the hip joint. As a consequence, results of various studies may appear to be contradictory when, in fact, testing conditions explain differing results. Some gender-related differences also have been found that explain differential findings.[32] It is best to examine muscle action at the hip joint in the context of specific functions such as single-limb support, posture, and gait. The next section will briefly review muscle function, but we will leave more detailed analyses for later in this and other chapters. Although the traditional action of each muscle on the distal femoral segment is described for the most part, it must be emphasized that any of the muscles are as likely (or more likely) to produce joint action by moving the proximal pelvic segment instead.

Flexors

The flexors of the hip joint function primarily as mobility muscles in open chain function; that is, they function primarily when the limb is not bearing weight to bring the lower extremity forward during ambulation or in various sports. The flexors may function secondarily to resist strong hip extension forces that occur as the body passes over the weight-bearing foot. Nine muscles have action lines crossing the anterior aspect of the hip joint. Of these, the primary muscles of hip flexion are the **iliopsoas, rectus femoris, tensor fascia lata,** and **sartorius.** The iliopsoas muscle is considered to be the most important of the primary hip flexors. It consists of two separate muscles, the **iliacus** muscle and the **psoas major** muscle, both of which attach to the femur by a common tendon. The two components of the iliopsoas have many points of origin, including the iliac fossa and the disks, bodies, and transverse processes of the lumbar vertebrae. The two muscles pass over the symphysis pubis but under the inguinal ligament

(Fig. 10–22). The attachment of the psoas major to the anterior vertebrae and the iliacus to the iliac fossa make it likely that activity or tension in these muscles would anteriorly tilt the pelvis (iliacus) and pull the lumbar vertebrae anteriorly (psoas major). In closed chain function (head vertical), these muscles are responsible for creating a lumbar lordosis as the trunk above the muscle attachments and the head extend to compensate for the anterior pelvic tilt and lower lumbar flexion. The role of the iliopsoas in hip flexion may be particularly critical when hip flexion from sitting position is required. Smith and colleagues[33] propose that the hip cannot be flexed beyond 90° when the iliopsoas is paralyzed because the other hip flexor muscles are effectively actively insuffi-

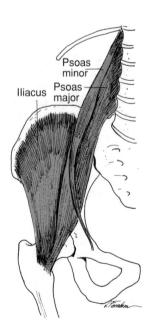

FIGURE 10–22. Anterior view of the right hip shows the attachments of the iliopsoas muscle.

cient in that position. Basmajian and DeLuca[31] summarize the often contradictory evidence of many investigations by concluding that both segments of the iliopsoas are active in various stages of hip flexion. Because the hip rotation function of the iliopsoas is frequently questioned, Basmajian and DeLuca also suggest that any concomitant medial or lateral rotatory function is at best weak and should be ignored.

The rectus femoris muscle is the only portion of the quadriceps muscle that crosses both the hip joint and knee joint. It originates on the anterior inferior iliac spine and inserts by way of a common tendon into the tibial tuberosity. The rectus femoris flexes the hip joint and extends the knee joint. As a two-joint hip flexor, the position of the knee during hip flexion will affect its ability to generate force at the hip. Simultaneous hip flexion and knee extension considerably shorten this muscle and increase the likelihood of active insufficiency. Consequently, the rectus femoris makes its best contribution to hip flexion when the knee is maintained in flexion.

The sartorius muscle is a straplike muscle originating on the anterior superior iliac spine. It crosses the anterior aspect of the femur to insert into the upper portion of the medial aspect of the tibia (Fig. 10–23). The sartorius is considered to be a flexor, abductor, and lateral rotator of the hip, as well as a flexor and medial rotator of the knee. Wheatley and Jahnke[34] proposed that the sartorius, although a two-joint muscle, should be relatively unaffected by the position of the knee given the relatively small proportional change in length with increased knee flexion. Its function is probably most important when the knee and hip need to be flexed simultaneously (as in climbing stairs) but its small cross-section would argue against a unique or critical role at the hip joint.[6]

The tensor fascia lata muscle originates more laterally than the sartorius. Its origin is on the anterolateral lip of the iliac crest. The muscle fibers extend only about one-quarter of the way down the lateral aspect of the thigh before inserting into the iliotibial band (see Fig. 10–23). The **iliotibial band** (**ITB**) or iliotibial tract is the thickened lateral portion of the fascia lata of the hip and thigh. The ITB attaches proximally to the iliac crest lateral to the tensor fascia lata. After the tensor attaches to the ITB, the ITB continues distally on the lateral thigh to insert into the lateral condyle of the tibia. The tensor fascia lata muscle is considered to flex,

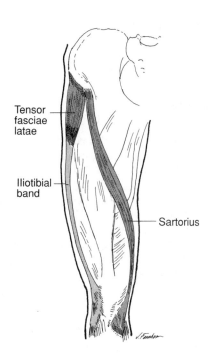

FIGURE 10–23. The anterior aspect of the right hip and knee shows the location of the tensor fascia lata and the sartorius. Both are two-joint muscles that act at the hip and the knee.

abduct, and medially rotate the femur at the hip,[31] although the tensor's contribution to hip abduction may be dependent on simultaneous hip flexion.[35] The most important contribution of the tensor fascia lata may be in maintaining tension in the ITB. The ITB assists in relieving the femur of some of the tensile stresses imposed on the shaft by weight-bearing forces[13,35] (see Fig. 10–14). Because bone more effectively resists compressive than tensile stresses, reduction of tensile stresses is important in maintaining integrity of the bone.[21] Functionally, the tensor fascia lata and ITB are expendable. The ITB may be removed and used for autogenous fascial transplants without any evident change in active or passive hip or knee function.[35]

The secondary hip flexors are the pectineus, adductor longus, adductor magnus, and the gracilis muscles. These muscles are described in the next section because they are predominantly adductors of the hip. Each, however, is capable of contributing to hip joint flexion but that contribution is hip joint position dependent. Kapandji[8] notes that these muscles contribute to flexion only between 40° to 50° of hip flexion. Once the femur is superior to the point of origin of a muscle, the muscle will become an extensor of the hip joint. The gracilis, a two-joint muscle, is active as a hip flexor when the knee is extended but not when the knee is flexed.[34]

Adductors

The hip adductor muscle group is generally considered to include the **pectineus, adductor brevis, adductor longus, adductor magnus,** and the **gracilis.** The pectineus muscle is a small muscle located medial to the iliopsoas (Fig. 10–24). The other adductors are also located anteromedially (Fig. 10–25). The adductors longus, brevis, and magnus muscles arise in a group from the body and inferior ramus of the pubis to insert along the linea aspera. The gracilis muscle is the only two-joint adductor. It originates on the symphysis pubis and pubic arch and inserts on the medial surface of the shaft of the tibia.

The contribution of the adductor muscles to hip joint function has been debated for many years. Basmajian and DeLuca[31] believe the variability in study findings supports the theory of Janda and Stara that the adductors function not as prime movers, but by reflex response to gait activities. As shall be seen in our discus-

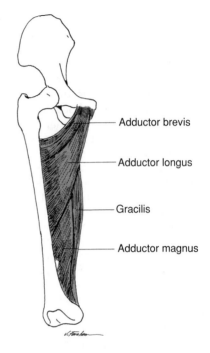

FIGURE 10–25. The adductors of the right hip.

sion of muscle function in bilateral stance, the adductors may be synergists to the abductor muscles when both feet are on the ground, enhancing side-to-side stabilization of the pelvis. Although the role of the adductor muscles may be less clear than that of other hip muscle groups, the relative importance of the adductors should not be underestimated. The adductors as a group contribute 22.5% to the total muscle mass of the lower extremity compared to only 18.4% for the flexors and 14.9% for the abductors.[36] The adductors are also capable of generating a maximum isometric torque greater than that of the abductors.[37]

Extensors

The one-joint **gluteus maximus** muscle and the two-joint **hamstrings** muscle group are the primary hip joint extensors. These muscles may receive assistance from the posterior fibers of the gluteus medius, from the superior fibers of the adductor magnus, and from the piriformis muscle. The gluteus maximus is a large, quadrangular muscle that originates from the posterior sacrum, dorsal sacroiliac ligaments, sacrotuberous ligament, and a small portion of the ilium. The maximus crosses the sacroiliac joint before its most su-

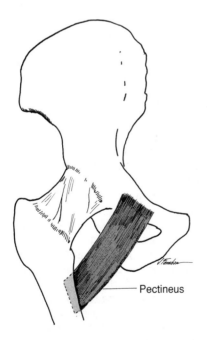

FIGURE 10–24. Anterior view of the right hip shows the attachments of the pectineus muscle. The pectineus is an adductor and a flexor of the hip.

perior fibers insert into the iliotibial band (as do the fibers of the tensor fascia lata) and its inferior fibers insert into the gluteal tuberosity (Fig. 10–26). The gluteus maximus is the largest of the lower extremity muscles, the muscle alone constituting 12.8% of the total muscle mass of the lower extremity.[36] The maximus is a strong hip extensor that appears to be active primarily against a resistance greater than the weight of the limb. Its moment arm (MA) for hip extension is considerably longer than that of either the hamstrings or the adductor magnus muscles and is maximal in the neutral hip joint position.[32] A favorable length-tension relationship, however, allows it to exert its peak extensor moment at 70° of hip flexion.[28] The maximus has a substantial capacity to laterally rotate the femur,[38] although it may reverse this function in extremes of range.[31]

The three two-joint extensors are the long head of the **biceps femoris,** the **semitendinosus,** and the **semimembranosus** muscles— known collectively as the **hamstrings.** Each of these three muscles originates on the ischial tuberosity. The biceps femoris crosses the posterior femur to insert into the head of the fibula and lateral aspect of the lateral tibial condyle. The other two hamstrings insert on the medial aspect of the tibia. All three muscles extend the hip with or without resistance, as well as being important knee flexors. The hamstrings in-

crease their MA for hip extension as the hip flexes to 35° and decrease it thereafter. The MA of the gluteus maximus is maximal at neutral and decreases with any hip flexion thereafter.[32] Regardless of these changes in MA with joint position, the MA of the combined hamstrings at the hip is smaller than that of the gluteus maximus at all points in the hip flexion/extension ROM. As two-joint muscles, the role of the hamstrings in hip extension is also strongly influenced by knee position. If the knee is flexed to 90° or more, the hamstrings may not be able to contribute much to hip extension force because of active insufficiency or approaching active insufficiency. Extension forces in the hip increase by 30% if the knee is extended during hip extension.[28] Unlike the semimembranosus and semitendinosus, the biceps femoris may contribute to lateral rotation of the hip.[31]

Abductors

Active abduction of the hip is brought about predominantly by the **gluteus medius** and the **gluteus minimus** muscles. The superior fibers of the gluteus maximus and the sartorius may assist when the hip is abducted against strong resistance. The tensor fascia lata is given variable credit for its contribution and may be effective as an abductor only during simultaneous hip flexion. The gluteus medius lies deep to the gluteus maximus. It originates on the lateral surface of the wing of the ilium and inserts into the greater trochanter. The gluteus medius has anterior, middle, and posterior parts that function asynchronously during movement at the hip.[39] Analogous to the deltoid muscle of the glenohumeral joint, the anterior fibers of the gluteus medius are active in hip flexion and medial rotation, whereas the posterior fibers function during extension and lateral rotation. All portions of the muscle abduct. The trochanteric bursa of the gluteus medius separates the distal tendon of the muscle from the trochanter over which it must slide. Under some conditions, this bursa may become inflamed and be a source of pain.[14]

The gluteus minimus muscle lies deep to the gluteus medius, arising from the outer surface of the ilium with its fibers converging on an aponeurosis that ends in a tendon on the greater trochanter. The trochanteric bursa of the gluteus minimus allows the tendon to slide over the trochanter. The gluteus minimus and

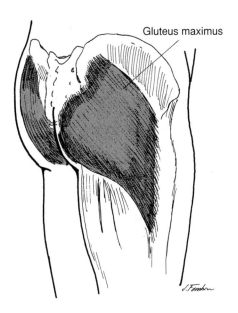

FIGURE 10–26. The gluteus maximus muscle.

medius muscles function together to either abduct the femur (distal level free) or, more importantly, to stabilize the pelvis (and superimposed HAT) in unilateral stance against the effects of gravity. As will be presented later, the gluteus medius and minimus muscles will offset the gravitation adduction torque on the pelvis around the stance hip (pelvis drop). The abductors are physiologically designed to work most effectively in a neutral or slightly adducted hip (slightly lengthened abductors).[40,41] Isometric abduction torque in the neutral hip position is 82% greater than abduction torque when the hip is in 25° of abduction (shortened abductors).[37]

Lateral Rotators

Six short muscles have lateral rotation as a primary function. These muscles are the **obturator internus** and **externus,** the **gemellus superior** and **inferior, quadratus femoris,** and the **piriformis** muscles. Other muscles that have fibers posterior to the axis of motion at the hip (the posterior fibers of the gluteus medius and minimus and superior fibers of the gluteus maximus) may produce lateral rotation combined with the primary action of the muscle. Of the primary lateral rotators, each inserts either on or in the vicinity of the greater trochanter (Fig.

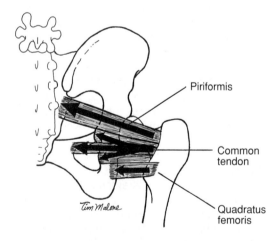

Piriformis

Common tendon

Quadratus femoris

Tim Malone

FIGURE 10–27. The lateral rotators of the hip joint have action lines that lie nearly perpendicular to the femoral shaft (making them excellent rotators) and parallel to the head and neck of the femur (making them excellent compressors). The common tendon is the shared insertion of the gemellus superior, gemellus inferior, and the obturator internus. The obturator externus is not shown. The proximal attachment of the piriformis is on the anterior sacrum.

10–27). The obturator internus muscle originates from the inside (posterior aspect) of the obturator foramen and emerges through the lesser sciatic foramen to insert on the medial aspect (inside) of the greater trochanter. The gemellus superior and gemellus inferior muscles arise from the ischium of the pelvis, just above and just below the point where the obturator internus passes through the lesser sciatic notch. Both gemelli follow and blend with the obturator internus tendon to insert with the internus tendon into the greater trochanter.

The obturator externus muscle is sometimes considered to be an anteromedial muscle of the thigh because it originates on the external (anterior) surface of the obturator foramen. However, it crosses the posterior aspect of the hip joint and inserts on the medial aspect of the greater trochanter in the trochanteric fossa. The quadratus femoris muscle is a small quadrangular muscle that originates on the ischial tuberosity and inserts on the posterior femur between the greater and lesser trochanters. The piriformis muscle originates largely on the anterior surface of the sacrum, passes through the greater sciatic notch, and follows the inferior border of the posterior gluteus medius to insert above the other lateral rotators into the medial aspect of the greater trochanter. The piriformis and gluteus maximus are the only two muscles that cross the sacroiliac joint. The sciatic nerve, the largest nerve in the body, enters the gluteal region just inferior to the piriformis muscle.

The lateral rotator muscles are positioned to perform their rotatory function effectively, given the nearly perpendicular orientation to the shaft of the femur (see Fig. 10–27). However, exploration of function of these muscles has been restricted because of the relatively limited access to electromyography (EMG) surface or wire electrodes. Like their rotator cuff counterpart at the glenohumeral joint, these muscles would certainly appear to be effective joint compressors because their combined action line parallels the head and neck of the femur. Hypothetically, the lines of pull of these deep one-joint muscles should make them ideal tonic stabilizers of the joint during most weight-bearing and non-weight-bearing hip joint activities. Their ability to perform lateral rotation may decrease with hip flexion,[38] although their line of pull into the acetabulum should not be particularly affected by hip position.

Medial Rotators

There are no muscles with the primary function of producing medial rotation of the hip joint. However, muscles with lines of pull anterior to the hip joint axis at some point in the ROM may contribute to this activity. The more consistent medial rotators are the anterior portion of the gluteus medius and the tensor fascia lata muscles. Although controversial, the weight of evidence appears to support the adductor muscles as medial rotators of the joint.[31,33] The ability of hip joint muscles to shift function with changing position of the hip joint is evident when examining medial rotation of the hip. There is a trend toward increased medial rotation torques (or decreased lateral rotation torques) with increased hip flexion among many of the hip joint muscles,[38] with three times more medial rotation torque in the flexed hip than in the extended hip.[33]

Muscle Function in Stance

Bilateral Stance

In erect bilateral stance, both hips are in neutral or slight hyperextension and weight is evenly distributed between both legs. The LOG falls just posterior to axis for flexion/extension of the hip joint. The posterior location of the LOG creates an extension moment of force around the hip that tends to posteriorly tilt the pelvis on the femoral heads. The gravitational extension moment is largely checked by passive tension in the hip joint capsuloligamentous structures, although slight or intermittent activity in the iliopsoas muscles in relaxed standing may assist the passive structures.[31]

In the frontal plane during bilateral stance, the superincumbent body weight is transmitted through the sacroiliac joints along the pelvic trabecular system to the right and left femoral heads. It is typically presumed that the weight of the HAT (two-thirds of body weight) is distributed so that each femoral head receives one-half of the superincumbent weight.[42] As shown in Figure 10–28, the joint axis of each hip lies at an equal distance from the LOG of HAT (DR = DL). Because the body weight (W) on each femoral head is the same (WR = WL), the magnitude of the gravitational torques around each hip must be identical (WR × DR = WL × DL). The two torques, however, occur in opposite directions. The weight of the body acting around the right hip tends to drop the pelvis

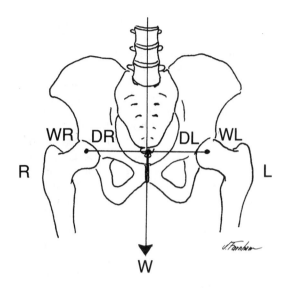

FIGURE 10–28. An anterior view of the pelvis in normal erect bilateral stance. The weight acting at the right (WR) times the distance from the right hip joint axis to the body's center of gravity (DR) is equal to the weight acting at the left hip (WL) times the distance from the left hip to the body's center of gravity (DL) (WR × DR = WL × DL).

down on the left (right adduction moment), whereas the weight acting around the left hip tends to drop the pelvis down on the right (left adduction moment). These two opposing gravitation moments of equal magnitude balance each other and the pelvis is maintained in equilibrium in the frontal plane without the assistance of active muscles. Assuming that muscular forces are not required to maintain either sagittal or frontal plane stability at the hip joint in bilateral stance, the compression across each hip joint in bilateral stance should simply be one-half the superimposed body weight (or one-third of HAT to each hip).

EXAMPLE 6: Using a hypothetical case of someone weighing 180 lb, the weight of HAT will be 120 lb (2/3 × 180 lb). Of that 120 lb, half will presumably be distributed through each hip. Because we are assuming no additional compressive force produced by hip muscle activity, the total hip joint compression at each hip in bilateral stance will be 60 lb; that is, total hip joint compression through each hip in bilateral stance is one-third of body weight.

Bergmann and colleagues[43] showed in several subjects with an instrumented pressure sensitive hip prostheses that the joint compression across each hip in bilateral stance was 80% to 100% of body weight, rather than one-third of body weight as commonly proposed. When they added a symmetrically distributed load to the subject's trunk, the hip joint forces both increased by the full weight of the load, rather than by half of the superimposed load as might be expected. Although the mechanics of a prosthetic hip may not fully represent normal hip joint forces, the findings of Bergmann and colleagues call to question the simplistic view of hip joint forces in bilateral stance. The slight activity in the iliopsoas may account for more joint compression than previously thought.

When bilateral stance is not symmetrical, frontal plane muscle activity will be required to either control the side-to-side motion or to return the hips to symmetrical stance. In Figure 10–18, the pelvis is shifted to the right, resulting in relative adduction of the right hip and abduction of the left hip. To return to neutral position, an active contraction of the right hip abductors would be expected. However, a contraction of the left hip adductors would accomplish the same goal. In bilateral stance, the contralateral abductors and adductors may function as synergists to control the frontal plane motion of the pelvis. *Under the condition that both extremities bear at least some of the superimposed body weight,* the adductors may assist the abductors in control of the pelvis against the force of gravity or the ground reaction force. In unilateral stance, activity of the adductors either in the weight-bearing or non-weight-bearing hip *cannot* contribute to stability of the stance limb. Hip joint stability in unilateral stance is the sole domain of the hip joint abductors. In the absence of adequate hip abductor function, the adductors can contribute to stability in bilateral stance.

Unilateral Stance

In Figure 10–29, the left leg has been lifted from the ground and the full superimposed body weight is being supported by the right hip joint. Rather than sharing the compressive force of the superimposed body weight with the left limb, the right hip joint must now carry the full burden. Additionally, the weight of the non-weight-bearing left limb that is hanging on the left side of the pelvis must be supported along with the weight of HAT. Of the one-third portion of the body weight found in the lower extremities, the nonsupporting limb must account for half of that, or one-sixth of the full

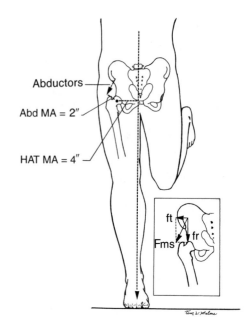

FIGURE 10–29. In right unilateral stance, the weight of HAT acts 4 inches from the right hip joint. The 4-inch moment arm slightly underestimates the location of the LOG because it ignores the weight of the hanging left limb. The hip abductors have a moment arm of approximately 2 inches. (Inset: The pull of the abductors |Fms| on the horizontally oriented pelvis will resolve into a translatory component |ft| that will pull the acetabulum into the center of the femoral head and a rotatory component |fr| that will pull the pelvis down on the superior aspect of the femoral head.)

body weight.[44] The magnitude of body weight (W) compressing the right hip joint in right unilateral stance, therefore, is

$$\text{Right hip joint compression}_{\text{body weight}}$$
$$= |2/3 \times W| + |1/6 \times W|$$

$$\text{Right hip joint compression}_{\text{body weight}}$$
$$= 5/6 \times W$$

EXAMPLE 7: Again using our hypothetical subject weighing 180 lb, HAT in this individual weighs 120 lb (two-thirds body weight). One lower extremity weighs one-sixth body weight, or 30 lb. Therefore, when this individual lifts one leg off the ground, the supporting hip joint will undergo 150 lb (or five-sixth body weight) of compression *from body weight alone.*

Although we have accounted for the increase in hip joint compression from body weight as one moves from double-limb support to single-limb support, the problem is more complex. The hip joint is not only being compressed by body weight (gravity) but that body weight is also concomitantly creating a torque around the hip joint.

The force of gravity acting on HAT and the non-weight-bearing lower limb (HATLL) will create an adduction torque around the supporting hip joint; that is, gravity will attempt to drop the pelvis around the right weight-bearing hip joint axis. The LOG can be estimated to lie 4 inches from the right hip joint axis (MA = 4 inches), although the actual distance will vary among individuals.[45] The 4-inch estimate is for symmetrical stance. The actual MA will be slightly greater because the weight of the hanging left leg will pull the center of gravity of the superimposed weight slightly to the left. For simplicity, this increase in MA will be ignored, but our torque calculation will *underestimate* the actual gravitation torque. In our simplified hypothetical example, the magnitude of the gravitational adduction torque at the right hip will be

$$\text{HATLL Torque}_{\text{adduction}} = 150 \text{ lb} \times 4 \text{ in}$$
$$= 600 \text{ in-lb}$$

To maintain the single-limb support position, there must be a countertorque (abduction moment) of equivalent magnitude or the pelvis will drop. If the trunk follows the pelvis, the person will fall to the unsupported side. The countertorque must be produced by the force of the hip abductors (gluteus medius and minimus) acting on the pelvis. Assuming that the abductor muscles act through a typical MA of 2 inches[45] and knowing that the muscles must generate an abduction torque equivalent to the adduction torque of gravity (600 in-lb), we can solve for the magnitude of muscle contraction (F_{ms}) needed to maintain equilibrium in our hypothetical example.

$$\text{Torque}_{\text{abduction}} = 600 \text{ in-lb} = 2 \text{ in} \times F_{ms}$$
$$F_{ms} = \frac{600 \text{ in-lb}}{2 \text{ in}} = 300 \text{ lb}$$

To prevent the pelvis from falling to the unsupported side, the abductors must generate a force of at least 300 lb (recall that we underestimated the gravitation torque). Assuming that all the muscular force is transmitted through the acetabulum to the femoral head, the 300-lb muscular compressive force is now added to the 150 lb of compression due to body weight passing through the supporting hip. Thus, the total hip joint compression, or joint reaction force, at the stance hip joint in unilateral sup-

port can be estimated for our hypothetical subject at

300 lb of muscular joint compression

+150 lb of body weight compression

total hip joint compression ≥ 450 lb

The location of the joint reaction force can be further defined by knowing the angle of pull of the hip abductors. The action line of the abductors has been estimated to average 22° to 30° from vertical,[42,46] yielding the force components shown in Figure 10–29 (inset). Assuming an angle of pull of approximately 30° from vertical, we can estimate that nearly two-thirds of the total hip abductor force (~200 lb) acting on the pelvis will bring the pelvis vertically downward on the femoral head, and one-third of the force (~100 lb) will pull the pelvis laterally into the femoral head. The vertically directed downward force of 200 lb will fall into the same line as the vertical force of the body weight (150 lb), resulting in a net force of approximately 350 lb through the primary weight-bearing areas of the acetabulum and femoral head. The remaining 100 lb of the total 450 lb of hip joint compression should be distributed more uniformly around the periphery of the femoral head as the femur and acetabulum are snugged together, recalling that the acetabular fossa and fovea of the femur are nonarticular and, therefore, non-weight-bearing.

The hypothetical figures used above oversimplify the forces involved in hip joint stresses as already noted. Total hip joint compression or joint reaction forces are generally considered to be 2.5 to 3 times body weight in static unilateral stance.[28,42,45] Investigators have calculated or measured forces of four and seven times body weight in, respectively, the beginning and end of the stance phase of gait,[47] and seven times the body weight in activities such as stair climbing.[48] Although weight loss can reduce the hip joint reaction force, the larger component of the joint reaction force is generated by the contraction of the hip abductors. The magnitude of hip abductor force required can be affected by individual differences in the angle of pull of the muscles, in the angle of inclination of the femoral head, and in the angle of femoral torsion. Physiologic and biomechanical factors necessitating increased force production by the hip abductor muscles over time may accelerate joint deterioration as a result of the abnormally large joint compressive forces that prevent normal compression and release of cartilage.

Reduction of Muscle Forces in Unilateral Stance

If the hip joint undergoes osteoarthritic changes leading to pain on weight-bearing, the joint reaction force must be reduced to avoid pain. If total joint compression in unilateral stance is approximately three times body weight, a loss of 1 lb of body weight will reduce the joint reaction force by 3 lb. For most painful hip joints, however, greater reductions in compression are generally required than can be realistically achieved through weight loss. The solution must be in a reduction of abductor muscle force requirements. If less muscular countertorque is needed to offset the effects of gravity, there will be a decrease in the amount of muscular compression across the joint although the body weight compression will remain unchanged. The need to diminish abductor force requirements also occurs when the abductor muscles are weakened through paralysis or through structural changes in the femur that reduce biomechanical efficiency of the muscles. In fact, paralysis of the hip abductor muscles (gluteus medius and gluteus minimus) is considered the most serious muscular disability in the hip region.[6] Hip abductor muscle weakness will inevitably affect gait, whereas paralysis of other hip joint muscles in the presence of intact abductors will permit someone to walk or even run with relatively little disability.

Several options are available when there is a need to decrease abductor muscle force requirements. Some compression reduction strategies occur automatically, but at a cost of extra energy expenditure and structural stress. Other strategies require intervention such as assistive devices, but minimize the energy cost.

COMPENSATORY LATERAL LEAN OF THE TRUNK

Gravitational torque at the pelvis is the product of body weight and the distance that the LOG lies from the hip joint axis (MA). If there is a need to reduce the torque of gravity in unilateral stance and if body weight cannot be reduced, the MA of the gravitational force can be reduced by laterally leaning the trunk over the pelvis *toward the side of pain or weakness* when in unilateral stance on the painful limb. Although leaning toward the side of pain might appear counterintuitive, the compensatory lateral lean of the trunk

toward the painful stance limb will swing the LOG closer to the hip joint, thereby reducing the gravitational MA. Because the weight of HATLL must pass through the weight-bearing hip joint regardless of trunk position, leaning toward the painful or weak supporting hip does not increase the joint compression due to body weight. However, it does reduce the gravitational torque. If there is a smaller gravitational adduction torque, there will be a proportional reduction in the need for an abductor countertorque. Although it is theoretically possible to laterally lean the trunk enough to bring the LOG *through* the supporting hip (reducing the torque to zero) or to the *opposite side* of the supporting hip (reversing the direction of the gravitational torque), these are relatively extreme motions that require high energy expenditure and would result in excessive wear and tear on the lumbar spine. More energy-efficient and less structurally stressful compensations can still yield dramatic reductions in the hip abductor force.

EXAMPLE 8: Returning to our hypothetical subject weighing 180 lb, let us assume that he can laterally lean to the right enough to bring the LOG within 1 inch of the right hip joint axis (Fig. 10–30). The gravitational adduction torque would now be

$$\text{HATLL Torque}_{\text{adduction}} = 5/6 \ (180 \ \text{lb}) \times 1 \ \text{in}$$

$$\text{HATLL Torque}_{\text{adduction}} = 150 \ \text{in-lb}$$

If only 150 in-lb of adduction torque were produced by the superimposed weight, the abductor force needed would be

$$\text{Torque}_{\text{abduction}} = 150 \ \text{in-lb} = 2 \ \text{in} \times F_{\text{ms}}$$

$$F_{\text{ms}} = \frac{150 \ \text{in-lb}}{2 \ \text{in}} = 75 \ \text{lb}$$

If only 75 lb of abductor force were required, the total hip joint compression in unilateral stance using the compensatory lateral lean would now be

75 lb of muscular joint compression

+150 lb of body weight compression

total hip joint compression $\geq$ 225 lb

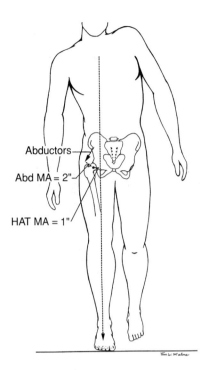

FIGURE 10–30. When the trunk is laterally flexed toward the stance limb, the moment arm of HAT is substantially reduced (e.g., 1 inch as compared to 4 inches with the neutral trunk), whereas that of the abductors remains unchanged (e.g., 2 inches). The result is a substantially diminished torque from HAT and, consequently, a substantially decreased need for hip abductor force to generate a countertorque.

The 225-lb joint reaction force estimated here is half the 450 lb of hip joint compression previously calculated for our hypothetical subject in single-limb support. This reduction is enough to relieve some of the pain symptoms experienced by someone with arthritic changes in the joint or to relieve a weak set of abductors of half their load. The compensatory lean is instinctive and commonly seen in people with hip joint disability. When a lateral trunk lean is seen during gait and is due to hip abductor muscle weakness, it is known as a **gluteus medius gait.** If the same compensation is due to hip joint pain, it is known as an **antalgic gait.** In some instances, the 75-lb abductor force we calculated as necessary to stabilize the pelvis is still beyond the work capacity of very weak or completely paralyzed hip abductors. In such cases of extreme abductor muscle weakness, the pelvis will drop to the unsupported side even in the presence of a lateral trunk lean to the supported side. If lateral lean and pelvic drop occur during walking, the gait

deviation is commonly referred to as a **Trendelenburg gait.** The lateral lean that accompanies the drop of the pelvis must be sufficient to keep the LOG within the supporting foot.

Whether a lateral trunk lean is due to muscular weakness or pain, a lateral lean of the trunk during walking still uses more energy than ordinarily required for single-limb support and may result in stress changes within the lumbar spine if used over an extended time period. Using a cane or some other assistive device offers a realistic alternative to the person with hip pain or weakness.

USE OF A CANE IPSILATERALLY

Pushing downward on a cane held in the hand on the *side of pain or weakness* would reduce the superimposed body weight by the amount of downward thrust; that is, some of the weight of HATLL would follow the arm to the cane, rather than arriving on the sacrum and the weight-bearing hip joint. Inman[28] suggested that it is realistic to expect that someone can push down on a cane with approximately 15% of his body weight. The proportion of body weight that passes through the cane will not pass through the hip joint and will not create an adduction torque around the supporting hip joint.

EXAMPLE 9: If our 180-lb subject can push down on the cane with 15% of his body weight, 27 lb of body weight (180 lb × 0.15) will pass through the cane. The magnitude of HATLL is reduced to 123 lb (150 lb − 27 lb). If the gravitational force of HATLL works through our estimated MA of 4 inches (remember, the cane is intended to avoid the trunk lean), the torque of gravity is reduced to 492 in-lb (123 lb × 4 in). With a gravitational adduction torque of 492 in-lb, the required force of the abductors acting through a 2-in MA is reduced to 246 lb (492 in-lb ÷ 2 inches). The new hip joint reaction force using a cane *ipsilaterally* would then be

| 246 lb of muscular joint compression |
| +123 lb of body weight compression |
| total hip joint compression ≥ 369 lb |

The 369 lb of hip joint compression when using a cane ipsilaterally provides some relief over the 450 lb of compression ordinarily seen in unilateral stance. It is still greater, however, than the 225 lb found with a compensatory lateral trunk lean. Although a cane used ipsilaterally provides some benefits in energy expenditure and structural stress reduction, it is not as effective in reducing hip joint compression as the undesirable lateral lean of the trunk. *Moving the cane to the opposite hand produces substantially different and better results.*

USE OF A CANE CONTRALATERALLY

When the cane is moved to the side *opposite the painful or weak hip joint*, the reduction in HATLL is the same as it is when the cane is used on the same side as the painful hip joint; that is, the superimposed body weight passing through the weight-bearing hip joint is reduced by approximately 15% of body weight. However, we now have the cane substantially farther from the painful supporting hip joint than it would be if used on the same side (Fig. 10–31); that is, in addition to relieving some of the superimposed body weight, the cane is now in a position to assist the abductor muscles in providing a countertorque to the torque of gravity.[49]

EXAMPLE 10: Our sample 180 lb patient has a superimposed body weight (HATLL) of 150 lb, of which 27 lb (W × 0.15) passes through the cane. Consequently, 123 lb of force will pass through the hip in left unilateral stance (Fig. 10–31) and will create a gravitation adduction torque of 492 in-lb. Please note again that these values only estimate the actual forces. If we assume an average MA of 20 inches between the cane in the right hand and the left weight-bearing hip joint (see Fig. 10–31), the cane would generate an opposing abduction torque of

Torque$_{cane}$ = 25 lb × 20 in = 500 in-lb

In our example, the torque of the cane appears to slightly exceed the torque produced by gravity. Recalling that the gravitational moment arm should be slightly greater than 4 inches, the gravitation torque we computed slightly *underestimated* the actual adduction torque. Let us assume, therefore, that the gravitation adduction torque and the countertorque provided by the cane offset each other. If the cane completely offset the effect of gravity, we would completely eliminate the need for a hip abductor muscle force. The total hip joint

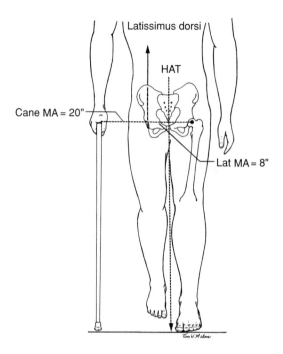

FIGURE 10–31. When a cane is placed in the hand opposite the painful supporting hip, the weight passing through the left hip is reduced, and activation of the right latissimus dorsi provides a countertorque to that of HAT and diminishes the need for a contraction of the left hip abductors. The moment arm of the cane is estimated to be 20 inches, whereas the moment arm of the latissimus dorsi is estimated to be 8 inches.

compression in unilateral stance using a cane in the opposite hand would be

0 lb of muscular joint compression

+123 lb of body weight compression

total hip joint compression ≥ 123 lb

The hip joint reaction force without muscular compression from the hip abductors would be due only to the body weight itself, or 123 lb. This is, of course, an improvement over our calculated total hip compression using a lateral lean (225 lb) and a greater improvement yet over joint compression in normal unilateral stance (450 lb). Unfortunately, the classic treatment of biomechanics of cane use also appears to substantially overestimate the effects of the cane. Krebs and colleagues[50] found a maximum of a 40% reduction in contact forces at one point on an instrumented femoral head prosthesis during cane-assisted gait, not the nearly 75% reduction the classic calculation would indicate. The discrepancy can be resolved by addressing how the force applied to the cane provides a countertorque to gravity.

We have just reviewed the classic description of how using a cane in the hand opposite to a painful or weak hip affects forces across that joint. A similar explanation can be found in numerous texts and journal articles. However, few address the question of *how* the downward thrust of the arm on the cane actually acts on the pelvis. As we saw in Chapter 1, the equilibrium of an object (such as the pelvis) can only be affected by forces actually applied to that object. The explanation for the effect of the cane lacks cohesiveness unless we can explain how the force on the cane translates to a force applied to the pelvis. Although conjectural, we propose that the force of the downward thrust on the cane arrives on the pelvis through a contraction of the latissimus dorsi muscle.

It is well established that the latissimus dorsi is a depressor of humerus[31] through both its humeral attachment and its more variable scapular attachment,[6] and has been classically defined as the "crutch-walking muscle."[33,51] Because the downward thrust on the cane is accomplished through shoulder depression just as crutch walking is, it is logical to assume that the latissimus dorsi is active when a cane is used. The latissimus dorsi attaches to the iliac crest of the pelvis. A contraction of the latissimus dorsi would result in an upward pull on the iliac crest on the side of the cane (opposite the weak or painful weight-bearing hip) as shown in Figure 10–31. An upward pull on the side of the pelvis opposite the supporting hip joint axis (hip hiking force) creates an abduction torque around the supporting hip joint. This abduction torque can offset the gravitational adduction torque around the same hip joint. It is reasonable to estimate that the magnitude of latissimus dorsi muscle contraction should be approximately the same as the downward thrust on the cane (27 lb) under the supposition that this muscle initiates the thrust. Measures of the MA of the pull of the latissimus dorsi on the pelvis are not readily available. However, the latissimus has an attachment to the pelvis on the posterior iliac crest lateral to the erector spinae.[6] Given this, let's assume that the line of pull of the muscle is applied to the pelvis approximately above the acetabulum. If we continue to assume that the gravitational force lies 4 inches from the acetabulae, the line of pull of the latissimus should lie about 8 inches from the acetabulum

of the weight-bearing hip joint (see Fig. 10–31). Now let's use the estimated upward pull of the latissimus dorsi and its estimated moment arm to calculate the total hip joint compression for our hypothetical hip patient using a cane in the contralateral hand.

EXAMPLE 11: We have a 180-lb patient with left hip pain using a cane in his right hand (see Fig. 10–31). If he pushes down on the cane in his right hand with a 27 lb force (15% of body weight), HATLL will have a magnitude of 123 lb and will create a gravitational adduction torque around the stance hip joint of 492 in-lb (123 lb × 4 inches). The countertorque (abduction around the stance left hip) produced by a contraction of the right latissimus dorsi is given by

$$\text{Torque}_{\text{Rt. Latissimus}} = 27 \text{ lb} \times 8 \text{ in}$$

$$= 216 \text{ in-lb}$$

If the gravitational adduction torque is 492 in-lb and the abduction torque produced by the right latissimus is 216 in-lb, there is still an unopposed adduction torque around the stance left hip of 276 in-lb. Consequently, a contraction of the left hip abductors is still needed. The magnitude of required abductor force will be

$$\text{Torque}_{\text{abduction}} = 276 \text{ in-lb} = 2 \text{ in} \times F_{ms}$$

$$F_{ms} = 276 \text{in-lb} \backslash 2 \text{ in} = 138 \text{ lb}$$

Given both a contraction of the right latissimus dorsi and the left hip abductors, total hip joint compression at the left stance hip would be:

138 lb of abductor muscle compression

+123 lb of body weight compression

total hip joint compression ≥ 261 lb

In the calculation of total hip joint compression in Example 11, we considered body weight compression and abductor muscle compression without adding in any compression from the contraction of the latissimus dorsi. The latissimus dorsi, unlike the hip abductor muscles, does not cross the hip and cannot create compression across the hip joint. Our new estimate of total hip joint compression (261 lb) using a cane contralaterally resulted in a higher estimated joint reaction force than the classic analysis (123 lb) first presented in this section. The higher estimate, however, is more in line with the findings of Krebs and colleagues[50] that a cane opposite a painful hip can relieve the affected hip of as much as 40% of its load. If we reduced the normal hip joint compression of our hypothetical patient (calculated earlier to be 450 lb) by 40%, we would still expect to find a compressive force of 270 lb (450 lb × 0.60) when a cane is used in the opposite hand. Our estimate of 261 lb of remaining joint compression with use of a cane is, therefore, within the maximum expected reduction.

ADJUSTMENT OF A CARRIED LOAD

When someone with hip joint pain or weakness carries a load in the hand or on the trunk (as with a backpack or purse), there is a potential to increase the demands on the hip abductors and increase the hip joint compression. The added external load will increase the superimposed weight acting through the affected supporting hip in unilateral stance. Concomitantly, the gravitational torque *may* increase, resulting in an increased demand on the supporting hip abductors for countertorque. Although the increase in superimposed weight when carrying a load cannot be avoided, it is possible to avoid the increase in gravitational torque on the side of a painful or weak hip. If the external load is carried in the arm or on the side of the trunk *ipsilateral* to the painful or weak hip, the asymmetrical external load will cause a shift in the combined body/external load COG *toward* the painful hip. Any shift of the COG (or resulting LOG) toward the painful hip will reduce the gravitational MA. If the external load is not too great, the reduction in the gravitational MA can result in a reduction in gravitational adduction torque around the stance hip joint. With a reduction in gravitational adduction torque, there is a reduced demand on the hip abductors to provide an offsetting countertorque, as well as a reduction in hip joint compression when in unilateral stance on the affected limb. Of course, the reverse effect will occur if the load is carried on the side *opposite* to the weak or painful hip. In that scenario, the external load both increases superimposed body weight *and* increases the gravitational moment arm around the weak or painful hip when in unilateral stance on that hip.

Neumann and Cook[52] measured EMG activity in the gluteus medius during varying load-carrying conditions. They found that a load of 10% of body weight carried on the right reduced the need for hip abductor activity when in right unilateral stance; that is, the increase in superimposed body weight was offset by the decrease in gravitational MA. When the load on the right was increased to 20% of body weight, the right abductor activity was statistically similar to the activity before the load was added. The increase in superimposed body weight and decrease in MA resulted in the same gravitational torque as when there was no load. When the load was carried in the left hand, there was a substantial increase in right abductor activity during right stance. This load condition increased the magnitude of HAT *and* displaced the LOG *away* from the hip joint, increasing the gravitational torque and the need for hip abductor activity. Whereas Neumann and Cook looked at gluteus medius activity to assess the results of a carried load, Bergmann and colleagues[43] estimated hip joint reaction forces in several subjects and measured actual forces in one subject with an instrumented femoral head prosthesis. They found that most of their subjects could carry loads of up to 25% of body weight in the right hand and still show a slight reduction in hip joint compression over the no-load condition when in right unilateral stance. They point out, however, that a typical compensatory shift of the trunk away from the load should be avoided if the goal is to reduce hip joint compression.

Carrying a moderate load (less than 25% of body weight) on the side of hip pain or hip abductor weakness may be a reasonable alternative for reducing hip joint pain or a gluteus medius gait if a person is resistant to using a cane. Carrying a load on the side opposite a weak or painful hip should be avoided.

Hip Joint Pathology

The foundation should be clearly laid at this point for an understanding of dysfunction at the hip joint. The very large active and passive forces crossing the joint make it susceptible to wear and tear of normal components and to failure of weakened components. Small changes in the biomechanics of the femur or the acetabulum can result in increases in passive forces above normal levels or in weakness of the dynamic joint stabilizers. Some of the more common problems and the underlying mechanisms are discussed in this section.

Arthrosis

The most common painful condition of the hip is due to deterioration of the articular cartilage and to subsequent related changes in articular tissues.[45] Known as **osteoarthritis, degenerative arthritis,** or perhaps most appropriately as **hip joint arthrosis,** prevalence rates are about 10% to 15% in those over 55 years of age, with approximately equal distribution among men and women.[53] Although trauma or malalignment such as femoral anteversion may be associated with occurrence,[46] 50% of the cases are considered to be idiopathic[5]; that is, half of the cases of hip joint arthrosis have no evident underlying pathology. Changes may be due to subtle deviations present from birth, to tissue changes inherent in aging, to the repetitive mechanical stress of loading the body weight on the hip joint over a prolonged period, or to interactions of each of these factors. The factors most closely associated with idiopathic hip joint arthrosis are increased age and increased weight/height ratio.[54] Lane and colleagues found no association between osteoarthritic changes and running status among older subjects.[55]

The mechanism for cartilaginous degeneration in the hip joint is not clear-cut. When a biomechanical problem is not evident, degenerative changes may be due not to excessive forces at the hip joint but to inadequate forces. This would explain why there is little or no association between increased activity level with sports or recreational activities and hip arthrosis.[56,57]

It may be that forces in excess of half the body weight are needed to fully compress the femoral head into congruent contact with the dome of the acetabulum.[3] Using a number of other studies as a base, Bullough and associates[3] hypothesized that we typically spend no more than 5% to 25% of our time in unilateral lower extremity weight-bearing activities where the load may be sufficient to compress the articular cartilage of the dome of the acetabulum. Lower loads and infrequent high joint forces may be inadequate to maintain flow of nutrients and wastes through the avascular cartilage. The theory of inadequate compression as a contributing factor to hip joint degeneration is supported by the more common degenerative changes in the femur being at the periphery of the head and the peri-

foveal area, rather than at the superior primary weight-bearing area.[3,24] The periphery of the head receives only about one-third the compressive force of the superior portion of the head,[42] whereas the superior portion of the head is compressed not only in standing but is also in contact with the posterior acetabulum during sitting activities.[24] The area of the femoral head around the fovea is most commonly in the non-weight-bearing acetabular notch and would undergo compression relatively infrequently. Wingstrand and associates[15] proposed that excessive intra-articular fluid from relatively benign synovitis or trauma may reduce articular congruence and the stabilizing effect of atmospheric pressure, resulting in microinstability and unfavorable cartilage loads.

Fracture

Although the weight-bearing forces coming through the hip joint may cause deterioration of the articular cartilage, the bony components must also be of sufficient strength to withstand the forces that are acting around and through the hip joint. As noted in the section on the weight-bearing structure of the hip joint, the vertical weight-bearing forces that pass down through the superior margin of the acetabulum in both unilateral and bilateral stance act at some distance from ground reaction force up the shaft of the femur. The result is a bending force across the femoral neck (see Fig. 10–14). Normally the trabecular systems are capable of resisting the bending forces, but abnormal increases in the magnitude of the force or weakening of the bone can lead to bony failure. The site of failure is likely to be in areas of thinner trabecular distribution such as the zone of weakness (see Fig. 10–13).

Bony failure in the femoral neck is uncommon in the child or young adult even with large applied loads. However, femoral neck fractures occur at the rate of about 98/100,000 people in the United States, with the average age of occurrence being in the seventies. Hip joint fractures occur among white adults at a much higher rate than among black adults.[58] There is a predominance of fractures in women, although this is certainly influenced by their greater longevity. In the middle-aged group, women actually suffer fewer hip fractures than do men, although the fractures in this age group are usually attributable to substantial trauma.[58] In 87% of cases of hip fracture among the elderly population, the precipitating factor appears to be moderate trauma such as that caused by a fall from standing, from a chair, or from bed. There is consensus that hip fracture is associated with, but not exclusively due to, diminished bone density.[53] Bone density decreases about 2% per year after age 50 and trabeculae clearly thin and disappear with aging.[59] Cummings and Nevitt[59] believe the exponential increase in hip fractures with age cannot be accounted for by decreased bone density alone and propose that the slowed gait characteristic of the elderly may play an important part. They contend that the slowing of gait makes it less likely that momentum will carry the body forward in a fall (generally on to an outstretched hand), and more likely that the fall will occur backward on to the hip area weakened by bone loss and no longer padded by the fat and muscle bulk of youth.

Hip fracture will continue to receive considerable attention because of the high health care costs of both conservative and operative treatment. Not only is the condition painful, but malunion of the fracture can lead to joint instability or cartilaginous deterioration (or both) due to poorly aligned bony segments. Although the femoral head may receive some blood supply via the ligament of the femoral head, an absent or diminished supply through the ligament of the head (as occurs with aging) means reliance on anastomoses from the circumflex arteries. This circumflex arterial supply may be disrupted by femoral neck fracture, leaving the femoral head susceptible to avascular necrosis and requiring replacement of the head of the femur with an artificial implant. Femoral neck fracture also has an associated mortality rate that may be as high as 20%.[58]

Bony Abnormalities of the Femur

When the bony structure of the femur is altered through abnormal angles of torsion or inclination, subsequent changes in the direction and magnitude of the forces acting around the hip can lead to other pathologic conditions such as increased likelihood of joint arthrosis, increased likelihood of femoral neck fracture, or muscular weakness. The normal angles of inclination and torsion appear to represent optimal balance of stresses and muscle alignment. Alterations may actually appear to result in advantages relative to some functions, but are always accompanied by concomitant disadvantages relative to others.

Coxa Valga/Coxa Vara

In coxa valga (see Fig. 10–5a) the angle of inclination in the femur is greater than the normal adult angle of 125°. The increased angle brings the vertical weight-bearing line closer to the shaft of the femur, diminishing the shear, or bending, force across the femoral neck. The reduction in force is actually reflected in a reduction in density of the lateral trabecular system.[25] However, the decreased distance between the femoral head and the greater trochanter also decreases the length of the MA of the hip abductor muscles. The decreased muscular MA results in an increased demand for muscular force generation to maintain sufficient abduction torque to counterbalance the gravitational adduction moment acting around the supporting hip joint during single-limb support. Either the additional muscular force requirement will increase the total joint reaction force within the hip joint, or the abductor muscles will be unable to meet the increased demand and will be functionally weakened. Although the abductors may be otherwise normal, the reduction in biomechanical effectiveness may produce the compensations typical of primary abductor muscle weakness. Coxa valga also decreases the amount of femoral articular surface in contact with the dome of the acetabulum. As the femoral head points more superiorly, there is a decreasing amount of coverage from the acetabulum superiorly. Consequently, coxa valga decreases the stability of the hip and predisposes the hip to dislocation.[8,10,21]

Coxa vara is considered to give the advantage of improved hip joint stability (if not too extreme an angle reduction). The apparent improvement in congruence occurs because the decreased angle between the neck and shaft of the femur will turn the femoral head deeper into the acetabulum, decreasing the amount of articular surface exposed superiorly and increasing coverage from the acetabulum. A varus femur, if not due to trauma, may also increase the length of the MA of the hip abductor muscles by increasing the distance between the femoral head and the greater trochanter.[12] The increased MA decreases the amount of force that must be generated by the abductor muscles in single-limb support and reduces the joint reaction force. However, coxa vara has the disadvantage of increasing the bending moment along the femoral head and neck. This increase in bending force can actually be seen by the increased density of trabeculae laterally in the femur, due to the increase in tensile stresses.[25] The increased shear force along the femoral neck will increase the predisposition toward femoral neck fracture.[10,21]

Coxa vara may increase the likelihood in the adolescent child that the femoral head will slide on the cartilaginous epiphysis of the head of the femur. In childhood, the epiphysis is fairly horizontal.[6] Consequently, the superimposed weight merely compresses the head into the epiphyseal plate. In adolescence, growth of the bone results in a more oblique orientation of the epiphyseal plate. The epiphyseal obliquity makes the plate more vulnerable to shear forces at a time when the plate is already weakened by the rapid growth that occurs during this period of life.[58] Weight-bearing forces may slide the femoral head inferiorly, resulting in a slipped capital femoral epiphysis. As is true for a hip fracture, the altered biomechanics and at-risk blood supply require that normal alignment be restored before secondary degenerative changes can occur.

Anteversion/Retroversion

Variations in the angle of torsion also affect hip biomechanics and function. Anteversion of the femoral head reduces hip joint stability because the femoral articular surface is more exposed anteriorly. The line of the hip abductors may fall more posterior to the joint, reducing the MA for abduction.[46] As is true for coxa valga, the resulting need for additional abductor muscle force may predispose the joint to arthrosis or may functionally weaken the joint, producing energy-consuming and wearing gait deviations. The effect of femoral anteversion may also be seen at the knee joint. When the femoral head is anteverted, pressure from the anterior capsuloligamentous structures and the anterior musculature may push the femoral head back into the acetabulum, causing the entire femur to medially rotate. Although the medial rotation of the femur improves the congruence in the acetabulum, the knee joint axis through the femoral condyles is now turned medially, altering the plane of knee flexion/extension and resulting in a toe-in gait. The abnormal position of the knee joint axis and toed-in gait are commonly labeled **medial femoral**

torsion. Medial femoral torsion and femoral anteversion are the *same* abnormal condition of the femur. The label designates whether the exaggerated twist in the femur is altering the mechanics at the hip joint (femoral anteversion) or at the knee joint (medial femoral torsion). As shall be seen in the next two chapters, an anteverted femur will also affect the biomechanics of the patellofemoral joint at the knee and of the subtalar joint in the foot.

Femoral retroversion is the opposite of anteversion and creates opposite problems from femoral anteversion.

Summary

The normal hip joint is well designed to withstand the forces that act through and around it, assisted by the trabecular systems, cartilaginous coverings, muscles, and ligaments. Alterations in the direction or magnitude of forces acting around the hip create abnormal concentrations of stress that predispose the joint structures to injury and degenerative changes. The degenerative changes, in turn, can create additional alterations in function that not only affect the hip joint's ability to support the body weight in standing, in locomotor activities, and other activities of daily living but may also result in adaptive changes at more proximal and distal joints. Consequently, the reader must understand both the dysfunction that might occur at the hip *and* the associated dysfunctions that may result in or from dysfunction elsewhere in the lower extremity and spine. The remaining chapters of this text will focus not only on primary dysfunction at a joint complex but on associated dysfunction related to proximal and distal joint problems.

REFERENCES

1. Moore, K, and Dalley, AI: Clinically Oriented Anatomy, ed 4. Lippincott Williams & Wilkins, Philadelphia, 1999.
2. Brinckmann, P, et al: Stress on the articular surface of the hip joint in healthy adults and persons with idiopathic osteoarthrosis of the hip joint. Biomechanics 14:149–156, 1981.
3. Bullough, P, et al: The relationship between degenerative changes and load-bearing in the human hip. J Bone Joint Surg 55B:746–758, 1973.
4. Adna, S, et al: The acetabular sector angle of the adult hip determined by computed tomography. Acta Radiol Diagn 27:443–447, 1986.
5. Brinckmann, P, et al: Sex differences in the skeletal

geometry of the human pelvis and hip joint. Biomechanics 1:427–430, 1981.

6. Williams, P (ed): Gray's Anatomy, ed 38. Churchill Livingstone, New York, 1995.

7. Svenningsen, S, et al: Regression of femoral anteversion. Acta Orthop Scand 60:170–173, 1989.

8. Kapandji, I: The Physiology of the Joints, Vol 2, ed 5. Williams & Wilkins, Baltimore, 1987.

9. Williams, P, and Warwick, R (eds): Gray's Anatomy, ed 37. WB Saunders, Philadelphia, 1985.

10. Singleton, HC, and LeVeau, BF: Stability and stress. A review. Phys Ther 55(9):957–973, 1975.

11. Rosse, C: The Musculoskeletal System in Health and Disease. Harper & Row, Hagerstown, MD, 1980.

12. Iglic, A, et al: Biomechanical study of various greater trochanter positions. Arch Orthop Trauma Surg 114:76–78, 1995.

13. Radin, E: Biomechanics of the human hip. Clin Orthop 152:28–34, 1980.

14. D'Ambrosia, R: Musculoskeletal Disorders: Regional Examination and Differential Diagnosis, ed 2. JB Lippincott, Philadelphia, 1986.

15. Wingstrand, H, et al: Intracasular and atmospheric pressure in the dynamics and stability of the hip. Acta Orthop Scand 61:231–235, 1990.

16. Chen, H-H, et al: Adaptations of ligamentum teres in ischemic necrosis of the human femoral head. Clin Orthop 328:268–275, 1996.

17. Fuss, F, and Bacher, A: New aspects of the morphology and function of the human hip joint ligaments. Am J Anat 192:1–13, 1991.

18. Crock, H: An atlas of the arterial supply of the head and neck of the femur in man. Clin Orthop 152: 7–27, 1980.

19. Tan, C, and Wong, W: Absence of the ligament of the head of femur in the human hip joint. Singapore Med J 31:360–363, 1990.

20. Yutani, Y, et al: Cartilaginous differentiation in the joint capsule. J Bone Miner Metab 17:7–10, 1999.

21. Radin, E, et al: Practical Biomechanics for the Orthopedic Surgeon. John Wiley & Sons, New York, 1979.

22. Pauwels, F: Biomechanics of the Normal and Diseased Hip. Springer-Verlag, Berlin, 1976.

23. Kummer, B: Is the Pauwels' theory of hip biomechanics still valid? A critical analysis, based on modern methods. Ann Anat 175:203–210, 1993.

24. Athanasiou, K, et al: Comparative study of the intrinsic mechanical properties of the human acetabular and femoral head cartilage. J Orthop Res 12:340–349, 1994.

25. Bombelli, R, et al: Mechanics of the normal and osteoarthritic hip: A new perspective. Clin Orthop 182:69–78, 1984.

26. Norkin, C, and White, D: Measurement of Joint Motion: A Guide to Goniometry, ed 2. FA Davis, Philadelphia, 1995.

27. Observational Gait Analysis Handbook Department, PaPT. Rancho Los Amigos Hospital, Downey, CA, 1989.

28. Inman, V, et al: Human Walking. Williams & Wilkins, Baltimore, 1981.

29. Kendall, F, et al: Muscles: Testing and Function, ed 4. Williams & Wilkins, Baltimore, 1993.

30. Gowitzke, B, and Milner, M: Scientific Bases of Human Movement, ed 3. Williams & Wilkins, Baltimore, 1988.

31. Basmajian, J, and DeLuca, C: Muscles Alive, ed 5. Williams & Wilkins, Baltimore, 1985.

32. Nemeth, G, and Ohlsen, H: In vivo moment arm lengths for hip extensor muscles at different angles of hip flexion. J Biomech 18:129–140, 1985.

33. Smith, L, et al: Brunnstrom's Clinical Kinesiology, ed 5. FA Davis, Philadelphia, 1996.

34. Wheatly, M, and Jahnke, W: Electromyographic study of the superficial thigh and hip muscles in normal individuals. Arch Phys Med 32:508, 1951.

35. Kaplan, E: The iliotibial tract. J Bone Joint Surg 40A:825–832, 1958.

36. Ito, J: Morphological analysis of the human lower extremity based on the relative muscle weight. Okajimas Folia Anat Jpn 73:247–252, 1996.

37. Murray, M, and Sepic, S: Maximum isometric torque of hip abductor and adductor muscles. Phys Ther 48:2, 1968.

38. Delp, S, et al: Variation of rotation moment arms with hip flexion. J Biomech 32:493–501, 1999.

39. Soderburg, GL, and Dostal, WF: Electromyographic study of three parts of the gluteus medius muscle during functional activities. Phys Ther 58(6):691–696.

40. Jensen, R, et al: A technique for obtaining measurements of force generated by hip muscles. Arch Phys Med 52:207, 1971.

41. Olson, V, et al: The maximum torque generated by the eccentric, isometric and concentric contractions of the hip abductor muscles. Phys Ther 52:2, 1972.

42. Nordin, M, and Frankel, V: Basic Biomechanics of the Skeletal System, ed 2. Lea & Febiger, Philadelphia, 1989.

43. Bergmann, G, et al: Hip joint forces during load carrying. Clin Orthop 335:190–201, 1997.

44. LeVeau, B: Williams and Lissner's Biomechanics of Human Motion, ed 3. WB Saunders, Philadelphia, 1992.

45. Cailliet, R: Soft Tissue Pain and Disability, ed 3. FA Davis, Philadelphia, 1996.

46. Clark, JM, and Haynor, DR: Anatomy of the abductor muscles of the hip as studied by computed tomography. J Bone Joint Surg 69A:1021–1031, 1987.

47. Paul, J, and McGrouther, D: Forces transmitted at the hip and knee joint of normal and disabled persons during a range of activities. Acta Orthop Belg (Suppl) 41:78–88, 1975.

48. Crowinshield, R, et al: A biomechanical investigation of the human hip. J Biomech 11:75, 1976.

49. Blount, W: Don't throw away the cane. J Bone Joint Surg 18A:3, 1956.

50. Krebs, D, et al: Hip biomechanics during gait. J Orthop Sports Phys Ther 28:51–59, 1998.

51. Schenkman, M, and DeCartaya, V: Kinesiology of the shoulder complex. J Orthop Sports Phys Ther 8:438–450, 1987.

52. Neumann, D, and Cook, T: Effect of load and carrying position on the electromyographic activity of the gluteus medius muscle during walking. Phys Ther 65:305–311, 1985.

53. Kelsey, J: The epidemiology of diseases of the hip: A review of the literature. Int J Epidemiol 6:269–280, 1977.

54. Pogrund, H, et al: Normal width of the adult hip joint: The relationship to age, sex and obesity. Skel Radiol 10:10–12, 1983.

55. Lane, N, et al: The relationship of running to osteoarthritis of the knee and hip and bone mineral density of the lumbar spine: A 9 year longitudinal study. J Rheumatol 25:334–341, 1998.

56. Lane, N, et al: Recreational physical activity and the risk of osteoarthritis of the hip in elderly women. J Rheumatol 26:849–854, 1999.

57. Panush, RS, and Brown, DG: Exercise and arthritis. Sports Med 4:54–64, 1987.

58. Lewinnek, G, et al: The significance and a comparative analysis of the epidemiology of hip fractures. Clin Orthop 152:35–43, 1980.
59. Cummings, S, and Nevitt, M: A hypothesis: The causes of hip fracture. J Gerontol Med Sci 44:M107-M111, 1989.

Study Questions

1. Which side of the femoral neck and which side of the femoral shaft are subjected to compressive stresses during weight-bearing? How does the bone respond to these stresses?

2. What is the primary weight-bearing area of the femoral head? Of the acetabulum? Where are degenerative changes most commonly found for the femoral head and acetabulum?

3. Describe why using a cane on the side opposite hip joint pain or weakness is more effective than using the cane on the same side.

4. Demonstrate how variations in the angle of inclination affect the MA of the hip abductors by drawing the following: a normal angle of inclination at the hip, the angle in coxa vara, and the angle in coxa valga. Please include the action line and the MA of the hip abductors in the diagram.

5. Describe what would happen to the pelvis in left unilateral stance when the left hip abductors are paralyzed. How is equilibrium maintained in this situation?

6. Describe motion at the right and left hip joints and at the lumbar spine during hiking of the pelvis in right limb stance, assuming that the person is to remain upright.

7. Contrast the close-packed versus maximally congruent position for the hip joint.

8. Calculate the minimum joint reaction force (total hip joint compression) at the right hip joint that would occur for a 200-lb person standing symmetrically on both legs versus one leg (assuming a gravitational MA of 4 inches and the abductor muscle MA of 2 inches).

9. Under what circumstances does the hip joint participate as part of an open chain? As part of a closed chain?

10. What bony abnormality or abnormalities of the femur or pelvis predispose the hip joint to the possibility of dislocation? Why?

11. Which structures at the hip joint, given their location, would appear likely to limit the extremes of motion in flexion? extension? lateral rotation? medial rotation? abduction and adduction?

12. Which muscles of the hip joint are affected by knee joint position? Which position of the knee makes these muscles less effective at the hip joint?

13. If someone was in a unilateral stance on the left limb, what hip joint motion would result from forward rotation of the pelvis?

14. If a person has a painful right hip, in which direction should she lean her trunk to reduce the forces on the right hip during right unilateral support? Explain the reasons for your answer.

15. What position does the hip joint tend to assume when there is joint pain? Why is this?

16. Identify several factors that might predispose someone to a femoral neck fracture.

17. How does the femoral head receive its blood supply? What problems might jeopardize that supply?

18. Relate femoral anteversion to medial femoral torsion.

19. Under what circumstances might the hip adductors work synergistically with the hip abductors?

20. Why is the acetabular notch nonarticular? In what ways does this serve hip joint function?

21. How would you advise a woman with hip joint pain to carry her purse? Why?

CHAPTER 11
THE KNEE COMPLEX

OBJECTIVES

Following the study of this chapter, the reader should be able to:

Describe

1. The articulating surfaces at the tibiofemoral and patellofemoral joints.
2. The joint capsule including the plicae and bursae.
3. The anatomic and mechanical axes of the knee.
4. Motion of the femoral condyles during flexion and extension in a closed kinematic chain.
5. Motion of the tibia in flexion and extension in an open kinematic chain.

Draw

1. The Q angle when given an illustration of the lower extremity.
2. Moment arm of the quadriceps at the following degrees of knee flexion: 90°, 130°, 30°, and 10°.
3. The action lines of the vastus lateralis and the vastus medialis oblique.

Locate

1. The attachments of all the muscles at the knee.
2. The bursae surrounding the knee.
3. The attachments of the ligaments of the medial and lateral compartments.

Identify

1. Structures that contribute to medial, lateral, and anterior-posterior stability of the knee, including dynamic and static stabilizers.
2. Structures that contribute to rotatory stability at the knee.
3. The normal forces that are acting at the knee.

Compare

1. The knee and the elbow joint on the basis of similarities/dissimilarities in structure and function.
2. The lateral with the medial meniscus on the basis of structure and function.
3. The forces on the patellofemoral joint in full flexion with full extension.
4. The action of the quadriceps in an open kinematic chain with that in a closed kinematic chain.
5. The effectiveness of the hamstring muscles as knee flexors in each of the following hip positions: hyperextension, 10° of flexion, and full flexion (open kinematic chain).
6. The effectiveness of the rectus femoris muscle as a knee extensor at 60° of knee flexion with its effectiveness at 10° of knee flexion.
7. The anterior cruciate ligament with the posterior cruciate ligament in regard to structure and function.

Explain

1. The function of the menisci.
2. How a tear of the medial collateral ligament may affect joint function.
3. The functions of the suprapatellar, gastrocnemius, infrapatellar, and prepatellar bursae.
4. Why the semiflexed position of the knee is the least painful position.
5. Why the knee may be more susceptible to injury than the hip joint.
6. The plicae and how they may affect knee structure and function.

· ·

Introduction

The knee complex is similar to the elbow complex in that flexion and extension of the knee produces a functional shortening and lengthening of the extremity. In addition to providing mobility, however, the knee complex plays a major role in supporting the body during dynamic and static activities. In a closed kinematic chain the knee joint works in conjunction with the hip joint and ankle to support the body weight in the static erect posture. Dynamically, the knee complex is responsible for moving and supporting the body in sitting and squatting activities and for supporting and transferring the body weight during locomotor activities. In an open kinematic chain the knee provides mobility for the foot in space. The fact that the knee must fulfill major stability as well as major mobility roles is reflected in its structure and function. The knee is not only one of the largest joints in the body but is also the most complex. The development of prostheses that are capable of simulating some of the functions of the knee joint has only occurred during the past 20 or 30 years.[1]

The knee complex is composed of two distinct articulations located within a single joint capsule: the tibiofemoral joint and the patellofemoral joint. The tibiofemoral joint is the articulation between the distal femur and the proximal tibia. The patellofemoral joint is the articulation between the patella and the femur. Although the patella serves the tibiofemoral mechanism, the characteristics, responses, and problems of the patellofemoral joint are distinct enough from the tibiofemoral joint to warrant separate attention. The superior tibiofibular joint is not considered to be a part of the knee complex because it is not contained within the knee joint capsule and is functionally related to the ankle joint; it will be discussed in Chapter 12.

Structure of the Tibiofemoral Joint

The tibiofemoral, or knee joint, is a double condyloid joint (defined by the medial and lateral articular surfaces) with 2° of freedom of motion.[2] Flexion and extension occur in the sagittal plane around a coronal axis; medial and lateral rotation occur in the transverse plane about a vertical axis. Careful examination of the articular surfaces and the relationship of the surfaces to each other will facilitate an understanding of the movements at the knee joint and both the functions and dysfunctions common to the joint.

Femoral Articular Surface

The large medial and lateral condyles on the distal femur form the proximal articular surfaces of the knee joint. The condyles have a large and very obvious curvature anteroposteriorly but are also each slightly convex in the frontal plane. The anteroposterior convexity of the condyles is not a consistent spherical shape but has a smaller radius of curvature posteriorly (Fig. 11–1). The two condyles are separated by the intercondylar notch or fossa through most of their length, but are joined anteriorly by an asymmetrical, shallow, saddle-shaped groove called the **patellar groove** or **surface;** the patellar surface is separated from the tibial articular surface by two slight grooves that run obliquely across the condyles (Fig. 11–2a).[2] The shaft of the femur is not vertical but is angled in such a way that the femoral condyles do not lie immediately below the femoral head, but somewhat medial. Given the obliquity of the shaft of the femur, the lateral condyle lies more directly in line with the shaft than does the medial condyle (Fig. 11–2b). The articular surface of the lateral condyle is also not as long as the articular surface of the medial femoral condyle.

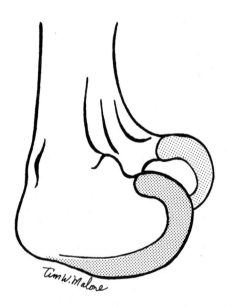

FIGURE 11–1. The arteroposterior convexity of the condyles is not consistently spherical, being more accentuated posteriorly.

When the femur is examined through an inferior view (see Fig. 11–2a), the lateral condyle would appear *at first glance* to be longer. However, when the patellofemoral surface is excluded, it can be seen that the lateral tibial surface stops before the medial. The medial femoral condyle is, on average, two-thirds of an inch longer than the lateral condyle.[3] The medial condyle extends further distally than the lateral so that, despite the angulation of the shaft of the femur, the distal end of the femur is essentially horizontal (see Fig. 11–2b).

Tibial Articular Surface

The articulating surfaces on the tibia that correspond to the femoral articulating surfaces are the two concave, asymmetrical medial and lateral tibial condyles or plateaus (Fig. 11–3a). The proximal tibia is enlarged as compared to the shaft and overhangs the shaft posteriorly (the lateral condyle more so than the medial). The articulating surface of the medial tibial condyle is 50% larger than that of the lateral condyle (corresponding to the larger medial femoral condyle) and the articular cartilage of the medial tibial condyle is three times thicker.[3] The two tibial condyles are separated by a roughened area and two bony spines called the **intercondylar tubercles.** These tubercles become lodged in the intercondylar notch of the femur during knee extension (Fig. 11–3b).

Tibiofemoral Articulation

When the large articular condyles of the femur are placed on the shallow concavities of the tibial condyle, the incongruence of the knee joint is evident. As has been true elsewhere in the body, articular incongruence at the knee is accompanied by an accessory joint structure that enhances congruence and assists in the balance between mobility and stability needed by the joint. Each of the condyles of the knee joint has its own accessory joint structure, together known as the **menisci** of the knee.

Menisci

Two asymmetrical fibrocartilaginous joint disks called menisci are located on the tibial condyles (Fig. 11–4). The medial meniscus is a semicircle; the lateral meniscus is four-fifths of a ring.[2] Both menisci are open toward the in-

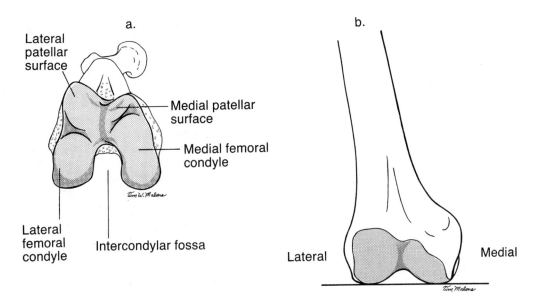

Lateral patellar surface

Medial patellar surface

Medial femoral condyle

Lateral femoral condyle

Intercondylar fossa

a.

b.

Lateral

Medial

FIGURE 11–2. (a) The patellar surface is separated from the tibial articular surface by two slight grooves that run obliquely across the condyles. The medial femoral condyle is longer than the lateral femoral condyle; the lateral lip of the patellar surface is larger than the medial lip of the patellar surface. (b) Given the obliquity of the shaft of the femur, the lateral femoral condyle lies more directly in line with the shaft than does the medial. The medial condyle is more prominent, however, resulting in a horizontal distal femoral surface despite the oblique shaft.

tercondylar area, thick peripherally and thin centrally, forming concavities into which the respective femoral condyles can sit (Fig. 11–5). The wedge- shaped menisci increase the radius of curvature of the tibial condyles and, therefore, joint congruence. By increasing congruence (articular contact), the menisci also play an important part in distributing weight-bearing forces, in reducing friction between the joint segments, and serving as shock absorbers.[4] The menisci have multiple attachments to surrounding structures, some common to both and some unique to each. Each meniscus is connected around its periphery to the tibial condyle by the **coronary ligaments,** which are composed of fibers from the knee joint capsule. Both menisci are also attached directly or indirectly to the patella via the so-called **patellomeniscal**[5,6] or **patellotibial ligaments,**[7] which are anterior capsular thickenings. The open ends of the menisci, which are attached to their respective tibial intercondylar tubercles, are

FIGURE 11–3. (a) A superior view of the articulating surfaces on the tibia illustrates differences in size and configuration between the medial and lateral tibial plateaus. (b) A view of the posterior aspect of the tibiofemoral joint illustrates how the tibial intercondylar tubercles become lodged in the femoral intercondylar fossa when the joint is fully extended.

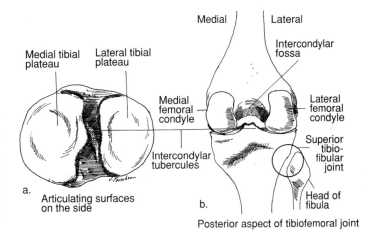

Medial tibial plateau

Lateral tibial plateau

Medial

Lateral

Intercondylar fossa

Medial femoral condyle

Lateral femoral condyle

Superior tibiofibular joint

Intercondylar tubercules

Head of fibula

a. Articulating surfaces on the side

b.

Posterior aspect of tibiofemoral joint

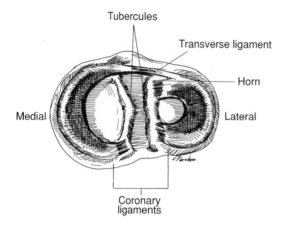

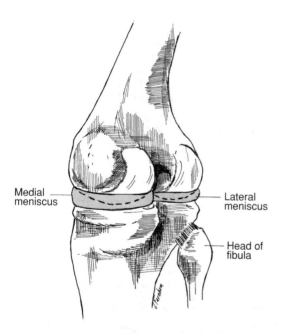

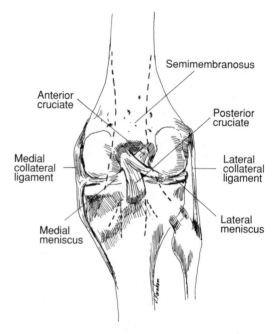

Tubercules

Transverse ligament

Horn

Medial

Lateral

Coronary
ligaments

FIGURE 11–4. Structure of the menisci. A superior view of the menisci illustrates differences in size and configuration between the medial and lateral menisci. The medial meniscus is C-shaped, whereas the lateral meniscus is shaped like a ring or circle.

called **horns.** Each meniscus has an anterior and a posterior horn. The anterior horns of the two menisci are joined to each other by the transverse ligament, which may be connected to the patella via the joint capsule.[5]

Benjamin and colleagues[8] found that the attachment site of the posterior horn of the more mobile lateral meniscus had a greater zone of uncalcified fibrocartilage than the attachment site of the posterior horn of the medial meniscus. These authors suggest that the findings are consistent with the premise that greater quantities of uncalcified fibrocartilage are found at mobile attachment sites. The attachment sites of the anterior horns of the two menisci also differed in that the attachment site of the anterior horn of the lateral meniscus had a thicker zone of cortical calcified cartilage than the anterior horn of the medial meniscus. The authors attributed this finding to the fact that forces transmitted through the anterior cruciate ligament are partly relayed to the tibia through the anterior horn of the lateral meniscus.

The lateral meniscus, in addition to the connections it shares with the medial meniscus, is attached to the **posterior cruciate ligament (PCL)** (Fig. 11–6) and **popliteus muscle** via the coronary ligaments and posterior capsule,[9] and to the somewhat variable posterior **menis-**

Medial
meniscus

Lateral
meniscus

Head of
fibula

FIGURE 11–5. A posteromedial view of an extended right tibiofemoral joint shows the menisci tightly interposed between the femur and the tibia. The dotted lines indicate the wedge shape of the menisci and show how the menisci deepen and contour the tibial articulating surface to accommodate the femoral condyles.

Semimembranosus

Anterior
cruciate

Posterior
cruciate

Medial
collateral
ligament

Lateral
collateral
ligament

Medial
meniscus

Lateral
meniscus

FIGURE 11–6. Meniscal attachments. The medial meniscus is shown with its attachments to the medial collateral ligament, anterior cruciate ligament (ACL), and the outline of the semimembranosus muscle. The lateral meniscus is shown with its attachments to the posterior cruciate ligament (PCL). Its attachments to the popliteus muscle are not shown in the drawing.

cofemoral ligaments.[2,10] Some fibers from the **anterior cruciate ligament (ACL)** may also join the anterior and posterior horns.[10] The connections of the lateral meniscus are considered to be fairly loose, leaving the lateral menisci a fair amount of mobility on the lateral tibial condyle.

The medial meniscus is attached to the medial collateral ligament (see Fig. 11–6) and to the **semimembranosus muscle** through its capsular connections.[2,11] The medial meniscus is more firmly attached and less movable on the tibial condyle than the lateral meniscus. Its lack of mobility may be one of several reasons why the medial meniscus is torn more frequently than the lateral meniscus. The meniscal attachments are summarized in Table 11–1.

The menisci and meniscoligamentous complex are well established in the 8-week-old embryo[12] and during the first year of life the menisci are well vascularized throughout. The vascularity of the meniscal body gradually recedes from 18 months to 18 years until only the outer 25% to 33% is vascularized by capillaries from the joint capsule and the synovial membrane. Over age 50 years only the periphery of the meniscal body is vascularized.[13] The horns remain completely vascularized throughout life.[14] In young children whose menisci have ample blood supply,[2,12] the incidence of meniscal injuries is low. In the adult only the peripheral vascularized region of the meniscal body is capable of inflammation, repair, and remodeling following a tearing injury. However, the newly formed tissue is not identical to the tissue before injury and is not as strong.[13]

The horns of the menisci and the peripheral vascularized portion of the meniscal bodies are well innervated with free nerve endings (nociceptors) and three different mechanoreceptors (Ruffini corpuscles, Pacinian corpuscles, and Golgi tendon organs). Innervation for the posterior horns is somewhat denser in comparison to the anterior horns which may be due to the fact that the posterior horns carry a greater proportion of the load.[8,13] The meniscal innervation pattern indicates that the menisci are a source of information about joint position, direction of movement, and velocity of movement as well as information about tissue deformation.

Tibiofemoral Alignment and Weight-Bearing Forces

The anatomic (longitudinal) axis of the femur, as already noted, is oblique, directed inferiorly and medially from its proximal to its distal end. The anatomic axis of the tibia is directed almost vertically. Consequently, the femoral and tibial longitudinal axes normally form an angle *medially* at the knee joint of 185° to 190° (Fig. 11–7); that is, the femur is angled off vertical 5° to 10°,[5,15] creating a physiologic (normal) valgus angle at the knee. Although this might appear to weight the lateral condyles more than the medial, this is not the case. The mechanical axis of the lower extremity is the weight-bearing line from the center of the head of the femur to the center of the superior surface of the head of the talus[16] (Fig. 11–8). This line normally passes through the center of the knee joint between the intercondylar tubercles and averages 3° from the vertical given the width of the hip joints as compared to spacing of the feet.[5] Because the weight-bearing line (ground reaction force) follows the mechanical rather than the anatomic axes, the weight-bearing stresses on the knee joint in *bilateral static stance* are equally distributed between the medial and

Table 11–1. **Meniscal Attachments**

Attachments	Medial and Lateral Menisci	
Common	Intercondylar tubercles of the tibia Tibial condyle via coronary ligaments Patella via patellomeniscal or patellofemoral ligaments Transverse ligaments Anterior cruciate ligament	
	Medial Meniscus	Lateral Meniscus
Unique	Medial collateral ligament Semitendinosus muscle	Anterior and posterior meniscofemoral ligaments Posterior cruciate ligament Popliteus muscle

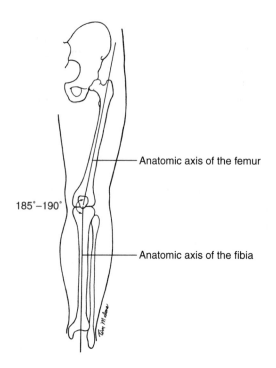

185°–190°

— Anatomic axis of the femur

— Anatomic axis of the fibia

FIGURE 11–7. The long axis of the femur and the long axis of the tibia intersect to create a physiologic valgus at the knee joint of 185° to 190°.

the dynamic knee joint ordinarily may reach two to three times body weight in normal gait[3] and five to six times body weight in activities such as running and stair climbing,[17] the menisci assume 40% to 60% of the imposed load.[18] If the menisci are removed, the magnitude of the average load per unit area on the articular cartilage nearly doubles on the femur and is six or seven times greater on the tibial condyle.[17] Elimination of any angulation between the femur and tibia (a mild genu varum) will increase the compression on the medial meniscus by 25%. Five degrees of genu varum (medial tibiofemoral angle of 175°) will increase the forces by 50%.[13]

Knee Joint Capsule

Given the incongruence of the knee joint, even with the compensation of the menisci, stability is heavily dependent on the surrounding joint structures. In knee flexion when surrounding passive structures tend to be lax, the incongruence of the joint permits at least some anterior

lateral condyles, without any concomitant horizontal shear forces.[16] This is not necessarily the case in unilateral stance or once *dynamic forces* are introduced to the joint. Deviations in normal force distribution may be caused, among other things, by an increase or decrease in the normal tibiofemoral angle.

If the *medial* tibiofemoral angle is greater than 195° (165° or less measured laterally), an abnormal condition called **genu valgum** ("knock knees") exists (Fig. 11–9). This condition will increase the compressive force on the lateral condyle while increasing the tensile stresses on the medial structures. If the medial tibiofemoral angle is 180° or less (exceeding 180° as measured laterally), the resulting abnormality is called **genu varum** ("bow legs") (Fig. 11–10). In this condition, the compressive stresses on the medial tibial condyle are increased, whereas the tensile stresses are increased laterally. In either genu valgum or genu varum, constant overloading of, respectively, the lateral or medial articular cartilage may result in damage to the cartilage.

The menisci of the knee are important in distributing and absorbing the large forces crossing the knee joint. Although compressive forces in

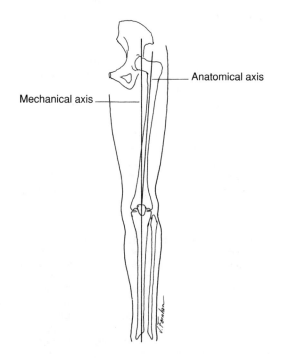

— Anatomical axis

Mechanical axis —

FIGURE 11–8. The mechanical axis (weight-bearing line) of the lower extremity passes through the hip, knee, and ankle joints. Because the mechanical axis lies more nearly vertical than the longitudinal (anatomic) axis, weight-bearing forces are about equally distributed between the medial and lateral condyles of the knee joint.

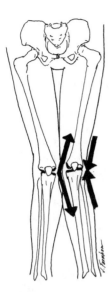

FIGURE 11–9. An increase in the normal medial valgus angle results in genu valgum or "knock knees." Arrows on the lateral aspect of the left tibiofemoral joint indicate the presence of compression forces, whereas the arrows on the medial aspect indicate the presence of distraction (tensile) forces.

displacement, posterior displacement, and rotation of the tibia beneath the femur.[19, 20] The knee joint capsule and its associated ligaments are critical to restricting such motions to main-tain joint integrity and normal joint function. Although muscles clearly play a role in stabilization (as we shall examine more closely later in the chapter), it is almost impossible to effectively stabilize the knee with active muscular forces alone in the presence of substantial disruption of passive restraining mechanisms.

The joint capsule that encloses the tibiofemoral and patellofemoral joints is large, complexly attached, and lax with several recesses (Fig. 11–11). Posteriorly, the capsule is attached proximally to the posterior margins of the femoral condyles and intercondylar notch and distally to the posterior tibial condyle. The capsule is reinforced posteriorly by a number of muscles and by the oblique popliteal and arcuate ligaments. Medially and laterally, the capsule begins proximally above the femoral condyles to continue distally to the margins of the tibial condyle. The collateral ligaments reinforce the sides of the capsule. Anteriorly, the patella, the tendon of the quadriceps muscles superiorly, and the patellar ligament inferiorly complete the anterior portion of the joint capsule. Anteromedially and anterolaterally, expansions from the vastus medialis and vastus lateralis muscles extend from the patella and patellar ligament to the corresponding collateral ligaments and tibial condyles.[2] The antero-

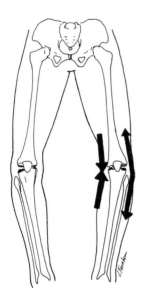

FIGURE 11–10. A decrease in the normal medial valgus angle results in genu varum or "bow legs." Arrows on the lateral aspect of the left tibiofemoral joint indicate the presence of distraction (tensile) forces, whereas arrows on the medial aspect of the joint indicate the presence of compression forces.

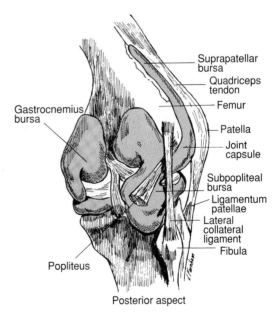

Posterior aspect

FIGURE 11–11. This view of the posterolateral aspect of the knee complex shows the synovial portion of the knee joint capsule and related bursae.

medial and anterolateral portions of the capsule are known as the **extensor retinaculum** or the **medial and lateral patellar retinacula.**[2]

Extensor Retinacula

The capsular and retinacular connections have been variously described and are the subject of some disagreement. There appear to be two layers, the deeper of the two having longitudinally oriented fibers connecting the capsule anteriorly to the menisci and tibia via the coronary ligaments.[6,7] These connections may be called the patellomeniscal[5] or the patellotibial bands.[7,21] The more superficial second layer consists of transversely oriented fibers of which the more proximal blend with fibers of the vastus medialis and lateralis muscles and the more distal continue to the posterior femoral condyles. The transverse fibers connecting the patella and the femoral condyles are known as the **patellofemoral ligaments.**[7,21,22] The lateral patellofemoral ligament is connected not only to the vastus lateralis muscle but also to the iliotibial band either directly[7,22] or indirectly via an iliopatellar band.[23,24] The iliotibial band and its associated fascia lata are accompanied posteriorly by the tendon of the biceps femoris muscle to provide superficial reinforcement to the capsular and retinacular layers.[10] According to Terry and coworkers,[25] the biceps femoris acts as both a static and dynamic stabilizer of the knee. These authors found that anterolateral/anteromedial rotatory knee instability is often associated with injury to the biceps femoris.

Synovial Lining

The intricacy of the fibrous layer of the knee joint capsule is surpassed by its synovial lining, the most extensive and involved in the body.[2] The synovium adheres to the inner wall of the fibrous layer except posteriorly where the synovium invaginates anteriorly following the contour of the femoral intercondylar notch. The invaginated synovium adheres to the anterior aspect and sides of the ACL and the PCL. The infolding of the synovial lining results in the ACL and the PLC being contained within the fibrous capsule but not within the synovial sleeve.[2] Embryonically, the synovial lining of the knee joint capsule is actually divided by septa into three separate compartments. There is initially a superior patellofemoral compartment and two separate medial and lateral tibiofemoral compartments. By 12 weeks of gestation, the synovial septa are resorbed to some degree, resulting in a single joint cavity, but retaining the posterior invagination of the synovium that forms some separation of the condyles.[26,27] The superior compartment continues to be recognizable as a superior recess of the capsule known as the **suprapatellar bursa.** The medial and lateral compartments, although not truly separate in the fully formed knee, are still referenced as a way of classifying joint structures that are considered to belong to one compartment or the other.[28,29] Posteriorly, the synovial lining may invaginate laterally between the popliteus muscle and lateral femoral condyle. It may also invaginate medially between the semimembranosus tendon, the medial head of the gastrocnemius muscle, and the medial femoral condyle.

When the synovial septa, which exist embryonically, are not completely resorbed but persist into adulthood, they exist as folds or pleats of synovial tissue known as **plicae** or **patellar plicae.**[30,31] These vestiges have been observed in 20% to 60% of the normal population[32] and are referred to, in order of most frequently to least frequently found, as the **inferior plica (infrapatellar plica),** the **superior plica (suprapatellar plica),** and the **medial plica (mediopatellar plica).** Dupont[30] also describes a lateral plica but states that it is rare. The inferior plica, which also has been described as the **infrapatellar fold or ligamentum mucosum,** is located below the patella anterior to the ACL. The inferior plica extends from the anterior portion of the intercondylar notch to attach to the infrapatellar fat pad.[30,31] According to *Gray's Anatomy,*[2] the infrapatellar fat pad that separates the synovial lining of the joint from the patellar ligament is itself covered with synovium. The synovial covering of the fat pad projects into the interior of the joint on either side of the patellar ligament (alar folds) and joins to form a single band, the inferior plica (infrapatellar fold or ligamentum mucosum) (Fig. 11–12). The superior plica is located between the suprapatellar bursa and the knee joint. This plica is often bilateral and symmetrical and extends from the synovial pouch at the anterior aspect of the femoral metaphysis area to attach to the posterior aspect of the quadriceps tendon above the patella. Dandy[33] identified 10 different configurations for the superior plica and found that 64.2% of knees examined either had no superior plica or a plica that extended one-third of the way across the suprapatellar pouch. In an examination of patients who were complaining of knee pain, swelling, or instability, Bae and associates[34] found that 88% of these patients had a superior plicae with complete septum. The medial plica arises from the medial wall of the pouch of the retinaculum and runs parallel to the medial edge of the patella to attach to the infrapatellar fat pad and synovium of the inferior plica.[30,31]

Many variations exist in the size, shape, and frequency of the plicae and consequently descriptions of the plica often vary among authors. For example, in a review of the literature Dupont[30] found that the superior plica was referred to by at least 4 different names and the medial plica by 19 different terms including among others the medial intra-articular band, alar ligament, semilunar fold, medial shelf, and patellar meniscus. Synovial plica, when they exist, are generally composed of loose, pliant, and elastic fibrous connective tissue that easily passes back and forth over the femoral condyles as the knee flexes and extends.[26,27] Occasionally, however, the plica may become irritated and inflamed, which leads to pain, ef-fusion, and changes in joint structure and function.[30,32,34] The plica syndrome generally does not arise from the most common infrapatellar plica, but from either the medial or superior plicae.[35]

The knee joint capsule is reinforced by a number of ligaments that play an important part not only in knee joint stability but, as we shall see, in knee joint mobility.

Knee Joint Ligaments

The roles of the various ligaments of the knee have received extensive attention, reflecting their importance to knee joint stability and the frequency with which function is disrupted through ligamentous injury. Given the lack of bony restraint to virtually any of the knee motions, the ligaments are credited with resisting or controlling:

1. Excessive knee extension
2. Varus and valgus stresses at the knee (attempted adduction or abduction of the tibia, respectively)
3. Anterior or posterior displacement of the tibia beneath the femur
4. Medial or lateral rotation of the tibia beneath the femur
5. Combinations of anteroposterior displacements and rotations of the tibia, known as rotatory stabilization

Although the tibial motions were, for the most part, cited in this list, it is also possible that the stresses may occur on the femur while the tibia is fixed (weight-bearing). In such instances, the anteroposterior displacements and rotations will reverse; that is, anterior displacement of the tibia is equivalent to posterior displacement of the femur and so forth.

The large body of literature available on ligamentous function of the knee joint can be confusing and appears contradictory. This may be due to some confusion in terms as to whether the tibia or the femur is being referenced, but it is more likely due to complex and variable functioning and to dissimilar testing conditions. It is clear that ligamentous function can change depending on the position of the knee joint, on how the stresses are applied, and on what active or passive structures are concomitantly intact. We will credit the ligaments with the ability to provide stabilization in those positions and directions on which there appears to be consensus.

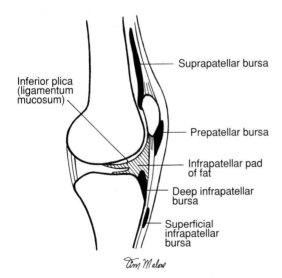

Inferior plica (ligamentum mucosum)

Suprapatellar bursa

Prepatellar bursa

Infrapatellar pad of fat

Deep infrapatellar bursa

Superficial infrapatellar bursa

Tim Malone

FIGURE 11–12. The infrapatellar pad of fat that separates the synovial lining of the joint from the patellar ligament is covered with synovium. The synovial covering of the pad of fat projects into the interior of the joint on either side of the patellar ligament and joins into a single band the inferior plica (ligamentum mucosum or infrapatellar fold).

Collateral Ligaments

The medial (tibial) collateral ligament (MCL) attaches to the medial aspect of the medial femoral epicondyle, sloping anteriorly to insert into the medial aspect of the proximal tibia (Fig. 11–13). The posterior medial fibers of the ligament blend with fibers of the joint capsule and some fibers extend medially to attach to the medial meniscus. The lateral (fibular) collateral ligament (LCL) is a strong cordlike structure extending from the lateral femoral epicondyle and attaching posteriorly to the head of the fibula (Fig. 11–14). Unlike the MCL, the LCL has no attachment either to the meniscus or to the joint capsule. Both collateral ligaments are taut in full extension and, therefore, help resist hyperextension of the knee joint.

MEDIAL COLLATERAL LIGAMENT

The MCL resists valgus stresses across the knee joint, being especially effective in the extended knee when the ligament is taut. However, it may play a more critical role in resisting valgus stresses in the slightly flexed knee when other structures make a lesser contribution. Grood and associates[36] found that the MCL carried 57% of the valgus stress when the knee was at 5° of flexion, but 78% of the load when the knee was flexed to 25°. The MCL is also aligned in such a way as to check lateral rotation of the tibia.[10] Nielsen and associates[37,38] found that the MCL made a major contribution throughout the knee joint range of motion

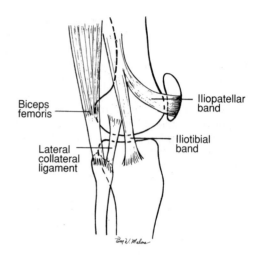

FIGURE 11–14. Lateral knee joint structures.

(ROM) to checking lateral rotation of the tibia combined with either anterior or posterior tibial displacement. The MCL is also a backup restraint to pure anterior displacement of the tibia when the primary restraint of the ACL is absent.[10]

LATERAL COLLATERAL LIGAMENT

The LCL resists varus stresses (attempted adduction of the tibia) across the knee. Given its alignment, it also appears to limit lateral rotation of the tibia, making its most substantial contribution at about 35° of flexion, in conjunction with the posterolateral capsule.[37,38] The LCL also resists combined lateral rotation with posterior displacement of the tibia in conjunction with the tendon of the popliteus muscle.[10]

ILIOTIBIAL BAND

The iliotibial band (ITB) or iliotibial tract is formed proximally from the fascia investing the tensor fascia lata, the gluteus maximus, and the gluteus medius muscles. The ITB continues distally to attach to the linea aspera of the femur via the lateral intermuscular septum and inserts into the lateral tubercle of the tibia, reinforcing the anterolateral aspect of the knee joint (see Fig. 11–14). Puniello [39]describes this portion of the ITB as the deep capsulo-osseous layer with fascial attachments to the gastrocnemius and plantaris muscles. Although there are muscular connections to the iliotibial band, Kaplan[40] considered the ITB to be essentially a passive structure at the knee joint be-

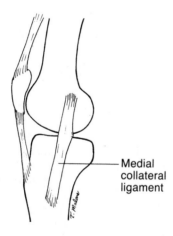

FIGURE 11–13. The medial collateral ligament (MCL) runs from the medial condyle of the femoral down and anteriorly to the right.

cause contraction of either the tensor fascia lata or the gluteus maximus muscles did not produce any longitudinal excursion of the distal ITB. The ITB appears to be consistently taut regardless of position of the hip joint or knee joint, although it falls anterior to the knee joint axis in extension and posterior to the axis in flexion.[9,41] According to Puniello,[39] the ITB is drawn posteriorly when the knee is flexed beyond 30°. The ITB is comparable to that of the MCL,[9] and its strength comparable to that of the ACL.[24] The fibrous connections of the ITB to the biceps femoris and vastus lateralis muscles through the lateral intermuscular septum form a sling behind the lateral femoral condyle, assisting the ACL in preventing posterior displacement of the femur when the tibia is fixed and the knee joint is near extension.[24] The ITB sends fibers from its anterior margin to attach to the patella, forming an iliopatellar band[24,40] that may be implicated in abnormal lateral forces on the patella.[41] When the ITB moves posteriorly in knee flexion it exerts a lateral pull on the patella resulting in a progressive laterally tilting as flexion increases.[39]

Cruciate Ligaments

The ACL and PCL are centrally located within the articular capsule but lie outside the synovial cavity. These ligaments are named according to their tibial attachments. The ACL arises from the anterior aspect of the tibia; the PCL arises from the posterior aspect of the tibia. Usually both ligaments are described as having main posterolateral and smaller anteromedial bands that behave differently in different movements[2]; however, the division of the cruciate ligaments into two separate bands may be an oversimplification because the structure and function of these ligaments is extremely complex.

The composition of the ligaments is similar to other ligaments because the major cell type found in the ligaments is the fibroblast and the major portion of both ligaments is composed of bundles of type I collagen that are separated by type III collagen fibrils. However, both ligaments contain zones that resemble fibrocartilage. In the ACL the fibrocartilaginous zone is located 5 to 10 mm proximal to the tibial ligament insertion in the anterior portion of the ligament. In the PCL the fibrocartilaginous zone is located in the middle third of the ligament. The pericellular collagen in these regions tests posi-

itive for type II cartilage and the cells in the area are chondrocytes. An avascular region is located within the fibrocartilaginous zone of the ACL where the ligament faces the anterior rim of the intercondylar fossa. The fibrocartilaginous zone of the PCL is also avascular. Shearing and compressive stress are considered to be stimuli for the development of fibrocartilaginous areas within dense connective tissue and in the ACL these stresses may develop when the ligament impinges on the anterior rim of the intercondylar fossa when the knee is fully extended. In the PCL the compressive and shear stress may result from twisting of the fiber bundles in the middle third of the ligament.[42]

ANTERIOR CRUCIATE LIGAMENT

The ACL attaches to the anterior tibia, passes under the transverse ligament,[10] and extends superiorly and posteriorly to attach to the posterior part of the inner aspect of the lateral femoral condyle (Fig. 11–15). Generally, the numerous fascicles of the ACL are grouped into an anteromedial band (AMB) and a posterolateral band (PLB), with the names taken again from the points of tibial origin. However, descriptions of the various bands vary considerably. For example, Fuss[43] describes a third intermediate band, and Livesay and associates[44] refer to anterior and posterior sections of the AMB. Changes in the lengths of the various bands or fibers during joint motion are used as indicators of the ligaments' functions. For example, when bands are shortest they are considered to be lax and to offer little restraint and when the band or bands are longest they are considered to be taut and to offer the most restraint. At 0° of knee flexion the AMB is at its shortest length (lax) while the PLB is at it longest length (taut).[45] Therefore at 0° the lax AMB would be able to offer the least restraint and the taut PLB would be able to offer the most restraint. At 30° of knee flexion the AMB has lengthened so that it is longer than the PLB.[45] At 90° of flexion the AMB is about 3.6 mm longer than it was at 0°, and the PLB is shorter than it was at 0°. Under valgus loading the length of both bands of the ACL increases as knee flexion increases. Anterior loading alone or combined with valgus loading causes an increase in length of all portions of the ACL with increases in knee flexion.[45] In anterior loading some portion of the ACL is tight throughout the knee joint range[46] (AMB lax in

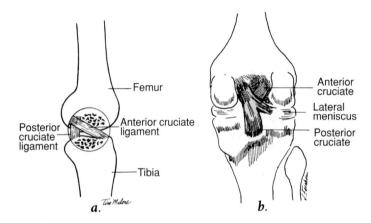

FIGURE 11–15. (a) A schematic drawing of the knee joint ignores the condyles to which each ligament attaches, but shows the longer and more oblique ACL as it crosses the shorter, thicker, and more vertically oriented PCL. (b) A posterior view of the knee joint shows the femoral condyles to which the ACL and PCL each attach.

extension while PLB is taut). In flexion, the AMB is taut (maximally tensed at 70° of flexion[41]) and the PLB is lax.[10,47,48] According to Fuss[43] the intermediate third band of fibers of the ACL is taut in all positions.

The ACL is generally considered the primary restraint to anterior displacement of the tibia on the femoral condyles. There would appear to be essentially no anterior translation of the tibia possible in full extension when many of the supporting passive structures of the knee are taut (including the PLB of the ACL). However, a cadaver study that used serial sectioning of ligaments and application of measured loads concluded that the ACL carried 87% of the load when an anterior translational force was applied to the extended knee.[49] Forces producing anterior translation of the tibia will result in maximal excursion of the tibia at about 30° of flexion[19] when neither of the ACL bands are particularly tensed.

Passive extension of the knee generated forces in the ACL only during the last 10° of extension. At 5° of hyperextension forces in the ACL ranged from 50 to 24 N. The highest forces generated in the ACL (133–370 N) occurred when 10 Newton-meters of medial tibial torque was applied to the hyperextended knee.[50]

The PLB checks and, therefore, tends to be injured with excessive knee hyperextension, whereas the AMB tends to be injured with trauma to the flexed knee.[47] The ACL would also appear to make at least a minor contribution to restraining both varus and valgus stresses across the knee joint.[36,37] When the MCL is damaged and the knee is flexed, the ACL will make a more major contribution to restraining varus and valgus stresses.[51] Experi-

mental excision of the ACL leads to an increase in anterior tibial translation between 0° and 90° flexion and an increase in valgus tibial rotation between 30° and 90° flexion. Also, the lateral tilt of the patella increases from a tilt of 6.3° to 9.0° between 0° and 90° flexion and the lateral shift of the patella changes from 2.9 mm at 15° of flexion to 5.9 mm at 90° of flexion.[52]

Both cruciate ligaments appear to play a role in producing and controlling rotation of the tibia. The ACL appears to twist around the PCL in medial rotation of the tibia, thus *checking* excessive medial rotation.[47] However, other investigators have also found that stress on the ACL produced by an anterior translational force on the tibia will *create* a concomitant medial rotation of the tibia.[10,19,20] When the ACL was sectioned experimentally in cadavers, anterior displacement increased and the amount of medial rotation decreased with the application of an anterior translational force.[20] When Lipke and associates[53] loaded an ACL-deficient cadaver limb under conditions simulating weight-bearing, they found both excessive anterior displacement of the tibia and excessive medial rotation. Unlike most other situations where motions of the free tibia (femur fixed) will be mirrored by reverse motions of the free femur (tibia fixed), tension in the ACL does not appear to produce rotation of the femur.[19] Regardless of the rotatory effect of the ACL on the tibia, injury to the ACL appears to occur most commonly when the knee is flexed and the tibia rotated *in either direction*. In flexion and medial rotation, the ACL is tensed as it winds around the PCL. In flexion and lateral rotation, the ACL is tensed as it is stretched over the lateral femoral condyle.[54] When attempting to determine whether there has been a tear of the ACL, the presence of *both* anteromedial and anterolateral instability is the most diagnostic. Of the knees presenting with instability in both directions, Terry and Hughston[55] found 100% to have confirmed torn or nonfunctional ACLs. Another consequence of a torn ACL is a loss of normal proprioception at the knee.[56]

An investigation of the effects of muscle activity on the ACL showed that quadriceps muscle activity significantly strained the ACL when the knee was in the range of 20° to 60° flexion. Essentially, the ACL acted as an antagonistic force to the quadriceps.[57] However, when the hamstrings were co-contracting with the quadriceps, in situ forces in the ACL at 15°, 30°, and 60° were reduced by 30%, 43%, and 44%, respectively.[58] Hamstring co-contraction also reduced anterior lateral tibial translation as well as tibial medial rotation at the same knee flexion angles between 15° and 60° of flexion.[59] Therefore, the hamstrings can be considered to act synergistically with the ACL.

POSTERIOR CRUCIATE LIGAMENT

The PCL, which runs superiorly and somewhat anteriorly from its posterior tibial origin to attach to the inner aspect of the medial femoral condyle, is shorter and less oblique than the ACL (see Fig.11–15b). The PCL cross-sectional area is only 120% to 150% of the ACL. The PCL increases in cross-sectional area proximally, whereas the ACL increases distally.[60] The PCL blends with the posterior capsule and periosteum as it crosses to its tibial attachment.[61] Saddler[61] did not find any evidence of two separate functional bands but rather multiple fibers of different lengths with a high proximal to distal sensitivity to length changes based on femoral attachments. However, the PCL usually is divided into an AMB and a PLB named by the tibial origin. The AMB is lax in extension, and the PLB is taut. At 80° to 90° of flexion, the AMB is maximally taut and the PLB is relaxed.[48] Harner and coworkers[60] determined that the AMB is larger and stronger than the PLB.

There is consensus that the PCL is the primary restraint to posterior displacement of the tibia beneath the femur, with little or no displacement possible in full extension. The PCL was found to carry 93% of the load in the extended knee when a posterior translational force was applied to the tibia.[49] In the flexed knee, maximal displacement of the tibia with a posterior translational force occurs at 75° to 90° of flexion, although sectioning of the PCL increased posterior translation at all angles of flexion.[20] The PCL also has some role in restraining varus and valgus stresses at the knee.[36,37]

As is true for the ACL, the PCL appears to play a role in both restraining and producing rotation of the tibia. Posterior translatory forces on the tibia are consistently accompanied by concomitant lateral rotation of the tibia,[20] with little or no rotation produced at the femur.[19] Tension in the PCL with knee extension may be instrumental in creating the lateral rotation of the tibia that is critical to locking of the knee for stabilization. The popliteus muscle shares the function of the PCL in resisting posteriorly directed forces on the tibia and contributes to knee stability when the PCL is absent.[62] Hamstring muscle contraction strains the PCL when the knee is flexed from 70° to110°. A contraction of the gastrocnemius muscle significantly strains the PCL at flexion angles greater than 40°, whereas quadriceps contraction reduces strain in the PCL at knee flexion angles between 20° and 60°.[58] The PCL, posterior joint capsule, lateral collateral ligaments, posterior oblique ligament, MCL with meniscus attached, posterior medial and posterior lateral meniscotibial bands, and posterior meniscofibular ligament comprise a complex restraining system for knee extension.[43]

Posterior Capsular Ligaments

The posteromedial aspect of the capsule is reinforced by the tendinous expansion of the semimembranosus muscle, which is known as the **oblique popliteal ligament** (Fig. 11–16). This ligament passes from a point posterior to the medial tibial condyle and attaches to the central part of the posterior aspect of the joint capsule. The posterolateral aspect of the capsule is reinforced by the **arcuate popliteal (arcuate) ligament** (see Fig. 11–16). The arcuate ligament arises from the posterior aspect of the head of the fibula and passes over the tendon of the popliteus muscle to attach to the intercondylar area of the tibia and to the lateral epicondyle of the femur. Both the oblique popliteal and the arcuate ligaments are taut in full extension and assist in checking hyperextension of the knee. The arcuate and oblique popliteal ligaments play an important role in

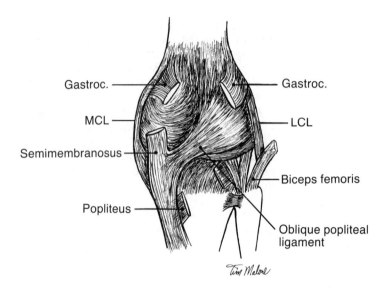

Gastroc.

Gastroc.

MCL

LCL

Semimembranosus

Biceps femoris

Popliteus

Oblique popliteal ligament

Tim Malone

FIGURE 11–16. A view of the posterior capsule of the knee joint shows the reinforcing oblique popliteal ligament. Also seen are the collateral ligaments (MCL and LCL) and some of the reinforcing posterior musculature (semimembranosus, biceps femoris, medial and lateral heads of the gastrocnemius, and the upper and lower sections of the popliteus).

checking varus and valgus stresses, respectively, in the extended knee[36,37] and in providing secondary restraint to other tibial motions.[37,38,53] The popliteofibular ligament becomes taut at 0°, 30°, 45°, and 90° and acts as a restraint to lateral rotation of the tibia when posterior force is applied to the knee. The ligament also helps to limit posterior translation of the tibia.[63]

Meniscofemoral Ligaments

The two meniscofemoral ligaments arise from the posterior horn of the lateral meniscus and insert on the lateral aspect of the medial femoral condyle near the insertion site of the PCL.[60,64] The ligament that runs anterior to the PCL is called either the **ligament of Humphrey** or **anterior meniscofemoral ligament.** The ligament that runs posterior to the PCL is called either the **ligament of Wrisberg** or **posterior meniscofemoral ligament.** According to Cailliet[31] the ligament of Wrisberg is also known as the **third cruciate ligament of Robert.** Cho and colleagues[65] determined that frequent variations occur in the location of both proximal and distal attachment sites of these ligaments and Kusayama[64] found considerable variation in the presence or absence of the ligaments. Cailliet found that ligaments are found in 76% of the people examined. Thirty-five percent of people examined had ligaments of Humphrey and an equal percent had ligaments of Wrisberg; only 6% had both ligaments.[31] The meniscofemoral ligaments work in conjunction with

the popliteus muscle and become taut during femoral lateral rotation and may prevent posterior translation of the tibia.

Knee Joint Bursae

The extensive ligamentous apparatus of the knee joint and the large excursion of the bony segments set up substantial frictional forces between muscular, ligamentous, and bony structures. However, numerous bursae prevent or limit such degenerative forces. Three bursae have already been mentioned in discussion of the knee joint capsule. These are the suprapatellar bursa, the subpopliteal bursa, and the gastrocnemius bursa. These bursae are not usually separate entities but are either invaginations of the synovium within the joint capsule (see Fig. 11–11) or communicate with the capsule through small openings.[66] The suprapatellar bursa lies between the quadriceps tendon and the anterior femur; the subpopliteal bursa lies between the tendon of the popliteus muscle and the lateral femoral condyle; and the gastrocnemius bursa lies between the tendon of the medial head of the gastrocnemius muscle and the medial femoral condyle. The gastrocnemius bursa may also continue beneath the tendon of the semimembranosus muscle to protect it from the medial femoral condyle.

The lubricating synovial fluid contained in the knee joint capsule moves from recess to recess during flexion and extension of the knee, lubricating the articular surfaces. In extension, the posterior capsule and ligaments are taut

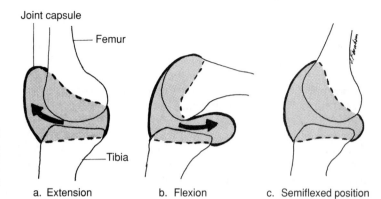

Joint capsule
Femur
Tibia

a. Extension

b. Flexion

c. Semiflexed position

FIGURE 11–17. (a) The synovial fluid is forced anteriorly during extension. (b) In flexion, the synovial fluid is forced posteriorly. (c) In the semi-flexed position, the capsule is under the least amount of tension.

and the gastrocnemius and subpopliteal bursae are compressed. This shifts the synovial fluid anteriorly[66] (Fig. 11–17a). In flexion, the suprapatellar bursa is compressed anteriorly by tension in the anterior structures and the fluid is forced posteriorly (Fig. 11–17b). When the joint is in the semiflexed position, the synovial fluid is under the least amount of tension (Fig. 11–17c). When there is an excess of fluid in the joint cavity due to injury or disease, the semi-flexed knee position helps to relieve tension in the capsule and therefore helps to reduce pain.

Several other bursae are associated with the knee but do not communicate with the synovial capsule (Fig. 11–18). The prepatellar bursa, located between the skin and the anterior surface of the patella, allows free movement of the skin over the patella during flexion and extension. The subcutaneous infrapatellar bursa lies between the patellar ligament and the overlying skin. The subcutaneous infrapatellar bursa and the prepatellar bursa may become inflamed as a result of direct trauma to the front of the knee or through activities like kneeling. The deep infrapatellar bursa, which is located between the patellar ligament and the tibial tuberosity, is separated from the synovial cavity of the joint by the infrapatellar pad of fat. The deep infrapatellar bursa helps to reduce friction between the patellar ligament and the tibial tuberosity.

There are also several small bursae that are associated with the ligaments of the knee joint. There is commonly a bursa between the LCL and the tendon of the biceps femoris muscle and between the LCL and the popliteus muscle. Also, there is a bursa deep to the MCL protecting it from the tibial condyle and one superficial to the MCL protecting it from the tendons of the semitendinosus and gracilis muscles that cross the MCL.

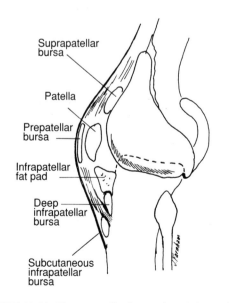

Suprapatellar bursa

Patella

Prepatellar bursa

Infrapatellar fat pad

Deep infrapatellar bursa

Subcutaneous infrapatellar bursa

FIGURE 11–18. The prepatellar bursa, deep infrapatellar bursa, and superficial infrapatellar bursa are separate from the knee joint cavity.

Knee Joint Function

Knee Joint Motion

The primary motions of the knee joint are flexion/extension and, to a lesser extent, medial/lateral rotation. These motions occur about changing but definable axes and serve the weight-bearing functions of the lower extremity. The knee joint can also undergo tibial or femoral displacement anteriorly and posteriorly and some abduction and adduction through varus and valgus forces. However, these movements are generally not considered part of the *function* of the joint but are, rather, part of the cost of the tremendous compromise between mobility and stability. The small amounts of anteroposterior displacement and varus/valgus forces that can occur in the normal flexed knee are the result of joint incongruence and variations in ligamentous elasticity. The magnitude of such motions varies among individuals and from side to side in the same individual.[10,19,20] Excessive amounts of such motions are abnormal and generally indicate ligamentous incompetence. We will focus on normal knee joint motions, including both osteokinematics (degrees of freedom) and arthokinematics (intra-articular movements within the joint).

Flexion/Extension

The axis for flexion and extension at the tibiofemoral joint passes horizontally through the femoral condyles at an angle to the mechanical and anatomic axes.[5] The obliquity of the axis (lower on the medial side of the joint) is similar to that found at the elbow, causing the tibia to move from a position slightly lateral to the femur in full extension to a position medial to the femur in full flexion (Fig. 11–19). However,

unlike the elbow, the axis of motion for flexion and extension at the knee is not relatively fixed, but moves to a considerable extent through the ROM. The instant axis of rotation (IAR) for each point in the knee joint ROM can be found in a series of roentgenograms and the path of these sequential centers plotted. The pathway of the IAR of the tibiofemoral joint for flexion and extension forms a semicircle, moving posteriorly and superiorly on the femoral condyles with increasing flexion (Fig. 11–20).[3]

Because many of the muscles associated with the knee are two-joint muscles that cross both the hip and the knee, hip joint position can influence knee ROM. Passive range of knee flexion is generally considered to be 130° to 140°.[67] Knee flexion may be limited to 120° or less when the hip joint is simultaneously hyperextended and the stretched rectus femoris muscle becomes passively insufficient.[2] Knee flexion may also reach as much as 160° in activities like squatting when the hip and knee are flexing at the same time and the body weight is superimposed on the joint.[2,5] Normal gait on level ground requires approximately 60° of knee flexion.[68] This requirement increases to about 80° for stair climbing[69] and to 90° or more for sitting down into a chair and arising from it. Activities beyond simple mobility tasks require 115° of knee flexion or more.[10] Knee joint extension (or hyperextension) of 5° to 10° is considered within normal limits.[2] Excessive knee hyperextension is termed **genu recurvatum.**

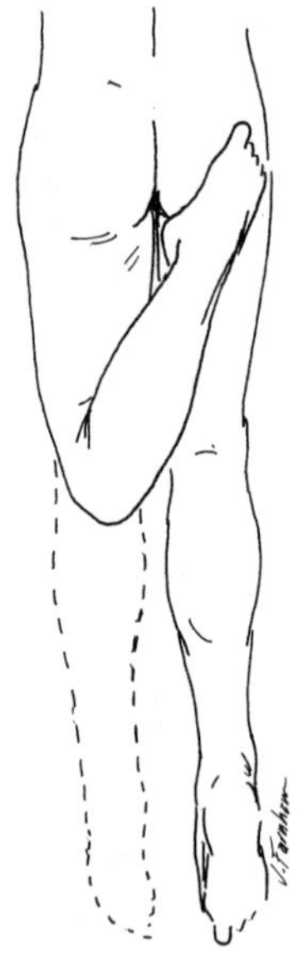

FIGURE 11–19. The tibia moves from a position slightly lateral to the femur in extension to a position slightly medial to the femur in flexion.

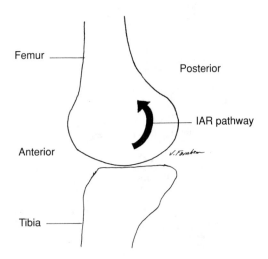

FIGURE 11–20. Schematic drawing of the knee joint. The arrow represents the path of the instantaneous axis of rotation (IAR) for the joint as it moves from extension into flexion.

When the lower extremity is weight-bearing and the knee is part of a closed kinematic chain, range limitations at the ankle joint may cause restriction in knee joint flexion or extension. For example, a limitation in ankle dorsiflexion (due to tight plantarflexors) may prevent the knee from being flexed; a limitation in plantarflexion (due to tight dorsiflexors) may restrict the ability of the knee to fully extend. If the ankle were fixed in the position shown in Figure 11–21, the knee would be unable to either flex or extend without lifting all or some part of the foot from the ground.

Rotation

The knee joint rotates in two different ways that are quite different both structurally and functionally. **Axial rotation** provides the second degree of freedom to the tibiofemoral joint. Alternatively, there is joint rotation involved in the locking mechanism of the knee joint, also known as **terminal** or **automatic rotation.** Rotation associated with the locking mechanism occurs with close-packing of the knee joint and does not contribute to degrees of freedom. Automatic rotation will be considered in the next section on joint arthrokinematics.

Axial rotation of the knee joint occurs around a longitudinal axis that runs through or close to the medial tibial intercondylar tubercle.[5,70] Medial and lateral rotation of the knee joint are named for the motion or relative motion of the tibia (unless motion of the femur is specified). The medial and lateral rotation available in axial rotation occur because of articular incongruence and ligamentous laxity. Consequently, the range of knee joint rotation depends on the position of the knee. When the knee is in full extension, it is in the close-packed (locked) position and the ligaments are taut; no axial rotation is possible. The tibial tubercles are lodged in the intercondylar notch and the menisci are tightly interposed between the articulating surfaces. As the knee flexes increasingly toward 90°, the capsule and ligaments become more lax. The tibial tubercles are no longer in the intercondylar notch and the condyles of the tibia and femur are free to move on each other. At 90° of knee flexion, approximately 60° to 70° of either active or passive rotation is possible.[2] The range for lateral rotation (0–40°) is slightly greater than the range for medial rotation (0–30°[3.,5,11]). The maximum range of axial rotation is available at 90° of knee flexion, with the magnitude of axial rotation diminishing as the knee approaches both full extension and full flexion.

Arthrokinematics

FLEXION/EXTENSION

The large articular surface of the femur and the relatively small tibial condyle create a potential problem as the femur begins to flex on the tibia. If the femoral condyles were permitted to roll posteriorly on the tibial condyle, the femur would run out of tibial condyle before much flexion had occurred. This would result in a limitation of flexion, or the femur would roll off the tibia (Fig. 11–22). For the femoral condyles to continue to roll with increased flexion of the femur, the condyles must simultaneously glide anteriorly on the tibial condyle to prevent them from rolling posteriorly off the tibial condyle (Fig. 11–23a). The first part of flexion of the femur from full extension (0–25°) is primarily rolling of the femoral condyles on the tibia,[71] bringing the contact of the femoral condyles posteriorly on the tibial condyle. As flexion continues, the rolling is accompanied by a simultaneous anterior glide just sufficient to create a nearly pure spin of the femur; that is, the magnitude of posterior displacement that would occur with the rolling of the condyles is offset by the magnitude of anterior glide, resulting in little linear displacement of the femoral condyles after 25° of flexion.

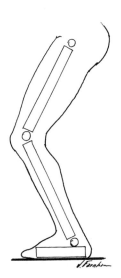

FIGURE 11–21. If the ankle were to be fused in dorsiflexion, knee flexion and extension could not occur without lifting some or all of the foot from the ground.

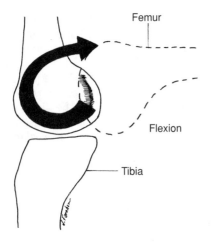

FIGURE 11–22. Schematic illustration of pure rolling of the femoral condyles on a fixed tibia shows the femur rolling off of the tibia.

The anterior glide of the femoral condyles results in part from the tension encountered in the ACL as the femur rolls posteriorly on the tibial condyle. The glide may be further facilitated by the menisci whose wedge shape forces the femoral condyle to roll "uphill" as the knee flexes. As shown in Figure 11–24, the oblique contact force of the wedged meniscus (meniscus-on-femur) creates an anterior shear (shear 1) on the femur. Similarly, the oblique reaction force of femur-on-meniscus (FM) also has a shear component (shear 2) that forces the menisci posteriorly on the tibial condyle. The result is that the menisci accompany the femoral condyles as the condyles move posteriorly on the tibial condyle, maintaining the increased

congruence the menisci provide in the fully extended knee. The menisci cannot move in their entirety because they are attached at their horns to the intercondylar tubercles of the tibial condyle. Rather, the posterior migration is a posterior distortion, with the anterior aspect of the menisci remaining relatively fixed. Given the closer attachment of the two horns of the lateral meniscus to each other, the lateral meniscus will distort slightly more than the medial.

Extension of the knee from flexion occurs initially as a rolling of the femoral condyles on the tibial condyle, displacing the femoral condyles anteriorly back to neutral position. After the initial forward rolling, the femoral condyles glide posteriorly just enough to continue extension of the femur as an almost pure spin (roll plus posterior glide) of the femoral condyles on the tibial condyles (see Fig. 11–23b). Tension in the PCL and the shape of the menisci facilitate the intra-articular movements of the femoral condyles during knee extension. The condyles are once again accompanied in displacement by distortion of the wedge-shaped menisci. As extension begins from full flexion, the posterior margins of the menisci return to their neutral position. As extension continues, the anterior margins of the menisci move anteriorly with the femoral condyles.

The motion (or distortion) of the menisci with flexion and extension are an important component of the motions. Given the need of the menisci to reduce friction and absorb forces of the large femoral condyles on the small tibial condyle, the menisci must remain beneath the femoral condyles to continue their

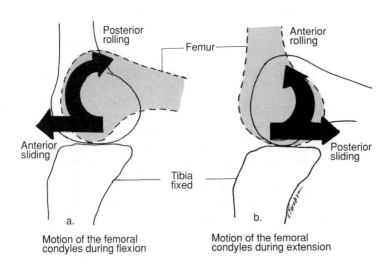

a. Motion of the femoral condyles during flexion

b. Motion of the femoral condyles during extension

FIGURE 11–23. (a) A schematic representation of rolling and sliding of the femoral condyles on a fixed tibia. The femoral condyles roll posteriorly while simultaneously sliding anteriorly. (b) Motion of the femoral condyles during extension. The femoral condyles roll anteriorly while simultaneously sliding posteriorly.

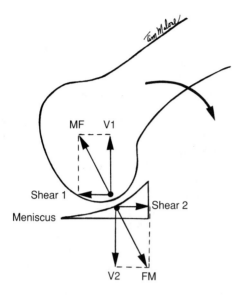

MF V1

Shear 1

Meniscus

V2 FM

Shear 2

FIGURE 11–24. Schematically represented, the oblique contact of the femur with the wedge-shaped meniscus results in the forces of **meniscus-on-femur** (MF) and **femur-on-meniscus** (FM). These can be resolved into vertical and shear components. Shear 1 assists the femur in its forward glide during flexion, and shear 2 assists in the posterior migration of the menisci that occurs with knee flexion.

of flexion, the shorter lateral femoral condyle completes its rolling-gliding motion. As extension continues, the longer medial condyle continues to roll and to glide posteriorly although the lateral condyle has halted. This continued motion of the medial femoral condyle results in medial rotation of the femur on tibia, pivoting about the fixed lateral condyle. The medial rotatory motion of the femur is most evident in the final 5° of extension.[2] Increasing tension in the knee joint ligaments as the knee approaches full extension may also contribute to the rotation within the joint.

Because the medial rotation of the femur that accompanies the final stages of knee extension is not voluntary or produced by muscular forces, it is referred to as **automatic** or **terminal rotation** of the knee joint. This rotation within the joint that accompanies the end of extension also brings the knee joint into the close-packed or locked position. The tibial tubercles are lodged in the intercondylar notch, the menisci are tightly interposed between the tibial and femoral condyles, and the ligaments are taut. Consequently, automatic rotation is also known as the **locking mechanism** or **screw home mechanism** of the knee. To initiate flexion, the knee must first be *unlocked*; that is, the medially rotated femur cannot flex in the sagittal plane, but must laterally rotate before flexion can proceed. A flexion force will *automatically* result in lateral rotation of the femur because the longer medial side will move before the shorter lateral side of the joint. If there is an external restraint to unlocking or derotation of the femur, the joint, ligaments, and menisci can be damaged as the femur is forced into flexion oblique to the sagittal plane in which its structures are oriented.

Automatic rotation or locking of the knee occurs in both open chain and closed chain knee joint function. In an open kinematic chain, the freely moving tibia *laterally rotates on the relatively fixed femur* during the last 30° of extension. Unlocking, consequently, is brought about by *medial rotation of the tibia on the femur* before flexion can proceed.

function. Failure of the menisci to distort in the proper direction can also result in limitation of joint motion. If the femur literally rolls up the wedge-shaped menisci in flexion (without either the anterior glide of the femur or the posterior distortion of the menisci), the increasing thickness of the menisci and the threat of rolling off the posterior margin will cause flexion to be limited. Similarly, failure of the menisci to distort anteriorly with the femoral condyles in extension will cause the thick anterior margins to become wedged between the femur and tibia as the segments are drawn together in the final stages of extension. The interposition of the menisci will prevent extension from being completed.

LOCKING AND UNLOCKING

Although the incongruence of the femoral condyles and tibial condyle results in a rolling and gliding of the condylar surfaces on each other, the asymmetry in the size of the medial and lateral condyles also causes complex intraarticular motions. Using weight-bearing closed chain motion as an example, extension of the femur on the relatively fixed tibia results in additional motions to those described in the previous section. As the femur extends to about 30°

AXIAL ROTATION

During axial rotation of the knee joint, the longitudinal axis for motion lies at the medial intercondylar tubercle. Consequently, the medial condyles act as the pivot point while the lateral condyles move through a greater arc of motion than the medial regardless of the direction of rotation. When lateral rotation of the tibia occurs at the knee joint (tibia free to move), the medial tibial condyle moves only slightly anteriorly on the relatively fixed medial femoral condyle while the lateral tibial condyle moves a large distance posteriorly on the relatively fixed lateral femoral condyle. In medial rotation the direction of motion of the tibial condyles reverses, with the medial tibial condyle moving only slightly posteriorly while the lateral condyle moves anteriorly through a larger arc of motion. When the tibia is fixed and the femur is free to move, lateral rotation of the femur (which is medial rotation of the knee joint) occurs as the lateral femoral condyle moves posteriorly on the lateral tibial condyle while the medial femoral condyle moves slightly anteriorly. Lateral rotation of the femur on the tibia produces an opposite set of motions.

When there is rotation between the femoral and tibial condyles (either in axial or automatic rotation), the menisci of the knee joint maintain their relationship to the femoral condyles just as they did in flexion and extension; that is, in rotation of the knee, the menisci will distort in the direction of movement of the corresponding femoral condyle. In medial rotation, the medial meniscus will distort anteriorly on the tibial condyle to remain beneath the anteriorly moving medial femoral condyle, and the lateral meniscus will distort posteriorly to remain beneath the posteriorly moving lateral femoral condyle. In this way, the menisci continue to reduce friction and distribute the forces the femoral condyles create on the tibial condyle *without restricting motion* of the femur as more solid or firmly attached structures would do.

The motions of the knee joint, exclusive of automatic rotation, are produced to a great extent by the muscles that cross the joint. We will complete our examination of the tibiofemoral joint by first examining the individual contribution of the muscles, emphasizing their mobility role in producing knee joint motion. We will then re-examine both the passive knee joint structures and the muscles in their combined role as stabilizers of this very complicated joint.

Muscles

Flexors

Seven muscles flex the knee. The knee flexors are the semimembranosus, semitendinosus, biceps femoris, sartorius, gracilis, popliteus,

and gastrocnemius muscles. All of the knee flexors, except for the short head of the biceps femoris and the popliteus, are two-joint muscles. As two-joint muscles, their ability to produce effective force can be influenced by the relative position of the two joints over which they pass. Four of the flexors (the popliteus, gracilis, semimembranosus, and semitendinosus muscles) are considered to medially rotate the tibia on the fixed femur, whereas the biceps femoris is considered to be a lateral rotator of the tibia.

The semitendinosus, semimembranosus, and the biceps femoris muscles are known collectively as the **hamstrings.** These muscles all originate on the ischial tuberosity of the pelvis. The semimembranosus and the semitendinosus insert on the posteromedial and anteromedial aspects of the tibia, respectively. The semimembranosus muscle has fibers that attach to the medial meniscus. This attachment assists in knee flexion by facilitating posterior motion of the medial meniscus during active knee flexion. The significance of this contribution will be discussed with the popliteus muscle. The semitendinosus muscle has a fibrous septum that separates it into distinct proximal and distal compartments.[72] This may give it some specificity of action at the hip joint and at the knee joint.

The biceps femoris muscle has two heads, both of which insert on the lateral condyle of the tibia and the head of the fibula (Fig. 11–25). The biceps femoris tendon may be attached to the iliotibial band and retinacular fibers of the lateral joint capsule, a set of attachments that implies that the biceps femoris has a stabilizing role at the posterolateral aspect of the joint. The short head of the biceps femoris does not cross the hip joint and, therefore, has a unique action at the knee joint.[73]

Most of the hamstrings, crossing both the hip (as extensors) and the knee (as flexors), work most effectively at the knee joint if they are lengthened over a flexed hip. Electromyographic (EMG) recordings of the biceps femoris show that there is a decrease in EMG activity as the muscle is lengthened and an increase in activity as the muscle is shortened. Because the muscle generates greater tension when it is elongated, fewer motor units are required to produce the same amount of torque. Shortening of the muscle causes it to approach active insufficiency and more motor units are required to produce the same torque. With active

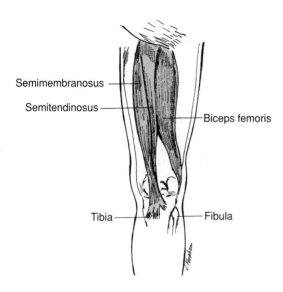

Semimembranosus

Semitendinosus

Biceps femoris

Tibia

Fibula

FIGURE 11–25. The hamstring muscles are shown in a posterior view of the knee. The arteromedial insertion site of the semitendinosus is not visible.

knee flexion with the body in the prone position, the hamstrings muscles are forced to attempt to shorten over both the hip (which will be extended) and over the knee. The hamstrings will weaken as knee flexion proceeds because the muscle group is approaching active insufficiency and must overcome the increasing tension in the rectus femoris, which is approaching passive insufficiency (Fig. 11–26).

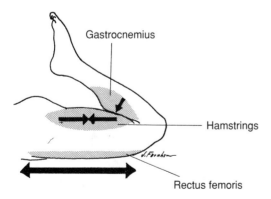

Gastrocnemius

Hamstrings

Rectus femoris

FIGURE 11–26. During active knee flexion in the prone position, the rectus femoris is stretched over the hip and the knee and becomes passively insufficient. The hamstrings are actively shortened over the hip and the knee and are likely to develop active insufficiency. In addition, the bulk of the contracting muscles (hamstrings and gastrocnemius) also limits the range of active knee flexion in the prone position.

The **gastrocnemius muscle** arises from the posterior aspects of the medial and lateral condyles of the femur by two heads. It inserts into the calcaneus by way of the calcaneal tendon. Except for the plantaris muscle (which is commonly absent), the gastrocnemius is the only muscle at the knee that crosses the ankle and the knee (Fig. 11–27). Although the gastrocnemius generates a large plantarflexor torque at the ankle, it makes a relatively small contribution to knee flexion. In fact, when someone goes up on the toes (plantarflexes their ankles) and then only slightly flexes the knee, the gastrocnemius will relax (leaving the maintenance of the position to the soleus muscle). Apparently the gastrocnemius becomes actively insufficient quite easily. Rather than working to produce knee flexion, the gastrocnemius appears to be effective in preventing knee joint hyperextension. Paralysis of the plantarflexors is classically accompanied by a snapping back of the knee into hyperextension in the final stages of single-limb support during walking. From observing this abnormal response, we can conclude that the gastrocnemius must contribute substantially to resisting the very large extension torque at the knee joint at this point in the gait cycle. The gas-

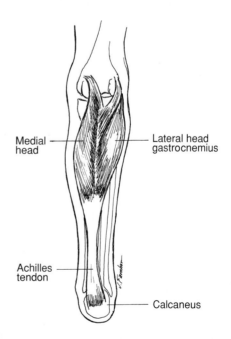

Medial head

Lateral head gastrocnemius

Achilles tendon

Calcaneus

FIGURE 11–27. The posterior aspect of the knee complex showing the gastrocnemius muscle. The gastrocnemius helps to provide support for the posterior aspect of the knee.

trocnemius appears to be less a mobility muscle at the knee joint than a dynamic stabilizer.

The **sartorius muscle** arises anteriorly from the anterior superior spine of the ilium and crosses the femur to insert into the anteromedial surface of the tibial shaft posterior to the tibial tuberosity. Although a potential flexor and medial rotator of the tibia, activity in the sartorius is more common with hip motion than with knee motion. It appears to be relatively impervious to active insufficiency, because it is equally active at the hip with the knee flexed and with the knee extended.[74] This may be accounted for somewhat by the fact that it consists of a large group of three or four fibers in series joined by fibrous septa,[72] rather than being a group of single fibers, continuous from proximal attachment to distal. Variations in distal attachment of the sartorius muscle are not uncommon. When attached just anterior to its more usual location, it may fall anterior to the knee joint axis, serving as a mild knee joint extensor rather than as a knee flexor.

The **gracilis muscle** arises from the inferior half of the symphysis pubis arch and inserts on the medial tibia by way of a common tendon with the sartorius and the semitendinosus muscles. It is not only a hip joint flexor and adductor, but it can also flex the knee joint and produce slight medial rotation of the tibia. The gracilis apparently becomes actively insufficient readily, however, ceasing activity if the hip and knee are permitted to flex simultaneously.[74]

The gracilis, semitendinosus, and sartorius muscles attach to the tibia by a common tendon on the anteromedial aspect of the tibia (Fig. 11–28). The common tendon is called the **pes anserinus** because of its shape (*pes anserinus* means "goose's foot"). The three muscles of the pes anserinus appear to function effectively as a group to stabilize the medial aspect of the knee joint.

The only other one-joint knee flexor besides the short head of the biceps femoris is the relatively small **popliteus muscle**. This muscle originates on the posterior aspect of the lateral femoral condyle and attaches on the medial aspect of the tibia. The fibers of the muscle run medially across the posterior aspect of the knee joint (Fig. 11–29). The popliteus muscle is a medial rotator of the tibia on the femur in an open kinematic chain (or a lateral rotator of the femur on the tibia in a closed kinematic chain). The active popliteus muscle is considered to

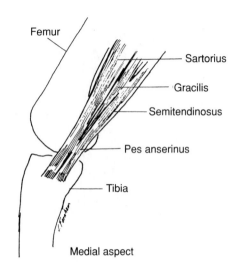

FIGURE 11–28. The sartorius, gracilis, and semitendinosus insert as a conjoined tendon known as the pes anserinus on the anteromedial aspect of the tibia.

play an important role in initiating unlocking of the knee because it reverses the direction of automatic rotation that occurred in the final stages of knee extension. It is important to note, however, that unlocking of the knee joint will still occur effectively if the knee flexion takes place passively.

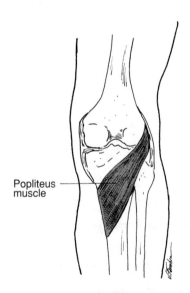

FIGURE 11–29. A posterior view of the knee joint showing the popliteus muscle (more superficial structures have been removed). The direction of pull will unlock the fully extended knee by medially rotating the tibia (open chain) or laterally rotating the femur (closed chain).

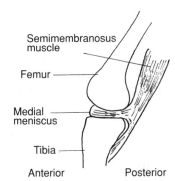

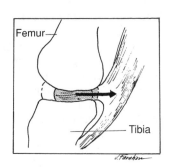

FIGURE 11–30. A schematic representation of the semimembranosus muscle and its attachment to the medial meniscus is shown. The arrow in the insert represents the direction of pull of the muscle on the medial meniscus during flexion.

The popliteus muscle is commonly attached to the lateral meniscus as the semimembranosus muscle is to the medial meniscus. Because both the semimembranosus and the popliteus are knee flexors, activity in these muscles will not only generate a flexion torque but will actively contribute to the posterior movement of the two menisci on the tibial condyles that should occur during knee flexion as the femur begins its rolling motion. The ability of the menisci to distort during motion ensures that the slippery surface is present throughout the femoral ROM. The medial meniscus is drawn posteriorly by tension in the semimembranosus muscle (Fig. 11–30). The lateral meniscus is drawn posteriorly by tension in the popliteus expansion. Although the menisci will move posteriorly on the tibial condyle even during passive flexion, the assistance of the semimembranosus and popliteus muscles reinforces the movement and minimizes the chance that the menisci will become entrapped and limit knee flexion.

Extensors

The four extensors of the knee are known collectively as the **quadriceps femoris** muscle. The only portion of the quadriceps that crosses two joints is the rectus femoris, which originates on the inferior spine of the ilium. The vastus intermedius, vastus lateralis, and vastus medialis muscles originate on the femur and merge into a common tendon, the quadriceps tendon (Fig. 11–31). The fibers of the quadriceps tendon continue distally as the patellar ligament. The patellar ligament runs from the apex of the patella, across the anterior surface of the patella, into the proximal portion of the tibial tubercle.[2] The vastus medialis and vastus lateralis also insert directly into the medial and lateral aspects of the patella by way of the retinacular fibers of the joint capsule.

Together, the muscles of the quadriceps femoris extend the knee. Lieb[75] found the resultant pull of the muscle fibers in relation to the long axis of the femur to be 7° to 10° medially and 3° to 5° anteriorly. The pull of the vastus lateralis alone was found to be 12° to 15° lateral to the long axis of the femur, with distal fibers more angulated yet. The pull of the vastus intermedius was parallel to the shaft of the femur, making it the purist knee extensor of the group. The angulation of the pull of the vastus medialis depended on which segment of the muscle was assessed. The upper fibers were angulated 15° to 18° medially to the femoral shaft, whereas the distal fibers were angulated as much as 50° to 55° medially. The drastically different orientation of lower fibers of the vastus medialis muscle has resulted in reference to the upper fibers as the **vastus medialis**

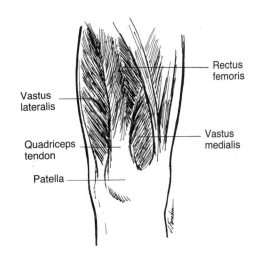

FIGURE 11–31. Three of the four segments of the quadriceps femoris can be seen in this anterior view of the knee joint as the muscles insert into the common quadriceps tendon.

longus (VML) and the lower fibers as the **vastus medialis oblique (VMO).**

Mechanically, the efficiency of the quadriceps muscle is affected by the patella; the patella lengthens the moment arm (MA) of the quadriceps by increasing the distance of the quadriceps tendon and patellar ligament from the axis of the knee joint. The patella, as an anatomic pulley, deflects the action line of the quadriceps femoris away from the joint, increasing the angle of pull and the ability of the muscle to generate a flexion torque. However, the patella does not function as a simple pulley because in a simple pulley the tension is equal in the rope on either side of the pulley. The tension in the quadriceps tendon at the superior aspect of the patella is not equal to the tension in the patellar ligament on the inferior aspect of the patella.[76–78] Evans and coworkers[79] found that the maximum force in the quadriceps tendon exceeds that in the patellar ligament by a ratio of 8:5. As Grelsamer and Klein[78] point out, the patella actually acts as a cam or eccentric pulley because the patella can both redirect and magnify force. Interposing the patella between the quadriceps tendon and the femoral condyles also reduces friction between the tendon and condyles.[21] The femoral condyles encounter not the quadriceps tendon, but the hyaline cartilage-covered posterior surface of the patella. The patella is tied to the tibial tuberosity by the patellar ligament, making the patella almost like an anterior wall to the tibia. As the femur flexes on the tibia, the patella remains essentially still while relatively sliding down the moving femoral condyles. The position of the patella relative to the joint axis

varies as the instantaneous axis shifts and as the contour of the femoral condyles changes. The effect of the patella on the MA of the quadriceps muscle, therefore, will vary through the knee joint ROM. Regardless of joint position, however, substantial decreases in the strength (torque) of the quadriceps of up to 49% have been found following removal of the patella[80] because the MA of the quadriceps is substantially reduced at most points in the ROM (Fig. 11–32).

Although increasing the magnitude of torque produced by the quadriceps muscle appears to serve function well, it does have a cost. Increasing the angle of pull of the quadriceps on the tibia and, thus, the size of the rotatory component of the pull of the quadriceps, also increases the magnitude of shear of that same component; that is, the rotatory component not only creates rotation of the tibia around an axis but also creates a translatory force that attempts to shear the tibia anteriorly beneath the femur. As shown in Chapter 1, Figure 1–62 , the anterior shear created by the quadriceps must be offset by a pull similar to that provided by the ACL. Increases and decreases in the angle of pull of the quadriceps are accompanied by concomitant increases and decreases in stress in the ACL. Wilk and coworkers[81] investigated anteroposterior shear force, compression force, and extensor torque in open versus closed chain exercises. These authors found that the anterior shear force, which stresses the ACL, was found in an open chain knee extension exercise when the knee was extending from 38° to 10°. The maximal anterior shear occurred be-

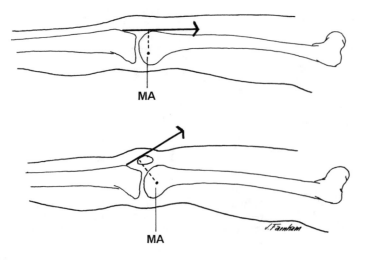

MA

MA

J. Farnham

FIGURE 11–32. The lower portion of the illustration shows a normal knee in extension with the patella positioned anterior to the tibiofemoral joint. The arrow indicates the action line of the quadriceps and the dotted line indicates the moment arm (MA) of the quadriceps. The top drawing shows a knee with the patella removed. The arrow indicates the changed action line of the quadriceps, and the dotted line indicates the decreased MA that results from removal of the patella.

tween 20° and 11°. In contrast, no anterior shear force was found in the closed chain exercises (squat and leg press). However, the authors[81] found that the posterior shear force, which stresses the PCL, was present throughout the entire ROM in closed chain exercises with a maximum force occurring between 83° and 105° of knee flexion. A posterior shear force was also found during open chain exercise, but this force was only present between 60° and 101° of flexion. Closed chain exercises are often prescribed following ACL or PCL injury on the premise that closed chain exercises are less stressful, more like functional movement, and safer than open chain exercises. However, this study demonstrated that the stress on the PCL that is present during some types of closed chain exercises may actually be detrimental to the healing process. In an investigation of isokinetic exercise, Kellis and Balzopoulous[82] found that the antagonistic effect appears to depend on the type of muscle action (eccentric or concentric) of the antagonist. The anterior shear force was not affected by antagonist activity, but posterior shear forces, patella tendon, and compressive forces were affected. Therefore, it would appear that the forces generated by antagonistic activity during isokinetic exercise need to be considered when using isokinetic exercise as part of the rehabilitation process following knee injuries.

The contribution of the patella to improving torque production by the quadriceps will vary with the joint ROM. In full knee flexion, the patella slides into the intercondylar notch of the femur, effectively eliminating the patella as a pulley. The rounded contour of the femoral condyles at this point, however, is already deflecting the muscle action line. Also, in full flexion the instantaneous axis of rotation has moved well posteriorly into the femoral condyles, further away from the action line of the quadriceps muscle. The movement of the IAR, therefore, already results in an increased MA for extension without the mediation of the patella.[15]

During knee extension, the MA of the quadriceps muscle lengthens as the patella leaves the intercondylar notch and must travel over the rounded femoral condyles. At about 60° of knee flexion, the patella is pushed by the rounded femoral condyles as far from the IAR as it will go. With continued extension, the MA once again begins to diminish. Evidence of the change in the MA is seen in the findings that the mean maximum isometric torque of the knee extensors is greater at 60° of knee flexion than at either 30° or 45°.[83] This is influenced, however, not only by the MA, but by the changing length-tension of the muscle and by the type of contraction. When peak torque is assessed during active isokinetic knee extension, the greatest amount of torque generated by the knee extensor muscles occurs at 45° of knee flexion.[83]

The decrease in the length of the MA of the quadriceps muscle and the decrease in the length-tension of the muscle during the last 15° of knee extension place the quadriceps at a mechanical and physiologic disadvantage. A 60% increase in quadriceps force over that needed in the rest of the ROM is required to complete the last 15° of knee joint extension.[74] Consequently, although the effect of the patella on improving the MA of the quadriceps femoris is diminished in the final stages of knee extension, the small improvement in MA provided by the patella may be most important here. Given the reduced ability of the muscle to generate active tension, the relative size of the MA is critical to torque production. Removal of the patella will have almost no effect on the strength of the quadriceps muscle as the muscle initiates extension from full flexion because the patella has little effect at this point in the range. Loss of the patella in the 60° to 30° range of flexion will produce a noticeable weakness in extension, but the roundness of the femoral condyles will still deflect the line of pull of the muscle and the length-tension is still favorable. Loss of the patella has its most profound effect in the last stages of joint extension when the decrease in MA may reduce torque to the point where knee extension cannot be completed by an active quadriceps muscle contraction alone.

The loss of the patella is most evident when the tibia is the moving segment and the quadriceps muscle must work against the resistance of gravity. In weight-bearing, however, the diminished quadriceps extensor function can be supplemented by other forces affecting the closed chain. In fact, patterns of quadriceps activity may appear quite different in the weight-bearing position. In weight-bearing, the quadriceps controls knee flexion (rather than creating extension) by acting eccentrically during activities. The quadriceps then works concentrically in extension to return the body to the erect posture. When the erect posture has been attained, activity of the extensors ceases. No knee extensor muscle activity is necessary to maintain knee extension in normal erect stance because the line of gravity (LOG) is located anterior to the axis of flexion and extension at the knee joint. The resulting gravitational torque created around the knee joint is sufficient to maintain the knee in extension. The posterior joint capsule, ligaments, and musculotendinous structures are able to maintain equilibrium at the knee by counterbalancing the gravitational torque and preventing hyperextension. If the LOG passes posterior to the knee joint axis, the gravitational torque will tend to cause knee flexion and activity of the knee extensor muscles is necessary to counterbalance the gravitational torque and maintain the knee joint in equilibrium. The extensor muscles, which have the responsibility of supporting the body weight and resisting the force of gravity, are about two times stronger than the flexor muscles.

In a closed kinematic chain, movement of the knee is accompanied by movement at the hip and ankle. Thus, knee flexion usually occurs in weight-bearing in conjunction with hip flexion and ankle dorsiflexion. Activity of the soleus muscle, which is continuously active in erect stance, exerts a posterior pull on the tibia as it acts in reverse action and contributes to knee joint stability in the erect posture. Secondary support may also be given to the knee in extension by the flexor muscles as they develop passive tension as a result of being stretched over the posterolateral and posteromedial aspects of the knee.

Further consideration of the effect of the quadriceps femoris muscles will be given in discussion of the patellofemoral joint. Although the patella primarily serves the quadriceps mechanism, the quadriceps mechanism can have a substantial effect on the ability of the patella to fulfill its function in an effective, pain-free way.

Stabilization

The supporting structures of the knee may be classified on the basis of *function, structure,* or *location.* Classification systems based on function use a static/dynamic differentiation, whereas those based on structure use a capsular/extracapsular method. Systems based on location use a compartmental approach, referring to the embryonic medial and lateral joint compartments. According to the functional classification sys-

tem, the **static stabilizers** include the passive structures such as the joint capsule and the ligaments. Included as static stabilizers are components of the joint capsule and associated structures such as the coronary ligaments and the meniscopatellar and patellofemoral ligaments. Ligaments that are static stabilizers include the MCL and LCL, the ACL and PCL, the oblique popliteal and arcuate, and the transverse ligament. Because the ITB is considered to be a passive force at the knee despite its muscular connections, we will consider it as part of the static stabilizers. The **dynamic stabilizers** of the knee include the following muscles and aponeuroses: the quadriceps femoris and extensor retinaculum, pes anserinus (semitendinosus, sartorius, and gracilis muscles), popliteus, biceps femoris, and the semimembranosus.[28]

According to the classification system based on location, the supporting structures of the knee joint that are located on the anteromedial, medial, and posteromedial aspects of the knee are **medial compartment structures.** Structures located in the same respective areas on the lateral aspect are **lateral compartment structures.**[28,29] The medial compartment structures include the following: the medial patellar retinaculum, MCL, oblique popliteal ligament, and the PCL. The medial compartment structures also include the medial head of the gastrocnemius, the pes anserinus, and the semimembranosus muscles. The **lateral compartment structures** include the following static and dynamic stabilizers: ITB; the biceps femoris and popliteus muscles; LCL; the meniscofemoral, arcuate, and ACL; and the lateral patellar retinaculum.

Regardless of the classification system used, attempting to credit structures with contributing primarily to one type of stabilization is extremely difficult and generally requires oversimplification of effect. The many studies and literature reviews already cited in this chapter make it clear that the contribution of both muscles and ligaments are dependent on joint position (not only of the knee joint, but of the surrounding joints), magnitude and direction of force, availability of reinforcing structures, and nature of the testing conditions. (Almost all knee joint structures can contribute to stability in all directions under specific normal or abnormal conditions.) The variations among individuals (and between knees in the same individual) also contribute to the variation in findings. The following summary should be considered, therefore, a reiteration of some (but not all) contributors to stability of the knee joint.

Some Contributors to Anterior-Posterior Stabilization

Anterior-posterior stability of the knee is provided by static and dynamic stabilizers and lateral and medial compartment structures. The contribution of the ligaments to anterior-posterior stability was discussed previously. Some stabilizers, however, are particularly critical and bear reiteration of function. The extensor retinaculum, which is composed of fibers from the quadriceps femoris, fuses with fibers of the joint capsule to provide dynamic support for the anteromedial and anterolateral aspects of the knee. The quadriceps femoris works synergistically with the PCL to resist forces attempting to displace the tibia posteriorly. The medial and lateral heads of the gastrocnemius reinforce the medial and lateral aspects of the posterior capsule. The popliteus is considered to be a particularly important posterolateral stabilizer, complementing the function of the PCL.[74] The meniscofemoral ligaments may act as secondary restraints to posterior translation of the tibia.[64] The ACL and the hamstrings work in a complementary manner to resist forces that are attempting to displace the tibia anteriorly or shear the femur posteriorly.[54] Such forces are exemplified by the pull of the quadriceps and by the effect of the ground reaction force on the tibia when the heel hits the ground.[84] Kaplan[9] placed particular emphasis on the semimembranosus, contending that the knee could not be stable in flexion unless this structure and its multiple connections remained intact.

The role of the patella itself cannot be ignored when examining anterior-posterior stability of the knee. The patella prevents the femur from sliding forward off the tibia, actually serving as part of the tibia connected by an elastic tendon. This combination of patella and tibia cradles the femur.[85]

Some Contributors to Medial-Lateral Stabilization

Medial-lateral stability at the knee is provided for by static and dynamic soft tissue structures and by the tibial tubercles and menisci when the knee is in full extension. The knee, like the elbow, is reinforced on its medial and lateral aspects by collateral ligaments. The collaterals clearly play a critical role in resisting varus-valgus stresses, especially in the more extended knee. Both cruciates contribute, although the magnitude and balance of the contribution varies with many factors. As knee flexion increases, the dynamic stability provided by the musculature such as the muscles of the pes anserinus on the medial aspect of the knee become increasingly important. Laterally, the iliotibial tract, LCL, popliteus tendon, and biceps tendon form a quadruple complex that contributes to stability.[9] The posterolateral capsule is particularly important in varus stability in extension, whereas the popliteus is a major stabilizer in 0° to 90° of flexion.[37]

The menisci are particularly important to medial-lateral stability because the knee remains stable in full extension regardless of sectioning of ligamentous structures.[37] Removing both menisci would appear to have its greatest effect on stabilization during varus and valgus stresses.[86]

Some Contributors to Rotational Stabilization

The complex nature of rotational stabilization of the knee makes it particularly difficult to isolate certain structures as major contributors. It would appear, however, that the role of the passive mechanisms predominate over the dynamic mechanisms. The cruciates are most often credited with rotational stability of the joint, especially in the extended knee.[20] However, rotational instability may occur even in the presence of intact cruciates.[38] Credit is also given to the MCL, LCL, posteromedial capsule, posterolateral capsule, and the popliteus tendon by investigators exploring rotational stability under varied conditions.[37,38,53] The meniscofemoral ligaments are credited with helping to restrain excessive lateral rotation.[31]

The Patellofemoral Joint

The role of the patella has been well covered in discussion of the quadriceps femoris. It is primarily an anatomic eccentric pulley and a mechanism to reduce friction between the quadriceps tendon and the femoral condyles. The ability of the patella to perform its functions without restricting knee motion depends on its mobility. The motions of the patella are shown in Figures 11–33, 11–34, and 11–35. The

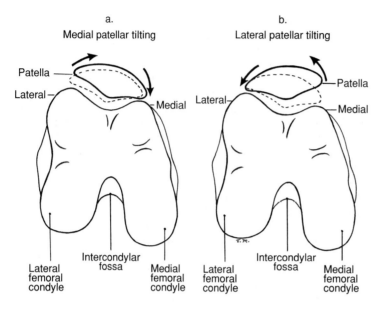

a.
Medial patellar tilting

b.
Lateral patellar tilting

FIGURE 11–33. (a) Medial patellar tilting. The diagram shows the distal end of a right femur. The dotted lines represent the normal resting position of the patella in full knee extension. The solid patellar outline shows the position of the patella in a medial patellar tilt. (b) Lateral patellar tilting. The patella may also tilt superiorly and inferiorly, but these motions are not shown in the diagram.

patella has the ability to slide on the femoral condyles while remaining seated between them. In full knee extension, the patella sits on the anterior surface on the distal femur. With knee flexion, the patella slides distally on the femoral condyles, seating itself between the femoral condyles. In full flexion, the patella sinks into the intercondylar notch. This sagittal plane motion of the patellar, called **patellar**

flexion, lags behind knee flexion.[87] Knee extension reverses the sliding of the patella and brings it back to the patella surface of the femur. This motion of the patella is referred to as **patellar extension.**[87] According to Heegaard,[88] the flexion/extension motions of the patella are completely determined by the configuration of the articular surfaces and the orientation of the extensor mechanism. As the

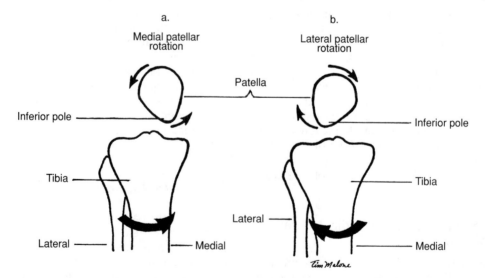

a.
Medial patellar rotation

b.
Lateral patellar rotation

FIGURE 11–34. (a) Medial rotation of the patella. The diagram shows the proximal end of a right tibia and fibula and a right patella. The femur has been removed to emphasize patellar motion. The inferior pole of the patella follows medial rotation of the tibia during both automatic and axial rotation. (b) Lateral rotation of the patella. The inferior pole of the patella follows the lateral rotation of the tibia during both automatic and axial rotation.

a.

Medial patellar
shift

b.

Lateral patellar
shift

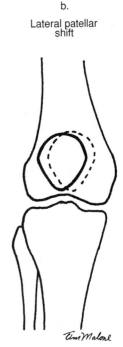

FIGURE 11–35. (a) Medial patellar shift. The dotted patellar outline shows the normal resting position of the patella in full knee extension. The solid patellar outline shows a medially shifted patella. (b) Lateral patellar shift. The solid patellar outline shows a laterally shifted patella.

patella travels (or "tracks") down the femur, it undergoes some rotation about its vertical axis (**patellar tilt**) (see Fig.11–33). The tilting motion helps the patella accommodate to some of the asymmetry of the femoral condyles. The patella tilts medially from 0° to 30°[87] (0–20°[88]) and over 100°.[88] Lateral tilting occurs between 20° (30°[87]) and 100°[88](130°[87]) of flexion. The patella also must rotate about an anteroposterior axis (rotation of the patella) to remain seated in the intercondylar notch as the femur undergoes either automatic or axial rotation. Because the inferior aspect of the patella is tied to the tibial tuberosity, the inferior patella continues to point to the tibial tuberosity while moving with the femur. In **medial rotation of the patella** the inferior pole of the patella follows medial rotation of the tibia while the femur laterally rotates on the tibia (see Fig.11–34 a). In **lateral rotation of the patella** the inferior patellar pole remains laterally with the tibia as the femur rotates medially on the tibia (see Fig11–34b).[89] The patella laterally rotates 6° to 7° as the knee flexes from 25° to 130°, with most of the rotation having occurred by 60° of knee flexion.[90] The mediolateral translation that the patella undergoes during knee joint movement is referred to as **patellar shift**.[87,88] The patella shifts medially with medial tibial rotation at all flexion angles (see Fig.11–35a)

and laterally with knee flexion (see Fig.11–35b). At full extension the average lateral shift equals 7.5 to 10 mm but this shift disappears by 30° flexion. Failure of the patella to slide, tilt, rotate, or shift appropriately can lead to restriction in knee joint ROM, to instability of the patellofemoral joint, or to pain caused by erosion of the patellofemoral surfaces. Therefore, the normal passive mobility of the patella is often assessed clinically. Manually produced displacement of the normal patella at 0° produced a medial shift of 9.6 mm and a lateral shift of 5.4 mm. At 35° flexion a medial shift of 9.4 mm and a lateral shift of 10.0 mm was obtained.[91]

We must closely examine the oddly shaped patella, the uneven surface on which it sits, and the tremendous forces to which the patella and patellofemoral surfaces are subject to understand the many potential problems encountered by the patella in performing what would appear to be a relatively simple function. A comprehension of the structures and forces that influence patellofemoral function leads readily to an understanding of the common clinical problems found at the patellofemoral joint.

Patellofemoral Articular Surfaces

The triangularly shaped patella is distinguished by being the largest sesamoid bone in the body. Together with the femoral surface on which it sits, the patellofemoral joint is also the least congruent joint in the body.[92] The total articular surface of the patella is much smaller than the femoral trochlear surface and the material properties of the patellar surface vary throughout the articular surface as well as from the properties of the apposing trochlear cartilage.[78] The posterior surface of the patella is covered by articular cartilage and divided by a vertical ridge. The ridge may be situated approximately in the center of the patella, dividing the articular surface into approximately equally sized medial and lateral patellar facets. Occasionally, the ridge may be situated slightly toward the medial border of the patella, making the medial facet smaller than the lateral.[93] Regardless of size, the medial and lateral facets are flat to slightly convex side to side and top to bottom. At least 30% of the patellae also have a second vertical ridge toward the medial border, separating the medial facet from an extreme medial edge known as the **odd facet** of the patella[92] (Fig. 11–36).

The patellar articulating surface of the femur is the intercondylar groove or femoral sulcus on the anterior aspect of the distal femur. The groove or sulcus corresponds to the vertical ridge on the patella, dividing the femoral surface into lateral and medial portions. The femoral surfaces are concave side to side, but convex top to bottom.[2] The lateral facet is slightly more convex than the medial surface and has a more highly developed lip than the medial surface (Fig. 11–37 and Fig. 11–2a). The angle formed by the medial and lateral facets (angle of the femoral sulcus) has been found to average 138°, but varies widely among individuals (116–151°).[94,95]

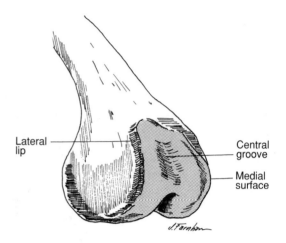

FIGURE 11–37. Articulating surfaces on the femur. Note the well-developed lateral lip on the lateral aspect of the articulating surface.

Patellofemoral Joint Congruence

In the fully extended or neutral knee, the patella lies on the femoral sulcus. The vertical position of the patella in the femoral sulcus is related to the length of the patellar tendon. Ordinarily, the ratio of the length of the tendon (LT) to the length of the patella (LP) is approximately 1:1. This ratio (LT/LP) is referred to as the **index of Insall and Salviti.**[96,97] It is specifically calculated by measuring LT from the apex of the patella to the small notch just proximal to the tibial tuberosity on lateral radiograph and the greatest diagonal LP.[96] The ratio may be affected by gender, with females having slightly larger ratios (or slightly longer patellar tendons).[94,98,99] The limit of normal for the ligament to patella ratio is 1.3,[96] or the ligament should not exceed the patella in length by more than 20%.[100] An excessively long tendon produces an abnormally high position of the patella on the femoral sulcus known as **patella alta.** (The ramifications of this will be seen later in the chapter.)

The patella in the neutral or extended knee has little or no contact with the femoral sulcus beneath it. There is *at most* only a narrow band of contact between the inferior pole of the patella and the femoral sulcus.[101] The first consistent contact of the patella is made at 10° to 20° of flexion on inferior margin of the patella across both medial and lateral facets. With increasing flexion, the area of contact increases and shifts from distal to proximal, spreading from the ridge separating the medial and odd

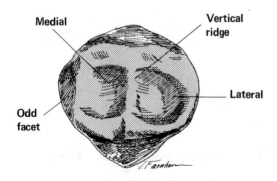

FIGURE 11–36. Articulating surfaces on the patella.

facet to the lateral facet. By 90° of knee flexion, all portions of the patella have experienced some (although inconsistent) contact, with the exception of the odd facet. As flexion continues past 90°, the medial facet enters the intercondylar notch, and the odd facet achieves contact for the first time.[102] At 135° of flexion, contact is on the lateral and odd facets,[89] with the medial facet completely out of contact.[103]

Overall, the medial patellar facet normally receives the most consistent contact with the femoral surfaces,[93,104] whereas the odd facet receives the least. Because any imbalance in compression and release of pressure on cartilage can lead to degenerative changes, it is not surprising that the most common cartilaginous changes on the patella are, in fact, found on the medial and odd facets. The changes, however, appear to be part of the normal aging process, are not necessarily progressive, and are commonly asymptomatic.[17,92,105] Although the lack of sufficient compression on the odd facet may be obvious (it is in contact only in full knee flexion), the excessive compression on the medial facet must be understood in the context of the patellofemoral joint reaction forces. Singerman and colleagues[106] found that the point of application on the patella of the resultant contact force (COP) migrated superiorly from 20° to 90° flexion. Above 90° the COP migrated inferiorly. However, the relationship between the different components of force and flexion angle exhibited a high degree of variability.

Patellofemoral Joint Reaction Forces

The patella is pulled on simultaneously by the quadriceps tendon superiorly and by the patella tendon inferiorly. When the pulls of these two structures are vertical or in line with each other, the patella may be suspended between them, making little or no contact with the femur. This is essentially the case when the knee joint is in full extension. Cadaver studies have confirmed that there is little or no contact between the patella and the femur in this position.[104] Even a strong contraction of the quadriceps in full extension will produce little or no patellofemoral compression. This is the rationale for use of straight leg-raising exercises as a way of improving quadriceps muscle strength without creating or exacerbating patellofemoral problems.

As knee flexion proceeds from full extension, the pull of the quadriceps tendon (F_Q) and the pull of the patellar ligament (F_{pl}) become increasingly oblique, compressing the patella into the femur (Fig. 11–38). According to Hirokawa and coworkers[107] the contact force on the lateral side always exceeds that of the medial side from 0° to 100° flexion. Hegaard[108] found that peak pressures during passive knee flexion were higher on the lateral facets near full flexion and full extension. An almost even distribution of pressure occurred in the midflexion range. Tensile stresses are found in the frontal plane beneath either the lateral or medial facets. The increasing compression caused by the quadriceps mechanism with increased joint flexion occurs whether the muscle is active or passive. If the quadriceps muscle is inactive, the elastic tension alone will increase with increased knee joint flexion. If the quadriceps muscle is active, both the active tension and passive elastic tension will contribute increasingly to compression as the knee flexion angle increases. The compression, of course, creates a joint reaction force across the patellofemoral joint. The total joint reaction force is influenced both by the magnitude of active and passive pull of the quadriceps and by the angle of knee flexion. High shear

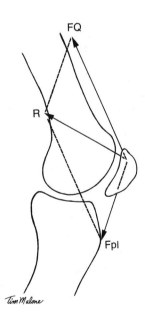

FIGURE 11–38. The combined pull of the quadriceps (F_Q) and the patellar ligaments (Fp_l) can be composed into a single resultant vector (R) that will clearly compress the patella into the femur. The magnitude of R will increase with an increase in magnitude of (F_Q) and (Fp_l) and with increased knee flexion.

stresses are found at the patella tendon insertion site where ossification of cartilage is accelerated in areas responding to high shear stresses. The highest tensile stress is concentrated beneath the patella ligament insertion.

The patellofemoral joint reaction force found in gait when the foot first contacts the ground and the knee flexes slightly to 10° to 15° is 50% of body weight.[102] The increased knee flexion and quadriceps muscle activity seen with stair climbing or with running hills may increase the patellofemoral joint reaction force to 3.3 times body weight at 60°.[21,102] The joint reaction force may reach 7.8 times the body weight at 130° of knee joint flexion in such activities as deep knee bends when knee flexion is extreme and a strong quadriceps contraction is required.[102] Although reaction forces at other lower-extremity joints may reach these same magnitudes, they do so over much more congruent joints; that is, the compressive forces are distributed over larger areas. At the normal patellofemoral joint, the medial facet bears the brunt of the compressive force. Several mechanisms help minimize or dissipate the patellofemoral joint compression on the patella in general and on the medial facet specifically.

Because there is essentially no compressive force on the patella in full extension, no compensatory mechanisms are necessary. As knee joint flexion proceeds, the area of patellar contact gradually increases, spreading out the increased compressive force. From 30° to 70° of flexion, contact occurs at the thick cartilage of medial facet near the central ridge. In fact, the cartilage of the medial facet is the thickest hyaline cartilage in the human body.[104] The thick cartilage can better withstand the substantial compressive forces. The greater thickness and higher permeability of the patellar joint surface may improve joint stability because the patella is able to seat more deeply in the trochlea. Within this same ROM, the patella has its greatest effect as a pulley, maximizing the MA of the quadriceps. With a large MA, less quadriceps muscle force (and less patellofemoral joint compression) is needed to produce the same torque. As flexion proceeds, the MA diminishes, necessitating an increase in force production by the quadriceps. Between 70° and 90°, however, the patella is no longer the only structure contacting the femoral condyles. At this point in the flexion range, the quadriceps tendon contacts the femoral condyles, dissi-

pating some of the patellofemoral compression.[102,103]

Conversely the joint reaction force increases as the knee extends from 90° to 45° and then decreases with increasing extension.[78] The adaptive mechanisms of the patella in dealing with the high joint reaction forces appear to be fairly successful. Although some cartilaginous deterioration is common at both the odd and the medial facet, it bears reiteration that these changes rarely cause problems.

Medial-Lateral Patellofemoral Joint Stability

In the extended knee, the patella perches precariously on the femoral sulcus. Until the patella begins sliding down the femoral condyles with knee joint flexion and is drawn into the intercondylar notch (at about 20° of flexion), medial-lateral stability rests solely on active and passive tension in the structures around the patella. Ficat[109] identified that the patellofemoral joint is under the permanent control of two restraining mechanisms that cross each other at right angles: a transverse group of stabilizers and a longitudinal group of stabilizers. The position of the patella and its mobility will be determined by the relative tension in these two stabilizing systems.

The transverse stabilizers of the patella have been variously described. The medial and lateral extensor (patellar) retinacula join the vastus medialis and lateralis muscles, respectively, directly to the patella.[2] Several investigators have described medial and lateral patellofemoral ligaments that may be part of or blend with the retinacular fibers.[7,21,22] The medial patellofemoral ligament is found to contribute an average of 53% of total force resisting displacement of the patella when the knee is in full extension. There may also be an iliopatellar band attaching the patella directly to the iliotibial tract.[23,24]

The longitudinal stabilizers of the patella are the patellar tendon inferiorly and the quadriceps tendon superiorly. The patellotibial ligaments are thickenings of the capsule anteriorly, which extend from the inferior border of the patella distally to the anterior coronary ligaments and anterior margins of the tibia on each side of the patellar tendon.[7,21] As has been demonstrated, the longitudinal structures can stabilize the patella through patellofemoral compression. The compression is essentially absent in the extended knee, leaving the patella relatively unstable in this knee joint position. When extension is exaggerated, as in genu recurvatum, the pull of the quadriceps muscle and patellar ligament may actually distract the patella from the femoral sulcus, further aggravating the instability of the patella. There are also other contributing longitudinal structures and other effects of the longitudinal structures to be examined. Both the transverse and the longitudinal structures will influence the medial-lateral positioning of the patella within the femoral sulcus and the so-called **patellar tracking** or path of the patella as it slides down the femoral condyles within the intercondylar notch.

Medial-Lateral Positioning of the Patella

All the passive and dynamic transverse and longitudinal stabilizing mechanisms of the patella can influence the medial-lateral position of the patella. The passive mobility of the patella and its medial-lateral positioning are largely governed by the passive and dynamic pulls of the structures surrounding it. When the knee is fully extended and the musculature relaxed, some investigators have concluded that the patella should be able to be passively displaced medially or laterally no more than one-half the width of the patella[110] and that the excursion should be symmetrical.[111] Others, however, have not found either relationship to hold true[91,112] or have found considerable variation among individuals.[22] Imbalance in passive tension or changes in the line of pull of the dynamic structures will substantially influence the patella. This is predominantly true when the knee joint is in extension and the patella sits on the relatively shallow femoral sulcus. Abnormal forces, however, may influence the excursion of the patella even in its more secure location within the intercondylar notch during knee flexion.

Medial-Lateral Forces on the Patella

During active extension or when the quadriceps muscle is passively stretched, the patella is pulled by the quadriceps. The force on the patella is determined by the resultant pull of the four segments of the quadriceps (F_Q) and by the pull of the patellar ligament (F_{pl}). Since the action lines of F_Q and F_{pl} do not coincide, the patella tends to be pulled slightly laterally by the two forces (Fig. 11–39). Anything that might increase the obliquity of the resultant

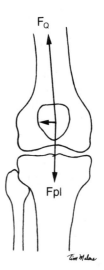

FIGURE 11–39. The pull of the quadriceps (F_Q) and the pull of the patellar ligament (F_{pl}) lie at a slight angle to each other, producing a slight lateral force on the patella.

pull of the quadriceps or the obliquity of the patellar ligament in the frontal plane may increase the lateral force on the patella. An increase in this lateral component may increase the compression on the lateral patellar facet as it pushes harder into the lateral lip of the femoral sulcus (in knee extension) or the lateral aspect of the intercondylar notch (in knee joint flexion). A large lateral force on the patella may actually cause it to sublux or dislocate off the lateral lip of the femoral sulcus when the knee is extended. However, even a very large lateral force on the patella would be unlikely to result in dislocation once the patella is in the intercondylar notch.

The pull of the vastus lateralis muscle is normally 12° to 15° lateral to the long axis of the femur with even greater obliquity in its lower fibers.[75] The pull of the vastus medialis longus muscle is approximately 15° to 18° medial to the femoral shaft, with the VMO pulling 50° to 55° medially.[75] Because these two muscles pull not only on the common quadriceps tendon but also exert a pull on the patella through their retinacular connections, complementary function is critical; that is, relative weakness of the vastus medialis muscle (especially the VMO fibers) may substantially increase the resultant lateral forces on the patella. The VMO appears to be extremely susceptible to the inhibitory effects of joint effusions and is often inhibited in cases of injury that are accompanied by inflammation and swelling. Generally the VMO inserts into the superomedial aspect of the patella about one-third to one-half of the way down on the medial border. However, in instances of patellar malalignment the VMO insertion site may be located less than a quarter of the way down on the patellas's medial aspect and as a result the VMO cannot effectively counteract the lateral motion of the patella.[78]

The obliquity of the pull of the quadriceps muscle and patellar tendon can increase with problems other than imbalance between the vastus lateralis and medialis. Genu valgum increases the obliquity of the femur and, concomitantly, the obliquity of the pull of the quadriceps. Femoral anteversion (internal femoral torsion) in the older child or adult generally results in the femoral condyles being turned in (medially rotated) relative to the tibia. This creates an increased obliquity in the patellar tendon that may also be seen with lateral tibial torsion. Each of these conditions can predispose the patella to excessive pressure laterally or to subluxation or dislocation.

The net effect of the pull of the quadriceps and the patellar ligament is commonly assessed clinically using the **Q (quadriceps) angle** of the knee. The Q angle is the angle formed between a line connecting the anterior superior iliac spine (ASIS) to the midpoint of the patella and a line connecting the tibial tubercle and the midpoint of the patella (Fig. 11–40). An angle of 10° to 15° measured with the knee either in full extension or slightly flexed is considered to be normal.[78] Some authors postulate that women have a slightly greater Q angle than men.[21,94] The increased angle among women has been attributed to the fact that they have a wider pelvis, increased femoral anteversion, and relative knee valgus. However, whether or not women have a greater Q angle than men is still a matter for debate.[78] The Q angle is usually measured with the knee in extension, because excessive lateral forces may be more of a problem here and because as the knee is flexed, the Q angle will reduce as the tibia rotates medially relative to the femur.[113]

A Q angle of 20° or more is considered to be abnormal, creating excessive lateral forces on the patella that may predispose the patella to pathologic changes.[105,114] Although an excessively large Q angle is usually an indicator of some structural misalignment, an apparently normal Q angle is *not* necessarily consistent

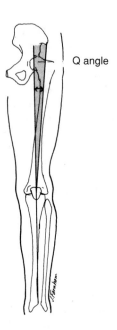

FIGURE 11–40. The Q angle is the angle between a line connecting the anterior superior iliac spine to the midpoint of the patella and the extension of line connecting the tibial tubercle and the midpoint of the patella.

with the absence of problems. The line between the ASIS of the pelvis and the midpatella is only an estimate of the line of pull of the quadriceps. If substantial imbalance exists between the vastus medialis and lateralis muscles, the Q angle may underestimate the lateral force on the patella because the actual pull of the quadriceps muscle is no longer on the estimated line. Similarly, a patella that is already subluxed or dislocated may be seen with an inaccurately small Q angle and be misinterpreted as normal.[115]

Forces other than the alignment and balance of the components of the quadriceps muscle may influence patellar positioning. Excessive tension in or adaptive shortening of the lateral retinaculum or stretch of the medial retinaculum have been implicated in patellar dysfunction. Excessive tension in the lateral retinaculum (or weakness in the VMO) may cause the patella to tilt laterally, thus increasing compression laterally and reducing it medially. There is some indication that the patellar connections to the ITB may exert an excessive lateral pull on the patella when the ITB band is tight.[116] It is unknown whether changes in the passive structures are primary or are secondary to changes in the dynamic stabilizers.

Any misalignment of the medial-lateral stabilizers of the patella may lead to excessive pressure on the lateral patellar facet. Even large lateral forces can be prevented from subluxing or dislocating the patella as long as the lateral lip of the femoral sulcus is of sufficient height. When it is underdeveloped, however, even relatively small lateral forces may create patellar subluxation or full dislocation. This may be a causative factor in the higher incidence of patellofemoral problems seen in adolescence, when the patellofemoral joint is still developing.[28] The height of the lateral lip of the femoral sulcus may also be a factor in patella alta. In this condition, the lateral lip is not necessarily underdeveloped (although it may be), but the high position of the patella places the patella proximal to the high lateral wall. The upper aspect of the femoral sulcus is less developed and, therefore, makes it easier to sublux the patella.

The result of changes in patellofemoral alignment or imbalance of forces across the joint will be discussed in the following section on injury and disease.

Effects of Injury and Disease

The joints of the knee complex, like other joints in the body, are subject to developmental defects, injury, and disease processes. However, a number of factors make the knee joint unique. The knee, unlike the shoulder, elbow, and wrist, must support the body weight and at the same time provide mobility. Although the hip and ankle joints similarly support the body weight, the knee is a more complex structure than either the hip or ankle. The knee joint also joins two of the longest levers in the body and is located in a more exposed position than either the hip or the ankle joints.

Knee Joint Injury

The interest and participation in physical fitness and sports activities currently in vogue among all age groups and both sexes is subjecting the knee complex to an increased risk of injury. Sports such as jogging, skating, skiing, football, and tennis may cause either direct or indirect injury. Injuries to the knee complex may involve the menisci, the ligaments, the bones, or the musculotendinous structures. Meniscal injuries, especially of the medial meniscus, are common and usually occur as a result of sudden rotation of the femur on the fixed tibia when the knee is in flexion.[117] Axial rotation in the flexed knee occurs with the medial meniscus as the pivot point. The more rigidly attached medial meniscus may tear under the sudden load.

Ligamentous injuries may occur as a result of a force that causes the joint to exceed its normal ROM. A blow to the lateral aspect of the knee joint or the tibia may cause a valgus stress that results in a tearing of the ligaments restraining valgus motion. Likewise, forced hyperextension of the knee may cause tearing of the posterior ligaments. Although excessive forces may cause ligamentous tears, lower-level forces may similarly cause disruption in ligaments weakened by aging, disease, immobilization, steroids, or vascular insufficiency. Each of these may affect the collagen or ground substance of the ligaments. Cyclic loading (whether short term and intense or over a prolonged period) may also affect viscoelasticity and stiffness.[54] A weakened ligament may take 10 months or more to return to normal stiffness once the underlying problem has been resolved.[47]

The bony and cartilaginous structures may be injured either by the application of a direct force, such as bumping the patella or falling on the knees, or by indirect forces that are exerted by abnormal ligamentous and muscular forces. Knee joint instability, as frequently seen in the knee following ACL injury, can lead to progressive changes in the articular cartilage, in the menisci, and in the other ligaments attempting to restrain the increased joint mobility.[84,118]

The numerous bursae and tendons at the knee are also subject to injury. The cause of injuries to these structures may be either a direct blow or prolonged compressive or tensile stresses. Bursitis most commonly occurs in the prepatellar bursa and the superficial infrapatellar bursa (known as **housemaid's knee**), but may also occur in high-friction areas such as at the bursa beneath the pes anserinus. The localized tenderness generally associated with bursitis may also be found if the fat pad between the patellar ligament and anterior synovial membrane becomes inflamed.[11]

Another potential source of pain and dysfunction in the knee joint is the presence of a patellar plica. Classic symptoms include pain with prolonged sitting, with stair climbing, and during resisted extension exercises. More than half the patients will also complain of a snapping sensation.[35] In flexion, the plica is drawn tightly over the medial femoral condyle and pressed under the patella. The resultant tension in the band may cause patellar misalignment (leading to pain) or the plica itself may become inflamed.[27,35] If the inflamed plica becomes fibrotic, it may create a secondary synovitis around the femoral condyle and deterioration of the condylar cartilage may occur.[26,27,35] A thickened or inflamed superior plica may erode the superior aspect of the medial facet of the patella.[31]

Patellofemoral Joint Injury

We have presented and discussed the mechanics of a number of problems that may predispose the knee to patellofemoral dysfunction. Any one problem in isolation, or various combinations of problems (which may include primary and secondary changes), may lead to excessive pressure on the lateral facets of the patella, to lateral subluxation, or to lateral dislocation. Whether excessive pressure, subluxation, and dislocation are separate clinical entities or part of a continuum of patellofemoral dysfunction is arguable.[115,119,120] Each, however, is commonly associated with knee pain, poor tolerance of sustained passive knee flexion (as in sitting for long periods), "giving way" of the knee and exacerbation of symptoms by repeated use of the quadriceps on a flexed knee. These symptoms are similar to the complex of symptoms found with patella plica, which may occur as a related disorder. Differentiation in symptomatology may occur, however, when patellar subluxation or dislocation is present. Tenderness of the medial retinaculum and medial border of the patella develop with repeated subluxation or dislocation. The medial retinaculum is stretched as the patella deviates toward or slips over the lateral lip of the femoral sulcus or condyle. The return of the patella into the intercondylar notch may affect the medial patella (occasionally causing osteochondral fracture).[28,109,110]

Until recently, cartilaginous changes seen on the lateral patellar facet were considered to be diagnostic of patellofemoral dysfunction, and the term **chondromalacia patella** (softening of the cartilage) assigned. With the knowledge that similar cartilaginous changes can be found in asymptomatic knees and that the medial patellar facet frequently shows greater change without symptoms or progressive carti-

lage deterioration, more general diagnoses have been used, including patellofemoral arthralgia or patellofemoral pain syndrome.[21] Although in fact cartilage changes on the medial patellar facet are more common, changes found on the lateral facet will more commonly progress to osteoarthritis.[17,105] The mechanism of pain is presumed to indicate the disruption of cartilage, the by-products of which irritate the synovium, which when inflamed, may cause stretching of sensitive surrounding structure.[92,101] Pain may also arise from the innervated subchondral bone, which is subjected to increased load as the cartilage deteriorates.[21] Such cartilage deterioration is generally found when there is substantial misalignment or instability. Minor structural, stability, or overuse problems typically found among adolescents and young adults may cause patellofemoral pain. In such instances, however, the pain frequently resolves spontaneously over time and will *not* necessarily progress to later osteoarthritic problems.[17] However, because cartilage is aneural, a lack of symptoms may indicate an early stage of chondromalacia that will become symptomatic only after additional trauma.[31]

Summary

A Model for Dysfunction

Given the range of possible problems that can occur in the knee joint, an exhaustive discussion is beyond the scope of this text. However, a thorough knowledge of normal structure and function can be used to predict or understand the immediate impact on the joint of a specific injury and the secondary effects on intact structures. An example of such an analysis is presented in Table 11–2, using the example of rupture of the MCL. The four aspects of normal structure and function to be considered are:

- The normal function that the structure is designed to serve
- The stresses that are present during normal situations
- Anatomic relationship of the structure to adjacent structures
- Functional relationship of the structure to other structures

Any injury or disease process can be considered by using the model and normal structure and function as the basis for analysis. The

Table 11–2. **Injury to the Medial Collateral Ligament of the Knee**

Normal Ligament	Effects of Injury
Normal Function 1. Medial stability. Provides resistance to tensile stress at the medial aspect of the tibiofemoral joint. 2. Rotatory stability. Provides resistance to rotation at the tibiofemoral joint.	**Lack of Normal Function** 1. Decrease in medial stability of tibiofemoral joint. 2. Decrease in rotatory stability at tibiofemoral joint in flexion. May lead to excessive lateral rotation of the tibia, which causes the medial tibial condyle to subluxate anteriorly.
Normal Stresses 1. Normal tibiofemoral valgus creates tensile stress on medial aspect of the knee.	**Abnormal Stresses** 1. Possible increase in physiologic valgus, increased tensile stress on medial aspect.
Normal Anatomic Relationships 1. Attachments to the joint capsule, medial meniscus, tibia and femur.	**Disturbed Anatomic Relationships** 1. Possible tear of joint capsule, medial meniscus, or avulsion of bony attachments to tibia or femur.
Normal Functional Relationships 1. Works in conjunction with cruciates to provide anteromedial and posteromedial rotatory stability. Works with medial compartment structures. 2. Helps to prevent excessive compressive stress on the lateral tibiofemoral joint surfaces by restraining the widening of the medial joint aspect.	**Altered Functional Relationships** 1. Increased tensile stress on cruciates and medial compartment structures because these structures must provide additional support. 2. Increased compressive forces on lateral aspect of the tibiofemoral joint.

model in Table 11–2 can also be applied to such injuries as a torn meniscus or torn cruciate ligament.

REFERENCES

1. Sonstegard, DA, et al: The surgical replacement of the human knee joint. Sci Am 238(1):44–51, 1978.
2. Williams, PL, and Warwick R (eds): Gray's Anatomy, ed 38. WB Saunders, Philadelphia, 1995.
3. Nordin, M, and Frankel, VH: Basic Biomechanics of the Skeletal System, ed 2. Lea & Febiger, Philadelphia, 1989.
4. Aagaard, H, and Verdonk, R: Function of the normal meniscus and consequences of meniscal resection. Scand J Med Sci Sports 9:134, 1999.
5. Kapandji, IA: The Physiology of the Joints, Vol. 2, ed 2. Williams & Wilkins, Baltimore, 1970.
6. Seebacher, JR, et al: Structure of the posterolateral aspect of the knee. J Bone Joint Surg (Am) 64:536–540, 1982.
7. Larson, RL, et al: Patellar compression syndrome: Surgical treatment by lateral retinacular release. Clin Orthop 134:158–167, 1970.
8. Benjamin, M, et al: Quantitative differences in the histology of the attachment zones of the meniscal horns in the knee joint of man. J Anat 177:121, 1991.
9. Kaplan, EB: Some aspects of functional anatomy of the human knee joint. Clin Orthop 23:18–29, 1962.
10. Nicholas, JA, and Hershman, EB: The Lower Extremity and Spine in Sports Medicine. CV Mosby, St. Louis, 1986.
11. Cailliet, R: Soft Tissue Pain and Disability, ed 3. FA Davis, Philadelphia, 1996.
12. Clark, CR, and Ogden, FA: Development of menisci of human knee joint. J Bone Joint Surg 65A:538–546, 1983.
13. Gray, JC: Neural and vascular anatomy of the menisci of the human knee. J Orthop Sports Phys Ther 29:29, 1999.
14. Petersen, W, and Tillman, B: Structure and vascularization of the knee joint menisci [abstract]. Z Othop Ihre Grenzgeb 137:31, 1999.
15. Reilly, DT: Dynamic loading of normal joints. Rheum Dis Clin North Am 14:497–502, 1988.
16. Johnson, F, et al: The distribution of the load across the knee: A comparison of static and dynamic measurements. J Bone Joint Surg 62B, 1980.
17. Radin, EL, et al: Role of the menisci in distribution of stress in the knee. Clin Orthop 185:290–293, 1984.
18. Seedhom, BB: Loadbearing function of the menisci. Physiotherapy 62:7, 1978.
19. Torzilli, PA, et al: An in vivo biomechanical evaluation of anterior-posterior motion of the knee. J Bone Joint Surg 63A:960–968, 1981.
20. Fukubayashi, T, et al: An in vitro biomechanical evaluation of anterior-posterior motion of the knee. J Bone Joint Surg 64A:258–264, 1982.
21. Cox, JS: Patellofemoral problems in runners. Clin Sports Med 4:699–715, 1985.
22. Paulos, L, et al: Patellar malalignment, a treatment rationale. Phys Ther 60:1624–1632, 1980.
23. Blauth, M, and Tillman, B: Stressing on the human femoro-patellar joint. Anat Embryol 168:117–123, 1983.
24. Terry, GC, et al: Anatomy of the iliopatellar band and iliotibial tract. Am J Sports Med 14:39–45, 1986.

25. Terry, GC, and La Orade, RF: The biceps femoris muscle complex at the knee. Am J Sports Med 24:2, 1996.

26. Bogdan, RF: Plicae syndrome of the knee. J Am Podiatr Soc 75:377–381, 1985.

27. Blackburn, TA, et al: An introduction to the plicae. J Orthop Sports Phys Ther 3:171–177, 1982.

28. Hughston, JC, et al: Classification of knee ligament instabilities, part I: The medial compartment and cruciate ligaments. J Bone Joint Surg (Am) 58(2):159, 1976.

29. Hughston, JC, et al: Classification of knee ligament instabilities, part II: The lateral compartment. J Bone Joint Surg (Am) 58(2):173, 1976.

30. Dupont, J-Y: Synovial plicae of the knee. Arthroscopic surgery. Part II: The knee clinics. Sports Med 16:87, 1997.

31. Cailliet, R: Knee Pain and Disability, ed 3. FA Davis, Philadelphia, 1992.

32. Deutsch, AL, et al: Synovial plicae of the knee. Radiology 141:627, 1981.

33. Dandy, DJ: Anatomy of the medial suprapatellar plica and medial synovial shelf. J Athrosc Rel Surg 6:79,1990.

34. Bae, DK, et al: The clinical significance of the complete type of suprapatellar membrane. Arthroscopy 14:830, 1998.

35. Hardaker, WT, et al: Diagnosis and treatment of the plicae syndrome of the knee. J Bone Joint Surg 62A:221–225, 1980.

36. Grood, ES, et al: Ligamentous and capsular restraints preventing straight medial and lateral laxity in intact human cadaver knees. J Bone Joint Surg 63A:1257–1269, 1981.

37. Nielsen, S, et al: Rotatory instability of cadaver knees after transection of collateral ligaments and capsule. Arch Orthop Trauma Surg 103:165–169, 1984.

38. Nielsen, S: Kinesiology of the knee joint: An experimental investigation of ligamentous and capsular restraints preventing knee instability. Dan Med Bull 34:297–309, 1987.

39. Puniello, MS: Iliotibial band tightness and medial patellar glide in patients with patellofemoral pain. J Orthop Sports Phys Ther 17:144, 1993.

40. Kaplan, EB: The iliotibial tract. J Bone Joint Surg 40A:817–832, 1958.

41. Jeffreys, TE: Recurrent dislocation of the patella due to abnormal attachment of ilio-tibial tract. J Bone Joint Surg 45B:740–743, 1963.

42. Petersen, W, and Tillman, B: Structure and vascularization of the cruciate ligaments of the human knee joint [abstract]. Anat Embryol (Berl) 200:325, 1999.

43. Fuss, FK: The restraining function of the cruciate ligaments on hyperextension and hyperflexion of the human knee joint. Anat Rec 230:283, 1991.

44. Livesay, GA, et al: Determination of the in situ forces and force distribution within the anterior cruciate ligamanet. Ann Biomed Eng 23:476, 1995.

45. Hollis, JM, et al: The effects of knee motion and external loading on the length of the anterior cruciate ligament. J Biomed Eng 113:208, 1991.

46. Arnoczky, SP: Anatomy of the anterior cruciate ligament. Clin Orthop 172:19–25, 1983.

47. Cabaud, HE: Biomechanics of the anterior cruciate ligament. Clin Orthop 172:26–30, 1983.

48. France, EP, et al: Simultaneous quantitation of knee ligament forces. J Biomech 16:553–564, 1983.

49. Piziali, RL, et al: The function of primary ligaments of the knee in anterior-posterior and medial- lateral motions. J Biomech 13:777–784, 1980.

50. Markolf, KL, et al: Direct measurement of resultant forces in the anterior cruciate ligament. An in vitro study performed with new experimental technology. J Bone Joint Surg 75:557, 1990.

51. Mills, OS, and Hull, ML: Rotational flexibility of the human knee due to varus/valgus and axial moments in vivo. J Biomech 24:673, 1991.

52. Hsieh, YF, et al: The effects of removal and reconstruction of the anterior cruciate ligament on patellofemoral kinematics. Am J Sports Med 26:201, 1994.

53. Lipke, JM, et al: Role of incompetence of the anterior cruciate and lateral ligaments in anterolateral and anteromedial stability. J Bone Joint Surg (Am) 63:954–959, 1981.

54. Feagin, JA, and Lambert, KL: Mechanism of injury and pathology of anterior cruciate ligament injuries. Orthop Clin North Am 16:41–45, 1985.

55. Terry, GC, and Hughston, JC: Associated joint pathology in the anterior cruciate ligament-deficient knee with emphasis on a classification system and injuries to the meniscocapsular ligament-musculotendinous unit complex. Orthop Clin North Am 16:29–38, 1985.

56. Frident, T, et al: Proprioceptive deficits after anterior cruciate ligament rupture. The relation to associated lesions and subjective knee function. Knee Surg Sports Traumatol Arthrosc 7:226, 1999.

57. Kurosawa, H, et al: Simultaneous measurement of changes in length of the cruciate ligaments during knee motion. Clin Orthop 265:233, 1991.

58. Dursalen, L, et al: The influence of muscle forces and external loads on cruciate ligament strain. Am J Sports Med 23:129, 1995.

59. Li, G, et al: The importance of quadriceps and hamstring loading on knee kinematics and in-situ forces in the anterior cruciate ligament. J Biomech 32:395, 1999.

60. Harner, CD, et al: The human posterior cruciate ligament complex: An interdisciplinary study, ligament morphology and biomechanical evaluation. Am J Sports Med 23:736, 1995.

61. Saddler, SC, et al: Posterior cruciate ligament anatomy and length-tension behavior of the posterior cruciate ligament surface fibers. Am J Knee Surg 9:194, 1996.

62. Harner, CD, et al: The effects of a popliteus muscle load on in-situ forces in the posterior cruciate ligament and on knee kinematics. A human cadaveric study. Am J Sports Med 26:669, 1998.

63. Veltri, DM, et al: The role of the popliteofibular ligament in stability of the human knee. Am J Sports Med 24:19, 1996.

64. Kusayama, T, et al: Anatomical and biomechanical characteristics of human meniscofemoral ligaments. Knee Surg Sports Traumatol Arthrosc 2:231, 1994.

65. Cho, JM, et al: Variations in meniscofemoral ligaments at anatomical study and MR imaging. Skeletal Radiol 28:189, 1999.

66. Rauschning, W: Anatomy and function of the communication between knee joint and popliteal bursae. Ann Rheum Dis 39:354–358, 1980.

67. Norkin, CC, and White, DW: Measurement of Joint Motion: A Guide to Goniometry. FA Davis, Philadelphia, 1985.

68. Pathokinesiology and Physical Therapy Department: Observational Gait Analysis Handbook. Rancho Los Amigos Medical Center, Professional Staff Association, Rancho Los Amigos Hospital, Downey, Calif., 1989.

69. Inman, VT, et al: Human Walking. Williams & Wilkins, Baltimore, 1981.

70. Lehmkuhl, LD, and Smith, LK: Brunnstrom's Clinical Kinesiology, ed 4. FA Davis, Philadelphia, 1983.

71. Wismans, J, et al: A three-dimensional mathematical model of the knee joint. J Biomech 13:677, 1980.

72. Wickiewics, TL, et al: Muscle architecture of the human lower limb. Clin Orthop 179:275–283, 1983.

73. Dunnen, JD, et al: Relationship between muscle length, muscle activity and torque of the hamstring muscles. Phys Ther 61:2, 1981.

74. Basmajian, JV, and DeLuca, CJ: Muscles Alive, ed 5. Williams & Wilkins, Baltimore, 1985.

75. Lieb, FJ, and Perry, J: Quadriceps function: An anatomical and mechanical study using amputated limbs. J Bone Joint Surg 50A:1535–1548, 1968.

76. Hehne, H-J: Biomechanics of the patellofemoral joint and its clinical relevance. Clin Orthop 258:73, 1990.

77. Heegaard, J, et al: The biomechanics of the human patella during passive knee flexion. J Biomech 28:1265, 1995.

78. Grelsamer, RP, and Klein, JR: The biomechanics of the patellofemoral joint. J Orthop Sports Phys Ther 28:286, 1998.

79. Evans, EJ et al: Fibrocartilage in the attachment zones of the quadriceps tendon and patellar ligament in man. J Anat 171:155, 1990.

80. Sutton, FS, et al: The effect of patellectomy on knee function. J Bone Joint Surg (Am) 58:537, 1976.

81. Wilk, K, et al: A comparison of tibiofemoral joint force and electromyographic activity during open and closed kinetic chain exercises. Am J Sports Med 24:518, 1996.

82. Kellis, E, and Balzopoulous, V: The effects of the antagonistic muscle force on intersegmental loading during isokinetic efforts of the knee extensors. J Biomech 32:19, 1999.

83. Murray, MP, et al: Strength of isometric and isokinetic contractions: Knee muscles of men aged 20–86. Phys Ther 60:412, 1980.

84. Tamea, CD, and Henning, CE: Pathomechanics of the pivot shift maneuver. Am J Sports Med 9:31–37, 1981.

85. McLeod, WD, and Hunter, S: Biomechanical analysis of the knee. Phys Ther 60:1561–1564, 1980.

86. Markolf, KL, et al: Role of joint load in knee stability. J Bone Joint Surg 63A:570–585, 1981.

87. Hefzy, MS, et al: Effects of tibial rotations on patellar tracking and patellofemoral contact areas. J Biomed Eng 14:329, 1991.

88. Heegaard, J, et al: Influence of soft structures on patellar three-dimensional tracking. Clin Orthop Rel Res 299:235, 1991.

89. Fujikawa, K, et al: Biomech of patello-femoral joint. Part I: A study of contact and congruity of the patellofemoral compartment and movement of the patella. Engr Med 12:3–11, 1983.

90. Sikorski, JM, et al: The importance of femoral rotation in chondromalacia patellae as shown by serial radiography. J Bone Joint Surg 61B, 1970.

91. Skalley, TC, et al: The quantitative measurement of normal passive medial and lateral patellar motion limits. Am J Sport Med 21:728, 1993.

92. Radin, EL: A rational approach to the treatment of patellofemoral pain. Clin Orthop 144:107–109, 1979.

93. Wiberg, G: Roentgenographic and anatomic studies on the femoropatellar joint. Acta Orthop Scand 12:319–409, 1941.

94. Aglietti, P, et al: Patellar pain and incongruence. Clin Orthop 176:217–223, 1983.

95. Merchant, AC, et al: Roentgenographic analysis of patellofemoral congruence. J Bone Joint Surg 56A:1391–1396, 1974.

96. Jacobsen, K, and Bertheussen, K: The vertical location of the patella. Acta Orthop Scand 45:436–445, 1974.

97. Insall, J, and Salvati, E: Patella position in the normal knee joint. Radiology 101:101–104, 1971.

98. Norman, O, et al: Vertical position of the patella. Acta Orthop Scand 54:908–913, 1983.

99. Runow, A: The dislocating patella: Etiology and prognosis in relation to generalized joint laxity and anatomy of the patellar articulation. Acta Orthop Scand Suppl 201:1–53, 1983.

100. Insall, J: Proximal realignment in the treatment of patellofemoral pain. In Pickett, JC, and Radin, EL (eds): Chondromalacia of the Patellae. Williams & Wilkins, Baltimore, 1983.

101. Goodfellow, J, et al: Patello-femoral joint mechanics and pathology: Chondromalacia patellae. J Bone Joint Surg 58B:291–299, 1976.

102. Hungerford, DS, and Barry, M: Biomechanics of the patellofemoral joint. Clin Orthop 144:9–15, 1979.

103. Hungerford, DS: Patellar subluxation and excessive lateral pressure as a cause of fibrillation. In Pickett, JC, and Radin, EL (eds): Chondromalacia of the Patellae. Williams & Wilkins, Baltimore, 1983.

104. Henche, R, et al: The areas of contact pressure in the patello-femoral joint. Int Orthop (SICOT) 4:279–281, 1981.

105. Insall, J, et al: Chondromalacia patellae: A prospective study. J Bone Joint Surg 58A:1–8, 1976.

106. Singerman, R, Rerilla, J, and Davy, DT: Direct in vitro determination of the patellofemoral contact force for normal knees. J Biomech Eng 117:8, 1995.

107. Kirokawa, S: Three-dimensional mathematical model analysis of the patellofemoral joint. J Biomech 24:659, 1991.

108. Heegaard, J, et al: The biomechanics of the human patella during passive knee flexion. J Biomech 28:1265, 1995.

109. Ficat, P: Lateral fascia release and lateral hyperpressure syndrome. In Pickett, JC, and Radin, EL (eds): Chondromalacia of the Patellae. Williams & Wilkins, Baltimore, 1983.

110. Carson, WG Jr, et al: Patellofemoral disorders: Physical and radiographic examination. Part 1. Clin Orthop 135:174, 1984.

111. Harwin, SF, and Stern, RE: Subcutaneous lateral retinacular release for chondromalacia patellae: A preliminary report. Clin Orthop 156:207–210, 1981.

112. Levangie, PK, et al: Assessment of medial and lateral patellar mobility in subjects with and without knee pain. Poster presentation, American Physical Therapy Association, Annual Conference, Nashville, Tenn., June 1989.

113. Hvid, I: Stability of the human patellofemoral joint. Engr Med 12:55–59, 1983.

114. Levine, J: Chondromalacia patellae. Phys Sports Med 7, 1979.

115. Kettelkamp, DB: Current concepts review: Management of patellar malalignment. J Bone Joint Surg 63A:1344–1348, 1981.

116. Ober, FR, et al: Recurrent dislocation of the patella. Am J Surg 43:497–500, 1939.

117. Derscheid, FL, and Malone, RT: Knee disorders. Phys Ther 60:12, 1980.

118. Noyes, FR, et al: Variable functional disability of the

anterior cruciate ligament-deficient knee. Orthop Clin North Am 16:47–67, 1985.

119. Abernethy, PJ, et al: Is chondromalacia patella a separate clinical entity? J Bone Joint Surg 60B:205–210, 1978.

120. Ficat, P: Lateral fascia release and lateral hyperpressure syndrome. In Pickett, JC, and Radin, EL (eds): Chondromalacia of the Patellae. Williams & Wilkins, Baltimore, 1983.

Study Questions

1. Describe the congruency of the tibiofemoral joint. What factors add to or detract from stability?

2. Describe the menisci of the knee, including shape, attachments, and function.

3. Describe the intra-articular movement of the femur on the tibia, as the femur moves from full extension into flexion. Where is the axis generally located and how does it change during the described motion?

4. Describe the locking mechanism of the knee, including the structure(s) responsible.

5. What happens to the menisci during motions of the knee? How do their attachments contribute to the movement?

6. Identify the bursae of the knee joint. Which of these are generally separate from and which are part of the capsule?

7. Which knee joint ligaments contribute to anterior-posterior stability of the knee joint and how does each make its contribution? To which compartment (medial or lateral) do each of the structures belong?

8. Which ligaments contribute to medial-lateral stability of the knee joint and how does each make its contribution? To which compartment do the structures belong?

9. What are the dynamic stabilizers of the knee, and in what plane do they contribute to stability?

10. What is the axis given for rotation of the knee joint? How does this differ between automatic and axial rotation? What implications does the location have for stress on the joint?

11. What is the normal physiologic angulation of the knee joint? What terms are used to describe pathologic increases or decreases in this angulation?

12. When is axial rotation of the knee greatest? Which muscles produce active medial rotation? Lateral rotation?

13. What is a patella plica and what implications does it have for knee joint dysfunction?

14. Describe the patellofemoral articulation, including the number and shape of the surfaces.

15. What function(s) does the patella serve at the knee joint?

16. How does the patella move in relation to the femur in normal motions? How would function be affected if the patella could not slide on the femur?

17. Describe the contact of the patella with the femur at rest in full extension. Describe the contact as knee flexion proceeds.

18. Is the patella equally effective as an anatomic pulley at all points in the knee ROM? At which point(s) is it most effective? Least effective?

19. Which facet(s) of the patella are subject to the earliest degenerative changes under normal conditions? Why?

20. Which facet of the patella is most likely to undergo excessive degenerative changes when there is misalignment? Describe the misalignment and the condition(s) that may predispose these changes.

21. What is the Q angle of the knee joint? How is it measured, and what implications does it have for patellofemoral problems?

22. What changes will the condition of genu recurvatum produce at the patellofemoral joint?

23. Why is ascending stairs commonly cited as producing knee pain? Relate this to patellofemoral joint compression.

24. Which aspect of the knee joint is most prone to injury? Why is this true, and what structures are most commonly involved?

CHAPTER 12

THE ANKLE AND FOOT COMPLEX

OBJECTIVES

Following the study of this chapter, the reader should be able to:

Define

1. The terminology unique to the ankle-foot complex, including supination/pronation, inversion/eversion, dorsiflexion/plantarflexion, flexion/extension, and adduction/abduction.

Describe

1. The compound articulations of the ankle, subtalar, talocalcaneonavicular, transverse tarsal, and tarsometatarsal joints.
2. The role of the tibiofibular joints and supporting ligaments.
3. The degrees of freedom and range of motion available at the joints of the ankle and foot.
4. The significant ligaments that support the ankle, subtalar, and transverse tarsal joints.
5. The triplanar nature of ankle joint motion.
6. The articular movements that occur in the weight-bearing subtalar joint during supination/pronation.
7. The relationship between tibial rotation and subtalar/talocalcaneonavicular supination/pronation.

8. The relationship between hindfoot supination/pronation and mobility/stability of the transverse tarsal joint.
9. The function of the tarsometatarsal joints, including when motion at these joints is called on.
10. Supination/pronation twist of the forefoot at the tarsometatarsal joints.
11. Distribution of weight within the foot.
12. The structure and function of the plantar arches, including the primary supporting structures.
13. When muscles supplement arch support, including those muscles that specifically contribute to arch support.
14. The effects of toe extension on the plantar arches.
15. The general function of the extrinsic muscles of the ankle-foot.
16. The general function of the intrinsic muscles of the foot.

Introduction

The ankle-foot complex is structurally analogous to the wrist-hand complex of the upper extremity. Although the hand is undeniably more critical to uniquely human functions, the ankle and foot receive more attention from both medical and lay communities. The interdependence of the ankle and foot with the more proximal joints of the lower extremities and the great weight-bearing stresses to which these joints are subjected have resulted in a greater frequency and diversity of difficulties in the joints of the ankle and foot than in its upper extremity counterpart. The prevalence of ankle-foot problems, in fact, has resulted in the formation of a branch of medicine, podiatry, that focuses on the correction and prevention of problems in structures distal to the knee. Specialists in orthopedics and sports medicine similarly find that ankle and foot problems or problems attributable to ankle or foot dysfunction make up a substantial percentage of their practice.

The frequency of ankle or foot problems can be traced readily to the foot's complex structure, to the need to sustain large weight-bearing stresses, and to the multiple and somewhat conflicting functions that the foot must perform. The ankle-foot complex must meet the stability demands of (1) providing a stable base of support for the body in a variety of weight-bearing postures without undue muscular activity and energy expenditure and (2) acting as a rigid lever for effective push-off during gait. The stability requirements can be contrasted to the mobility demands of (1) dampening of rotations imposed by the more proximal joints of the lower limbs, (2) being flexible enough to absorb the shock of the superimposed body weight as the foot hits the ground, and (3) permitting the foot to conform to the changing and varied terrain on which the foot is placed.[1] The ankle-foot complex meets its diverse requirements through its 28 bones that form 25 component joints. These joints include the proximal and distal tibiofibular joints, the talocrural or ankle joint, the talocalcaneal or subtalar joint, the talonavicular and the calcaneocuboid joints, the five tarsometatarsal joints, five metatarsophalangeal joints, and nine interphalangeal joints.

To facilitate description and understanding of the ankle-foot complex, the bones of the foot are traditionally divided into three functional segments. These are the **hindfoot** (posterior segment), composed of the talus and calcaneus; the **midfoot** (middle segment), composed of the navicular, cuboid, and three cuneiforms; and the **forefoot** (anterior segment), composed of the metatarsals and the phalanges (Fig. 12–1).[2] These terms are commonly used when describing ankle or foot dysfunction or deformity and are similarly useful in understanding normal ankle and foot function.

Ankle Joint

The term **ankle** specifically refers to the **talocrural joint;** that is, the articulation between the talus and the distal tibia (tibiotalar surface) and the talus and fibula (talofibular

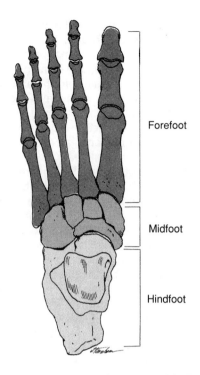

FIGURE 12–1. Functional segments of the foot.

Forefoot

Midfoot

Hindfoot

surface) (Fig. 12–2). The ankle is a synovial hinge joint with a joint capsule and associated ligaments. It is generally considered to have a single oblique axis with 1° of freedom: dorsiflexion/plantarflexion.

Ankle Joint Structure

Proximal Articular Surface

The proximal segment of the ankle is composed of the concave surface of the distal tibia and of the tibial and fibular malleoli. These three facets form an almost continuous concave joint surface that extends more distally on the fibular (lateral) side (see Fig. 12–2a) and on

the posterior margin of the tibia (see Fig. 12–2b). The structure of the distal tibia and the malleoli resembles and is referred to as a **mortise.** A common example of a mortise is the gripping part of a wrench. The wrench can either be fixed (fitting a bolt of only one size) or it can be adjustable (permitting use of the wrench on a variety of bolt sizes). The adjustable mortise is more complex than a fixed mortise because it combines mobility and stability functions. The mortise of the ankle is adjustable, relying on the **proximal** and **distal tibiofibular joints** to both permit and control the changes in the mortise.

The proximal and distal tibiofibular joints (Fig. 12–3) are anatomically distinct from the ankle joint, but these two linked joints function exclusively to serve the ankle. Unlike their upper extremity counterparts, the proximal and distal radioulnar joints, the tibiofibular joints do not add any degrees of freedom to the more distal segments of the extremity. However, fusion of the radioulnar joints would have little functional effect on the more distally located wrist function, whereas fusion of the tibiofibular joints may impair normal ankle function.

PROXIMAL TIBIOFIBULAR JOINT

The proximal tibiofibular joint is a plane synovial joint formed by the articulation of the head of the fibula with the posterolateral aspect of the tibia. Although the facets are fairly flat and vary in configuration among individuals, a slight convexity to the tibial facet and slight concavity to the fibular facet seem to predominate.[3] The inclination of the facets may vary from nearly vertical to nearly horizontal in orientation.[3,4] Each proximal tibiofibular joint is surrounded by a joint capsule that is reinforced by **anterior and posterior tibiofibular ligaments.** Most typically, the proximal tibiofibular joint is anatomically separate from the knee joint.[3] Motion at the proximal

FIGURE 12–2. The ankle joint. (a) Anterior view showing the mortise astride the body of the talus and the superior-inferior inclination of the ankle axis. (b) Lateral view of the talus and cross-section of the tibia showing the large lateral articulation on the talus for the fibular malleolus.

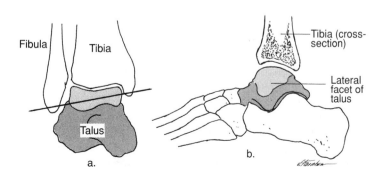

Fibula Tibia

Talus

a.

Tibia (cross-section)

Lateral facet of talus

b.

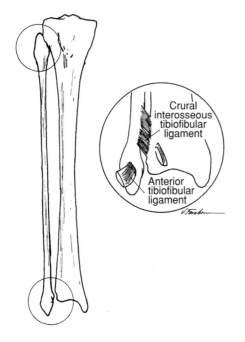

FIGURE 12–3. Proximal and distal tibiofibular joints. Inset shows the ligaments of the distal tibiofibular joint.

tibiofibular joint is variable but consistently small; it has been described as superior and inferior sliding of the fibula and as fibular rotation.[4,5] The relevance of motion at the proximal tibiofibular joint will be seen when the ankle articulation is examined more closely.

DISTAL TIBIOFIBULAR JOINT

The distal tibiofibular joint is a syndesmosis, or fibrous union, between the concave facet of the tibia and the convex facet of the fibula. The tibia and fibula do not actually come into contact with each other at this point but are separated by fibroadipose tissue. Although there is no joint capsule, there are several associated ligaments at the distal tibiofibular joint. Because the proximal and distal joints are linked, all the ligaments that lie between the tibia and fibular contribute to stability at both joints.

The ligaments of the distal tibiofibular joint are primarily responsible for maintaining a stable mortise. Rocce[6] concluded that the strongest and most important of the ligaments of the distal tibiofibular joint is the **crural tibiofibular interosseous ligament** (see Fig. 12–3, inset). Its oblique fibers run for a short distance between the tibia and fibula, maintaining proximity of the bones. The other ligamentous structures that support the distal tibiofibular joint are the **ante-**

rior and posterior tibiofibular ligaments and the **interosseous membrane.** The interosseous membrane directly supports both proximal and distal tibiofibular articulations. The distal tibiofibular joint is an extremely strong articulation. Stresses that tend to move the talus excessively in the mortise may tear the ankle collaterals first. Continued force may fracture the fibula proximal to the distal tibiofibular ligaments before the tibiofibular ligaments will tear.[7]

The function of the ankle (talocrural) joint depends on stability of the tibiofibular mortise. The tibia and fibula would be unable to grasp and hold on to the talus if the tibia and fibular were permitted to separate or if one side of the mortise were missing. The analogous mortise of a wrench could not perform its function of grasping a bolt if the two pincer segments moved apart every time a force was applied to the wrench. Conversely, the mortise must have some mobility between its two segments or the ankle joint would be better served by a single fused arch. The fibula would appear to serve the mobility function for the mortise. It has, in fact, little weight-bearing function, with no more than 10% of the weight that comes through the femur being transmitted through the fibula.[8,9] Given the relatively small weight-bearing function of the fibula, the hyaline cartilage of the proximal tibiofibular joint would appear to be dependent on joint motion to maintain nutrition of the cartilage. Therefore, the presence of an intact proximal and distal tibiofibular joint confirms mobility between these two bones. We will examine this motion in more detail when we examine ankle joint arthrokinematics.

Distal Articular Surface

The distal articular surface of the ankle joint is formed by the body of the talus. The body of the talus has three articular surfaces: a large lateral facet, a smaller medial facet, and a **trochlear** or superior facet. The large convex trochlear surface has a central groove that runs at a slight angle to the head and neck of the talus. The body of the talus also appears wider anteriorly than posteriorly, giving it a wedge shape (Fig. 12–4a). The degree of wedging may vary among individuals, with no wedging at all in some and a 25% decrease in width anteriorly to posteriorly in others.[10] The articular cartilage covering the trochlea is continuous with the cartilage covering the more extensive lateral (fibular)

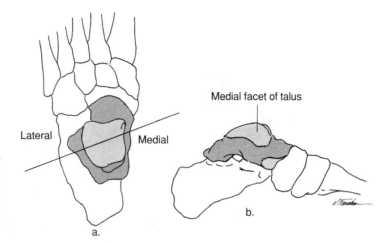

FIGURE 12–4. (a) Superior view of the talus shows its wedge-shaped trochlea and the anteroposterior inclination of the ankle axis. (b) Medial view of the talus shows the small medial facet for articulation with the tibial malleolus.

facet (see Fig. 12–2b) and the smaller medial (tibial) facet (Fig. 12–4b).

The ankle joint is the most congruent joint in the human body.[6] The structural integrity is maintained throughout the range of motion (ROM) of the joint by a number of important ligaments.

Ligaments

The capsule of the ankle joint is fairly thin and especially weak anteriorly and posteriorly. Therefore, the stability of the ankle depends on an intact ligamentous structure. The ligaments that support the proximal and distal tibiofibular joints (the crural tibiofibular interosseous ligament, the anterior and posterior tibiofibular ligaments, and the tibiofibular interosseous membrane) are important for stability of the mortise and, therefore, for stability of the ankle. Two other major ligaments maintain contact and congruence of the mortise and talus and control medial-lateral joint stability. These are the **medial collateral ligament** (**MCL**) and the **lateral collateral ligament** (**LCL**). Portions of the extensor and peroneal retinacula of the ankle are also credited with contributing to stability at the ankle joint.

The MCL is most commonly called the **deltoid ligament.** As its name implies, it is a fan-shaped ligament. It has both superficial and deep fibers that arise from the borders of the tibial malleolus and insert in a continuous line on the navicular anteriorly and on the talus and calcaneus distally and posteriorly (Fig. 12–5). Although the deltoid ligament is typically referred to in its entirely, Earll and colleagues[11]

found the tibiocalcaneal fibers of the superficial deltoid to be more critical than the other bands for maintaining normal ankle joint contact forces. The deltoid ligament as a whole is extremely strong. Forces that would open the medial side of the ankle may actually fracture off (avulse) the tibial malleolus before the deltoid ligament tears. This ligament not only helps to control medial distraction stresses on the joint but also helps check motion at the extremes of joint range.

The LCL is composed of three separate bands that are commonly referred to as separate ligaments. These are the **anterior** and **posterior talofibular** ligaments and the **calcaneofibular** ligament (Fig. 12–6). The **inferior extensor retinaculum** (Fig. 12–7) may also contribute to stability of the ankle joint.[12] Two additional structures that lie close and parallel to the calcaneofibular ligament appear to rein-

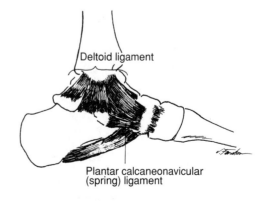

FIGURE 12–5. Medial ligaments of the posterior ankle-foot complex.

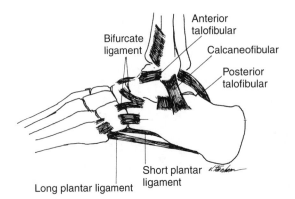

FIGURE 12–6. Lateral ligaments of the posterior ankle-foot complex.

force that ligament and serve a similar function. These are the inferior band of the **superior peroneal retinaculum** (see Fig. 12–7) and the much more variable **lateral talocalcaneal ligament.**[12–14]

Generally, the components of the LCL are weaker and more prone to injury than those of the MCL. The LCL helps to control varus stresses resulting in lateral distraction of the joint (talar tilt) and to check extremes of joint ROM. Many experiments have been conducted on serial sectioning of the lateral ligaments, with differing results that may be attributed not only to testing strategies but to individual variability. There is consensus, however, on several factors:

1. The contribution of the various segments of the LCL to checking dorsiflexion/plantarflexion, talar tilt (anteroposterior axis), or talar rotation (vertical axis) depends on the position of the ankle joint.[13,15–18]

2. The anterior talofibular ligament is the weakest and most commonly torn of the LCLs, followed by tears in the calcaneofibular ligament. Rupture of the anterior talofibular ligament invariably results in anterolateral rotatory instability of the ankle.[17,19,20]

3. The posterior talofibular ligament is the strongest of the collaterals and is rarely torn in isolation.[19,20]

The ankle collaterals and the retinacula also contribute to stability of the subtalar joint and will be revisited when we discuss that joint.

Ankle Joint Function

The ankle joint is classically considered to move around a single axis, contributing 1° of freedom to the foot when the foot is free to move, or to the tibia and fibula when the foot is weight-bearing. The primary motion is **dorsiflexion/plantarflexion.** However, many investigators have concluded from both in vivo and in vitro investigations that the ankle joint is capable of some rotation of the talus within the mortise in both the transverse plane around a vertical axis (**talar rotation** or **abduction/adduction**) and in the frontal plane around an anteroposterior axis (**talar tilt** or **inversion/eversion**).[19,21,23] Such motions result in a moving or instantaneous axis of rotation for the ankle joint. Rasmussen and Tovborg-Jensen[19] measured transverse plane talar motion (ligaments intact) to be as much as 7° of medial rotation and 10° of lateral rotation, while talar tilt (anteroposterior axis) averaged 5°. Lundberg and associates[22–24] found similar motions in their studies of the weight-bearing

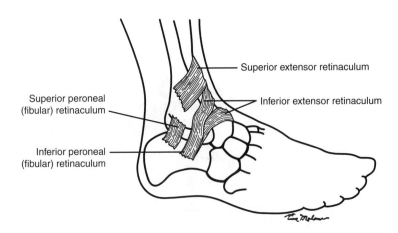

FIGURE 12–7. The superior and inferior extensor retinacula; the superior and inferior peroneal retinacula.

foot in vivo, although the magnitudes were smaller and depended on the position of the talus in the mortise.[22–24]

Although there may be some argument as to how fixed the ankle joint axis remains during motion or what accessory motions may exist at the joint, there is consensus among investigators that the primary ankle motion of dorsiflexion/plantarflexion occurs around an oblique axis that causes the foot to move across all three planes.

Axis

In neutral position of the ankle joint, the joint axis passes approximately through the fibular malleolus and the body of the talus, and through or just below the tibial malleolus.[25] The fibular malleolus, however, extends more distally than does the tibial malleolus and lies more posteriorly. This more posterior position of the fibular malleolus is due to the normal torsion or twist that exists in the distal tibia relative to its proximal plateau. The torsion in the tibia is similar to the torsion found in the shaft of the femur, although reversed in direction. The distal tibia is twisted laterally compared with its proximal portion, accounting for the toe-out position of the foot in normal standing. Given the relationship of the malleoli, the axis of the ankle is considered to be rotated laterally 20° to 30° in the transverse plane (see Fig. 12–4a) and inclined 10° down on the lateral side (see Fig. 12–2a).[4,26] However, individual differences may cause the axis to change, with the change in the transverse plane being as much as 30° on either side of the average values.[27]

Stiehl[27] used a simple hinged model with a level indicator to demonstrate how an axis inclined more distally and more posteriorly on the lateral side will create a triplanar motion. He showed that dorsiflexion around a typically inclined ankle axis will not only bring the foot up, but will simultaneously bring it slightly lateral to the leg (increased toe-out) and turn it longitudinally away from the midline (so-called pronation or eversion). Conversely, plantarflexion around the same single oblique ankle axis will result in the foot going down, moving medial to the leg (increased toe-in) and turning of the foot longitudinally toward the midline (so-called supination or inversion). When the foot is fixed, the same relative pattern of motion exists between the leg and foot, with the leg moving medial to the fixed foot in weight-bearing dorsiflexion (Fig.

12–8). Although Stiehl's model explains the relationship between the ankle and foot that we see functionally, it does not take into account the mobile mortise or, consequently, the need for the tibiofibular joints. Talar structure and joint arthrokinematics can give us additional insight into the demands of the normal ankle joint.

Arthrokinematics

The shape of the body of the talus is complex. The trochlea is wider anteriorly than posteriorly. The lateral (fibular) facet is substantially larger than the medial (tibial) facet and its surface is oriented slightly obliquely to that of the medial facet. Inman[28] proposed that the body of the talus can be thought of as a segment of a cone lying on its side with its base directed laterally. The cone should be visualized as "truncated" or cut off on either end at slightly different angles[29] (Fig. 12–9). Given this representation, it can be seen that the fibula moving on the lateral facet of the talus must have a

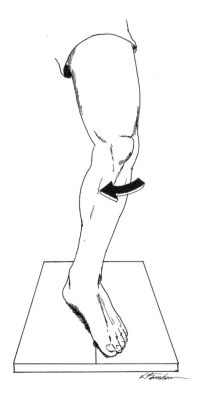

FIGURE 12–8. Given the triplanar ankle joint axis, dorsiflexion of the leg on the fixed foot results in the leg moving medial to the long axis of the foot and appearing to be medially rotated relative to the foot.

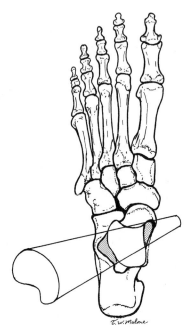

Truncated cone

FIGURE 12–9. The trochlea, smaller medial facet, and larger lateral facet of the talus can be pictured as part of a conical surface, with ends of the cone cut off (the larger end of the cone facing laterally).

greater displacement than the tibial malleolus moving on the smaller medial facet of the talus. The greater excursion of the lateral malleolus results in the imposition of motion on the fibula in several directions through the ankle ROM including lateral motion (widening or narrowing of the intermalleolar space), superior/inferior motion and medial/lateral rotation. Johnson,[30] in reviewing the research literature, found the motions to be consistently small in magnitude but variable in direction among individuals and with different loading conditions. Individual differences in fibular motion may be related to orientation of the proximal tibiofibular facet, with more mobility available in those facets that are more vertical,[3] or to factors such as tibiofibular ligamentous elasticity. Such individual differences may account for the variations in effect on ankle dorsiflexion/plantarflexion ROM that are seen when surgical tibiofibular fixation is necessary.[30] In general, however, mobility of the fibula at the tibiofibular joints should be considered a component of normal ankle motion. One also should find the magnitude of proximal tibiofibular motion to exceed that of the

distal tibiofibular joint as motion at one end of the fibula would produce a larger swing of motion at the opposite end of the bone. This presumably accounts for the proximal joint being synovial while the distal joint is a comparatively less mobile syndesmosis joint.

Given that the lateral malleolus must move more than the medial in ankle joint motion, the ankle joint axis cannot be fixed as it would be in a true hinge joint but must change from dorsiflexion to plantarflexion.[3,25,31] Scott and Winter,[32] however, used biomechanical modeling to determine that the ankle can be represented effectively as a simple (monocentric) hinge joint in gait, although they noted that the joint may be more variable under lower compressive loads. Similarly, Stiehl's model[27] seems to result in a functionally effective representation of ankle joint motion (minus the role of the fibula). It is important to note that the triplanar ankle joint motion occurs whether or not a fixed axis with a single degree of freedom is assumed. If the ankle axis shifts somewhat through the range, the motion outside the sagittal plane may increase.

With the large and congruent articular surfaces of the ankle, the ankle is able to withstand compression forces during gait of as much as 450% of body weight with little incidence of primary (nontraumatic) degenerative arthritis.[33–35] Greenwald and Matejczyk[36] demonstrated changes in contact across the joint surfaces with ankle motion and hypothesized that some incongruence in the ankle is necessary for normal load distribution, cartilage nutrition, and lubrication of the ankle joint.

Range of Motion

The normal ankle joint range is generally given as 20° of dorsiflexion from neutral, and a more variable 30° to 50° of plantarflexion from neutral.[5,19] However, ankle joint measurements made in living subjects in the weight-bearing position showed plantarflexion to be limited to 23° to 28°,[22,31] whereas active non-weight-bearing dorsiflexion was limited to an average of just over 4°.[37] Lundberg and colleagues[22] found the range of total foot plantarflexion to vary among individuals, with anywhere from 60% to 90% of that motion attributable to the ankle joint with the remainder occurring at more distal joints.

Normal checks to ankle dorsiflexion and plantarflexion are primarily muscular. Active or passive tension in the triceps surae (**gastroc-nemius** and **soleus muscles**) are the main checks to dorsiflexion, with dorsiflexion more limited with knee extension than with knee flexion.[37] Tension in the **tibialis anterior**, **extensor hallucis longus**, and **extensor digitorum longus** muscles is the primary check to plantarflexion. Although the ligaments of the ankle assist in checking dorsiflexion and plantarflexion,[37] a more important function appears to be in minimizing side-to-side movement or rotation of the mortise on the talus. The ligaments are assisted in that function by the muscles that pass on either side of the ankle. The **tibialis posterior, flexor hallucis longus,** and **flexor digitorum longus** muscles help protect the medial aspect of the ankle; the **peroneus longus** and **peroneus brevis** muscles protect the lateral aspect. Bony checks to any of the potential ankle motions are rarely encountered unless there is extreme hypermobility (as may be found among gymnasts or dancers) or a failure of one or more of the other restraint systems. A more complete analysis of the function of the muscles crossing the ankle will be presented later, because all muscles of the ankle cross at least two and generally three or more joints of the ankle and foot.

The Subtalar Joint

The **talocalcaneal,** or **subtalar,** joint is a composite joint formed by three separate plane articulations between the talus superiorly and the calcaneus inferiorly. Together, the three surfaces provide a triplanar movement around a single joint axis. Function at the weight-bearing subtalar joint is critical for dampening the rotational forces imposed by the body weight while maintaining contact of the foot with the supporting surface.

Subtalar Joint Structure

The posterior talocalcaneal articulation is the largest of the three articulations found between the talus and calcaneus. The posterior articulation is formed by a concave facet on the undersurface of the body of the talus and a convex facet on the body of the calcaneus. The smaller anterior and middle talocalcaneal articulations are formed by two convex facets on the inferior body and neck of the talus and two concave facets on the calcaneus. The anterior

and middle articulations, therefore, have an intra-articular configuration that is the reverse of that found at the posterior facet. Between the posterior articulation and the anterior and middle articulations, there is a bony tunnel formed by a **sulcus** (concave groove) in the inferior talus and superior calcaneus. This funnel-shaped tunnel, known as the **tarsal canal,** runs obliquely across the foot. Its large end (the **sinus tarsi**) lies just anterior to the fibular malleolus; its small end lies posteriorly below the tibial malleolus and above a bony outcropping on the calcaneus called the **sustentaculum tali.** The tarsal canal and ligaments running the length of the tarsal canal divide the posterior articulation and the anterior and middle articulation into two separate noncommunicating joint cavities.[38] The posterior articulation has its own capsule; the anterior and middle articulations share a capsule with the talonavicular joint.

Like the ankle joint, the subtalar joint rarely undergoes degenerative change. Wang and colleagues[34] found that the subtalar articular surfaces, though smaller than those of the ankle, showed a similar proportion of contact across surfaces under similar conditions. They found that the posterior facet received 75% of the force transmitted through the subtalar joint, but also determined that the pressure in the posterior facet was similar to that at the medial and anterior facet given its larger contact area.

Ligaments

The subtalar joint is a stable joint that rarely dislocates. It receives ligamentous support from the ligamentous structures that support the ankle,[15] as well as from ligamentous structures that cross the subtalar joint alone. Harper[39] described a number of structures as contributing to the lateral support of the subtalar joint. These included, from superficial to deep, the calcaneofibular ligament and the lateral talocalcaneal ligament (variously present[14]), the **cervical ligament,** and the **interosseous talocalcaneal ligament.** The cervical ligament (Fig. 12–10), is the strongest of the talocalcaneal structures.[12,39] It lies in the anterior sinus tarsi and joins the neck of the talus to the neck of the calcaneus (hence, its name). The interosseous talocalcaneal ligament lies more medially within the tarsal canal, is more oblique (see Fig. 12–10), and has been described as having anterior and posterior bands.[5] Harper[39] also described the fairly com-

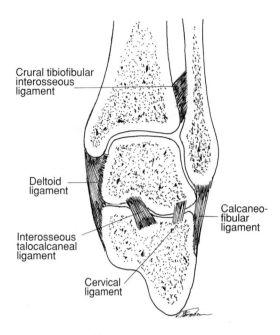

Crural tibiofibular
interosseous
ligament

Deltoid
ligament

Calcaneo-
fibular
ligament

Interosseous
talocalcaneal
ligament

Cervical
ligament

FIGURE 12–10. Ligaments of the subtalar joint (cross section, posterior view).

plex connections of the inferior extensor retinaculum that provides subtalar support superficially and within the tarsal canal. Although the roles of the cervical and interosseous ligaments in maintaining talocalcaneal stability are obvious, the contributions of the collaterals should not be underestimated.[13,14,40]

Subtalar Joint Function

Arthrokinematics

Although the subtalar joint is composed of three articulations, the alternating convex-concave facets limit the potential mobility of the joint. When the talus moves on the posterior facet of the calcaneus, the articular surface of the talus should slide in the same direction as the bone moves (concave surface moving on a stable convex surface). However, at the middle and anterior joints, the talar surfaces should glide in a direction opposite to movement of the bone (convex surface moving on a stable concave surface). Motion of the talus, therefore, is a complex twisting (or screwlike motion) that can continue only until the posterior and the anterior and middle facets can no longer accommodate simultaneous and opposite motions. The result is a triplanar motion of the talus around a single oblique joint axis. The

subtalar joint is, therefore, a uniaxial joint with 1° of freedom: **supination/pronation.**

The Subtalar Axis

The axis for subtalar supination/pronation has been the subject of many investigations. Studies have shown that large differences exist among apparently normal individuals. Manter[41] found the axis inclined 42° upward and anteriorly from the transverse plane (with a broad interindividual range of 29–47°), and inclined medially 16° from the sagittal plane (with, again, a broad interindividual range of 8–24°) (Fig. 12–11). The obliquity of the axis indicates that the motion around it will cross all three planes. Supination/pronation, like the triplanar ankle motion, can be modeled by a single oblique hinge joint,[42,43] and described by its component motions in each of the three planes. It should be understood, however, that subtalar motion is more complex than that of the ankle joint and that subtalar component motions *cannot and do not occur independently*. The components occur simultaneously as the calcaneus (or talus) twists across its three articular surfaces. Although some of the component motions can be observed more readily than others, the motions *always occur together*.

To understand subtalar pronation/supination, we must first identify the planes and names of the component motions. If the subtalar joint axis were vertical, the motion around that axis would be described as **abduction/adduction**; if the subtalar axis were longitudinal (anteroposterior), the motion would be described as **inversion/eversion**; and if the subtalar axis were coronal, the motion would be described as **plantarflexion/dorsiflexion**. In reality, the subtalar axis lies about half way between being longitudinal and being vertical. Consequently, the component motions of eversion/inversion (longitudinal axis) and abduction/adduction (vertical axis) are about equal in magnitude. The subtalar axis is inclined only slightly toward being coronal and therefore has only a small component of dorsiflexion/plantarflexion. It is important to note that the contribution of each of the component movements to supination or pronation will vary with individual differences in inclination of the subtalar axis. If the subtalar axis is inclined upwardly only 30° (rather than the average of 42°), the axis will be less vertical and more longitudinal. In such a foot, the component contributions to supination and pronation would consist of nearly twice as much inversion/ever-

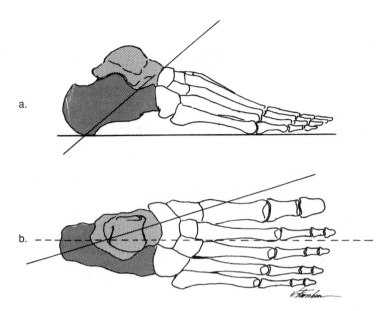

FIGURE 12–11. Axis of the subtalar joint. (a) Inclined up anteriorly, approximately 42°. (b) Inclined in medially, approximately 16°.

sion as there is adduction/abduction. We must now examine how, given the subtalar axis, the component motions aggregate to make up pronation/supination.

Non-Weight-Bearing Subtalar Joint Motion

Supination/pronation of the subtalar joint will first be described by motion of its distal non-weight-bearing segment (the calcaneus) as has been done each time we initially described a joint's motion. Supination is composed of the component calcaneal motions of adduction (vertical axis); inversion (anteroposterior or longitudinal axis); and plantarflexion (coronal axis). Pronation of the non-weight-bearing calcaneus is composed of the component motions of abduction (vertical axis), eversion (anteroposterior or longitudinal axis), and dorsiflexion

(coronal axis). The three components of calcaneal motion that make up supination (adduction, inversion, and plantarflexion,) and pronation (abduction, eversion, and dorsiflexion) are an obligatory combination of motions that can not be separated. However, when the posterior aspect of the calcaneus is observed (as from behind the person), the calcaneal component of inversion/eversion (varus-valgus angulation of the calcaneus with respect to the tibia) can be readily observed. The eversion component of calcaneal pronation is seen as an increase in the medial angulation between the long axis of the tibia and an axis through the tuberosity of the calcaneus (Fig. 12–12a). The calcaneal component of eversion is, therefore, equivalent to valgus of the calcaneus and the terms may be used interchangeably. Consequently, subtalar pronation may also be described as having the calcaneal components of abduction, valgus and

FIGURE 12–12. (a) Subtalar pronation is accompanied by eversion of the calcaneus. This can be seen in a posterior view as an increase in the medial angle formed by a line through the leg and through the tuber of the calcaneus (calcaneovalgus). (b) Subtalar supination is accompanied by inversion of the calcaneus. This can be seen in a posterior view as a decrease in the medial angle formed by a line trough the leg and through the tuber of the calcaneus (calcaneovarus).

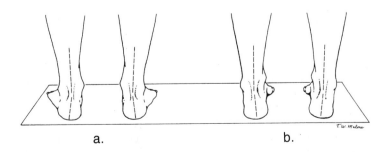

a.

Calcaneovalgus

b.

Calcaneovarus

dorsiflexion. When the posterior aspect of the calcaneus is viewed in subtalar supination, calcaneal inversion is observable as a varus angulation between the calcaneus and the tibia (Fig. 12–12b). Consequently subtalar supination may also be described as having the calcaneal components of adduction, varus, and plantarflexion. Although one can more easily observe the inversion/eversion (or varus/valgus) component of calcaneal motion, it must be recalled that this calcaneal motion *cannot* occur in isolation, but can only occur simultaneously with the less visible components of calcaneal abduction/adduction and calcaneal dorsiflexion/plantarflexion. Because of the complex nature of the subtalar joint surfaces, the component motions that constitute subtalar supination and pronation cannot occur independently.

Weight-Bearing Subtalar Joint Motion

When the foot is non-weight-bearing, the motion across the subtalar joint is accomplished by the distal calcaneal segment. When the calcaneus is on the ground and weight-bearing, it is *not* free to accomplish each of the component motions. The calcaneus can still evert and invert (valgus and varus motions, respectively), although this will result in some side-to-side motion of the foot on the ground. However, the calcaneus cannot dorsiflex/plantarflex or abduct/adduct while it is bearing weight because the superimposed body weight effectively prevents these movements. Because subtalar motion cannot consist of inversion/eversion in isolation, the other two components of the subtalar motion are accomplished by the proximal talar segment of the joint rather than by the distal calcaneal segment.

The motion accomplished at a joint remains unchanged whether the distal segment of the joint moves or whether the proximal segment moves. When the proximal segment is referenced rather than the distal, however, the motion of the proximal segment will be the opposite of what was described in the distal segment. In weight-bearing subtalar motion, the direction of movement for the talus is the opposite of that described for the calcaneus to produce the same motion between the segments. In weight-bearing supination, the calcaneus retains its ability to invert. However, the calcaneus cannot adduct and plantarflex in weight-bearing, so the same joint motion is obtained by abduction and dorsiflexion of the talus. Weight-bearing subtalar supination, therefore, is accomplished by the component

movements of inversion (varus) of the calcaneus and dorsiflexion and abduction of the talus. Weight-bearing subtalar pronation is accomplished by the component movement of eversion (valgus) that the calcaneus retains, as well as by plantarflexion and adduction of the talus. The component motions of abduction and adduction of the talus occur around a vertical axis and are sometimes referred to as lateral rotation and medial rotation of the talus, respectively.

Although understanding non-weight-bearing subtalar pronation/supination begins our understanding of this complex joint, the most critical functions of the foot occur in weight-bearing. We must also recognize that when the foot is weight-bearing, there is effectively a closed chain formed for the lower extremity (assuming either bilateral stance or the head fixed in the upright position). Consequently, the kinematics and kinetics of the subtalar joint will affect and be affected by more proximal and distal joints. The first consequence of closed chain subtalar function can be seen in its interdependence with lower extremity or leg rotation.

WEIGHT-BEARING SUBTALAR JOINT MOTION AND ITS AFFECT ON THE LEG

During weight-bearing subtalar supination/pronation, the components of dorsiflexion and plantarflexion of the talus may be absorbed by the ankle joint as the body of the talus slides within the tibiofibular mortise (posteriorly in dorsiflexion and anteriorly in plantarflexion). The tibia remains unaffected by the talar dorsiflexion/plantarflexion as long as the ankle joint is free to move. However, the component motion of abduction/adduction of the talus that must occur as part of weight-bearing supination/pronation cannot be absorbed by the ankle joint. When the talus must rotate (abduct/adduct) as part of weight-bearing subtalar motion, the body of the talus cannot rotate within the mortise more than a few degrees. Consequently, the talus will carry the superimposed mortise with it. When the subtalar joint supinates in weight-bearing, the talus must abduct (laterally rotate). In doing so, it carries the tibia and fibula that form the mortise with it, producing lateral rotation of the leg. Weight-bearing subtalar pronation causes adduction of the talus; talar adduction carries the tibia and fibula into medial rotation.

Through the component movements of abduction and adduction of the talus, weight-bearing subtalar joint motion directly influences the segments and joints superior to it. A weight-bearing subtalar joint maintained in pronation (e.g., a flat foot) creates a medial rotatory force on the leg that may influence the knee joint, and potentially the hip, in a number of ways.

EXAMPLE 1: When one foot is maintained in pronation during weight-bearing, there is a sustained medial rotatory force on the lower extremity. That force may create a rotatory stress at the knee joint, or it may cause medial rotation at the hip joint. Hip joint medial rotation will cause the knee to face somewhat medially, resulting in an increased Q angle and the potential for increased lateral subluxing forces on the patellofemoral joint.

Just as the subtalar joint may create rotatory forces on the leg, so too may rotation of the leg influence the subtalar joint. When a lateral rotatory force is imposed on the leg (as in rotating to the right around a planted right foot), the lateral motion of the tibia carries the mortise and its mated body of the talus laterally as well. The talus cannot be rotated laterally (abducted) without also causing the other component movements that are part of subtalar supination. When the talus is abducted by the rotating leg, therefore, the talus also will dorsiflex in the mortise and the calcaneus will move into inversion. A medial rotatory force imposed on the leg will necessarily result in subtalar pronation as the talus is medially rotated (adducted) by the rotating tibiofibular mortise. The interdependence of the leg and talus were mechanically represented by Inman and Mann[44] using the concept of the subtalar joint as a mitered hinge. Figure 12–13 presents a good visualization of this concept.

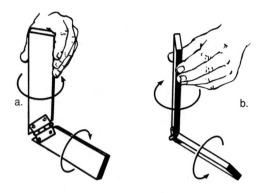

FIGURE 12–13. The subtalar joint can be visualized as a mitered hinge between the leg and the foot. (a) Medial rotation of the leg proximally imposes pronation on the distally located foot. (b) Lateral rotation of the leg proximally imposes supination on the distally located foot. (From Mann, RA: Biomechanics of running. In Mann, RA [ed]: Surgery of the Foot, ed 5. CV Mosby, St Louis, 1986, p 19, with permission.)

One of the primary functions of the subtalar joint is seen in the interdependence of the subtalar joint and the leg. When the foot is weight-bearing, the subtalar joint motion absorbs the imposed lower-extremity rotations that would otherwise either spin the foot on the ground or disrupt the ankle joint by rotating the talus within the mortise. When the subtalar joint is non-weight-bearing (in an open chain), the motions of the subtalar joint and the leg are independent and do not influence each other. Table 12–1 summarizes non-weight-bearing and weight-bearing subtalar component movements.

ROM and Subtalar Neutral

The range of subtalar supination and pronation are difficult to assess because of the triplanar nature and because the component contribu-

Table 12–1. **Summary of Subtalar Component Motions**

	COMPONENT MOVEMENTS OF SUBTALAR SUPINATION/PRONATION	
	Non–Weight-Bearing	**Weight-Bearing**
Supination	Calcaneal inversion (or varus)	Calcaneal inversion (or varus)
	Calcaneal adduction	Talar abduction (or lateral rotation)
	Calcaneal plantarflexion	Talar dorsiflexion
		Tibiofibular lateral rotation
Pronation	Calcaneal eversion (or valgus)	Calcaneal eversion (or valgus)
	Calcaneal abduction	Talar adduction (or medial rotation)
	Calcaneal dorsiflexion	Talar plantarflexion
		Tibiofibular medial rotation

tions vary with the inclination of the subtalar axis. The calcaneal component of subtalar motion (the varus-valgus angulation of the posterior calcaneus with the posterior midline of the leg), however, is relatively easy to measure in both weight-bearing and non-weight-bearing movements. The available range of the component of eversion (valgus) of the calcaneus has been measured as 5° to 10° and inversion (varus) as 20° to 30° for a total range of 35° to 40°.[14,45,46] Although the total range of inversion/eversion is not controversial, the ranges of inversion and eversion depend on what one takes to be the neutral or 0° position for the calcaneus. The so-called **subtalar neutral position** has been defined differently by different investigators, with some issues raised as to the appropriateness of the measurement techniques.

The definition of subtalar neutral has important implications for assessment of foot function. Subtalar neutral is used to assess the position of the hindfoot to assess its potential role in dysfunction of more proximal and distal joints and is similarly used as a reference point for assessing position of the forefoot. The ability to identify the neutral position of the subtalar joint, therefore, would appear to have important implications for assessment of lower extremity function. Subtalar neutral was defined by Root and colleagues[46] as the point from which the calcaneus will invert twice as many degrees as it will evert. Subtalar neutral is found by first fully supinating the subtalar joint (or, more correctly, maximally inverting the calcaneus) and then carrying the calcaneus two-thirds of the way through to maximum subtalar pronation (maximal calcaneal eversion). Baily and colleagues[47] used radiologic evidence to demonstrate that the neutral position of the subtalar joint was quite varied among individuals. It was not always found two-thirds of the way from maximum supination, although the average neutral subtalar position for their subjects was close to this value. Åstrom and Arvidson[45] used the technique of Elveru and colleagues[48] to find subtalar neutral by palpating the head of the talus in 121 subjects with no known foot problems. This technique presumably allows for individual variations in subtalar axis position. Åstrom and Arvidson found the average position of the calcaneus in the palpated "subtalar neutral" position to be 2° of calcaneal valgus (relative to the midline of the calf). When Åstrom and Arvidson used the method of Root and colleagues,

the "subtalar neutral" position was 1° of calcaneal varus. McPoil and Cornwall[49] used palpation of the talar head to determine subtalar neutral among normal subjects and found an average position of 1.5° of calcaneal varus. However, when the calcaneal position was assessed during the stance phase of gait, McPoil and Cornwall found that the calcaneus typically did not reach the predetermined subtalar neutral position in most individuals. This would appear contradictory to the nearly universal belief that the subtalar joint in normal gait pronates as stance begins, returns to neutral during midstance, and then supinates by the end of stance. McPoil and Cornwall[49] concluded that, among normal subjects, the neutral subtalar joint was probably better represented by the position of the calcaneus in relaxed bilateral stance, a position that averaged approximately 3.5° of calcaneal valgus (eversion) in their subjects. Their data would appear to support the conclusion of Åstrom and Arvidson that the normal weight-bearing foot is more pronated than previously thought and that reliance on the palpated subtalar neutral position could lead to overdiagnosis of excessive subtalar pronation.[45]

Although the end range positions of calcaneal inversion/eversion are clinically reproducible measures, the talar dorsiflexion/plantarflexion component of weight-bearing subtalar motion cannot be measured other than in static radiographs. The talar abduction/adduction component, however, has been estimated by measuring the tibial rotation that accompanies abduction/adduction of the talus. Close and colleagues[50] measured approximately 10° of tibial rotation during the stance phase of gait. This 10° range would represent the best estimate of the amount of abduction/adduction of the talus that occurs during the weight-bearing portion of gait. Root and colleagues[46] measured a similar magnitude of calcaneal eversion/inversion during gait. The equivalence of the subtalar ranges of eversion/inversion and abduction/adduction during gait do not represent the full available motion, but are in agreement with the 4:4:1 contribution of eversion/inversion, abduction/adduction, and dorsiflexion/plantarflexion projected by Sgarlato[51] for an average subtalar joint axis. That is, for every 4° of calcaneal eversion, one should see 4° of adduction of the talus (4° of medial rotation of the tibia) and 1° of plantarflexion of the talus with the typical subtalar axis.

Although there is not consensus on many aspects of subtalar function, there is general agreement that full supination is the close-packed or locked position for the subtalar joint, and pronation is a position of relative mobility. In supination, ligamentous tension draws the talocalcaneal joint surfaces together, resulting in locking of the articular surfaces. Conversely, the adduction and plantarflexion of the talus that occurs in weight-bearing pronation causes a splaying (spreading) of the adjacent tarsal bones that permits some intertarsal mobility. Not surprisingly, the role of the ligaments at the subtalar joint is controversial. The cervical ligament and interosseous talocalcaneal ligament are variously credited with checking pronation or supination.[2,14,38,52] Sarrafian[14] believes the position of the ligaments to be along the subtalar axis, causing the ligaments to remain tight in both positions. Using his premise, individual shifts in location of the axis or of the ligaments could account for discrepant findings of other investigators.

Examination of the subtalar joint is not complete and an understanding of its role as the determinative joint of the foot[6] cannot be obtained without examining the fact that the talus moves in weight-bearing subtalar motion not only on the calcaneus below it, but also on the navicular just anterior to it and on the ligament that helps support the talar head. The linkage of the talus to the structures below it and anterior to it have led to the anatomic and functional concept of the **talocalcaneonavicular joint.**

Talocalcaneonavicular Joint

In weight-bearing subtalar motion, the talar component motions (abduction/adduction and plantarflexion/dorsiflexion) move the talus on the calcaneus and on the relatively immobile navicular.[53] The articulation of the talus with the navicular, the **talonavicular joint,** is classically considered part of the **transverse tarsal joint.** However, an understanding of hindfoot function can best be obtained by first examining the talonavicular joint as part of the expanded concept of the talocalcaneonavicular joint, or the **TCN.**

TCN Joint Structure

The TCN joint name ties together the talonavicular and the subtalar (talocalcaneal) joints

that are both anatomically and functionally related. The talonavicular articulation is formed proximally by the anterior portion of the head of the talus and distally by the concave posterior navicular. The talar head, however, also articulates inferiorly with the anterior and medial facets of the calcaneus and with the **plantar calcaneonavicular ligament** that spans the gap between the calcaneus and navicular below the talar head. Consequently, we can visualize the TCN as a ball-and-socket joint where the large convexity of the head of the talus is received by a large "socket" formed by the concavity of the navicular, the concavities of the anterior and medial calcaneal facets, by the plantar calcaneonavicular ligament, and by the deltoid ligament medially and the **bifurcate ligaments** laterally (Fig. 12–14). The plantar calcaneonavicular ligament, most commonly referred to as the **spring ligament,** is a triangular sheet of ligamentous connective tissue arising from the sustentaculum tali of the calcaneus and inserting on the inferior navicular. It is continuous medially with a portion of the deltoid ligament of the ankle and joins laterally with the medial band of the bifurcate ligament (also known as the lateral calcaneonavicular ligament). Davis and colleagues[54] found the plantar calcaneonavicular ligament to have two distinct segments, each of which contributed to the talar "acetabulum." The larger compo-

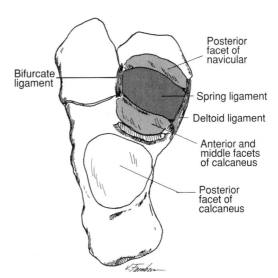

FIGURE 12–14. Superior view looking into the talocalcaneonavicular joint. The talus as been removed, showing the enlarged concavity formed by the navicular, the deltoid ligament, and the medial band of the bifurcate ligament.

nent of the ligament was the superomedial portion of the calcaneonavicular ligament or the **SMCN ligament.** The SMCN ligament was found to be intimately associated with the superficial deltoid ligament and formed a medial and plantar articular sling for the head of the talus, including a triangular-shaped avascular articular facet where the talar head rested on the ligament.[54] The concept that the SMCN ligament was part of the actual articulation rather than simply holding together the calcaneal and navicular facets was supported by the presence of fibers indicating that the ligament resisted bending as well as tensile stresses. Davis and colleagues[54] also described a second component of the calcaneonavicular ligament, referred to as the inferior calcaneonavicular ligament or **ICN ligament.** This ligament was plantar and lateral to the SMCN portion, with a composition that suggested it resisted tensile stresses only and had no tissue that appeared to be articular. They also confirmed the findings of other investigators[55] that the ligament has little or no elasticity and so is better described as a "sling" than as a spring.

The head of the talus and its large socket are enclosed by a single capsule that encompasses the TCN. Within that capsule lie the anterior and middle facets of the subtalar joint and the talonavicular joint. The floor of the capsule is formed by the SMCN and ICN ligaments and the sides by the deltoid and bifurcate ligaments. It should be recalled that the large posterior facet of the subtalar joint is contained within its own capsule. The capsules of the posterior subtalar joint and the TCN are physically separated by the tarsal canal and by the ligaments found within that canal.

The TCN joint shares the ligamentous support of the subtalar joint, including the medial and lateral collateral ligaments, the inferior extensor retinacular structures, and the cervical and interosseous talocalcaneal ligaments. Of course, the TCN is also supported by those ligaments that help to compose it (SMCN, ICN, and bifurcate ligaments) and by the **dorsal talonavicular ligament.** Additional support is also received from the ligaments that reinforce the adjacent **calcaneocuboid joint** because, as we shall see in our discussion of the transverse tarsal joint, the talonavicular and calcaneocuboid joints are functionally linked.

TCN Joint Function

The talus acts as a ball-bearing placed between the tibiofibular mortise superiorly, the calcaneus inferiorly, and the navicular anteriorly. Motion of the weight-bearing talus at one articulation *must* cause motion at each of its inferior articulations.

The TCN joint, therefore, like its subtalar component that contributes to it, is a triplanar joint with 1° of freedom: supination/pronation. The axis for TCN supination and pronation is inclined 40° upward and anteriorly and 30° medially and anteriorly (Fig. 12–15).[55] This is, as one would expect, essentially the same as the

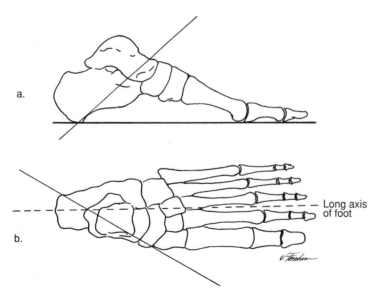

a.

b.

Long axis of foot

FIGURE 12–15. Talocalcaneonavicular joint axis. (a) Inclined up anteriorly, approximately 40°. (b) Inclined in anteriorly, approximately 30°.

axis for the subtalar joint alone. The axis of the talonavicular joint, however, is inclined medially more than the subtalar joint axis, which gives the TCN joint more dorsiflexion/plantarflexion than attributed to the subtalar joint. TCN joint motions may have a slightly greater range than those of the subtalar joint alone, but the movements of the talus and calcaneus and the weight-bearing relationship to the tibia are virtually identical to those presented in discussion of the subtalar joint.

Functionally, the articulations that make up the subtalar and talonavicular joints exist as components of the more complete TCN joint. This relationship is evident not only kinematically as we have already seen, but also kinetically. Forces transmitted through the leg to the talus are shared by each of the articular surfaces that make up the TCN. Reeck and colleagues[56] looked at force transmission through applied loads on the tibia and fibula, as well as tensile loading of extrinsic muscles on cadaver specimens. They found that the transmitted forces were greatest at the posterior subtalar facet, following in decreasing order by the talonavicular, anterior and medial subtalar, and SMCN ligament articulations. However, given the similarly decreasing contact areas of each articulation, the pressures were similar at each articulation in most foot positions. Although the pressures at each articular surface increased as the foot moved toward toe-off, the pressure at the posterior subtalar facet exceeded that of the others at the end of the stance phase of gait.[56]

Terminology for motions of the subtalar and TCN joints, like that for many joints we have examined, is not universally accepted. In this text, we have chosen to use supination/pronation as the composite (triplanar) motions that include the frontal plane (anteroposterior axis) components of inversion/eversion. Readers may find others reversing this usage; that is, using inversion/eversion as the composite triplanar motions and supination/pronation as the frontal plane components. Although pronation/supination and inversion/eversion are often substituted for each other, there is consensus across the literature in using varus-valgus of the calcaneus to refer to the frontal plane component of subtalar motion. Regardless of how the terms are used, it should be noted that subtalar supination is invariably linked with subtalar inversion and calcaneovarus, whereas subtalar pronation is invariably linked with subtalar eversion and calcaneovalgus. Mandatory coupling of the components as part of a single composite triplanar motion may make the terminology controversy moot to those who understand foot function, but failure to define terms can lead to confusion among less sophisticated readers. Terms used in research and published literature should carefully be defined to impart the most and clearest information.

The TCN *joint is the key to foot function.* The bones and joints distal to the TCN essentially form a single elastic unit that, for the most part, moves in response to and as compensation for movement of the talus and the calcaneus.[50,55,57] This compensatory motion occurs largely at the transverse tarsal joint.

Transverse Tarsal Joint

The transverse tarsal (midtarsal) joint is a compound joint formed by the talonavicular and calcaneocuboid joints (Fig. 12–16). Because the talonavicular joint is classically considered to be part of the transverse tarsal joint, it belongs to two joint complexes: the TCN joint and the transverse tarsal joint. The other component of the transverse tarsal joint is the calcaneocuboid joint. The two joints together present an S-shaped joint line that transects

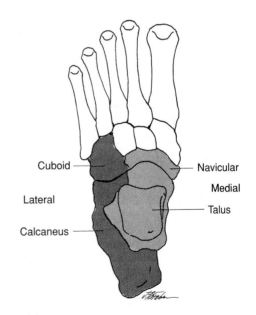

FIGURE 12–16. Talonavicular joint and calcaneocuboid joint form a compound joint known as the transverse tarsal joint line that transects the foot.

the foot horizontally, dividing the hindfoot from the midfoot and forefoot. Like the navicular, the cuboid is considered essentially immobile in the weight-bearing foot. Transverse tarsal joint motion, therefore, is considered to be motion of the talus and of the calcaneus on the relatively fixed naviculocuboid unit.[53,58] Motion at the compound transverse tarsal joint, however, is more complex than the simple joint line might suggest and occurs predominantly in response to action at the TCN.

Transverse Tarsal Joint Structure

The structure of the talonavicular joint has already been presented as part of the TCN joint. The calcaneocuboid joint is formed proximally by the anterior calcaneus, and distally by the posterior cuboid (see Fig. 12–16). The articular surfaces of both the calcaneus and the cuboid are complex, being reciprocally concave/convex across both dimensions. The reciprocal shape makes available motion at the calcaneocuboid joint more restricted than that of the ball-and-socket-shaped talonavicular joint; the calcaneus as it moves at the subtalar joint in weight-bearing must meet the conflicting arthrokinematic demands of the saddle-shaped surfaces, resulting in a twisting motion. The calcaneocuboid articulation has its own capsule that is reinforced by several major ligaments. These are the lateral band of the bifurcate ligament (also known as the **calcaneocuboid ligament**); the **dorsal calcaneocuboid ligament;** and the **plantar calca-**

neocuboid (short plantar) and the **long plantar ligaments** (see Fig. 12–6). The long plantar ligament is the most important of these ligaments, because it extends inferiorly between the calcaneus and the cuboid and then continues on distally to the bases of the second, third, and fourth metatarsals. It makes a significant contribution both to transverse tarsal joint stability and to related support of the longitudinal arch of the foot. Important support for the transverse tarsal joint is also provided by the extrinsic muscles of the foot as they pass medial and lateral to the joint, as well as by the intrinsic foot muscles located inferiorly.

Transverse Tarsal Joint Function

Axes

The transverse tarsal joint has been analyzed in a number of different ways, usually resulting in function around two independent axes. Manter[41] and Hicks[26] both proposed longitudinal and oblique axes around which the talus and calcaneous move on the relatively fixed naviculocuboid unit. The longitudinal (or anteroposterio) axis is nearly horizontal, being only slightly inclined upward and medially anteriorly (Fig. 12–17). Motion around this axis is triplanar, producing supination/pronation as seen at the subtalar/TCN joints. Unlike the axis of the subtalar/TCN joint, the longitudinal axis of the transverse tarsal joint approaches a true anteroposterior axis, so the inversion/eversion

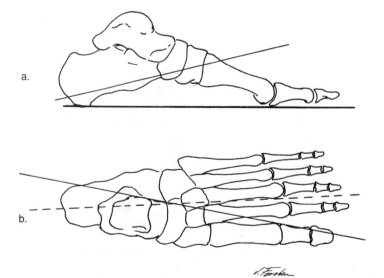

a.

b.

V. Forshen

FIGURE 12–17. Longitudinal axis of the transverse tarsal joint.

components of the movement predominate. The oblique (transverse) axis of the transverse tarsal joint nearly parallels the axis of the TCN joint, providing triplanar supination/pronation with predominating dorsiflexion/plantarflexion and abduction/adduction components. Motion around this axis is more restricted than motion around the longitudinal axis because the axis is more inclined across all three planes. The longitudinal and oblique axes together provide a total range of supination/pronation that is one-third to one-half of the range available at the TCN joint.[26] Root[46] has proposed that the longitudinal axis around which most of the movement can occur provides less than 10° of inversion/eversion. The two joints of the transverse tarsal joint can function somewhat independently, although motion at one is generally accompanied by at least some motion of the other.

The TCN joint and the transverse tarsal joint are mechanically linked by the shared talonavicular joint. Any subtalar, and therefore, TCN, motion must include motion at the talonavicular joint. Because talonavicular motion is interdependent with calcaneocuboid motion, subtalar/TCN motion will involve the entire transverse tarsal joint. As the TCN supinates, its linkage to the transverse tarsal joint carries the calcaneocuboid with it via the talonavicular joint. When the TCN is fully supinated and locked (bony surfaces drawn together), the transverse tarsal joint is also carried into full supination and its bony surfaces drawn together into a locked position. When the TCN is pronated and loose packed, the transverse tarsal joint is also mobile and loose-packed.

Action

The transverse joint is the transitional link between the hindfoot and the forefoot serving (1) to add to the supination/pronation range of the TCN joint and (2) to compensate the forefoot for hindfoot position. Compensation in this context refers to the ability of the forefoot to remain flat on the ground while the hindfoot is in varus or valgus. The first of the transverse tarsal joint functions can occur either in the weight-bearing or in the non-weight-bearing foot and is self-explanatory. The second function requires closer analysis.

In the weight-bearing position, medial rotation of the tibia imposes pronation on the TCN

joint. If the pronation force continued distally through the foot, the lateral border of the foot would tend to lift from the ground, diminishing the stability of the base of support and resulting in unequal weight-bearing. This undesirable effect of TCN pronation may be avoided when the transverse tarsal joint can absorb the rotation; that is, the talus and calcaneus move on the essentially fixed naviculocuboid unit, resulting in a relative supination of the forefoot distal to the transverse tarsal joint. The transverse tarsal joint maintains normal weight-bearing forces on the forefoot while allowing the hindfoot to absorb the rotation of the lower limb (Fig. 12–18).

As long as the hindfoot is pronated (and the TCN joint is mobile), the transverse tarsal joint is free to compensate for hindfoot position and to accommodate to the demands of the supporting surface. In static bilateral stance on level ground, both the TCN and the transverse tarsal joints pronate. As a person moves into single-limb support and begins to walk, the TCN will continue to pronate while the transverse tarsal joint will supinate approximately an equal amount to maintain proper weight-bearing in the forefoot. A rock under the medial forefoot may require even greater supination of the transverse tarsal joint to maintain appropriate contact of the forefoot with the ground, if additional supination range is available. If the range is not available at the transverse tarsal joint, the rock may force the hindfoot

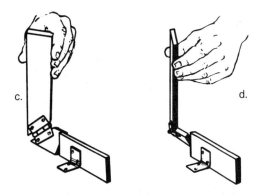

FIGURE 12–18. The transverse tarsal joint permits the forefoot to remain evenly on the ground, absorbing the pronation occurring at the subtalar joint through medial rotation of the leg (a) or the supination occurring at the subtalar joint through lateral rotation of the leg (b). (From Mann, RA: Biomechanics of running. In Mann, RA [ed]: Surgery of the Foot, ed 5. CV Mosby, St Louis, 1986, p. 15, with permission.)

into supination as well. With other surface demands such as standing sideways on a steep hill, the uphill foot must pronate substantially to maintain contact; pronation may be required at both the TCN and the transverse tarsal joints. When the hindfoot (TCN) is pronated, the joints of both the hindfoot and midfoot are mobile and free to make necessary compensatory changes required to maintain contact of the foot with the ground within the limits of the joint ROM.

Supination of the hindfoot (TCN) restricts the ability of the transverse tarsal joint to compensate or counterrotate the forefoot. The transverse tarsal joint is carried into increasing supination with increasing TCN supination. Consequently, transverse tarsal joint mobility is increasingly restricted as the TCN moves toward increasing supination. In full TCN supination, such as when the tibia is laterally rotated on the weight-bearing foot, supination locks not only the TCN but the transverse tarsal joint as well. Although the tarsometatarsal joints are capable of minor compensatory changes, the forefoot may follow into supination depending on the magnitude of the imposed force.

In normal gait, hindfoot supination occurs at a time when the foot is required to serve as a rigid lever (during the second half of the stance phase). The locking of the subtalar/TCN and the transverse tarsal joints facilitates transfer of weight through the tarsometatarsal joints to the forefoot by converting the foot to a rigid lever. Locking of the hindfoot and midfoot may be undesirable, however, if the hindfoot has been supinated by uneven terrain. The entire medial border of the foot may lift, and, unless the muscles on the lateral side of the foot are active, a supination sprain of the lateral ligaments will result. When the locked TCN and transverse tarsal joints are unable to absorb the rotation superimposed by the weight-bearing limb or by uneven ground, the forces must be dissipated at the ankle and may result in injury to the ankle joint structures.

Tarsometatarsal Joints

Tarsometatarsal Joint Structure

The tarsometatarsal (TMT) joints are plane synovial joints formed by the distal tarsal row posteriorly and by the bases of the metatarsals anteriorly (Fig. 12–19). The first TMT joint is the

articulation between the base of the first metatarsal and the medial cuneiform. It has its own articular capsule. The second TMT joint is the articulation of the base of the second metatarsal with a mortise formed by the middle cuneiform and the sides of the medial and lateral cuneiforms. This joint is set back more posteriorly than the other TMT joints; it is stronger and its motion more restricted. The third TMT joint, formed by the third metatarsal and the lateral cuneiform, shares a capsule with the second TMT joint. The fourth and fifth TMT joints are formed by the bases of the fourth and fifth metatarsals with the cuboid. These two joints also share a joint capsule. There are also small plane articulations between the bases of the metatarsals to permit motion of one metatarsal on the next. Each tarsometatarsal joint is reinforced by numerous dorsal, plantar, and interosseous ligaments. Additionally, stability is contributed by the **deep transverse metatarsal ligament,** similar to that found in the hand, that prevents splaying of the metatarsal heads at the TMT joints.[59]

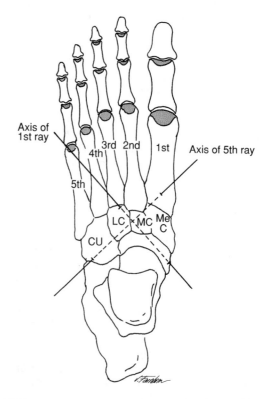

FIGURE 12–19. Tarsometatarsal, metatarsophalangeal, and interphalangeal joints of the foot (CU, cuboid; MeC, medial cuneiform; MC, middle cuneiform; LC, lateral cuneiform).

Tarsometatarsal Joint Function

Function of the TMT joint is primarily a continuation of the function of the transverse tarsal joint; that is, these joints attempt to regulate position of the metatarsals and phalanges relative to the weight-bearing surface. As long as transverse tarsal joint motion is adequate to compensate for the hindfoot position, TMT joint motion is not required. However, when the hindfoot position is extreme and the transverse tarsal joint is inadequate to provide full compensation, the TMT joints may rotate to provide further adjustment of forefoot position.[46]

Axes

Each TMT joint is considered to have a unique, although not fully independent axis of motion. Hicks[26] examined the axes for the five rays. A **ray** is a functional unit formed by a metatarsal and its associated cuneiform (first through third rays). The cunieforms are included as parts of a movement unit because the small amount of motion contributed by the cunionavicular joints has not been accounted for in some other way. The cuneonavicular motion, therefore, becomes functionally part of the available TMT motions. Where there is not an associated cuneiform, the ray is formed by the metatarsal alone (fourth and fifth rays) as it moves on the cuboid.

The axes for the first and fifth rays are shown in Figure 12–19. Each is oblique and, therefore, triplanar. ROM of the first ray is the largest of the metatarsals. The axis of the first ray is inclined so that dorsiflexion (extension) of the first ray is accompanied by inversion and adduction, while plantarflexion (flexion) is accompanied by eversion and abduction. The abduction/adduction components normally are minimal. Movements of the fifth ray around its axis are more restricted and occur with the opposite arrangement of components: dorsiflexion is accompanied by eversion and abduction and plantarflexion by inversion and adduction. The TMT joint motions are not considered to be pronation/supination movements because the components are not as consistent as the composite supination/pronation motions of the TCN and transverse tarsal joints.

The axis for the third ray nearly coincides with a coronal axis; the predominant motion, therefore, is dorsiflexion/plantarflexion. The axes for the second and fourth rays were not determined by Hicks[26] but were considered to be intermediate between the adjacent axes for the first and fifth rays, respectively. The second ray moves around an axis that is inclined toward, but is not as oblique as, the first axis. The fourth ray moves around an axis that is similar to, but not as steep as, the fifth axis. The second ray is considered to be the least mobile of the five. Table 12–2 provides a summary of the motions of the five rays during TMT dorsiflexion and plantarflexion.

Actions

The motions of the TMT joints are somewhat interdependent, as are the motions of the carpometacarpal (CMC) joints in the hand. The TMT joints also contribute to hollowing and flattening of the foot, just as the CMC joints do for the hand. An active dorsiflexion force across the non-weight-bearing TMTs will simultaneously extend the five metatarsals while also creating inversion at the first two rays and eversion at the last two rays. The opposite motions accompanying TMT dorsiflexion flatten the contour of the plantar surface of the foot. An active plantarflexion force across the non-weight-bearing TMTs will flex the TMTs while everting the first two rays and inverting the last two. This action increases the "cupping" of the plantar surface of the foot. However, the relevance of TMT joint motions is not found in the free foot (open chain) but in the weight-bearing foot (closed chain).

SUPINATION TWIST

When the hindfoot pronates to any substantial degree in weight-bearing, the transverse tarsal joint will generally supinate to counterrotate the forefoot. If the range of transverse tarsal supination is not sufficient to meet the de-

Table 12–2. **Summary of Motions of the Rays of the Foot**

	Dorsiflexion	Plantarflexion
First ray	Inversion	Eversion
	Slight adduction	Slight abduction
Second ray	Slight inversion	Slight eversion
Third ray	—	—
Fourth ray	Slight eversion	Slight inversion
Fifth ray	Eversion	Inversion
	Slight abduction	Slight adduction

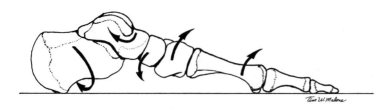

FIGURE 12–20. Extreme pronation of the foot is accompanied by adduction of the head of the talus, eversion of the calcaneus, and pronation at the transverse tarsal joint (not mandatory). If the forefoot is to remain on the ground, the tarsometatarsal joints must undergo a counteracting supination twist.

mands of the pronating force, the medial forefoot will press into the ground, and the lateral side will tend to lift. The first and second ray will be pushed into dorsiflexion while the fourth and fifth rays will plantarflex in an attempt to maintain contact with the ground. The component rotation that accompanies dorsiflexion of the first and second rays and plantarflexion of the fourth and fifth rays is inversion. Consequently, the entire forefoot undergoes an inversion rotation around a hypothetical axis at the second ray. This rotation is referred to as **supination twist** of the TMT joints.[26] As an example of supination twist of the forefoot, Figure 12–20 shows the response of the segments of the foot to a strong pronation torque across the TCN. The transverse tarsal joint can only supinate to a limited degree in response to the hindfoot motion and requires a supination twist of the TMT joints to fully adjust the forefoot. The configuration of the forefoot in a supination twist is not constant but can vary according to the weight-bearing needs of the foot and the terrain.

PRONATION TWIST

When the hindfoot and the transverse tarsal joints are both locked in supination, the adjustment of forefoot position must be left entirely to the TMT joints. With hindfoot supination, the forefoot tends to lift on its medial side and press into the ground on its lateral side. The first and second ray will plantarflex to maintain contact with the ground

while the fourth and fifth rays are forced into dorsiflexion. Because eversion accompanies plantarflexion of the first and second ray and dorsiflexion of the fourth and fifth ray, the forefoot as a whole undergoes a **pronation twist.**[26]

Pronation twist, like supination twist, can vary in configuration. Although the pronation twist may provide adequate counterrotation for moderate hindfoot supination, it may be inadequate to maintain forefoot stability in extreme supination. Figure 12–21 shows the rotations imposed on the weight-bearing foot by lateral rotation initiated in the lower extremity or by supination initiated at the TCN joint.

Pronation and supination twist of the TMT joints occur only when the transverse tarsal joint function is inadequate; that is, when the transverse tarsal joint is unable to counterrotate or its range is insufficient to fully compensate for hindfoot position.

Metatarsophalangeal Joints

The five metatarsophalangeal (MTP) joints (see Fig. 12–19) are condyloid synovial joints with 2° of freedom: extension/flexion (or dorsiflexion/plantarflexion) and abduction/adduction. Although both degrees of freedom might be useful to the MTP joints in the rare instances the foot participates in grasplike activities, flexion and extension are the predominant functional movements at these joints. In the weight-bearing foot, toe extension permits the

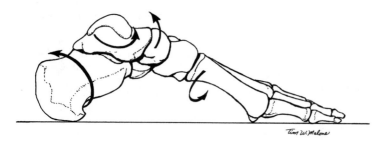

FIGURE 12–21. Extreme supination of the foot is accompanied by abduction of the head of the talus, inversion of the calcaneus, and mandatory supination of the transverse tarsal joint. If the forefoot is to remain on the ground, the tarsometatarsal joints must undergo a counteracting pronation twist.

body to pass over the foot while the toes dynamically balance the superimposed body weight as they press into the supporting surface through activity of the toe flexors.

MTP Joint Structure

The MTP joints are formed proximally by the heads of the metatarsals and distally by the bases of the proximal phalanges. The metatarsals may vary in length. In 56% of individuals, the second metatarsal is the longest of the metatarsals, with the first metatarsal being next, followed in order by the third through fifth metatarsals. This pattern of metatarsal length is referred to as an **index minus** foot. In 28% of the individuals, the first metatarsal is equivalent in length to the second metatarsal, a pattern identified as an **index plus minus** foot. The second metatarsal is shorter than the first in 16% of individuals (referred to as an **index plus** foot).[60] The pattern of metatarsal length may predispose an individual to a particular set of problems with the MTP joints and the toes.

The MTP joints of the foot are structurally analogous to the MCP joints of the hands, although there are some exceptions to the analogy. Unlike what we see at the MCP joints, the MTP extension range exceeds the flexion range. The heads of the metatarsals each bear weight in stance. Consequently, the articular cartilage must stop short of the weight-bearing surface on the plantar aspect of the metatarsal head. This restricts the available range of MTP flexion. Because there is no opposition available at the first TMT joint, the first toe (hallux) moves in the same plane as the other four digits. The first MTP joint, like the first MCP joint, has two sesamoid bones located at the joint. In neutral MTP position, the sesamoid bones lie in two grooves separated by the intersesamoid ridge. The ligaments associated with the sesamoid bones form a triangular mass that stabilizes the sesamoids within their grooves.[61] The sesamoid bones serve as anatomic pulleys for the flexor hallucis brevis muscle and protect the tendon of the flexor hallucis longus muscle from weight-bearing trauma as it passes through a tunnel formed by the sesamoid bones and the intersesamoidal ligament that connects their plantar surfaces.[61] Unlike those of the hand, the sesamoid bones of the foot share in weight-bearing with the relatively large quadrilaterally shaped head of the first

metatarsal.[62,63] In toe extension greater than 10°, the sesamoids no longer lie in their grooves and may become unstable. Chronic lateral instability may lead to MTP deformity.[62]

Stability of the MTP joints is provided by the **plantar plates** or plantar pad, the **collateral ligaments,** and the deep transverse metatarsal ligament. The plantar plates are structurally similar to the volar plates in the hand. These fibrocartilaginous structures in the four lesser toes are connected distally to the base of the proximal phalanges and proximally blend with the joint capsules and with the interconnecting deep transverse metatarsal ligament. The collateral ligaments have two components: a proper or phalangeal portion that parallels the metatarsal and phalange and an accessory component that runs obliquely from the metatarsal head to the plantar plate.[64] The plantar plates protect the weight-bearing surface of the metatarsal heads and, with the collaterals, contribute to stability of the MTP joints.[65] Deland and colleagues[64] noted that the plate and collaterals form a "substantial soft tissue box" connected to the sides of the metatarsal heads and supporting the MTP joints. They also noted that the long flexor tendons run in grooves in the plates that help maintain tendon position as the MTP are crossed. The sesamoids and thick plantar capsule of the first MTP joint replace the plantar plates found at the other toes.[61]

MTP Joint Function

Although the MTP joints have 2° of freedom, flexion/extension is clearly more important than abduction/adduction. The first MTP joint was found in one study to have 82° of extension and 17° of flexion.[66] The range will vary somewhat depending on the relative lengths of the metatarsals and whether the motions occur in weight-bearing or non-weight-bearing activities. The ROM of the first MTP has also been found to be influenced by the degree of dorsiflexion or plantarflexion of the TMT joints and to be more restricted with increasing age.[66] The MTP joints serve primarily to allow the foot to "hinge" at the toes so that the heel may rise off the ground while still maintaining the small but dynamic base of support afforded by the toes and the toe musculature. This function is enhanced by two structural aspects of the MTP joints: the **metatarsal break** and the effect of MTP extension on the **plantar aponeurosis.**

Extension

THE METATARSAL BREAK

The metatarsal break refers to the single oblique axis that lies through the second to fifth metatarsal heads and around which weight-bearing toe extension occurs. The inclination of the axis is produced by the diminishing lengths of the metatarsals from the second through the fifth toes and varies among individuals. The metatarsal break may range from 54° to 73° compared to the long axis of the foot.[1] It is called the break because it is where the foot hinges as the heel rises in weight-bearing.

For the weight-bearing heel to rise, there must be an active contraction of ankle plantarflexor musculature. Most of these muscles, as shall be discussed later, contribute to supination of the hindfoot and directly, or indirectly through the TCN, to transverse tarsal supination. The musculature cannot normally lift the body weight unless the joints of the hindfoot and midfoot are fully supinated and locked; that is, the heel will rise when the foot has become a rigid lever from the calcaneus through the metatarsals. The rigid lever will rotate around the metatarsal break (the MTP axis) (Fig. 12–22). During this period of MTP extension, the metatarsal heads glide in a posterior and plantar direction on the plantar plates and phalanges that are stabilized by the supporting surface. The toes become the base of support and the line of gravity of the body must move within this base to remain stable. The obliquity of the combined MTP joint axis serves the particular purpose of more evenly distributing the body weight across the toes than would occur if the axis were truly coronal. If the body weight passed forward through the foot and the foot lifted around a *coronal* MTP axis, an excessive amount of weight would be placed on the first metatarsal head and on the long second metatarsal. These two toes would also require a disproportionately large extension range. The obliquity of the metatarsal break shifts the weight laterally, minimizing the large load on the first two digits.

THE PLANTAR APONEUROSIS

The plantar aponeurosis is a dense fascia that runs nearly the entire length of the foot. It begins posteriorly on the calcaneus and continues anteriorly to attach by digitations to the plantar plates and then, via the plates, on to the proximal phalanx of each toe.[59,64] When the toes are extended at the MTP joints (regardless of whether the motion is active or passive, weight-bearing or non-weight-bearing), the aponeurosis is pulled increasingly tight as the proximal phalanges glide dorsally in relation to the metatarsals. The large metatarsal heads end up acting as pulleys around which the plantar aponeurosis is tightened. This role of the aponeurosis is supported by the finding of Deland and colleagues[64] that the fibrocartilage of the plantar plates is organized not only to resist weight-bearing compressive forces, but also to resist tensile stresses presumably applied through the tensed plantar aponeurosis. The tension in the plantar aponeurosis can contribute to supination of the foot as the heel is drawn toward the toes by its action (Fig. 12–23). When the joints of the hindfoot and midfoot supinate and lock through a strong active plantarflexion force in weight-bearing, continued force will cause the heel to lift and the toes to extend at the metatarsal break. The plantar aponeurosis will tighten as the MTPs extend, supporting the locked hindfoot and midfoot structures through which the body weight must pass to reach the toes. The tightened aponeurosis will also resist excessive toe extension by creating a passive flexor force across the MTP joint

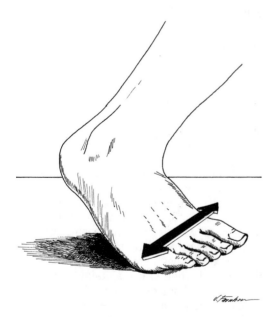

FIGURE 12–22. The metatarsal break distributes weight across the metatarsal heads as the heel lifts.

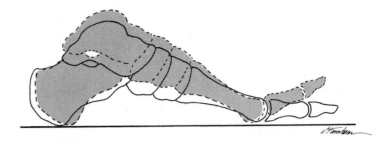

FIGURE 12–23. Elevation of the arch with toe extension occurs through the windlass effect of the metatarsophalangeal joints on the plantar aponeurosis.

as the structure tightens. The passive flexor force will assist the active toe musculature in pressing the toes into the ground to support the body weight on its now diminished base of support. The mechanism of the plantar aponeurosis is considered to be most effective at the first MTP and progressively less effective from the second to fifth MTPs.[67] The effect of MTP extension on the plantar aponeurosis will be further discussed when the arches of the foot are presented.

Flexion, Abduction, and Adduction

Flexion of the MTPs from neutral can occur to a limited degree but has relatively little use in the weight-bearing foot other than when the supporting terrain drops away distal to the metatarsal heads. Most MTP flexion occurs as a return to neutral from extension. Similarly, MTP abduction and adduction do not serve an obvious function. The joint motions apparently remain to absorb some of the force that would be imposed on the toes by the metatarsals as they move in a pronation or supination twist. The first toe is normally adducted on the first metatarsal about 15°.[62] An increase in this normal valgus angulation of the first MTP joint is referred to as **hallux valgus. Hallux valgus** may be associated with an index minus foot or with one of several other conditions, including a varus positioning of the first metatarsal (metatarsus varus). It can result in a reduction in ROM, gradual lateral subluxation of the flexor tendons crossing the first MTP and consequential shift of the weight-bearing load away from the first ray and toward the lesser toes. Exaggerated MTP abducted or adducted positions of the toes may also be seen when there are abduction or adduction deformities in bones or joints further back in the foot. The resultant MTP deviations may be an attempt to compensate toe position to prevent excessive weight on any one toe while also maintaining

the metatarsal break in an appropriate position for gait.

Interphalangeal Joints

The interphalangeal (IP) joints of the toes are synovial hinge joints with 1° of freedom: flexion/extension. There are five proximal IP joints and four distal IP joints. Each phalanx is virtually identical in structure to its counterpart in the hand, although substantially shorter in length. The toes function to smooth the weight shift to the opposite foot in gait and help maintain stability by pressing against the ground both in static posture when necessary, and in gait. The relative lengths of the toes may vary. The most common pattern is to find the first toe longer than the others (69% of individuals). The second toe may be longer than the first in 22% of the people, with 9% having first and second toes of equal lengths.[60] Viladot[60] has proposed that each configuration predisposes the foot to different problems, although the best configuration for modern footwear might be the index minus foot (second metatarsal shorter than the first) and a longer second toe.

Plantar Arches

The bony and ligamentous configuration of the TCN joint, the transverse tarsal joint, and the TMT joints combine to produce a structural vault within the foot. The MTP joints and toes are not part of the vault but, as shall be seen, may indirectly affect the shape of the vault when the plantar aponeurosis is tightened with MTP extension. Although we have examined the function of the joints of the foot individually and discussed the effect of each joint on contiguous joints, combined function is best investigated by looking at the behavior of the archlike structure of the foot.

The arch, or arches, of the foot can be described as a single twisted osteoligamentous plate (Fig. 12–24). The anterior margin of the plate (formed by the metatarsal heads) is horizontal and in full contact with the ground. The posterior margin of the plate (the posterior calcaneus) is vertical. The resulting twist in the plate between its horizontal and vertical margins imposes both longitudinal and transverse arcs.[1,68] Loading the plate (weight-bearing) will tend to untwist the plate, flattening the arches slightly. As the plate is unloaded (body weight removed), the resilient arches return to their original shape.

The actual mechanism of twisting and untwisting of the osteoligamentous plate occurs through motion at the TCN, transverse tarsal, and TMT joints that link the bones of the plate. The twisted plate, through its contributing joints, is a supporting mechanism designed to facilitate absorption and distribution of the superimposed body weight through the foot under changing weight-bearing conditions and changing terrain. Simkin and Leichter[69] note that the foot is capable of storing strain energy and releasing it in a "quasi-elastic" recoil that protects the bones of the lower limbs from stress fractures. The counterrotations that occur in twisting and untwisting of the plate appear to help maintain the superimposed leg in a vertical position while shock absorption takes place.[43] The adult configuration of the

arch is not present at birth, but evolves with the progression of weight-bearing. Gould and associates[70] found a flattened arch in all children examined between 11 and 14 months of age. By 5 years of age, as children approach more adult-like gait parameters, the majority of the children had developed an adult-like arch.

Structure

Although the concept of a single, twisted osteoligamentous plate gives the best representation of the vault of the adult foot, the vault more traditionally is considered to be composed of two different arches, the longitudinal and the transverse arches of the foot. The longitudinal arch has been described as an arch based posteriorly at the calcaneus and anteriorly at the metatarsal heads. The arch is continuous both medially and laterally through the foot, but because the arch is higher medially, the medial side is usually the side of reference (Fig. 12–25).

The transverse arch, like the longitudinal, is a continuous structure. It is easiest to visualize at the level of the anterior tarsals and at the bases of the metatarsals. At the anterior tarsals (Fig. 12–26a), the middle cuneiform forms the keystone of the arch. The arch continues distally to the metatarsals with slightly less curvature (Fig. 12–26b). The second metatarsal, recessed into its mortise, is at the apex of this arc. At the level of the metatarsal heads, the transverse arch is completely reduced with all metatarsal heads parallel to the weight-bearing surface.

The shape and arrangement of the bones are partially responsible for stability of the plantar arches. However, without additional support, the linkages of the arch would collapse and the plate would untwist. Because the plate can be thought of as one continuous set of interdependent linkages, support at one point in the plate may contribute to support throughout the plate. The plantar calcaneonavicular (spring) ligament, the interosseous talocalcaneal ligament, and the plantar aponeurosis have been credited with providing key passive support to the plate.[71,72] Because the superomedial portion of the calcaneonavicular ligament appears to directly support the head of the talus[54] and the cervical ligament (sometimes included as part of the interosseous talocalcaneal ligament) is thicker and stronger than its more medially located counterpart, we might add these

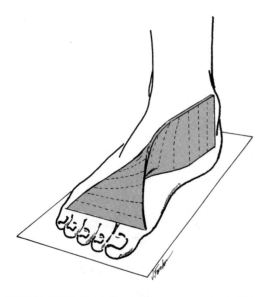

FIGURE 12–24. Twisted osteoligamentous plate of the foot, resulting in longitudinal and transverse arches.[18]

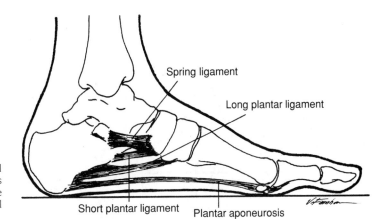

FIGURE 12–25. Medial longitudinal arch with its associated ligamentous support. (The plantar ligaments are projected through from the lateral side of the foot.)

structures to key supporting elements. Support from the long and short plantar ligaments appeared to be less influential.[71] The secondary supporting role of the long and short plantar ligaments may be because the weight-bearing compression through the calcaneocuboid joint crossed by these ligaments is only half that encountered by the talonavicular joint.[73]

Although other passive structures contribute to arch support, the role of the plantar aponeurosis is unique. The plantar aponeurosis spans the entire length of the twisted plate as it runs from posterior calcaneus to the bases of the proximal phalanges of the toes. The function of the aponeurosis has been likened to the function of a tie-rod on a truss.[55] The truss and the tie-rod form a triangle; the two struts of the truss form the sides of the triangle and the tie-rod is the bottom. The talus and calcaneus form the posterior strut, and the anterior strut is formed by the remaining tarsal and the metatarsals (Fig. 12–27). The plantar aponeurosis, as does the tie-rod, holds together the anterior and posterior struts when the body weight is loaded on the triangle. The struts in weight-bearing are subjected to compression forces while the tie-rod is subjected to tension forces. Increasing the load on the truss, or actually causing flattening of the triangle, will increase tension in the tie-rod.

The tension in the plantar aponeurosis in the loaded foot is evident if active or passive MTP extension is attempted while the triangle is flattened. The range of MTP extension will be limited. Conversely, raising the height of the triangle independent of the truss can unload the tie-rod. For example, when the tibia is subjected to a lateral rotatory force, the hindfoot will supinate and the plantar aponeurosis will be unloaded. With the reduction in tension in the plantar aponeurosis, the range of available toe hyperextension will increase. Finally, increasing tension in the tie-rod independent of loading the foot will draw the two struts of the truss together, shortening and raising the triangle. This phenomenon can occur when the MTP joints are extended. Whether the toes are extending with the distal lever free or the toes are

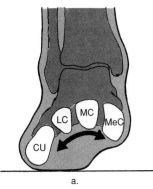
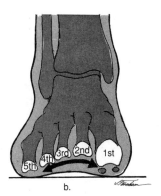

FIGURE 12–26. The transverse arch. (a) At the level of the anterior tarsals. (b) At the level of the middle of the metatarsals. (CU, cuboid; MeC, medial cuneiform; MC, middle cuneiform; LC, lateral cuneiform.)

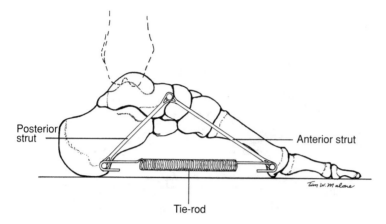

Posterior strut

Anterior strut

Tie-rod

FIGURE 12–27. The foot can be considered to function as a truss and tie-rod, with the calcaneus and talus serving as the posterior strut, the remainder of the tarsals and the metatarsals serving as the anterior strut, and the plantar aponeurosis serving as a tensed tie-rod. Weighting of the foot will compress the struts and create additional tension in the tie-rod.

being extended as the heel rises in weight-bearing, the aponeurosis is pulled tighter and the arch can be raised simply through an increase in passive tension in the aponeurosis. Through the mechanism of the plantar aponeurosis, the MTP joints (not actually part of the osteoligamentous plate) act interdependently with the joints of the hindfoot and may contribute to supination of the foot through the effect of MTP extension on the plantar aponeurosis.

Muscle activity appears to contribute little support to the osteoligamentous plate in the normal *static* foot.[68] In gait, however, both the longitudinally and transversely oriented muscles become active and contribute to support of the twisted plate. Key muscular support appears to be provided during gait by the tibialis posterior, with contributions also made by the flexor digitorum longus, the flexor hallucis longus, and the peroneous longus.[72] Muscle activity can either concentrically increase the twist in the plate or eccentrically control some untwisting of the resilient plate to absorb shock and allow the foot to conform to an uneven supporting surface.

Function

Although the archlike structure of the foot is similar to the structure of the palmar arches of the hand, the purpose served by each of these systems is quite different. The arches of the hand are predominantly structured to facilitate grasp and manipulation, but must also assist the hand in some weight-bearing functions. In contrast, the foot in most individuals is rarely called on to perform any grasp activities. The plantar arches are adapted exclusively to serve the weight-bearing functions of the foot. The

following *stability* functions could be performed by a foot with a fixed arch structure: (1) distribution of weight through the foot for proper weight-bearing and (2) conversion of the foot to a rigid lever. However, the following *mobility* functions can only be performed by a nonrigid structure: (1) dampening the shock of weight-bearing; (2) adapting to changes in the supporting surface; and (3) dampening superimposed rotations.

Weight Distribution

Because the foot is *not* a fixed arch, the distribution of body weight through the foot depends on the shape of the arch and the location of the line of gravity at a given moment. Consistently, however, distribution of superimposed body weight begins with the talus, because the body of the talus receives all the weight that passes down through the leg. In bilateral stance each talus receives 50% of the body weight; in unilateral stance, the weight-bearing talus receives 100% of the superimposed body weight. In static unilateral or bilateral stance, at least 50% of the weight received by the talus passes through the posterior subtalar articulation to the calcaneus, and 50% or less passes anteriorly through the TCN and calcaneocuboid joints to the forefoot. The pattern of weight distribution can be seen easily by looking at the trabeculae in the bones of the foot (Fig. 12–28). Because of the more medial location of the talar head, twice as much weight passes through the talonavicular joint as through the calcaneocuboid. The weight-bearing at the anterior margin of the osteoligamentous plate follows a similar pattern. In static standing, the distribution of weight at

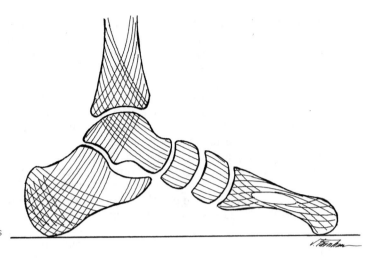

FIGURE 12–28. Trabeculae of the bones on the medial aspect of the foot.

the metatarsal heads occurs in a 2:1:1:1:1 proportion from the first ray medially to the fifth ray laterally.[74] The load-bearing function of the metatarsal heads changes during gait, although with considerable variability. Weight-bearing at each head increases as the metatarsal break is approached,[32] with weight on the second through fourth metatarsal heads generally exceeding that on the first and fifth.[75]

The large amount of weight imposed on the calcaneus in both static standing and in gait is partially dissipated by the heel pad, which lies on the plantar surface of the calcaneus. The heel pad is composed of fat cells that are located in chambers formed by fibrous septa attached to the calcaneus above and the skin below. The role of the heel pad is even more critical in gait when the loads on the calcaneus at contact of the heel will vary from 85% to 100% of body weight. Running may increase this force to 250% of body weight. The effectiveness of the cushioning action of the heel pad decreases with age and with concomitant loss of collagen, elastic tissue, and water. The change is evident in most people past 40 years of age.[10,76]

Mobility

The mobility component of weight distribution through the foot (shock absorption) and adaptation to the terrain can be seen in the response of the linkages and supporting structures of the arches to loading of the foot. In non-weight-bearing position, the subtalar/TCN joint is normally slightly supinated and the transverse tarsal joint is neutral. With weight-bearing, the osteoligamentous plate is loaded. The response to loading of the plate is eversion (valgus) of the calcaneus and adduction and plantarflexion of the head of the talus. The talar motion causes slight depression (anterior/inferior movement) of the navicular. Further depression of the talar head is checked by tension in the supporting structures of the arch. If no more than the body weight is introduced (such as in static bilateral stance), the TCN joint pronates to a neutral position and the transverse tarsal joint pronates fully.[46] The net effect is to absorb some of the shock of the superimposed weight through compression of cartilage at the weight-bearing joints, through untwisting of the plate and through elasticity of supporting structures. If the ground is not level and forefoot pronation is required, pronation twist of the forefoot at the TMTs can be called on before the hindfoot is forced to pronate further (maximally untwisting the plate). If there is a supination demand on the forefoot, both the transverse tarsal and TMT joints are available to respond before the hindfoot must begin to reverse its pronation position. Given the resiliency of the supporting structures of the arches, unloading the foot will restore the original arch and joint alignment once again.

The ability of the foot to absorb rotations of the leg is considered a mobility function. This is clear when twist of the tibia is a medial rotatory force. Not only does the TCN pronate in response, but the foot retains its ability to contour itself to other possible demands of the terrain. However, when the tibia is torsioned laterally, the absorption response of the TCN simultaneously locks the foot and severely limits the foot's ability to respond to changes in the terrain. The TCN joint will supinate as will the transverse tarsal joint. The TMT joint will undergo a pronation twist to maintain the metatarsal heads on the ground and the osteoligamentous plate will increase its twist. Although the tibial rotation has been absorbed, the plate cannot be twisted any further and is not mobile. The TMTs are free to respond *only* to a change in terrain requiring a supination twist that would unwind the plate slightly. Any other terrain change would tip the entire twisted plate laterally or require unlocking of the hindfoot and reversal of the lateral rotatory force on the tibia.

Muscles of the Ankle and Foot

There are no muscles in the ankle or foot that cross and act on only one joint. All act on at least two joints or joint complexes. Muscle activity will produce joint actions that are dependent on the angle of pull of the muscle in relation to the joint axis. In the foot, a joint may be intersected by two axes, and the instantaneous axis of rotation may vary considerably between extremes of joint range. Muscle action is further complicated by the interdependent nature of the ankle-foot joints. Therefore, although a brief review of muscle function is presented, muscle activity is best examined in the context of actual function in posture and in gait.

Extrinsic Musculature

Ankle Plantarflexors

The gastrocnemius muscle arises from two heads of origin on the condyles of the femur and inserts via the achilles (calcaneal) tendon into the most posterior aspect of the calcaneus. The soleus muscle is deep to the gastrocnemius, originating on the tibia and fibula and inserting with the gastrocnemius into the posterior calcaneus. The two heads of the gastrocnemius and the soleus muscles together are known as the **triceps surae** and are the main plantarflexors of the ankle. The achilles tendon occupies a position on the calcaneus that is far from the ankle axis and provides a large moment arm (MA) for plantarflexion. The achilles tendon also crosses the TCN joint and, therefore, acts on it. The resultant combined action line of the gastrocnemius and soleus muscles is generally considered

to pass just medial to the axes of the subtalarTCN joints, with activity of the gastrocnemius and soleus muscle each producing strong hindfoot supination.[2,5,35,76] Activity of the gastrocnemius and soleus on the weight-bearing foot will lock the foot into a rigid lever both through direct supination of the TCN and through indirect supination of the transverse tarsal joint. Continued plantarflexion force will raise the heel and cause elevation of the arch. The elevation of the arch by the triceps surae is easily observable in most people when they actively plantarflex the weight-bearing foot (Fig. 12–29). Elevation of the arch occurs through the twisting of the osteoligamentous plate as the hindfoot is supinated and through tightening of the plantar aponeurosis with MTP joint extension.

Some controversy about the role of the triceps surae at the TCN exists. Klein and colleagues[77] found a large intraindividual variation in the moment arm size and relative position of the line of pull of the triceps surae to the subtalar axis. They concluded in their cadaver study that the triceps surae were supinators when the subtalar joint was pronated and pronators when the subtalar joint was supinated. Thordarson and colleagues,[72] also using cadavers, attrib-

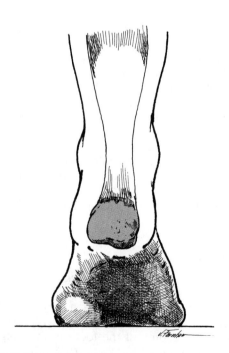

FIGURE 12–29. Activity of the triceps surae muscles on the fixed foot will cause ankle plantarflexion, talocalcaneonavicular supination, and elevation of the longitudinal arch.

uted an arch flattening effect to the triceps surae. Although activity of the triceps surae in living individuals appears to be consistently associated with TCN supination, it must be acknowledged that function of the triceps surae at the TCN may differ among individuals, especially if the TCN is abnormally pronated or supinated.

The other ankle plantarflexion muscles are the **plantaris,** the tibialis posterior, the flexor hallucis longus, the flexor digitorum longus, and the peroneus longus and brevis muscles. Although each of these muscles passes posterior to the ankle axis, the MA for plantarflexion for these muscles is so small that they provide only 5% of the total plantarflexor force at the ankle.[2] The plantaris muscle is so weak that its function can essentially be disregarded.

The tibialis posterior muscle is predominantly a supinator of the foot. It has a large MA for both TCN and transverse tarsal joint supination,[77] although its relatively small cross-sectional area enables it to produce only half the supination torque of the soleus muscle.[76] The tibialis posterior is credited with a being an important dynamic contributor to arch support and with having a significant role in controlling and reversing the pronation of the foot that occurs during gait.[2,72,77] Tibialis posterior dysfunction may be a key element leading to acquired flatfoot.[72]

The flexor hallucis longus and the flexor digitorum longus muscles both span the medial longitudinal arch and help support the arch during gait. These muscles attach to the distal phalanges of each digit and, through their actions, cause the toes to flex. Flexion of the IP joint of the hallux by the flexor hallucis longus muscles produces a press of the toe against the ground (Fig. 12–30a). Flexion of the distal and proximal IP joints of the four lesser toes by the flexor digitorum longus causes a gripping action that may produce a clawing (MTP extension with IP flexion) similar to what occurs in the fingers when the proximal phalanx is not stabilized by intrinsic musculature (Fig. 12–30b). As is true in the hand, activity of the interossei muscles can stabilize the MTP joint and prevent MTP hyperextension.

The peroneus longus and brevis muscles are the primary pronators of the TCN, each having a significant MA.[77] Although the MA for subtalar pronation is small, the peroneus longus will plantarflex and pronate the first ray to which it attaches. This action facilitates transfer of weight from the lateral to the medial side of the foot and stabilizes the first ray as the ground reaction force attempts to dorsiflex it. The peroneus longus muscle is also credited with support of the transverse and lateral longitudinal arches.[35] This appears to be contradictory to its function as a pronator, but the tendon of the peroneus longus spans the tarsals transversely and passes under the cuboid, thus helping to limit its depression (Fig. 12–31). Similarly, the peroneus longus can assist with pronation twist of the forefoot when the hindfoot is supinated; this increases the twist in the osteoligamentous plate. The stability of each of the peroneal tendons depends on integrity of the superior and inferior peroneal retinacula. Sprains of the lateral ankle structures may affect the peroneal retinacula that contribute to lateral ankle and subtalar support. Laxity of the superior retinaculum in particular may lead to subluxation of peroneal tendons and to splitting of the peroneus brevis from its unchecked excursion over the fibular malleolus.[13]

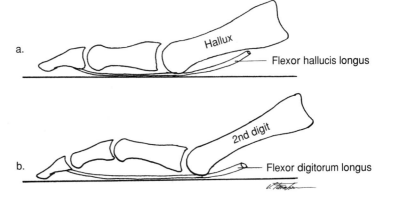

FIGURE 12–30. (a) Action of the flexor hallucis longus causes the distal phalanx of the hallux to press against the ground. (b) Activity of the flexor digitorum longus causes the four lesser toes to grip the ground.

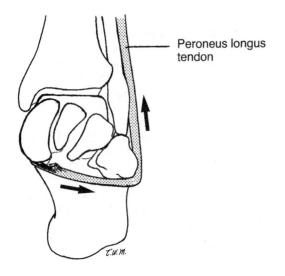

Peroneus longus
tendon

FIGURE 12–31. The tendon of the peroneus longus passes transversely beneath the foot. An active contraction of the muscle can support the transverse arch of the foot and therefore the twisted osteoligamentous plate.

Ankle Dorsiflexors

The dorsiflexor muscles of the ankle are the tibialis anterior, the extensor hallucis longus, the extensor digitorum longus, and the **peroneus tertius** muscles. The tibialis anterior and the extensor hallucis longus muscles are both strong dorsiflexors of the ankle and may also weakly supinate the TCN joint. The tibialis anterior and extensor hallucis longus are the only supinators that are active when the heel first contacts the ground in gait, a period when there is a strong pronation force on the hindfoot. The tibialis anterior, however, can exert only slightly more than half the supination force of the tibialis posterior.[76] The extensor hallucis longus is a weaker supinator than is the tibialis anterior.[5] The supination action of the tibialis anterior muscle may reverse if the line of pull falls to the lateral side of the subtalar joint axis, as it may in excessive foot pronation. The extensor hallucis longus also extends the MTP joints of the hallux. When the extensor hallucis longus attempts to dorsiflex the foot without the assistance of the tibialis anterior, the first toe will tend to claw simultaneously.

The extensor digitorum longus and the peroneus tertius muscles are relatively weak dorsiflexors of the ankle and pronators of the foot. The extensor digitorum longus also extends the MTP joints of the lesser toes. Its structure and function at the MTP and IP joints are identical to that of the extensor digitorum of the hand. Taken together, the musculature that produces supination of the foot is stronger than that producing pronation. This is why the relaxed and unweighted foot returns to a posi-

Table 12–3. **Intrinsic Muscles of the Foot**

Muscle	Function	Analog in Hand
Extensor digitorum brevis	Extends the MTP joints	None
Abductor hallucis	Abducts and flexes MTP of hallux	Abductor pollicis brevis
Flexor digitorum brevis	Flexes PIP of four lesser toes	Flexor digitorum superficialis*
Abductor digiti minimi	Abducts and flexes small toe	Abductor digiti minimi
Quadratus plantae	Adjusts oblique pull of flexor digitorum longus into line with long axes of digits	None
Lumbricals	Flex MTPs, extend IPs of four lesser toes	Lumbricals
Flexor hallucis brevis	Flexes MTP of hallux	Flexor pollicis brevis
Adductor hallucis	Oblique head: adducts and flexes MTP of hallux	Adductor pollicis
	Transverse head: adducts metatarsal heads transversely	
Flexor digiti minimi	Flexes MTP of small toe	Flexor digiti minimi
Plantar interossei	Adduct MTPs of 3rd–5th toes, flex MTPs, extend IPs of four lesser toes	Volar interossei
Dorsal interossei	Abduct MTPs of 2nd toe (either way), abduct MTPs, 3rd and 4th toes, flex MTPs, extend IPs of four lesser toes	Dorsal interossei

*The flexor digitorum superficialis is an extrinsic muscle, whereas the flexor digitorum brevis is an intrinsic foot muscle. MTP, metatarsophalangeal; PIP, proximal interphalangeal; IP, interphalangeal.

tion of slight subtalar inversion and a neutral transverse tarsal joint.

Intrinsic Musculature

The function of the intrinsic muscles of the foot can best be understood and appreciated by comparing each foot muscle with its corresponding hand muscle. Although most people are not able to use the muscles of the foot with the facility of those in the hand, the potential for similar function is limited only by the unopposable hallux and the length of the digits. The intrinsic muscles of the foot most often are relegated to their roles as stabilizers of the toes and as *important dynamic supporters of the transverse and longitudinal arches during gait*. The intrinsics of the hallux attach either directly or indirectly to the sesamoids and contribute to the stabilization of these weight-bearing bones.[61] The extensor mechanism of the toes is essentially the same as that of the fingers. The extensor digitorum longus and brevis are MTP extensors. Activity in the **lumbricals** and the **dorsal and plantar interossei musculature** maintains or produces IP extension. Perhaps more importantly, the toe intrinsics (as MTP flexors) can eccentrically assist in control of the toe extension produced indirectly by the ankle plantarflexors.[78] Table 12–3 summarizes the functions of the intrinsic muscles of the foot.

Deviations from Normal Structure and Function

The complex interdependency of the joints of the ankle and foot make it almost impossible to have dysfunction or abnormality in only one joint or structure. Once present, deviations from normal will affect both proximal and distal joints. The large number of congenital and acquired problems cannot each be described, but two examples of the "domino effect" of deformity will be given.

Flatfoot (Pes Planus)

The key to the foot in both function and dysfunction are the joints of the hindfoot. A pronated or flat foot (**pes valgus** or **pes planus**) is marked by excessive unwinding of the osteoligamentous plate with weight-bearing. The pronated position of the TCN-subtalar and the

transverse tarsal joints create (or result from) a medial rotatory stress on the leg. The medial rotatory stress or position of excessive medial rotation of the leg may result in several possible problems around the knee joint, including excessive angulation of the patellar tendon and excessive pressure on the lateral patellar facet. The lowering of the arch that accompanies TCN and transverse tarsal joint pronation may result in a functional leg length inequality if the problem is asymmetrical. Pronation of the subtalar joint can lower the ankle joint axis and result in a slight reduction in overall limb length.[79] Lowering the arch also tenses the plantar ligaments and the plantar aponeurosis (the tie-rods of the triangle). Prolonged stress on these structures can result in a cycle of microtears, pain, and inflammation.

With hindfoot pronation, the forefoot must adjust by supinating at the TMT joints. If adaptive tissue changes result in a sustained TMT supination, this is known as **forefoot varus** (effectively the same as supination twist). Forefoot varus is presumably diagnosed by assessing the position of the forefoot *relative to* the transverse plane in the subtalar neutral position of the hindfoot (typically in non-weight-bearing). Using this method of assessment, however, led some investigators to a diagnosis of forefoot varus in the majority of a large sample of normal individuals.[45,80] This finding calls to question either the method of ascertaining subtalar neutral (as noted earlier in this chapter) or argues against presuming that the forefoot should have a fixed relationship to the hindfoot for a foot to be considered normal.[45,80]

With the forefoot varus (supination twist) that might be expected to accompany an excessively pronated hindfoot, excessive dorsiflexion of the first ray may prevent shift of some of its normal weight-bearing support to the more laterally located rays.[60] The supinated position of the first ray that occurs with first ray dorsiflexion may also create additional valgus stress at the first MTP, resulting in a hallux valgus. Hallux valgus, in turn, changes the line of pull of the flexor muscles of the first toe and may affect the power of push-off in the final stages of stance.

The most common form of flatfoot is termed a **flexible flatfoot** and is marked by an arch that reappears when the foot is non-weight-bearing. Treatment is focused around prevention of excessive pronation when the foot is loaded by controlling valgus (eversion) of the calcaneus.

If this can be done, the cycle of tension in the passive structures can be interrupted and the effects on other segments of the closed chain reduced or eradicated.

Supinated Foot (Pes Cavus)

A less common but potentially more serious problem exists when the weight-bearing foot is excessively supinated (a cavus foot). In a cavus foot, the TCN-subtalar and transverse tarsal joints may be locked into supination, prohibiting these joints from participating in shock absorption or in adapting to uneven terrain. The hindfoot supination that results in added twist in the osteoligamentous plate may cause or be caused by a lateral rotatory stress on the leg. The lateral rotatory stress may, in turn, affect knee joint structures. The inability to absorb additional limb rotations across the hindfoot puts a strain on the ankle joint structures, especially the lateral collateral ligaments. The plantar aponeurosis remains slack and may adaptively shorten over time. The TMTs must undergo a pronation twist to maintain appropriate weight-bearing of the forefoot. This may result in chronic plantarflexion of the first ray. There is not an effective conservative intervention for a cavus foot as there is for a flexible flatfoot. The only exception would be in an instance where there is a correctable rotatory deficit in one of the superimposed leg segments and where secondary changes in the bones or soft tissue structures of the foot have not occurred.

Summary

Both function and dysfunction of the numerous structures and joints making up the foot and ankle are complex. It is frequently difficult to determine whether problems are primary or are secondary to problems proximal or distal to the site of pain. Regardless, increased participation in sports will inevitably result in an increased number of people seeking medical attention for foot and ankle problems. Offsetting this trend somewhat is the improving research and technology associated with footwear. It is unlikely, however, that even the most sophisticated footwear will be able to take into simultaneous consideration the many mobility and stability demands of the joints of the lower extremity, including the large number of individ-

ual differences. We will come back to the ankle and foot again as we examine the influence of these joints on both posture and gait.

REFERENCES

1. Morris, J: Biomechanics of the foot and ankle. Clin Orthop 122:10, 1977.
2. Cailliet, R: Foot and Ankle Pain, ed 3. FA Davis, Philadelphia, 1997.
3. Eichenblat, M, and Nathan, H: The proximal tibiofibular joint. Int Orthop (SICOT) 7:31–39, 1983.
4. Barnett, C, and Napier, J: The axis of rotation at the ankle joint in man: Its influence upon the form of the talus and mobility of the fibula. J Anat 86:1, 1952.
5. Kapandji, I: The Physiology of the Joints, Vol. 2, ed 5. Williams & Wilkins, Baltimore, 1987.
6. Rosse, D, and Clawson, DE: The leg, ankle and foot. In The Musculoskeletal System in Health and Disease. Harper & Row, Hagerstown, Md., 1980.
7. Rasmussen, O, et al: Distal tibiofibular ligaments. Acta Orthop Scand 53:681–686, 1982.
8. Takebe, K, et al: Role of the fibula in weight-bearing. Clin Orthop 184:2899–2892, 1984.
9. Segal, D, et al: The role of the lateral malleolus as a stabilizing factor of the ankle joint: A preliminary report. Foot Ankle 2:25–29, 1981.
10. Nuber, G: Biomechanics of the foot and ankle during gait. Clin Sports Med 7:1–12, 1988.
11. Earll, M, et al: Contribution of the deltoid ligament to ankle joint contact characteristics: A cadaver study. Clin Sports Med 17:317–324, 1996.
12. Stephens, M, and Sammarco, G: The stabilizing role of the lateral ligament complex around the ankle and subtalar joints. Foot Ankle 13:130–136, 1992.
13. Geppert, M, et al: Lateral ankle instability as a cause of superior peroneal retinacular laxity: An anatomic and biomechanical study of cadaveric feet. Foot Ankle 14:330–334, 1993.
14. Sarrafian, S: Biomechanics of the subtalar joint. Clin Orthop 290:17–26, 1993.
15. Kjaersgaard-Anderson, P, et al: Lateral talocalcaneal instability following section of the calcaneofibular ligament: A kinesiologic study. Foot Ankle 7:355–361, 1987.
16. Johnson, E, and Markolf, K: The contribution of the anterior talofibular ligament to ankle laxity. J Bone Joint Surg 44A:81–88, 1983.
17. Rasmussen, O, and Kromann-Andersen, C: Experimental ankle injuries. Acta Orthop Scand 54:356–362, 1983.
18. Bahr, R, et al: Ligament force and joint motion in the intact ankle: A cadaveric study. Knee Surg Sports Traumatol Arthrosc 6:115–121, 1998.
19. Rasmussen, O, and Touberg-Jensen, I: Mobility of the ankle joint: recording of rotatory movements in the talocrural joint in vitro with and without the lateral collateral ligaments of the ankle. Acta Orthop Scand 53:155–160, 1982.
20. Rasmussen, O, et al: An analysis of the function of the posterior talofibular ligament. Int Orthop (SICOT) 7:41–48, 1983.
21. Siegler, S, et al: The three dimensional kinematics and flexibility characteristics of the human ankle and sutalar joints—part I. Biomech Eng 110:364–373, 1988.
22. Lundberg, A: Kinematics of the ankle/foot complex: Plantarflexion and dorsiflexion. Foot Ankle 9:194–200, 1989.
23. Lundberg, A, et al: Kinematics of the ankle/foot com-

plex—part 3: Influence of leg rotation. Foot Ankle 9:304–309, 1989.

24. Lundberg, A, et al: Kinematics of the ankle/foot complex—part 2: Pronation and supination. Foot Ankle 9:245–253, 1989.

25. Lundberg, A, et al: The axis of rotation of the ankle joint. J Bone Joint Surg 71B(1):194–200, 1989.

26. Hicks, J: Mechanics of the foot I: The joints. J Anat 87:345, 1953.

27. Stiehl, J. Biomechanics of the ankle joint. In Stiehl, J (ed): Inman's Joints of the Ankle. Williams & Wilkins, Baltimore, 1991.

28. Inman, V, and Mann R: Biomechanics of the foot and ankle. In Mann, R (ed): Duvries Surgery of the Foot. CV Mosby, St. Louis, 1978.

29. Stiehl, J. Anthropomorphic studies of the ankle joint. In Stiehl, J (ed): Inman's Joints of the Ankle. Williams & Wilkins, Baltimore, 1991.

30. Johnson, J. Shape of the trochlea and mobility of the lateral malleolus. In Stiehl, J (ed): Inman's Joints of the Ankle. Williams & Wilkins, Baltimore, 1991.

31. Sammarcho, W, et al: Biomechanics of the ankle: A kinematic study. Orthop Clin North Am 4:76, 1973.

32. Scott, S, and Winter, D: Biomechanic model of the human foot: Kinematics and kinetics during the stance phase of walking. J Biomech 26:1091–1104, 1993.

33. Stauffer, R, et al: Force and motion analysis of normal, diseased and prosthetic ankle joints. Clin Orthop 127:189, 1977.

34. Wang, C, et al: Contact areas and pressure distributions in the subtalar joint. J Biomech 28:269–279, 1995.

35. Czerniecki, J: Foot and ankle biomechanics in walking and running. Am J Phys Med Rehabil 67(6):246–252, 1988.

36. Greenwald, AS, and Matejczyk, MB: Pathomechanics of the human ankle joint. Bull Hosp Joint Dis 38:105, 1977.

37. Hornsby, T, et al: Effect of inherent muscle length on isometric plantar flexion torque in healthy women. Phys Ther 67:1191–1196, 1987.

38. Viladot, A, et al: The subtalar joint: Embryology and morphology. Foot Ankle 5:54–65, 1984.

39. Harper, M: The lateral ligamentous support of the subtalar joint. Foot Ankle 11:354–358, 1991.

40. Martin, L, et al: Elongation behavior of the calcaneofibular and cervical ligaments during inversion loads applied in an open kinetic chain. Foot Ankle Int 19:232–239, 1998.

41. Manter, J: Movements of the subtalar and transverse tarsal joints. Anat Rec 80:397, 1941.

42. Sangeorzan, B: In Stiehl, J (ed): Inman's Joints of the Ankle. Williams & Wilkins, Baltimore, 1991.

43. Scott, S, and Winter, D: Talocrural and talocalcaneal joint kinematics and kinetcs during the stance phase of walking. J Biomech 24:743–752, 1991.

44. Inman, J: Joints of the Ankle. Williams & Wilkins, Baltimore, 1976.

45. Åstrom, M, and Arvidson, T: Alignment and joint motion in the normal foot. J Orthop Sports Phys Ther 22:216–222, 1995.

46. Root, M, et al: Normal and Abnormal Function of the Foot: Clinical Biomechanics, Vol II. Clinical Biomechanics Corp, Los Angeles, 1977.

47. Bailey, D, et al: Subtalar joint neutral. J Am Podiatr Assoc 74:59–64, 1984.

48. Elveru, R, et al: Goniometric reliability in a clinical setting. Subtalar and ankle joint measurements. Phys Ther 6:672–677, 1988.

49. McPoil, T, and Cornwall, M: Relationship between neutral subtalar joint position and pattern of rearfoot motion during walking. Foot Ankle 15:141–145, 1994.

50. Close, J, et al: The function of the subtalar joint. Clin Orthop 50:59, 1967.

51. Sgarlato, T: The angle of gait. Phys Ther 55:645, 1965.

52. Williams, P (ed): Gray's Anatomy, ed 38. Churchill Livingstone, New York, 1995.

53. Elftman, H: The transverse tarsal joint and its control. Clin Orthop 16:41–45, 1960.

54. Davis, W, et al: Gross, histological, and microvascular anatomy and biomechanical testing of the spring ligament complex. Foot Ankle 17:95–102, 1996.

55. Lapidus, P: Kinesiology and mechanical anatomy of the transverse tarsal joints. Clin Orthop 30:20, 1963.

56. Reeck, J, et al: Support of the talus: a biomechanical investigation of the contributions of the talonavicular and talocalcaneal joints, and the superomedial calcaneonavicular ligament. Foot Ankle Int 19:674–682, 1998.

57. Inkster, R: Inversion and eversion of the foot and the transverse tarsal joints. J Anat 72:612, 1938.

58. Lewis, O: The joints of the evolving foot. Part II: The intrinsic joints. J Anat 130:833–857, 1980.

59. Stainsby, G: Pathological anatomy and dynamic effect of the dsiplaced plantar plate and the importance of the integrity of the plantar plate-deep transverse metatarsal ligament tie-bar. Ann R Coll Surg Engl 79:58–68, 1997.

60. Viladot, A: Metatarsalgia due to biomechanical alterations of the forefoot. Orthop Clin North Am 4:165–178, 1973.

61. McCarthy, D, and Grode, SE: The anatomical relationships of the first metatarsophalangeal joint: A cryomicrotomy study. J Am Podiatr Assoc 70:493–504, 1980.

62. Yoshioka, Y, et al: Geometry of the first metatarsophalangeal joint. J Orthop Res 6:878–885, 1988.

63. Shereff, M: Pathophysiology, anatomy and biomechanics of hallux valgus. Orthopaedics 13:939–945, 1990.

64. Deland, J, et al: Anatomy of the plantar plate and its attachments in the lesser metatarsal phalangeal joint. Foot Ankle 16:480–486, 1995.

65. Bhatia, E, et al: Anatomical restraints to dislocation of the second metatarsophalangeal joint and assessment of a repair technique. J Bone Joint Surg 76A:1371–1375, 1994.

66. Buell, T, et al: Measurement of the first metatarsophalangeal joint range of motion. J Am Podiatr Med Assoc 78:439–448, 1988.

67. Mann, R: Foot problems in adults. AAOS Instructional Course Lectures 31:167–180, 1982.

68. MacConaill, M, and Basmajian, J: Muscles and Movement: A Basis for Human Kinesiology. Williams & Wilkins, Baltimore, 1969.

69. Simkin, A, Leichter, I: Role of the calcaneal inclination in the energy storage capacity of the human foot—a biomechanical model. Med Biol Eng Comput 28:149–152, 1990.

70. Gould, N, et al: Development of the child's arch. Foot Ankle 9:241–245, 1989.

71. Kitaoka, H, et al: Stability of the arch of the foot. Foot Ankle Int 1:644–648, 1997.

72. Thordarson, D, et al: Dynamic support of the human longitudinal arch. Clin Orthop 316:165–172, 1995.

73. Sarrafian, S: Functional characteristics of the foot and plantar aponeurosis under tibiotalar loading. Foot Ankle 8:4–18, 1987.

74. Manter, J: Distribution of compression forces in joint of the human foot. Anat Rec 96:313, 1946.

75. Luger, E, et al: Patterns of weight distribution under the metatarsal heads. J Bone Joint Surg 81B:199–202, 1999.
76. Perry, J: Anatomy and biomechanics of the hind foot. Clin Orthop 177:7–15, 1983.
77. Klein, P, et al: Moment arm length variations of selected muscles acting on talocrural and subtalar joints during movement: an in vitro study. J Biomech 29:21–30, 1996.
78. Kalin, P, and Hirsch, B: The origins and function of the interosseous muscles of the foot. J Anat 152:83–91, 1987.
79. Sanner, W, et al: A study of ankle joint height changes with subtalar joint motion. J Am Podiatr Soc 71:156–161, 1981.
80. Garbalosa, J, et al: The frontal plane relationship of the forefoot to the rearfoot in an asymptomatic population. J Orthop Sports Phys Ther 20:200–206, 1994.

Study Questions

1. Identify the proximal and distal articular surfaces that comprise the ankle (talocrural) joint. What is the joint classification?
2. Describe the proximal and distal tibiofibular joints, including classification and their composite function.
3. Identify the ligaments that support the tibiofibular joints.
4. Describe the ligaments that support the ankle joint, including the names of components, when relevant.
5. Why is ankle joint motion considered triplanar?
6. Why does the fibula move during dorsiflexion/plantarflexion of the ankle?
7. What are the primary checks to ankle joint motion?
8. Which muscles crossing the ankle are single-joint muscles?
9. Describe the three articular surfaces of the subtalar joint, including the capsular arrangement.
10. Which ligaments support the subtalar joint?
11. Describe the axis for subtalar motion. What movements take place around that axis and how are these motions defined?
12. When the foot is weight-bearing, the calcaneus (the distal segment) of the subtalar joint is not free to move in all directions. Describe the movements that take place during weight-bearing subtalar supination/pronation.
13. What is the close-packed position for the subtalar joint? Which motion of the tibia will lock the weight-bearing subtalar joint?
14. Describe the relationship between the subtalar and the TCN joint with regard to articular surfaces, axes, and available motion.
15. Describe the articulations of the transverse tarsal joint.
16. What is the general function of the transverse tarsal joint in relation to the subtalar joint?
17. What are the TMT rays? Describe the axis for each ray and the movements that occur around each axis.
18. What is the function of the TMT joints in relation to the TCN and the transverse tarsal joints?
19. How does pronation twist of the TMT joints relate to supination of the subtalar joint?
20. What ligaments contribute to support of the osteoligamentous arch of the foot?
21. What is the weight distribution through the various joints from the ankle through the metatarsal heads in unilateral stance?
22. How does extension of the MTPs contribute to stability of the foot?
23. In terms of structure, compare the MTPs of the foot to the MCPs of the fingers.
24. What is the metatarsal break? What function does it serve and when does this function occur?
25. What is the role of the triceps surae muscle group at each joint it crosses?
26. What is the non-weight-bearing posture of the subtalar (TCN) and transverse tarsal joints?
27. What other muscles besides the triceps surae exert a plantarflexion influence at the ankle? What is the primary function of each of these muscles?
28. Which muscles may contribute to support of the arch(es) of the foot?
29. What is the function of the quadratus plantae? What is the analog of this muscle in the hand?
30. Drawing an analogy between the foot and the hand, describe the function of each of the intrinsic and extrinsic foot muscles.
31. If a person has a pes planus, describe two possible causes for this condition.
32. Identify at least three possible effects of pes planus.

CHAPTER 13
POSTURE

OBJECTIVES
Following the study of this chapter, the reader should be able to:

Describe

1. The position of the hip, knee, and ankle joints in optimal erect posture.
2. The position of the LOG in optimal erect posture, using appropriate points of reference.
3. The "sway envelope."
4. The base of support.
5. The basic elements of postural control including ankle, hip, head, and stepping/grasping strategies.
6. The body's COP and its relation to the ground reaction force.
7. The gravitational moments acting around the vertebral column, pelvis, hip, knee, and the ankle in optimal erect posture.
8. The effects of moments on body segments in optimal erect posture.
9. Muscle and ligamentous structures that counterbalance moments in optimal erect posture.
10. The following postural deviations: pes planus, hallux valgus, pes cavus, forward head, genu varum and genu valgum, kyphosis, lordosis and idiopathic scoliosis.
11. The effects of the above postural deviations on body structures, that is, ligaments, joints, and muscles.
12. The effects of age on posture.

Explain

1. How the following postural deviations will affect either the magnitude or the direction of gravitational moments: genu valgum, forward head, genu recurvatum, kyphosis, and scoliosis.
2. How changes in alignment will affect supporting structures such as ligaments, joint capsules, muscles, various joint structures, and articular surfaces.

. . . .

Introduction

The basic elements of individual joint structures and associated muscles have been explored in the preceding chapters. The principles of biomechanics and knowledge of muscle physiology have been applied to various body segments for the purpose of gaining an understanding of joint and muscle function. In this chapter, the focus is on discovering how the various body structures are integrated into a system of levers that permits effective and efficient functioning of the body as a whole. Knowledge of individual joint and muscle structure and function is used as the basis for determining how each structure contributes to stability of the body in posture.

Static and Dynamic Posture

Posture can be either static or dynamic. In static postures the body and its segments are aligned and maintained in certain positions. Examples of static postures include standing, kneeling, lying, and sitting. Dynamic posture refers to postures in which the body or its segments are moving—walking, running, jumping, throwing, and lifting. An understanding of static posture forms the basis for understanding dynamic posture. Therefore, static posture will be emphasized in this chapter. The dynamic postures of walking and running are discussed in Chapter 14.

The study of any particular posture includes kinetic and kinematic analyses of all body segments. Humans and other living creatures have the ability to arrange and to rearrange body segments to form a large variety of postures, but maintenance of erect bipedal stance is unique to humans. The erect posture allows persons to use their upper extremities for the performance of large and small motor tasks. When the upper extremities are engaged by the use of crutches, canes, or other assistive devices to maintain the erect posture, an important human attribute is either severely compromised or lost.

Erect bipedal stance gives us freedom for the upper extremities, but in comparison with the quadrupedal posture, erect stance has certain disadvantages. Erect bipedal stance increases the work of the heart; places increased stress on the vertebral column, pelvis, and lower extremities; and reduces stability. In the quadruped posture the body weight is distributed between the upper and lower extremities. In human stance the body weight is borne exclusively by the two lower extremities. The human species' **base of support** (**BOS**), defined by an area bounded posteriorly by the tips of the heels and anteriorly by a line joining the tips of the toes, is considerably smaller than the quadrupedal base[1] (Fig. 13–1). The human's **center of gravity** (**COG**), which is sometimes referred to as the

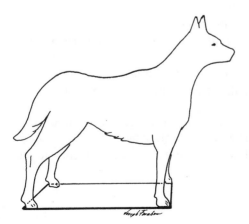

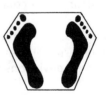

FIGURE 13–1. Bases of support. The quadripedal stance and the erect bidpedal stance.

body's center of mass, is located within the body approximately at the level of the second sacral segment, a location that is relatively distant from the BOS. Despite the instability caused by a small BOS and a high COG, maintaining stability in the static erect posture requires very little energy expenditure in the form of muscle contraction. The bones, joints, and ligaments are able to provide the major torques needed to counteract gravity and frequent changes in body position assist in promoting circulatory return.

Postural Control

Although only a minimal amount of muscular activity is required to maintain a stable erect standing posture, the control of posture is complex and is a part of the body's motor control system. The focus of this text is not on the motor control aspects of human function; however, a discussion of some features of postural control is necessary for an understanding of posture.

Postural control, which can be either static or dynamic, refers to a person's ability to maintain stability of the body and body segments in response to forces that threaten to disturb the body's structural equilibrium. According to Horak,[2] the ability to maintain stability in the erect standing posture is a skill that the **central nervous system** (**CNS**) learns using information from passive biomechanical elements, sensory systems, and muscles. The CNS interprets and organizes inputs from the various structures and systems and selects responses based on past experience and the goal of the response. **Reactive**[2] (**compensatory**[3]) responses occur as reactions to external forces that displace the body's COG. **Proactive**[2] (**anticipatory**[3]) responses occur in anticipation of internally generated destabilizing forces such as raising one's arms to catch a ball or bending forward to tie one's shoes.

Major Goals and Basic Elements of Control

The major goals of postural control in the erect position are to control the body's orientation in space; maintain the body's COG over the BOS, and stabilize the head with respect to the vertical so that the eye gaze is appropriately oriented. According to DiFabio,[4] stabilizing the head with respect to the vertical is the primary goal of postural regulation. Maintenance and control of posture depends on the integrity of the CNS, visual system, vestibular system, and the musculoskeletal system. In addition, postural control depends on information from receptors located in and around the joints (in joint capsules, tendons, and ligaments) as well as on the soles of the feet. The CNS must be able to detect and predict instability and must be able to respond to all of this input with appropriate output to maintain the equilibrium of the body. Furthermore, the joints in the musculoskeletal system must have a range of motion (ROM) that is adequate for responding to specific tasks, and the muscles must be able to respond with appropriate speeds and forces.

Absent or Altered Inputs and Outputs

When inputs are altered or absent, the control system must respond to incomplete or distorted data and thus the person's posture may be altered and stability compromised. Altered or absent inputs may occur either in the absence of the normal gravitational force in weightless conditions during space flight, or when someone has decreased sensation in the lower extremities.

EXAMPLE 1: The astronauts aboard the US Space Shuttle *Discovery* in June 1985 demonstrated erect postures, both in space and immediately on their return to earth, that were very different from their normal preflight postures. When the astronauts' feet were fastened to the floor in space, and immediately on their return to earth, the astronauts assumed a position in which the neck, hip, and knee were flexed significantly more than in preflight posture. The observed postural changes have been attributed to alterations in tactile, articular, and proprioceptive cues.[5]

In a more recent study of postural instabilities observed in astronauts returning from space flight, investigators concluded that the astronauts exhibited a large variety of changes in multijoint coordination. The investigators attributed these changes to a reweighting of vestibular inputs in the gravity diminished situation, which subsequently caused changes in postural control.[6] A more common example of altered inputs occurs when one attempts to attain and then maintain the erect standing posture when one's foot has "fallen asleep." Attempts at standing may result in a fall because input regarding the position of the foot and ankle as well as information from contact of the "asleep" foot with the supporting surface are missing.

Another instance in which inputs may be disturbed is following injury. A disturbance in the kinesthetic sense about the ankle and foot following ankle sprains has been implicated as a cause of poor balance or loss of stability.[7] Forkin and colleagues[8] in a study of gymnasts 1 to 12 months after an ankle sprain found that these individuals were less able to detect passive ROM in the previously injured ankle than they were in the uninjured ankle. The gymnasts in the study also reported that they believed that they were less stable in the standing posture than before their injury. Bernier and Perrin[9] also identified a group of men and women who had chronic functional instability following an ankle sprain.

In addition to altered inputs, a person's ability to maintain the erect posture may be affected by altered outputs such as the inability of the muscles to respond appropriately to signals from the CNS. For example, the muscles of a person with peripheral nerve damage may be paralyzed or partially paralyzed and not able to respond. In elderly persons, muscles that have atrophied through disuse may not be able to respond with the appropriate amount of force to counteract an opposing force. In persons with neuromuscular disorders both agonists and antagonists may respond at the same time, thus reducing the effectiveness of the response.

Muscle Synergies

Investigators of postural control have suggested that for any particular task many different combinations of muscles may be activated to complete the task. A normally functioning CNS selects the appropriate combination of muscles to complete the task based on an analysis of sensory inputs. Dietz[10] suggests that afferent input from Golgi tendon organs in the leg extensors signals changes in the projection of the body's COG with respect to the feet. Variations in an individual's past experience and customary patterns of muscle activity will also affect the response. Allum and coworkers[11] suggest that proprioceptive input from the hip or trunk may be more important than input from the legs in signaling and initiating responses. According to these authors, muscle activation is based primarily on input

from the hip and trunk proprioceptors. A second level of input includes cues from the vestibular system and proprioceptive input from all body segments.[11]

Monitoring of muscle activity patterns through electromyography (EMG) and determinations of muscle peak torque and power outputs are used to study postural responses during perturbations of upright postural stability. A **perturbation** is any sudden change in conditions that displaces the body posture away from equilibrium.[2] The perturbation can be sensory or mechanical. A **sensory perturbation** might be caused by altering of visual input such as might occur when one's eyes are covered unexpectedly. **Mechanical perturbations** are displacements that involve direct changes in the relationship of COG to the base of support. These displacements may be caused either by movements of body segments or of the entire body. One method of producing mechanical perturbations experimentally is by placing subjects on a movable platform. The platform can be moved forward or backward or from side to side. Some platforms can be tipped and the velocity of platform motion can be varied. The postural responses to perturbations caused by either platform movement or by pushes and pulls are **reactive** or **compensatory responses** in that they are **involuntary reactions.** These postural responses are referred to in the literature as either **synergies**[2] or **strategies**.[3] Therefore in this text the terms will be used interchangeably. The synergies are task specific and appear to vary with a number of factors including amount and direction of motion of the supporting surface; location, magnitude, and velocity of the perturbing force; and initial posture of the individual at the time of the perturbation.

FIXED-SUPPORT SYNERGIES

Horak and associates[2] describe synergies as centrally organized patterns of muscle activity that occur in response to perturbations of standing postures. **Fixed-support synergies** are patterns of muscle activity in which the BOS remains fixed during the perturbation and recovery of equilibrium. Stability is regained through movements of parts of the body but the feet remain fixed on the BOS. Two examples of fixed-support synergies are the ankle synergy and the hip synergy.

The **ankle synergy** consists of discrete bursts of muscle activity on either the anterior or pos-

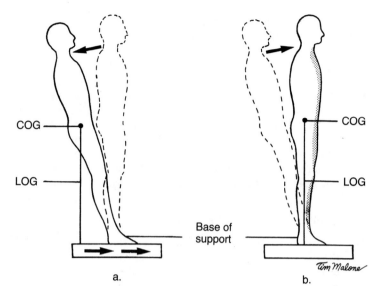

FIGURE 13–2. Perturbation of erect stance equilibrium by forward horizontal platform movement. (a) Anterior (forward) movement of the platform causes posterior (backward) movement of the body and, as a consequence, displacement of the body's center of gravity (COG) posterior to the base of support. (b) Use of the ankle strategy (activation of dorsiflexors, hip flexors, abdominals, and neck flexors) brings the body's COG back over the base of support and reestablishes stability.

terior aspects of the body that occur in a distal-to-proximal pattern in response to forward and backward movements of the supporting platform, respectively. Forward motion of the platform results in a relative displacement of the line of gravity (LOG) posteriorly (Fig. 13–2a). The muscles respond in an attempt to restore the LOG to a position within the BOS. Bursts of muscle activity occur in the ankle dorsiflexors,

hip flexors, abdominal muscles, and neck flexors. The tibialis anterior contributes to the restoration of stability by pulling the tibia anteriorly (reverse muscle action) and hence the body forward so that the line of gravity (LOG) remains or centers within the BOS (Fig. 13–2b). Backward motion of the platform results in a relative displacement of the LOG anteriorly. The muscles respond in an attempt to restore

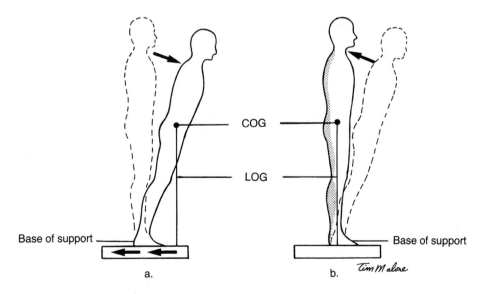

FIGURE 13–3. Perturbation of erect stance equilibrium by backward horizontal platform movement. (a) Posterior movement of the platform causes anterior movement of the body and, as a consequence, displacement of the body's COG anterior to the base of support. (b) Use of the ankle strategy (activation of the plantarflexors, hip extensors, back and neck extensors) brings the body's COG over the base of support and reestablishes stability.

the LOG to a position within the BOS (see Fig.13–3a). Bursts of activity in the plantarflexors, hip extensors, trunk extensors, and neck extensors are used to restore the LOG over the base of support (see Fig. 13–3b). The **hip synergy** consists of discrete bursts of muscle activity on the side of the body opposite to the ankle pattern in a proximal-to-distal pattern of activation.[12] Maki and McIlroy[3] suggest that the fixed-support hip synergy may be used primarily in situations where **change-in-support strategies (stepping** or **grasping synergies)** are not available.

CHANGE-IN-SUPPORT STRATEGIES

The change-in-support strategies include stepping (forward, backward or sidewise) and grasping (using one's hands to grab a bar or other fixed support) in response to movements of the platform. Stepping and grasping differ from fixed-support synergies because stepping/grasping moves or enlarges the body's BOS so that it remains under the body's COG (Fig. 13–4).[12, 13] Previously it was thought that the stepping synergy was used only as a last resort, being initiated when ankle and hip strategies were insufficient to bring and maintain the COG over the base of support.[12,14] However, Maki and McIlroy suggest that change-in-support strategies are common responses to perturbations among both the young and the old.[3] Furthermore, these authors observed that change-in-support synergies are the only synergies that are successful in maintaining stability in the instance of a large perturbation.[3] Comparisons of the stepping strategies used by the young and old show that the younger subjects have a tendency to take only one step, whereas the elderly subjects have a tendency to take multiple steps that are shorter and of less height than their younger counterparts.[3,15] However, no differences are apparent in the speed at which the young and elderly initiate the change-in-support stepping strategy. Luchies and associates[16] found that older subjects lifted their feet just as quickly as the younger subjects.

HEAD STABILIZING STRATEGIES

Recently two head stabilizing strategies have been described by DiFabio and Emasithi.[4] These proactive strategies differ from the previously described reactive strategies because head stabilizing strategies occur in anticipation of the initiation of internally generated forces. Furthermore the head strategies are used to maintain the head during sustained movement of the body, such as walking, whereas the previously described strategies are used to maintain the body in a static equilibrium situation. The authors describe the following two strategies for maintaining the vertical stability of the head: **head stabilization in space (HSS)** and **head stabilization on trunk (HST).**[4] The HSS strategy is a modification of head position in anticipation of displacements of the body's COG. The anticipatory adjustments to head position are independent of trunk motion. The HST strategy is one in which the head and trunk move as a single unit.

Kinetics and Kinematics of Posture

The muscle activity patterns described in response to perturbations are used to counteract forces that affect the equilibrium of the body in the erect standing posture. The following section examines the effects of both external and internal forces on the body and body segments to understand how static postures are maintained. The external forces that will be considered are **inertia, gravity,** and **ground reaction forces (GRFs).** The internal forces are produced by muscle activity and passive tension in ligaments, tendons, joint capsules, and other soft-tissue structures. According to the definition of equilibrium presented in Chapter 1, the external

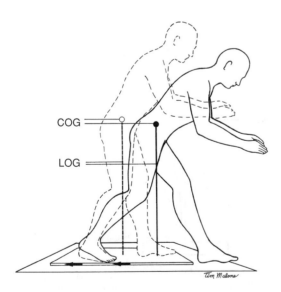

FIGURE 13–4. Perturbation of erect stance equilibrium by backward platform movement. The person in this illustration is using a stepping strategy to keep from falling forward in response to backward movement of the platform. Stepping forward brings the body's COG over a new base of support.

and internal forces must be balanced and the sum of all the forces and torques acting on the body and its segments must be equal to zero for the body to be in equilibrium. The body attempts to attain and maintain a state of equilibrium in erect standing with a minimum of energy expenditure as it attempts to keep the body's COG over the BOS and the head in a position that permits gaze to be appropriately oriented.

Inertial and Gravitational Forces

Generally, inertial forces are ignored in static postures because little or no acceleration is occurring except during postural sway. In the erect standing posture the body undergoes a constant swaying motion called **postural sway** or **sway envelope.**[13] The extent of the sway envelope for a normal individual standing with about 4 inches between the feet can be as large as 12° in the sagittal plane and 16° in the frontal plane.[13] The inertial forces that may result from this swaying motion usually are not considered in the analysis of forces for static postures.[17] However, inertial forces must be considered in postural analysis of all dynamic postures such as walking, running, and jogging.

Gravitational forces act downward from the body's COG. In the static erect standing posture the vertical projection of the body's COG (the LOG) falls within the BOS, which is typically the space defined by the two feet (see Fig. 13–1). In dynamic postures such as walking and running, the LOG falls outside of the borders of the feet during a large portion of the activity, thus making the body unstable during that portion of the task. The LOG must fall within the borders of the feet to maintain equilibrium in the static erect posture.[13]

Ground Reaction Forces

Whenever the body contacts the ground, the ground pushes back on the body. This force is known as the ground reaction force or GRF. The GRF is a composite (or resultant) force typically described as having three components: a vertical component force and two force components directed horizontally. One of the two horizontal forces is in a medial-lateral direction, whereas the other horizontal force is in an anterior-posterior direction along the ground. The **composite or resultant ground reaction force vector** (**GRFV**) is equal in magnitude but opposite in direction to the gravitational force in the erect static standing posture.[19] The GRFV

indicates the magnitude and direction of loading applied to the foot.[20] The point of application of the GRFV is at the body's **center of pressure** (**COP**), which is located in the foot in unilateral stance and between the feet in bilateral standing postures. If one were doing a handstand, the COP would be located between the hands. The COP, like the COG, is the theoretical point where the force is considered to act, although the body surface that is in contact with the ground may have forces acting over a large portion of its surface area.[21] The path of the COP that defines the extent of the sway envelope can be determined by plotting the COP at regular intervals when a person is standing on a force plate system (Fig. 13–5).[18, 22]

The GRFV and the LOG have coincident action lines in the static erect posture.[17] In Figure 1–27 (see Chap. 1), the GRFV "scale on man" and the LOG are part of the same linear force system. In many dynamic postures, the intersection of the LOG with the supporting surface may not coincide with the point of application of the GRFV. The horizontal distance from the point on the supporting surface where the LOG intersects the ground and the COP (where the GRFV acts) indicates the magnitude of the moment that must be opposed to maintain a posture and keep the person from falling.

The technology required to obtain GRFs, COP, and muscle activity is expensive and may not be available to the average evaluator of human function. Therefore, in the following sections a simplified method of analyzing posture will be presented using diagrams and the combined action of the LOG and the GRFV as a reference.

Coincident Action Lines

In an ideal erect posture, body segments are aligned so that the torques and stresses on body segments are minimized and standing can be maintained with a minimal amount of energy expenditure. The coincident action lines formed by the GRFV and the LOG serve as a reference for the analysis of the effects of these forces on body segments (Fig. 13–6). When the LOG and the GRFV coincide as they do in static posture, we can assess the effects at each joint using one or the other. We will use the LOG in the remainder of this chapter. The location of the LOG shifts continually (as does the COP) because of the postural sway. As a result of the continuous motion of the LOG, the moments acting around the joints are continually changing. Receptors in and around the joints of body

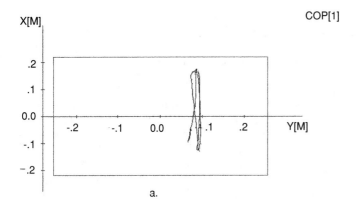

a.

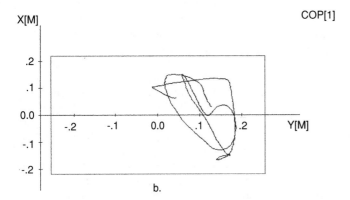

b.

FIGURE 13–5. Path of the center of pressure (COP) in erect stance. (a) A COP tracing plotted for a person standing on a force plate. The rectangle represents the outline of the force plate. The tracing shows a normal rhythmic anterior-posterior "sway envelope" during approximately 30 seconds of stance. (b) A COP tracing showing relatively uncontrolled postural sway. (COP tracings courtesy of Leonard Elbaum, Director of Research at the Physical Therapy Laboratory, Florida International University, Miami, Fla. Data were collected with an AMTI Force Platform, Newton, Mass. Analysis and display software were provided by Ariel Life Systems, Inc, La Jolla, Calif.)

segments and on the soles of the feet detect these changes and relay this information to the CNS. The CNS analyzes the inputs and under normal conditions makes an appropriate response to maintain postural stability.

Sagittal Plane

The effect of forces on body segments in the sagittal plane is determined by the location of the LOG relative to the axis of motion of body segments. When the LOG passes directly through a joint axis, no gravitational torque is created around that joint. However, if the LOG passes at a distance from the axis, a gravitational torque is created. This torque will cause rotation of the superimposed body segments around that joint axis unless the gravitational torque is opposed by a counterbalancing torque. The magnitude of the gravitational moment of force increases as the distance between the LOG and the joint axis increases. The direction of the gravitational moment of force depends on the location of the gravity line relative to a particular joint axis. If the gravity line is located *anterior* to the joint axis, the torque will tend to cause anterior motion of the proximal

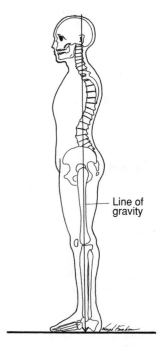

FIGURE 13–6. The location of the combined action line formed by the ground reaction force vector (GRFV) and the line of gravity (LOG) in optimal erect posture.

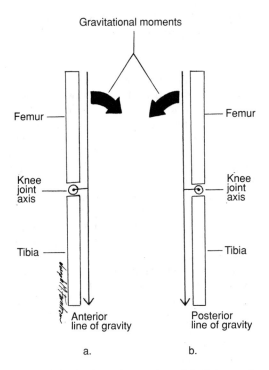

FIGURE 13–7. A schematic representation of the gravitational moments in the lower extremities of a person facing to the viewer's right. (a) The gravitation moment tends to move the proximal segment (femur) anteriorly when the LOG passes anterior to the joint axis. (b) The gravitational moment tends to move the proximal segment (femur) posteriorly when the LOG is located posterior to the joint axis.

segment of the body supported by that joint (Fig. 13–7a). If the gravity line falls *posterior* to the joint axis, the torque will tend to cause motion of the proximal segment in a posterior direction (Fig. 13–7b). In a postural analysis, gravitational moments producing sagittal plane motion of the proximal joint segment are referred to as either flexion or extension moments.

EXAMPLE 2: If the LOG passes anterior to the ankle joint axis, the gravitational torque will tend to rotate the tibia (proximal segment) in an anterior direction (Fig. 13–8). Anterior motion of the tibia on the fixed foot will result in dorsiflexion of the ankle. Therefore, the moment of force is called a dorsiflexion moment.

EXAMPLE 3: If the LOG passes anterior to the axis of rotation of the knee joint, the gravitational torque will tend to rotate the femur (proximal segment) in an anterior direction (Fig. 13–9). An anterior movement of the femur will cause extension of the knee. In this instance the moment of force is called an extension moment.

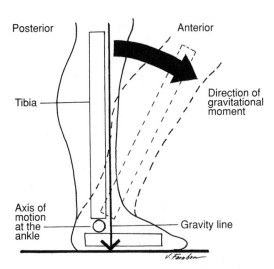

FIGURE 13–8. The anterior location of the LOG relative to the ankle joint axis creates a dorsiflexion moment. The arrow indicates the direction of the dorsiflexion moment. The dotted line indicates the direction in which the tibia would move if the dorsiflexion moment is unopposed.

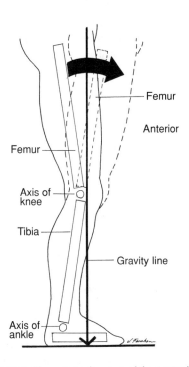

FIGURE 13–9. The anterior location of the LOG relative to the knee joint axis creates an extension moment. The arrow indicates the direction of the extension moment. The dotted line indicates the direction in which the femur would move if the gravitational moment were unopposed.

Optimal or Ideal Posture

Because the force of gravity is constantly acting on the body, an ideal posture is one in which the body segments are aligned vertically and the LOG passes through all joint axes. Normal body structure makes such an ideal posture impossible to achieve, but it is possible to attain a posture that is close to the ideal. In normal optimal standing posture, the LOG falls close to, but not through, most joint axes.[23] Therefore, in the normal optimal standing posture the gravitational torques are small and can be balanced by countertorques generated by passive ligamentous tension, passive muscle tension, and a minimal amount of muscle activity. The body segments in the normal optimal posture are in or near vertical alignment; the compression forces are distributed optimally over the weight-bearing surfaces of the joints; and no excessive tension is exerted on the ligaments or required by muscles. Slight deviations from the optimal posture are to be expected in a normal population because of the many individual variations found in body structure. However, deviations from the ideal posture that are large enough to either create unbalanced forces around joints or to cause other parts of the body to compensate for the deviations need to be identified and remedial action taken. If faulty postures are habitual and assumed continually on a daily basis, the body will not recognize these faulty postures as abnormal and over time structural adaptations will occur.

Analysis of Posture

Skilled observational analysis of posture involves identification of the location of body segments relative to the LOG. A **plumb line,** or line with a weight on one end, is used to represent the LOG. Evaluators of posture should be able to determine if a body segment or joint deviates from the normal optimal postural alignment by using their observational skills. Body segments on either side of the LOG should be symmetrical. More sophisticated analyses may be performed using radiography, photography, EMG, electrogoniometry, force plates, or three-dimensional computer analysis. However, a skilled observational analysis yields large amounts of information without the use of any instrumentation but a plumb line.

Lateral View—Optimal Alignment in the Sagittal Plane

Ankle

In the optimal erect posture the ankle joint is in the neutral position, or midway between dorsiflexion and plantarflexion. The LOG falls slightly anterior to the lateral malleolus and, therefore, anterior to the ankle joint axis.[24, 25] The anterior position of the LOG relative to the ankle joint axis creates a dorsiflexion moment. In the neutral ankle position there are no ligamentous checks capable of counterbalancing the dorsiflexion moment; therefore, muscle activity of the plantarflexors is necessary to prevent forward motion of the tibia. The soleus muscle acting in reverse action exerts a posterior pull on the tibia and in this way is able to oppose the dorsiflexion moment (Fig. 13–10).

Electromyographic studies have demonstrated that soleus[26, 27] and gastrocnemius[27] activity is fairly continuous in normal subjects during erect standing. This activity suggests that these muscles are exerting a minimal but constant torque about the ankles to oppose

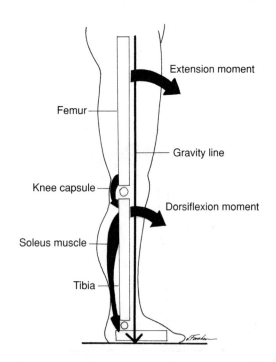

FIGURE 13–10. The extension moment acting around the knee joint is balanced by an opposing moment created by passive tension in the posterior joint capsule. The dorsiflexion moment at the ankle is counterbalanced by activity of the soleus muscle.

the gravitational dorsiflexion moment that exists at the ankle. Ankle joint muscles that have shown inconsistent activity in EMG recordings during standing are the tibialis anterior, peroneals, and tibialis posterior.[28] The tibialis anterior, tibialis posterior, and peroneals have primary actions other than plantarflexion at the ankle joint. Therefore, it is probable that these muscles are helping to provide transverse stability in the foot during postural sway rather than acting to oppose the gravitational moment at the ankle joint.

Knee

The knee joint is in full extension and the LOG passes anterior to the midline of the knee and posterior to the patella. This places the LOG just anterior to the knee joint axis. The anterior location of the gravitational line relative to the knee joint axis creates an extension moment.[25] Passive tension in the posterior joint capsule and associated ligaments is sufficient to balance the gravitational moment and prevent knee hyperextension. Little or no muscle activity is required to maintain the knee in extension in the optimal erect posture. However, a small amount of activity has been identified in the hamstrings. Activity of the soleus muscle may augment the gravitational extension moment at the knee through its posterior pull on the tibia as it acts at the ankle joint. In contrast, activity of the gastrocnemius may tend to oppose the gravitational extension moment because the muscle crosses the knee posterior to the knee joint axis.

Hip and Pelvis

In optimal posture, according to Kendall and McCreary,[29] the hip is in a neutral position and the pelvis is level with no anterior or posterior tilt (Fig. 13–11a). In a level pelvis position, lines connecting the symphysis pubis and the anterior superior iliac spines are vertical; and the lines connecting the anterior superior iliac and posterior superior iliac spines are horizontal.[29] In this optimal position, the LOG passes slightly posterior to the axis of the hip joint, through the greater trochanter.[23, 25, 30, 31] The posterior location of the gravitational line relative to the hip joint axis creates an extension moment at the hip that tends to rotate the pelvis (proximal segment) posteriorly on the femoral heads[32] (Fig. 13–11b). EMG studies have shown activity of the iliopsoas muscle during standing,[33] and it is possible that the iliopsoas is acting to create a balancing flexion moment at the hip. If the gravitational extension moment at the hip were allowed to act without muscular balance, as in a so-called relaxed standing posture, hip hyperextension ultimately would be checked by passive tension in the iliofemoral, pubofemoral, and ischiofemoral ligaments. The relaxed standing posture does not require any muscle activity at the hip but causes an increase in the tension stresses on the anterior hip ligaments. The relaxed standing posture may also increase the magnitude of the gravitational torque at other joints in the body.

Lumbosacral and Sacroiliac Joints

The optimal lumbosacral angle is about 30°.[34] Anterior tilting of the sacrum increases the lum-

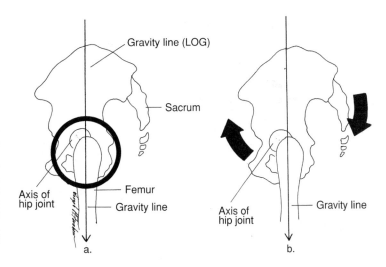

FIGURE 13–11. The location of the LOG relative to the axis of the hip joint. (a) The LOG passes through the greater trochanter and posterior to the axis of the hip joint. (b) The posterior location of the gravity line creates an extension moment at the hip, which tends to rotate the pelvis posteriorly on the femoral heads. The arrows indicate the direction of the gravitational moment.

bosacral angle and results in an increase in the shearing stress at the lumbosacral joint and may result in an increase in the anterior lumbar convexity in standing (Fig. 13–12a). However, the nature of the relationship between sacral inclination and lumbar lordosis remains controversial. Youdas et al.[35] in a study of 90 male and female subjects found only a weak association between lumbar lordosis and sacral inclination. On the other hand, Kosovessis and coworkers,[36,37] using x-ray evaluations of erect posture, found that the sacral inclination correlated strongly with both thoracic kyphosis and lumbar lordosis.[36]

In the ideal posture the LOG passes through the body of the fifth lumbar vertebra and close to the axis of rotation of the lumbosacral joint.[35] Gravity, therefore, creates a very slight extension moment at L5 to S1 that is opposed by the anterior longitudinal ligament. When the sacrum is in the optimal position, the LOG passes slightly anterior to the sacroiliac joints. The gravitational moment that is created at the sacroiliac joints tends to cause the anterior superior portion of the sacrum to rotate anteriorly and inferiorly while the posterior inferior portion tends to move posteriorly and superiorly (Fig. 13–12b). Tension in the sacrospinous and sacrotuberous ligaments counterbalances the gravitational torque and prevents the inferior portion of the sacrum from moving posteriorly. The superior portion of the sacrum is kept from being thrust anteriorly by the sacroiliac ligaments.[38]

Vertebral Column

The curves of the vertebral column should represent the normal configuration described in Chapter 4. When the vertebral curves are in optimal alignment, the LOG will pass through the midline of the trunk (Fig. 13–13). The location of the LOG relative to the vertebrae above the fifth lumbar level is controversial. Cailliet[39] reports that the LOG transects the vertebral bodies at the level of T1 and T12 vertebrae and at the odontoid process of the C2 vertebra. Duval-Beaupre[30] using x-ray examinations of the vertebral columns of 17 young adults found that the LOG in these individuals was located anterior to the anterior aspect of the T8 to T10 vertebrae. According to Bogduk[40] the LOG passes anterior to L4 and thus anterior to the lumbar spine in many individuals. In this instance a flexion moment would be present that would tend to pull the thorax and upper lumbar spine anteriorly. Activity of the erector spinae would be necessary to counteract the moment and maintain the body in equilibrium.

When Cailliet's frame of reference is used, the LOG will pass posterior to the axes of rotation of the cervical and lumbar vertebrae, anterior to the thoracic vertebrae, and through the body of the fifth lumbar vertebra. In this situation, the gravitational moments tend to increase the natural curves in the lumbar, thoracic, and cervical regions. The maximal gravitational torque occurs at the apex of each curve at C5, T8, and L3, because the apical vertebrae would be farthest from the LOG. According to Kendall,[29] the LOG passes through the bodies of the lumbar and cervical vertebrae and anterior to the thoracic vertebrae in the optimal posture.[30] In this instance, the stress on the supporting structures would be greatest in the thoracic area, where the LOG would fall at a distance from the vertebrae. Stress

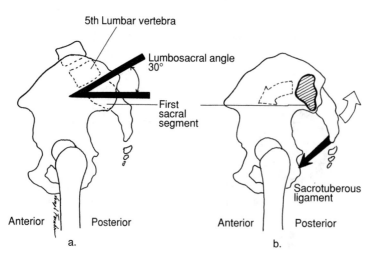

5th Lumbar vertebra

Lumbosacral angle 30°

First sacral segment

Sacrotuberous ligament

Anterior   Posterior

a.

Anterior   Posterior

b.

FIGURE 13–12. (a) The lumbosacral angle in optimal erect posture is about 30°. (b) The gravitational moment tends to rotate the superior portion of the sacrum anteriorly. Consequently, the inferior portion tends to thrust posteriorly. Passive tension in the sacrotuberous ligament prevents posterior motion of the inferior sacral segment.

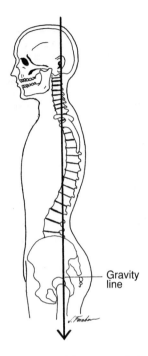

FIGURE 13–13. Location of the LOG in relation to the trunk.

in the lumbar and cervical regions would be comparatively less because the LOG falls close to or through the joint axes of these regions.

Although not confirming either Cailliet's or Kendall's hypotheses, EMG studies have shown that the longissimus dorsi, rotatores, and neck extensor muscles exhibit intermittent electrical activity during normal standing.[41] This evidence suggests that ligamentous structures and passive muscle tension are unable to provide enough force to oppose all gravitational moments acting around the joint axes of the vertebral column. In the lumbar region, where minimal muscle activity appears to occur, tension in the anterior longitudinal ligament and passive tension in the trunk flexors apparently is sufficient to balance the gravitational extension moment.

Head

The LOG relative to the head passes through the external auditory meatus, posterior to the coronal suture and through the odontoid process. Therefore, the LOG falls slightly anterior to the transverse (coronal) axis of rotation for flexion and extension of the head and creates a flexion moment (Fig. 13–14). The gravitational moment, which tends to tilt the head forward, is counteracted by tension in the ligamentum nuchae, tectorial membrane, posterior aspect of the zygapophyseal joint capsules, and posterior fibers of the annulus pulposus, and by activity of the capital extensors.[42,43] When a postural analysis is being performed, the plumb line should pass through the lobe of the ear and the head should be directly over the body's COG at S2.[43] A summary of the relationship of the LOG to various body segments in normal alignment in the sagittal plane is presented in Table 13–1.

Summary

The swaying motion that occurs in the normal erect posture will change the position of the LOG relative to individual joint axes. The COP also will move during swaying. For example, during forward sway of the body the LOG may move from the optimal posterior location relative to the hip joint axis to a position anterior to the hip joint axis (if the amount of swaying is sufficient). The COP will move anteriorly toward the toes. The flexion moment created by the change in position of the LOG may be counteracted by a brief burst of activity of the hip extensors, which will move the LOG and

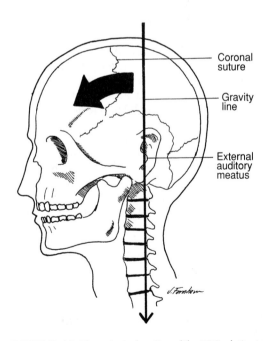

FIGURE 13–14. The anterior location of the LOG relative to the transverse axis for flexion and extension of the head creates a flexion moment.

Table 13–1. **Normal Alignment in the Sagittal Plane**

Joints	Line of Gravity	Gravitational Moment	Opposing Forces Passive Opposing Forces	Opposing Forces Active Opposing Forces
Atlanto-occipital	Anterior Anterior to transverse axis for flexion and extension	Flexion	1. Ligamentum nuchae 2. Tectorial membrane	Posterior neck muscles
Cervical	Posterior	Extension	1. Anterior longitudinal ligament	
Thoracic	Anterior	Flexion	1. Posterior longitudinal ligament 2. Ligamentum flavum 3. Supraspinous ligament	Extensors
Lumbar	Posterior	Extension	1. Anterior longitudinal ligament	
Sacroiliac joint	Anterior	Flexion type motion	1. Sacrotuberous ligament 2. Sacrospinous ligament 3. Sacroiliac ligament	
Hip joint	Posterior	Extension	1. Iliofemoral ligament	Iliopsoas
Knee joint	Anterior	Extension	1. Posterior joint capsule	
Ankle joint	Anterior	Dorsiflexion		Soleus

COP posteriorly. On the other hand, a burst of activity in the soleus muscles rather than the hip extensors might be used to bring the entire body and thus the LOG back into a position posterior to the hip joint axis.

A sudden backward movement of the supporting surface causes a similar but much larger and more forceful movement of the LOG as the body is thrust forward. Flexion moments are created at the neck and head; cervical, thoracic, and lumbar spine; hip; and ankle. To counteract these moments, the neck, back, hip extensors, and ankle plantarflexors may have to contract. The CNS responds with activation of a muscle or pattern of muscles that will counteract the inertial and flexion moments, bring the LOG back over the COG, and re-establish static erect equilibrium. These responses include the fixed-support and change-in-support strategies discussed in the first part of this chapter.

Lateral View—Deviations from Optimal Alignment

Minimizing energy expenditure and stress on supporting structures is one of the primary goals of any posture. Any change in position or malalignment of one body segment will cause changes to occur in adjacent segments as well as changes in other segments as the body seeks to adjust or compensate for the malalignment (closed chain response to keep the head over the sacrum). Changes from optimal alignment increase stress or increase force per unit area on body structures. If stresses are maintained over long periods of time, the body structures may be altered. Muscles may lose sarcomeres if held in shortened positions for extended periods. Such adaptive shortening may accentuate and perpetuate the abnormal posture, as well as prevent full ROM from occurring. Muscles may add sarcomeres if maintained in a lengthened position and as a consequence the muscle's length-tension relationship will be altered. Shortening of the ligaments will limit normal ROM, whereas stretching of ligamentous structures will reduce the ligament's ability to provide sufficient tension to stabilize and protect the joints. Prolonged weight-bearing stresses on the joint surfaces increase cartilage deformation and may interfere with the nutrition of the cartilage. As a result, the joint surfaces may become susceptible to early degenerative changes. The following examples illustrate how deviation from normal alignment of one or two body segments causes changes in other segments and increases the amount of energy required to maintain erect standing posture. Postural problems may originate in any part of the body and cause increased stresses and strains in throughout the musculoskeletal system. Postures that represent an attempt to either improve function or normalize appearance are called **compensatory postures**,[44] Evaluators of posture need to not only identify the deviation, but also to determine the cause of the deviation, compensatory postures, and possible effects of the deviation on bones, joints, ligaments, and muscles supporting the affected structures.

Foot and Toes

CLAW TOES

Claw toes is a deformity of the toes characterized by hyperextension of the metatarsophalangeal joint (MTP) combined with flexion of the proximal (PIP) and distal (DIP) interphalangeal joints.[45–51] Sometimes the proximal phalanx may subluxate dorsally on the metatarsal head (Fig.13–15a).[45] A callus may develop on the dorsal aspects of the flexed phalanges.

A few of the many suggested etiologies for this condition are as follows: the restrictive effect of shoes, a cavus-type foot, muscular imbalance, ineffectiveness of intrinsic foot muscles, neuromuscular disorders, and age-related deficiencies in the plantar structures. Valmassey[50] suggests that claw toe deformity is actu-

ally the same condition as hammer toe because the only difference in the conditions is that claw toe deformity affects all toes (second through fifth), whereas hammer toe usually affects only one or two toes.

HAMMER TOE

Generally, hammer toe is described as a deformity characterized by hyperextension of the MTP joint, flexion of the PIP joint, and hyperextension of the DIP joint (Fig. 13–15b).[45–49,51] Callosities (painless thickenings of the epidermis) may be found on the superior surface of the PIP joints over the heads of the first phalanges as a result of pressure from shoes or on the tips of the distal phalanges because of abnormal weight-bearing. The flexor muscles are stretched over the MTP joint and shortened over the IP joint. The extensor muscles are shortened over the MTP joint and stretched over the IP joint. If the long and short toe extensors and lumbricales are selectively paralyzed, the intrinsic and extrinsic toe flexors acting unopposed will buckle the PIP and DIP joints and cause a hammer toe deformity.

Knee

FLEXED KNEE POSTURE

In the flexed knee standing posture the LOG falls posterior to the knee joint axes. The posterior location of the LOG creates a flexion moment at the knees that must be balanced by activity of the quadriceps muscles to maintain the erect position. The quadriceps force re-

FIGURE 13–15. Claw toes and hammer toes. (a) The drawing of claw toes shows hyperextension at the metatarsophalangeal joint and flexion of the interphalangeal joints. The abnormal distribution of weight may result in callus formation either under the heads of the metatarsals or under the end of the distal phalanx. Abnormal pressure between the superior surfaces of the flexed interphalangeal joint and the lining of the shoe also may result in callus formation. (b) Hammer toes are characterized by hypertension of the metatarsophalangal and distal interphalangeal joints and flexion of the proximal interphalangeal joints. Callus formation caused by the pressure of the shoe develops on the superior surface of the proximal interphalangeal joints.

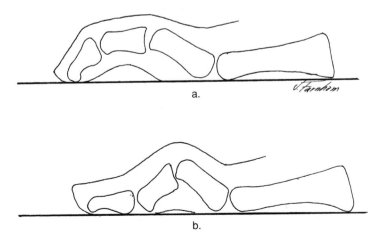

a.

b.

quired to maintain equilibrium at the knee in erect stance increases from zero with the knee extended to 22% of a maximum voluntary contraction (MVC) with the knee in 15° of flexion. A rapid rise in the amount of quadriceps force is required between 15° and 30° of knee flexion. When the knee reaches 30° of flexion, the necessary quadriceps force rises to 51% of a MVC.[52] The increase in muscle activity needed to maintain a flexed knee posture subjects the tibiofemoral and patellofemoral joints to greater than normal compressive stress.

Other consequences of a knee flexed erect standing posture are related to the ankle and hip. Because knee flexion in upright stance is accompanied by hip flexion and ankle dorsiflexion, the location of the LOG also will be altered in relation to these joint axes. At the hip, the LOG will fall anterior to the hip joint axes. Activity of the hip extensors may be necessary to balance the gravitational flexion moment acting around the hip, and increased soleus muscle activity may be required to counteract the increased gravitational dorsiflexion moment at the ankle (Fig. 13–16). The additional muscle activity subjects the hip and ankle joints to greater-than-normal compression

stress. Overall, the increased need for quadriceps, gastrocnemius, soleus and, perhaps, hip extensor activity would appear to substantially increase the energy requirements for stance. However, the hypothesized increase in energy expenditure caused by the posture may be overestimated when stiffness in muscle or joint structures reduces the need for active muscle contraction.

HYPEREXTENDED KNEE POSTURE (GENU RECURVATUM)

The hyperextended knee posture (Fig. 13–17) is one in which the LOG is located considerably anterior to the knee joint axis. The anterior location of the LOG causes an increase in the gravitational extensor moment acting at the knee, which tends to increase the hyperextension deviation and put the posterior joint capsule under considerable tension stress. A continual adoption of the hyperextended knee posture is likely to result in adaptive lengthening of the posterior capsule. The anterior joint surfaces on the femoral condyles and anterior portion of the tibial plateaus are subject to abnormal compression and are subject to degenerative changes of the cartilaginous joint sur-

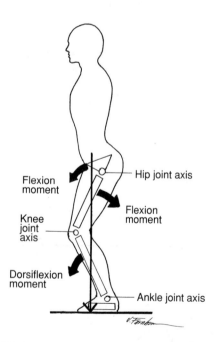

FIGURE 13–16. Gravitation moments in a flexed knee posture. Flexion moments are present, acting around the hip and knee joints, while a dorsiflexion moment is acting around the ankle.

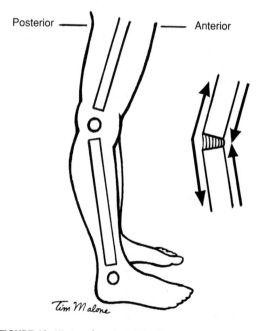

FIGURE 13–17. In a hyperextended knee posture, the anterior aspect of the knee is subjected to abnormal compressive forces while the posterior aspect is subjected to abnormal tensile forces. Note the limitation of dorsiflexion at the ankle.

faces. The length-tension relationship of the anterior and posterior muscles also may be altered and the muscles may not be able to provide the force necessary to provide adequate joint stability and mobility.

Hyperextension at the knee is usually caused by limited dorsiflexion at the ankle or a fixed plantarflexion position of the foot and ankle called **equinus.** It may also be the result of habits formed in childhood in which the child or adolescent stands with hips and knees hyperextended.

Pelvis

EXCESSIVE ANTERIOR PELVIC TILT

In a posture in which the pelvis is excessively tilted anteriorly, the lower lumbar vertebrae are forced anteriorly. The upper lumbar vertebrae move posteriorly to keep the head over the sacrum, thereby increasing the lumbar anterior convexity (lordotic curve). The LOG, therefore, is at a greater distance from the lumbar joint axes than is optimal and the extension moment in the lumbar spine is increased. The posterior convexity of the thoracic curve increases and becomes kyphotic to balance the lordotic lumbar curve and maintain the head over the sacrum. Similarly, the anterior convexity of the cervical curve increases to bring the head back over the sacrum (Fig. 13–18). Table 13–2 illustrates the changes that may result from an excessive anterior tilt.

In the optimal posture the lumbar disks are subject to anterior tension and posterior compression in erect standing. A greater diffusion of nutrients into the anterior compared to the posterior portion of the disk occurs in the optimal erect posture. Increases in the anterior convexity of the lumbar curve during erect standing increases the compressive forces on the posterior annuli and may adversely affect the nutrition of the posterior portion of the intervertebral disks. Also excessive compressive forces may be applied to the zygapophyseal joints.[53,54]

Vertebral Column

LORDOSIS

The term lordosis refers to an abnormal increase in the normal anterior convexities in either the cervical or lumbar regions of the vertebral column. As described in the section on

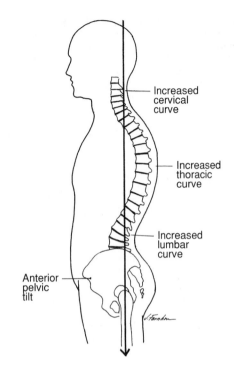

FIGURE 13–18. An excessive anterior pelvic tilt results in an increase in the lumbar anterior convexity. To compensate for the increased lumbar convexity, there is an increase in the posterior convexity of the thoracic region and an increase in the anterior convexity of the cervical curve.

anterior pelvic tilt, an increase in the lumbar curve may be accompanied by a compensatory increase in both the anterior convexity of the cervical curve and in the posterior convexity of the thoracic curve.

KYPHOSIS

The term kyphosis refers to an abnormal increase in the normal posterior convexity of the thoracic vertebral column. Sometimes kyphosis may develop as a compensation for an increase in the lumbar lordosis as seen in Figure 13–18 or the kyphosis may develop as a result of poor postural habits. Diseases such as tuberculosis or ankylosing spondylosis also may cause increases in the posterior convexity of the thoracic region. For example, **Gibbus** or **humpback deformity,** may occur as a result of tuberculosis, which causes vertebral fractures. Gibbus or humpback deformity is easily recognized by the Gibbus (hump) which forms a sharp posterior angulation in the upper thoracic vertebral column.[45] **Dowager's hump** is another easily recognizable kyphotic condition that is found most often in postmenopausal

Table 13–2. **Effects on Body Structures**

Deviation	Compression	Distraction	Stretching	Shortening
Excessive anterior tilt of pelvis	Posterior vertebral bodies Interdiskal pressure L5–S1 increased	Lumbosacral angle increased Shearing forces at L5–S1 Likelihood of forward slippage of L5 on S1 increased	Abdominals	Iliopsoas
Excessive lumbar lordosis	Posterior vertebral bodies and facet joints Interdiskal pressures increased Intervertebral foramina narrowed	Anterior annulus fibers	Anterior longitudinal ligament	Posterior longitudinal ligament Interspinous ligaments Ligamentum flavum Lumbar extensors
Excessive dorsal kyphosis	Anterior vertebral bodies Intradiskal pressures increased	Facet joint capsules and posterior annulus fibers	Dorsal back extensors Posterior ligaments Scapular muscles	Anterior longitudinal ligament Upper abdominals Anterior shoulder girdle musculature
Excessive cervical lordosis	Posterior vertebral bodies and facet joints Interdiskal pressure increased Intervertebral foramina narrowed	Anterior annulus fibers	Anterior longitudinal ligament	Posterior ligaments Neck extensors

women who have osteoporosis.[45] The anterior aspect of the bodies of a series of vertebrae collapse due to osteoporotic weakening. The vertebral body collapse causes an immediate lack of anterior support for the vertebral column, which bends forward causing an increase in the posterior convexity of the thoracic area (the hump) and an increase in compression on the anterior aspect of the vertebral bodies.

Head

FORWARD HEAD POSTURE

A forward head posture is one in which the head is positioned anteriorly at an increased distance from the LOG and the normal anterior cervical convexity is also increased with the apex of the lordotic curve at a considerable distance from the LOG compared to optimal posture (Fig 13–19). The constant assumption of a forward head posture causes unrelieved increased compression on the posterior zygapophyseal joints and posterior portions of the intervertebral disks and narrowing of the intervertebral foramina in the lordotic areas of the cervical region. The cervical extensor muscles may become ischemic because of the constant isometric contraction required to maintain the head in its forward position. The posterior aspect of the zygapophyseal joint capsules may become adaptively shortened and the narrowed intervertebral foramen may cause nerve root compression. In addition, the structure of the temporomandibular joint may become altered by the forward head posture and as a result the joint's function may be dis-

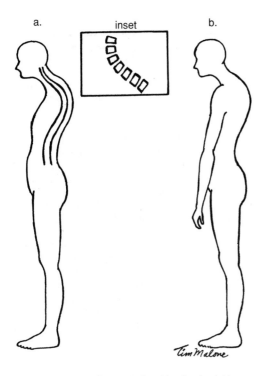

FIGURE 13–19. (a) The cervical and lumbar lordotic curves show an increase in the normal anterior convexity. The thoracic region shows an increase in the normal posterior convexity. The inset shows how the increase in the cervical lordotic curve creates compressive forces posteriorly and narrows the intervertebral foramen. (b) The drawing shows the forward shoulder position (arms medially rotated) that often accompanies a forward head posture.

turbed. In the forward head posture the scapulae may rotate medially, a thoracic kyphosis may develop, the thoracic cavity may be diminished, vital capacity can be reduced, and overall body height may be shortened (Table 13–3).

Anterior-Posterior View—Optimal Alignment

In an anterior view the LOG bisects the body into two symmetrical halves (Fig. 13–20). The head is straight with no tilting or rotation evident. The LOG bisects the face into two equal halves. The eyes, clavicles, and shoulders should be level (parallel to the ground). In a posterior view the inferior angles of the scapulae should be parallel and equidistant from the LOG. The waist angles and gluteal folds should be equal and the anterior superior iliac spine (ASIS) and posterior superior iliac spine (PSIS) should lie on a parallel line with the ground as well as being equidistant from the LOG. The joint axes of the hip, knee, and

ankle are equidistant from the LOG, and the gravitational line transects the central portion of the vertebral bodies. When postural alignment is optimal, little or no muscle activity is required to maintain medial-lateral stability. The gravitational torques acting on one side of the body are opposed by equal torques acting on the other side of the body (Tables 13–4 and 13–5).

Anterior-Posterior View—Deviations from Optimal Alignment

Any asymmetry of body segments caused either by movement of a body segment or by a unilateral postural deviation will disturb optimal muscular and ligamentous balance. Symmetrical postural deviations, such as bilateral **genu valgum (knock knee),** that disturb the optimal vertical alignment of body segments, cause an abnormal distribution of weight-bearing or compressive forces on one side of a joint and increased tensile forces on the other side. The increased gravitational torques that may occur require increased muscular activity and cause ligamentous stress.

Foot and Toes

PES PLANUS (FLATFOOT)

An evaluation of standing posture from the anterior-posterior aspect should include a careful evaluation of the feet. Normally the plumb line should lie equidistant from the malleoli, and the malleoli should appear to be of equal size and directly opposite from one another. When one malleolus appears more prominent or lower than the other and calcaneal eversion is present, it is possible that a common foot problem known as pes planus, or flatfoot, may be present. Calcaneal eversion of 5° to10° is normal in toddlers, but by 7 years of age no calcaneal eversion should be present.[50]

Flatfoot, which is characterized by a reduced or absent arch, may be either rigid or flexible. A rigid flatfoot is a structural deformity that may be hereditary. In the rigid flatfoot the medial longitudinal arch is absent in non-weight-bearing, toe standing, and normal weight-bearing situations. In the flexible flatfoot, the arch is reduced during normal weight-bearing situations, but reappears during toe standing or non-weight-bearing situations.

In either the rigid or flexible type of pes planus, the talar head is displaced anteriorly, medially, and inferiorly. The displacement of the

Table 13–3. **Forward Head Posture**

Deviation	Structural Components	Long-Term Effects on Structural Function
Forward head	Anterior location of LOG causes an increase in the flexion moment, which requires constant isometric muscle tension to support head	Muscle ischemia, pain, and fatigue and possible protrusion of nucleus pulposus
Increase in cervical lordosis	Narrowing of intervertebral foramen and compression of nerve roots	Damage to spinal cord and or nerve roots leading to paralysis
	Compression of zygapophyseal joint surfaces and increase in weight-bearing	Damage to cartilage and increased possibility of arthritic changes; adaptive shortening and possible formation of adhesions of joint capsules with subsequent loss of ROM
	Compression of posterior annulus fibrosus	
	Adaptive shortening of the posterior ligaments	Changes in collagen and early disk degeneration; diminished ROM at the intervertebral joints
	Adaptive lengthening of anterior ligaments	Decrease in cervical flexion ROM
	Increase in compression on posterior vertebral bodies at apex of cervical curve	Decrease in cervical extension ROM and decrease in anterior stability
		Osteophyte formation
Medial rotation of the scapula	Adaptive lengthening of upper posterior back muscles	Increase in dorsal kyphosis and loss of height
	Adaptive shortening of anterior shoulder muscles	Decrease in vital capacity and ROM of shoulder and arm

talus causes depression of the navicular, tension in the plantar calcaneonavicular (spring) ligament and lengthening of the tibialis posterior muscle (Fig. 13–21). The degree of flatfoot may be estimated by noting the location of the navicular relative to the head of the first metatarsal. Normally the navicular should be intersected by the Feiss line (Fig. 13–22). If the navicular is depressed, it will lie below the Feiss line and may even rest on the floor in a severe degree of flatfoot. The pronated flatfoot results in a relatively overmobile foot that may require muscular contraction to support the osteoligamentous arches during standing. It also may result in increased weight-bearing on the second through fourth metatarsal heads with subsequent plantar callus formation, especially at the second metatarsal. The rigid form of flatfoot interferes with push-off during walking because the foot is unable to assume the supinated position and become a rigid lever for push-off in gait. Weight-bearing pronation in the erect standing posture also causes medial rotation of the tibia and may affect knee joint function.

PES CAVUS

The medial longitudinal arch of the foot instead of being low (as in flatfoot) may be un-

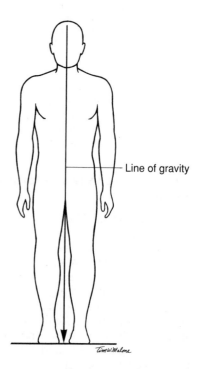

FIGURE 13–20. In anterior view of the human body, the LOG, in optimal posture, divides the body into two symmetrical parts.

Table 13–4. *Optimal Alignment: Anterior Aspect*

Body Segment	LOG Location	Observation
Head	Passes through middle of the forehead, nose and chin.	Eyes and ears should be level and symmetrical.
Neck/shoulders		Right and left angles between shoulders and neck should be symmetrical. Clavicles also should be symmetrical.
Chest	Passes through the middle of the xyphoid process.	Ribs on each side should be symmetrical.
Abdomen/hips	Passes through the umbilicus (navel).	Right and left waist angles should be symmetrical.
Hips/pelvis	Passes on a line equidistant from the right and left anterior superior iliac spines. Passes through the symphysis pubis.	Anterior superior iliac spines should be level.
Knees	Passes between knees equidistant from medial femoral condyles.	Patella should be symmetrical and facing straight ahead.
Ankles/feet	Passes between ankles equidistant from the medial maleoli.	Malleoli should be symmetrical, and feet should be parallel. Toes should not be curled, overlapping or deviated to one side.

Table 13–5. *Optimal Alignment: Posterior Aspect*

Body Segment	LOG Location	Observation
Head	Passes through middle of head.	Head should be straight with no lateral tilting. Angles between shoulders and neck should be equal.
Arms		Arms should hang naturally so that the palms of the hands are facing the sides of the body.
Shoulders/spine	Passes along vertebral column in a straight line, which should bisect the back into two symmetrical halves.	Scapulae should lie flat against the rib cage, be equidistant from the LOG and be separated by about 4 inches in the adult.
Hips/pelvis	Passes through gluteal cleft of buttocks and should be equidistant from posterior superior iliac spines.	The posterior superior iliac spines should be level. The gluteal folds should be level and symmetrical.
Knees	Passes between the knees equidistant from medial joint aspects.	Look to see that the knees are level.
Ankles/feet	Passes between ankles equidistant from the medial malleoli.	The heel cords should be vertical and the malleoli should be level and symmetrical.

usually high. A high arch is called **pes cavus** (Fig. 13–23). Pes cavus is a more stable position of the foot than pes planus. The weight in pes cavus is borne on the lateral borders of the foot and the lateral ligaments and the peroneus longus muscle may be stretched. In walking, the cavus foot is unable to adapt to the supporting surface because the subtalar and transverse tarsal joints tend to be near or at the locked supinated position.

HALLUX VALGUS

Hallux valgus is a fairly common deformity in which there is a medial deviation of the first

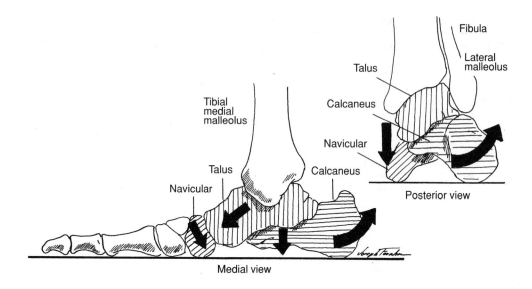

FIGURE 13–21. In pes planus ("flatfoot") there is displacement of the talus anteriorly, medially, and inferiorly; depression and pronation of the calcaneus; and depression of the navicular.

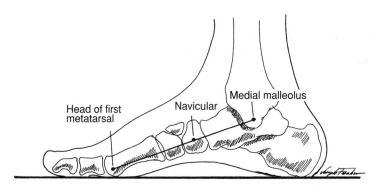

FIGURE 13–22. In the normal foot the medial malleolus, tuberosity of the navicular, and the head of the first metatarsal lie in a straight line called the Feiss line.

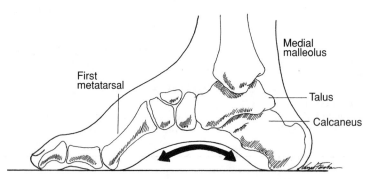

FIGURE 13–23. Pes cavus.

metatarsal at the tarsometatarsal joint and a lateral deviation of the phalanges at the metatarsophalangeal joint (Fig. 13–24). The bursa on the media aspect of the first metatarsal head may become inflamed and form a **bunion** in response to an increase in contact forces between the shoe and the side of the first MTP joint. In addition, bony overgrowth may occur on the medial aspect of the joint in an attempt by the body to increase the joint surface area. The combination of excess bone and bunion formation and possible MTP dislocation not only enlarge

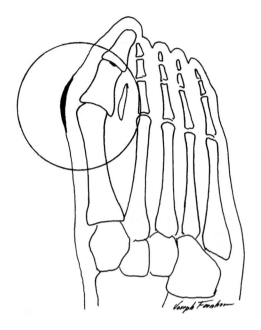

FIGURE 13–24. Hallux valgus.

the joint but are a source of pain and may require surgical intervention.

The most common cause of hallux valgus is abnormal pronation in combination with forefoot adductus, which leads to a hypermobile first ray. Flexor muscles are stretched over the MTP joints and shortened over the PIP joints. The extensor muscles are shortened over the MTP joints and stretched over the PIP joints. The sequence of events in the development of hallux valgus is summarized in Table 13–6.

Knees

Genu valgum (knock knees) is considered to be a normal alignment of the lower extremity in children from 2 to 6 years of age.[46] However, by about 6 or 7 years of age the physiologic valgus should begin to decrease, and by young adulthood the degree of valgus angulation at the knee should be only about 5° to 7°. In genu valgum the mechanical axes of the lower extremities are displaced laterally. If the degree of genu valgum exceeds 30° and persists beyond 8 years of age structural changes may occur. As a result of the increased torque acting around the knee, the medial knee joint structures are subjected to abnormal tensile or distraction stress, and the lateral structures are subjected to abnormal compressive stress (Fig.13–25). The patella may be laterally displaced and therefore predisposed to subluxation.

The foot also is affected as the gravitational torque acting on the foot in genu valgum tends to produce pronation of the foot with an accompanying stress on the medial longitudinal arch and its supporting structures as well as abnormal weight-bearing on the posterior medial aspect of the calcaneus (valgus torque). Additional related changes may include flatfloot, lateral tibial torsion, lateral patellar subluxation, and lumbar spine contralateral rotation.[44]

Genu varum (bow legs) is a condition in which the knees are widely separated when the feet are together and the malleoli are touching (see Fig.11–10 in Chap. 11). Some degree of genu varum is normal at birth and during infancy up to 3 or 4 years of age.[46, 50] Physiologic bowing is symmetrical and involves both the femur and the tibia. Cortical thickening on the medial concavity of both the femur and tibia may be present as a result of the increased compressive forces[46] and the patellae may be displaced medially. Some of the more commonly suggested cause of genu varum are vitamin D deficiency, renal rickets, osteochondritis, or epiphyseal injury.

Squinting or cross-eyed patella (in-facing patella) is a tilted/rotated position of the patella in which the superior medial pole of the patella faces medially and the inferior pole points laterally (Fig.13–26a). This altered patella position may be present in one or both knees and may be a sign of increased medial femoral torsion[50] (excessive femoral anteversion) or medial tibial rotation.[45] The Q angle may be increased in this condition and patella tracking may be adversely affected.

Grasshopper eyes patella refers to a high, laterally displaced position of the patella in which the patella faces upward and outward (Fig.13–26b). An abnormally long patella ligament may be responsible for the higher than normal position of the patella (patella alta). The medially rotated position of the patella is due to either femoral retroversion or lateral tibial torsion. Grasshopper eyes patella leads to abnormal patellar tracking and a decrease in the stability of the patella.

Vertebral Column

SCOLIOSIS

Another segment of the body that requires special consideration when evaluating posture from the anterior or posterior view is the vertebral column. Normally, when viewed from the

Table 13–6. *Sequence of Events: Development of Hallux Valgus*

Stage 1

Etiology		Osseous Change
Abnormal pronation in a forefoot adductus type of foot leads to a hypermobile 1st ray. The transverse head of the adductor hallicis muscle is unable to adequately stabilize the 1st metatarsal phalangeal (MTP) joint and the 1st metatarsal begins to move away from the proximal phalanx.	Instability in the 1st ray allows the transverse head of the adductor hallicis longus to pull the base of the proximal phalanx away from the head of the 1st metatarsal. The lateral sesamoid. bone is displaced laterally. The abductor hallicis muscle slides under the 1st metatarsal causing pronation of the hallux.	Bone absorption takes place on the medial joint aspect due to a decrease in the normal compression forces between the base of the proximal phalanx and the head of the 1st metatarsal. Bone deposition takes place on the lateral aspect of the joint in an attempt to maintain contact between articular surfaces of the MTP joint.

Stage 2

The extensor hallicis longus and flexor hallicis longus tendons are displaced laterally in relation to the MTP joint axis. The change in action lines of these muscles creates an adduction force against the 1st metatarsal and an abduction force against the hallux.	The transverse head of the adductor hallicus longus continues to pull the base of the proximal phalanx away from the 1st metatarsal head. The changed relationships of the bony components cause the intrinsic muscles to also pull the proximal phalanx away from the metatarsal head. Both sesamoid bones shift laterally and a bunion begins to form on the medial aspect of the MTP joint.	Bone absorption continues laterally on dorsal and distal margins of the 1st metatarsal head. Bone deposition continues on distal medial aspect of 1st metatarsal head as joint space widens.

Stage 3

The extensor hallicis longus and the flexor hallicus longus tendons are placed in a more lateral position in relation to the MTP joint axis so bowstring effect is increased and 1st metatarsal head is pulled further laterally. Increase in the space between the 1st and 2nd metatarsal.	The 1st metatarsal and 1st cuneiform are forced to deviate medially due to retrograde force generated by hallux pressing against 2nd digit. The tibial sesamoid bone is displaced to a position lateral to the metatarsal head and intrinsic muscles are unable to stabilize lateral joint aspect. The bunion on the medial joint aspect enlarges.	Continued deposition of bone on dorsolateral aspect of 1st metatarsal head in an attempt to maintain articular relationship between joint surfaces at the 1st MTP joint. The head enlarges even though bone continues be reabsorbed on the lateral aspect.

Stage 4

In this stage subluxation and/or dislocation of the 1st MTP joint may occur. The 1st metatarsal head displaces medially; the hallux is displaced laterally and may either override or underride the 2nd digit.	Usually, progression to subluxation of the 1st metatarsal joint is not seen unless the hallux valgus is accompanied by rheumatic inflammatory disease.	15–20% of patients have dislocation of the 2nd toe caused by pressure from underriding phalanges of 1st toe.[24]

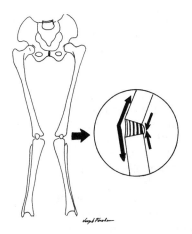

FIGURE 13–25. In genu valgum ("knock knees") the medial aspect of the knee complex is subjected to tensile stress and the lateral aspect is subjected to compressive stress.

posterior aspect, the vertebral column is vertically aligned and perfectly bisected by the LOG and the structures on either side of the column are symmetrical. The LOG falls through the midline of the occiput, through the spinous processes of all vertebrae, and directly through the gluteal cleft. In an optimal posture the vertebral structures, ligaments, and muscles are able to maintain the column in vertical alignment with little stress or energy expenditure. If one or more of the medial-lateral structures fails to provide adequate support, the column will bend to the side. The lateral bending will

be accompanied by rotation of the vertebrae because lateral flexion and rotation are coupled motions below the level of the second cervical vertebra.

Consistent lateral deviations of a series of vertebrae from the LOG in one or more regions of the spine may indicate the presence of a lateral spinal curvature called a **scoliosis** (Fig. 13–27). There are different types of scoliosis, but the **adolescent idiopathic** type makes up 80% of all scolioses.[55] The term idiopathic means that the cause of the condition is unknown. Idiopathic scoliotic curves are defined as structural curves[56] (Fig. 13–28). These curves involve changes in the structure of the vertebral bodies, transverse and spinous processes, intervertebral disks, ligaments, and muscles. Asymmetrical growth and development of the vertebral bodies leads to **wedging** of the vertebrae. Growth on the compressed side (concavity) is inhibited or slower than on the side of the convexity of the curve. Nonstructural scoliotic curves are called **functional curves** in that they can be reversed if the cause of the curve is corrected and structural changes are, by definition, not present. These curves are the result of correctable imbalances such as a leg length discrepancy or a muscle spasm. The curves in scoliosis are named according to the direction of the convexity and location of the curve. If the curve is convex to the left in the cervical area, the curve is designated as a left cervical scoliosis. If more than one region of the vertebral col-

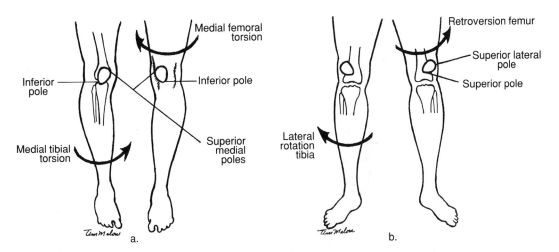

FIGURE 13–26. (a) In squinting or cross-eyed patella the superior medial pole of the patella faces medially while the inferior patellar pole faces laterally. (b) In grasshopper eyes patella the patellae are high, laterally situated, and face upward and outward.

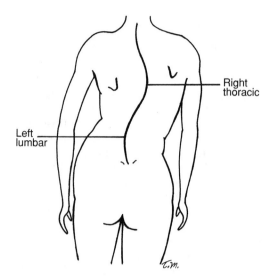

FIGURE 13–27. A lateral curvature of the vertebral column that is convex to the right in the thoracic region and convex to the left in the lumbar region.

umn is involved, the superior segment is named first. The curve shown in Figure 13–27 is a structural curve called a right thoracic, left lumbar scoliosis.

Investigators have postulated that adolescent idiopathic scoliosis may result from a dysfunction in the vestibular system,[57] a disturbance in control of the muscle spindle,[58] an inherited connective tissue disorder,[59] subcortical brain stem abnormalities,[60-62] or developmental instability.[63,64] Lidstrom[22] found differences in postural sway in 100 children aged 10 to 14 years; 35 of the children were siblings of scoliotic patients and 65 were control subjects.[22] This finding implicates the vestibular system and the possibility of a genetic component. As of this writing however, no evidence has been presented that unequivocally points to a single etiology for adolescent idiopathic scoliosis.[65]

Despite the ambiguity surrounding the cause or causes of adolescent idiopathic scoliosis the effects of unequal torques on the structures of the body are dramatic and can be devastating to those affected. The following example depicts a hypothetical series of events for adolescent idiopathic scoliosis. The first step in the process is unknown because researchers have been unable to identify the supporting structure involved in the initial failure. Therefore, it is just as possible that the sequence of events begins with a developmental disturbance that results in asymmetrical growth of the vertebrae rather than a failure in the muscular or ligamentous support system as suggested in the model.

Hypothetical Series of Events in Adolescent Idiopathic Scoliosis

1. Possible failure of support due to defect in muscular and/or ligamentous support systems
2. Creation of a lateral flexion moment
3. Deviation of the vertebrae with rotation
4. Compression of the vertebral body on the side of the concavity of the curve
5. Inhibition of growth of vertebral body on the side of the concavity of the curve in a still immature spine
6. Wedging of the vertebra in a still immature spine
7. Head out of line with sacrum
8. Compensatory curve
9. Adaptive shortening of trunk musculature on the concavity
10. Stretching of muscles, ligaments, and joint capsules on the convexity

These structural changes may progress to produce a severe deformity as growth proceeds unless intervention occurs at the appropriate time. Deformities can interfere with breathing and other internal organs as well as being cosmetically unacceptable. It has been estimated

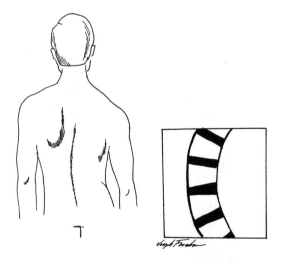

FIGURE 13–28. A lateral curvature of the vertebral column that is convex to the left in the thoracic region. Wedging of the vertebrae may be seen in the portion of the curve shown in the inset. This wedging illustrates one of the structural changes observed in idiopathic scoliosis.

that about 10% of the adolescent population in the United States have some degree of scoliosis. About 25% of this group has a curvature that will need intervention in the form of observation, bracing, or surgery. Adolescents whose vertebral columns are still immature and who have curves between 25° and 40° are considered to be at high risk because curves of this degree tend to progress.[66] According to Roach,[66] bracing is successful in preventing additional progression of the curve in 70% to 80% of the cases in which it is used. Curves that have progressed beyond 40° may require surgical intervention to prevent further progression. If a curvature is recognized early in its development, then measures may be instituted either to correct the curve or to prevent its increase.[67] According to the second phase of the Utah study in which a visual assessment (scoliosis screening) was performed of 3000 college-aged women (19–21 years of age) in 34 states and 5 foreign countries, 12% of this population had a previously undetected lateral deviation of the spine.[68]

In consideration of the fact that adolescent idiopathic scoliosis may be progressive in some cases and lead to a considerable amount of deformity without treatment, the initiation of screening programs in the schools appears to be important. However, as reported in 1986 only 20 states required screening programs for scoliosis.[56] Screening procedures are relatively simple to use and many evaluators rapidly become adept at identifying the changes that occur in scoliosis. The vertebral deviations in scoliosis cause asymmetrical changes in body structures and several of these changes may be detected through simple observation of body contours. Typical screening programs usually are designed for identification of the following features: unequal waist angles (Fig. 13–29a); unequal shoulder levels or unequal scapulae (Fig. 13–29b); rib hump; and obvious lateral spinal curvature (Fig. 13–29c).

Effects of Age, Pregnancy, Occupation, and Recreation on Posture

Age

Infants and Children

Postural control in infants develops progressively during the first year of life from control of the head, to control of the body in a sitting posture, to control of the body in a standing posture. Stability in a posture or the ability to fix and hold a posture in relation to gravity must be accomplished before the child is able to move within a posture. The child learns to maintain a certain posture usually through co-contraction of antagonist and agonist muscles around a joint and then is able to move in and out of the posture (sit to stand and stand to sit). Once stability is established, the child proceeds to controlled mobility and skill. Controlled mobility refers to the ability to move within the posture, for example, weight shifting in the standing posture. Skill refers to performance of activities like walking, running, and hopping, which are dynamic postural activities.[69]

The erect standing posture in infancy and early childhood differs somewhat from postural alignment in adults, but by the time a

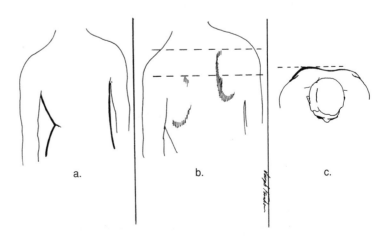

FIGURE 13–29. Typical changes in body contours used in scoliosis screening programs. (a) Uneven waist angles or difference in arm to body space. (b) Unequal shoulder height or unequal scapula level. (c) A rib hump during forward trunk flexion.

a.

b.

c.

child reaches the age of 10 or 11 years of age, postural alignment in the erect standing position should be similar to adult alignment (Table 13–7).[70] However, poor postural alignment in a 7- or 8-year-old child can be recognized because it is similar to poor postural alignment in adults. For example, the poor posture may include forward head, kyphosis, lordosis, and hyperextended knees.[29,70] According to Woollacott,[71] by the time a child reaches 7 to 10 years of age postural responses to platform perturbations are less variable and also comparable to adults in patterns of muscle activity and timing of responses. Responses of children younger than 7 years of age included greater coactivation of agonists and antagonists and slower response times for muscle activation than adults or older children.[71] Newell and colleagues[72] investigated COP motion (sway) in different age groups from 3 years to 92 years of age. The young adult group of students in their twenties had the least amount of movement of the COP; the individuals in the youngest and oldest groups had the greatest amount of COP motion.

Elderly

Postural alignment in the elderly often shows a more flexed posture than in the young adult (Fig.13–30); however, elderly individuals in their seventies and eighties may still demonstrate a close to optimal posture. The flexed posture observed in some elderly is probably due to a number of factors that may be attrib-

uted to the aging process, to a sedentary lifestyle, or to a combination of aging and sedentary lifestyle. Conditions such as osteoporosis also may affect the elderly posture. Osteoporosis (abnormal rarefaction of bone) weakens the vertebral bodies and makes them liable to fracture. Following the collapse of a series of the anterior portions of the weakened vertebrae, the normal posterior convexity of the thoracic curve increases (kyphosis). In kyphosis the anterior trunk flexor muscles shorten as the posteriorly located trunk extensors lengthen. Teramoto and coworkers[73] evaluated the effects of kyphosis in subjects from 20 to 90 years of age. The authors found that the degree of kyphosis significantly decreased lung volume and maximal inspiratory pressure in the elderly subjects.

Additional characteristics of posture in the elderly may be a forward head, which causes an increase in flexion in the cervical region and increase in extension at the atlanto-occipital joint. The ROM at the knees, hips, ankles, and trunk may be restricted because of muscle shortening and disuse atrophy. Furthermore, as voluntary postural response times in the elderly appear to be longer than in the young, the elderly may elect to stand with a wide BOS to have a margin of safety. Postural responses of older adults, aged 61 to 78 years, to platform perturbations show differences in timing and amplitude and include greater coactivation of antagonist and agonist muscles when compared to younger subjects, aged 19 to 38 years. Iverson and associates,[74] who tested noninstitutional-

Table 13–7. **Erect Stance: Normal Lower Extremity Alignment in Children**

Segment	Alignment	Degrees	Age
Knee			
	Genu varum	15–30°	1–2 y[45]
			1–4 y[50]
			1–3 y[24]
	Genu valgum	15°–30°	2–4 y[45,50]
			2–6 y[24]
	Lateral position of patella		1–6 y[50]
Foot			
	Pes planus		9 mo–2 or 4 y[50]
			2–6 y[24]
	Calcaneal eversion	5–10°	1 y
		5°	2 y
		4°	3 y
		0°	7 y

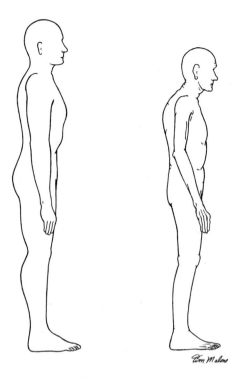

FIGURE 13–30. Changes in posture as a result of aging.

ized men 60 to 90 years of age on two types of balance tests that involved one-legged stance, found that balance time and torque production decreased significantly with age.[74] In some of the tests, the authors found that torque production was a significant predictor of balance time; that is, the greater the torque production, the longer the balance time. These authors also found that men who exercised five to six times per week had greater torque production than men who exercised less frequently. This finding suggests that high levels of fitness and activity may have beneficial effects on the aging person's ability to perform one-legged balancing activities that are needed for activities of daily living such as walking.[74]

Pregnancy

Normal pregnancies are accompanied by a weight gain, an increase in weight distribution in the breasts and abdomen, and softening of the ligamentous and connective tissue. The location of the woman's COG changes because of the increase in weight and its distribution anteriorly. Consequently, postural changes in pregnancy include an increase in the lordotic curves in the cervical and lumbar areas of the vertebral column, protraction of the shoulder girdle, and hyperextension of the knees. Franklin and Conner-Kerr[75] compared postural evaluations of 12 pregnant volunteers in their first trimester with evaluations of the same women in their third trimester. These investigators found changes in lumbar angle, head position, and anterior pelvic tilt. The lumbar angle increased by an average of 5.9°, the anterior pelvic tilt increased by an average of 4°, and the head become more posterior as pregnancy progressed from the first through the third trimester.[76] These changes in posture represent adaptations that help to maintain the COG centered over the BOS. Softening of ligamentous and connective tissues especially in the pelvis, sacroiliac joints, pubic symphyses, and abdomen change the support and protection offered by these structures and predispose pregnant women to strains in supporting structures.[76] Many women experience backache during pregnancy and all of the women in a study by Franklin and Conner-Kerr complained of backache.[75]

Occupation and Recreation

The static and dynamic postures assumed at work and during recreational activities may have adverse effects on joint structure and function. Injuries to joints and their supporting structures can lead to impaired function, decreased productivity, absences from work, and sometimes loss of job and permanent disability. Recognition by the medical profession that postures assumed at work and during recreational activities produce unique injuries requiring specialized knowledge for management has led to the establishment of medical specialties in the following areas: industrial or occupational medicine, performing arts medicine or simply "arts medicine," and sports medicine.

Each particular occupational and recreational activity has unique postures and resulting associated injuries. Bricklayers, surgeons, carpenters, and cashiers assume and perform tasks in standing postures for a majority of the working day. Others, such as secretaries, accountants, computer operators, and receptionists, assume sitting postures for a large proportion of the day. Performing artists often assume asymmetrical postures while playing a musical instrument, dancing, or acting. Running, jogging, and long distance walking are dynamic postures that have very specific associated injuries.

The high incidence of back problems in the population has led to a large amount of research related to lifting and stooping postures and to the development of various treatment programs.[77–84] Different sitting postures and their effects on intradiskal pressures in the lumbar spine have been analyzed.[81] Wheelchair postures and the effects of different degrees of anterior-posterior and lateral pelvic tilt on the vertebral column and trunk muscle activity in sitting and standing postures in selected work activities also have been investigated.[85] A large portion of the research suggests that many back problems are preventable because they result from mechanical stresses produced by prolonged static postures in the forward stooping or sitting positions and the repeated lifting of heavy loads.

Many of the injuries sustained during both occupational and recreational activities fall into the category of "overuse injuries." This type of injury is caused by repetitive stress that exceeds the physiologic limits of the tissues. Muscles, ligaments, and tendons are especially vulnerable to the effects of repetitive tensile forces, whereas bones and cartilage are susceptible to injury from the application of excessive compressive forces. A random sample of professional musicians in New York found that violin, piano, cello, and bass players were frequently affected by back and neck problems.[86] In a larger study involving 485 musicians, the authors found that 64% had painful overuse syndromes. The majority of problems were associated with the musculotendinous unit, and others involved bones, joints, bursae, and muscle. String players experienced shoulder and neck problems caused by the maintenance of abnormal head and neck positions, whereas flute players had shoulder problems associated with maintaining an externally rotated shoulder position that has to be assumed for prolonged periods during performances and practices.[87]

Each occupational and recreational activity requires a detailed biomechanical analysis of the specific postures involved to determine how abnormal and excessive stresses can be relieved. Sometimes the analysis involves not only a person's posture but also features of the work site such as chair or table height, weight of objects to be lifted or carried, and weight and shape of a musical instrument or tool. Treatment may involve a combination of modifications of the environment, adaptations of the instrument or tools, and modifications of posture.

Summary

Knowledge of biomechanics and normal human structure and function forms the basis for determining the potentially harmful effects of asymmetrical postures on joint structure and function in static and dynamic postures. This chapter has provided an introduction to the basic features of normal postural alignment in the erect standing position. The probable causes and possible effects of some of the more common postural malalignments have been analyzed and discussed. Also some of the basic elements of postural control have been introduced. This chapter and the previous chapters have provided the reader with basic kinematic and kinetic information that is required to analyze static erect human posture. Using the information contained in the chapter the reader should be able to recognize abnormal or extreme postures and the potentially harmful effects of these postures on body structures. The knowledge gained in this chapter forms a basis for analyzing dynamic posture of gait.

REFRERENCES

1. Schenck, JM, and Cordova, FK: Introductory Biomechanics, ed 2. FA Davis, Philadelphia, 1980.
2. Horak, FB, et al: Postural perturbations: New insights for treatment of balance disorders. Phys Ther 77:517, 1997.
3. Maki, BE, and McIlroy, WE: The role of limb movements in maintaining upright stance: The "change-in-support strategy." Phys Ther 77:489, 1997.
4. DiFabio, RP, and Emasithi, A: Aging and the mechanisms underlying head and postural control during voluntary motion. Phys Ther 77:458, 1997.
5. Clement, G, and Lestienne, F: Adaptive modifications of postural attitude in conditions of weightlessness. Exp Brain Res 72:381–389,1988.
6. Speers, RA, et al: Multivariate changes in coordination of postural control following spaceflight. J Biomech 31:883, 1998.
7. Garn, SN, and Newton, RA: Kinesthetic awareness in subjects with multiple ankle sprains. Phys Ther 68:1667–1671, 1988.
8. Forkin, DM, et al: Evaluation of kinesthetic defects indicative of balance control in gymnasts with unilateral chronic ankle sprains. Phys Ther 23:245, 1996.
9. Bernier, JN, and Perrin, DH: Effect of coordination training on proprioception of the functionally unstable ankle. J Orthop Sports Phys Ther 27:264, 1998.
10. Dietz, V: Evidence for a load receptor contribution to the control of posture and locomotion. Neurosci Biobehav Rev 22:495, 1998.

11. Allum, JH, et al: Proprioceptive control of posture: a review of new concepts. Gait Posture 8:214, 1998.
12. Horak, FB: Measurement of movement patterns to study postural coordination. Proceedings of the 10th Annual Eugene Michels Research Forum, APTA Section on Research, New Orleans, La., 1990.
13. Nashner, LM: Sensory, neuromuscular and biomechanical contributions to human balance. Proceedings of the APTA Forum, APTA, Alexandria, Va., 1990.
14. Keshner, EA: Reflex, voluntary and mechanical processes in postural stabilization. Proceedings of the APTA Forum, APTA, Alexandria, Va., 1990.
15. Luchies, CW, et al: Stepping responses of young and old adults to postural disturbances: Kinematics. J Am Geriatr Soc 42:506, 1994.
16. Luchies, CW, et al: Effects of age on balance assessment using voluntary and involuntary step tasks. J Gerontol Biol Med Sci 54:M140, 1999.
17. Schenkman, M: Interrelationship of neurological and mechanical factors in balance control. Proceedings of the APTA Forum Balance APTA, Alexandria, Va., 1990.
18. Patla, AE, et al: Identification of age-related changes in the balance-control system. Proceedings of the APTA Forum, APTA, Alexandria, Va., 1990.
19. Whipple, R, and Wolfson, LI: Abnormalities of balance, gait and sensorimotor function in the elderly population. Proceedings of the APTA Forum, APTA, Alexandria, Va., 1990.
20. Rogers, M: Dynamic biomechanics of normal foot and ankle during walking and running. Phys Ther 68:1822–1830,1988.
21. Rogers, M, and Cavanaugh, PR: Glossary of biomechanical terms, concepts and units. Phys Ther 64:82–98,1984.
22. Lidstrom, J, et al: Postural control in siblings to scoliosis patients and scoliosis patients. Spine 13:1070–1074, 1988.
23. Cailliet, R: Soft Tissue Pain and Disability, ed 3. FA Davis, Philadelphia, 1996.
24. Cailliet, R: Foot and Ankle Pain, ed 3. FA Davis, Philadelphia, 1997.
25. Danis, CG, et al: Relationship between standing posture and stability. Phys Ther 78:502, 1998.
26. Carlsoo, S: The static muscle load in different work positions: An electromyographic study. Ergonomics 4:193,1961.
27. Soames, RW, and Atha, J: The role of antigravity muscles during quiet standing in man. Appl Phys 47:159–167,1981.
28. Gray, ER: The role of the leg muscles in variations of the arches in normal and flat feet. Phys Ther 49:1084–1088, 1969.
29. Kendall, F, and McCreary, EK: Muscles: Testing and Function, ed 4. Williams & Wilkins, Baltimore, 1983.
30. Duval-Beaupere, G, et al: A barycentremetric study of the sagittal shape of spine and pelvis: The conditions required for an economic standing position. Ann Biomed Eng 20:451, 1992.
31. Kagaya, H, et al: Ankle, knee, and hip moments during standing with and without joint contractures. Am J Phys Med Rehabil 77:49, 1998.
32. Don Tigny, RL: Dysfunction of the sacroiliac joint and its treatment. J Orthop Sports Phys Ther 1:1,1979.
33. Basmajian, JV: Muscles Alive, ed 4. Williams & Wilkins, Baltimore, 1978.
34. Cailliet, R: Low Back Pain Syndrome, ed 5. FA Davis, Philadelphia, 1995.
35. Youdas, JW, et al: Lumbar lordosis and pelvic inclination of asymptomatic adults. Phys Ther 76:1066, 1996.
36. Korovessis, PG, et al: Reciprocal angulation of vertebral bodies in the sagittal plane in an asymptomatic Greek population. Spine 23:700, 1998.
37. Korovessis, P, et al: Segmental roentgenographic analysis of vertebral inclination on sagittal plane in asymptomatic versus chronic low back pain patients. J Spinal Disord 12:131, 1999.
38. Grieve, GP: The sacroiliac joint. Physiotherapy 62:12, 1976.
39. Cailliet, R: Neck and Arm Pain, ed 3. FA Davis, Philadelphia, 1991.
40. Bogduk, N: Clinical Anatomy of the Lumbar Spine and Sacrum, ed 3. Churchill Livingstone, New York, 1997.
41. Morris, JM, et al: An electromyographic study of intrinsic muscles of the back in man. J Anat 96:509,1962.
42. Kapandji, IA: The Physiology of the Joints, Vol 3. Churchill Livingstone, Edinburgh, 1974.
43. Cailliet, R: Head and Face Pain Syndromes. FA Davis, Philadelphia, 1992.
44. Riegger-Krugh, C, and Keysor, JJ: Skeletal malalignments of the lower quarter: Correlated and compensatory motions and postures. Phys Ther 23:164, 1996.
45. Magee, DJ: Othopedic Physical Assessment, ed 2. WB Saunders, Philadelphia, 1992.
46. Cailliet, R: Knee Pain and Disability, ed 3. FA Davis, Philadelphia, 1992.
47. Richardson, JK, and Iglarsh, ZA: Clinical Orthopaedic Physical Therapy. WB Saunders, Philadelphia, 1994.
48. Starkey, C, and Ryan, J: Evaluation of Orthopedic and Athletic Injuries. FA Davis, Philadelphia, 1996.
49. Malone, TR, et al: Orthopedic and Sports Physical Therapy, ed 3. CV Mosby, St. Louis, 1997.
50. Valmassy, RL: Clinical Biomechanics of the Lower Extremities. CV Mosby, St. Louis, 1996.
51. Myerson, MS, and Shereff, MJ: The pathological anatomy of claw and hammer toes. J Bone Joint Surg 71A:45–49,1989.
52. Perry, J, et al: Analysis of knee joint forces during flexed-knee stance. J Bone Joint Surg 57A:7, 1975.
53. Adams, MA, and Hutton, WC: The effect of posture on the diffusion into lumbar intervertebral discs. J Anat 147:121–134, 1986.
54. Adams, MA, and Hutton, WC: The effect of posture on the lumbar spine. J Bone Joint Surg 47B:625–629,1985.
55. Cailliet, R: Scoliosis. FA Davis, Philadelphia, 1975.
56. National Scoliosis Foundation: States that Require Postural Screening for Scoliosis. Belmont, Mass., July, 1986.
57. Jensen, GM, and Wilson KB: Horizontal postrotatory nystagamus response in female subjects with adolescent idiopathic scoliosis. Phys Ther 59:10,1979.
58. Yekutiel, M, et al: Proprioceptive function in children with adolescent scoliosis. Spine 6:560–566, 1981.
59. Miller, NH, et al: Genetic analysis of structural elastic fiber and collagen genes in familial adolescent idiopathic scoliosis. J Orthop Res 14:994, 1996.
60. Dretakis, EK, et al: Electroencephalographic study of schoolchildren with adolescent idiopathic scoliosis. Spine 13:143–145,1988.
61. Geissele, AE, et al : Magnetic resonance imaging of the brain stem in adolescent idiopathic scoliosis. Spine 16:761, 1991.
62. Machida, M, et al: Pathogenesis of idiopathic scoliosis: SEP's in chicken with experimentally induced scoliosis and in patients with idiopathic scoliosis. J Pediatr Orthop 14:329, 1994.

63. Goldberg, CJ, et al: Adolescent idiopathic scoliosis as developmental instability. Genetica 96:247, 1995.

64. Goldberg, CJ, et al: Scoliosis and developmental theory: Adolescent idiopathic scoliosis. Spine 22:2228, 1997.

65. Murray, DW, and Bulstrode, CJ: The development of adolescent idiopathic scoliosis. Eur Spine J 5:251, 1996

66. Roach JW: Adolescent Idiopathic Scoliosis. Othop Clin North Am 30:353, 1999.

67. Winter, RB, and Moe, JH: A plea for routine school examination of children for spinal deformity. Minn Med 57:419,1974.

68. Francis, RS: Scoliosis screening of 3,000 college-aged women: The Utah study. Phase 2. Phys Ther 68:1513–1516,1988.

69. O'Sullivan, SB: Motor control assessment. In O'Sullivan, S, and Schmitz, T (eds): Physical Rehabilitation: Assessment and Treatment, ed 3. FA Davis, Philadelphia,1994.

70. Connolly, B: Postural applications in the child and adult. In Kraus, S (ed): Clinics in Physical Therapy, Vol 11. Churchill Livingstone, New York, 1988.

71. Woollacott, M: Postural control mechanisms in the young and old. Proceedings of the APTA Forum, APTA, Alexandria, Va., 1990.

72. Newell, KM, et al: Short-term non-stationarity and the development of postural control. Gait-Posture 6:56, 1997.

73. Teramoto, S, et al: Influence of kyphosis on the age-related decline in pulmonary function. Adstract Nippon Ronen Igakkai Zasshi 35:23, 1998.

74. Iverson, B, et al: Balance performance, force production and activity levels in non-institutionalized men 60–90 years of age. Phys Ther 70:348–355,1990.

75. Franklin, ME, and Conner-Kerr, T: An analysis of posture and back pain in the first and third trimesters of pregnancy. J Orthop Sports Phys Ther 28:133, 1998.

76. Gleeson, PB, and Pauls, JA: Obstetrical physical therapy: Review of literature. Phys Ther 68:1699–1702,1988.

77. Platts, RGS: Spinal mechanics. Physiotherapy 63: 7,1977.

78. Hall, H: The Canadian back education unit. Physiotherapy 66:4,1980.

79. Studenski, S, et al: The role of instability in falls among older persons. Proceedings of the APTA Forum, APTA, Alexandria, Va., 1990.

80. Edgar, M: Pathologies associated with lifting. Physiotherapy 65:245, 1979.

81. Anderson, GBJ, et al: Analysis and measurement of the loads on the lumbar spine during work at a table. J Biomech 17:513,1979.

82. Matmiller, AW: The California back school. Physiotherapy 66:4,1980.

83. Kennedy, B: An Australian programme for management of back problems. Physiotherapy 66:4,1980.

84. Forsell, MZ: The Swedish back school. Physiotherapy 66:4,1980.

85. Borello-France, DF, et al: Modification of sitting posture of patients with hemiplegia using seat boards and backboards. Phys Ther 68:67–71,1988.

86. Brody, JE: For artists and musicians creativity can mean illness and injury. New York Times, October 17, 1989.

87. Lockwood, AH: Medical problems of performing artists. N Engl J Med 320:221, 1989.

Study Questions

1. What is a "sway envelope"?

2. Is quadriceps muscle activity necessary to maintain knee extension in static erect stance? Explain your answer.

3. Is activity of the abdominal muscles necessary to keep the pelvis level in static standing posture? Explain your answer.

4. What is the function of the sacrotuberous ligament in the erect standing posture?

5. In which areas of the vertebral column would you expect to find the most stress in the erect standing posture?

6. In the erect standing posture identify the type of stresses that would be affecting the following structures: apophyseal joints in the lumbar region, apophyseal joint capsules in the thoracic region, annulus fibrosus L5 to S1, anterior longitudinal ligament in the thoracic region, and the sacroiliac joints.

7. What effect might tight hamstrings have on the alignment of the following structures during erect stance: pelvis, lumbosacral angle, hip joint, knee joint, and the lumbar region of the vertebral column?

8. How would you describe a typical idiopathic lateral curvature of the vertebral column?

9. Describe the moments that would be acting at all body segments as a result of an unexpected forward movement of a supporting surface. Describe the muscle activity that would be necessary to bring the body's LOG over the COP.

10. Identify the changes in body segments that are commonly used in scoliosis screening programs.

11. Compare hammer toes with claw toes.

12. How do postural responses to perturbations of the erect standing posture in the elderly compare with responses of children who are 1 to 6 years of age?

13. Compare a flexed lumbar spine posture with an extended posture in terms of the nutrition of the disks and stresses on ligaments and joint structures.

14. What is the relationship between the GRFV, LOG, and COG in the erect static posture?

15. Explain how a hallux valgus deformity develops.

16. Describe the effects of a forward head posture on the zygapophyseal joints and capsules, intervertebral disks, vertebral column ligaments and muscles.

CHAPTER 14

GAIT

OBJECTIVES

Following the study of this chapter, the reader should be able to:

Define

1. The stance, swing, and double support phases of walking gait.
2. The subdivisions of the stance and swing phases of walking gait.
3. The time and distance parameters of walking gait.

Describe

1. Joint motion at the hip, knee, and ankle for one extremity during a walking and running gait cycle.
2. The location of the ground reaction force vector in relation to the hip, knee, and ankle joints during the stance phase of walking gait.
3. The moments of force acting at the hip, knee, and ankle joints during the stance phase of walking gait.

Explain

1. Muscle activity at the hip, knee, and ankle throughout the walking gait cycle, including why and when a particular muscle is active and the type of contraction required.
2. The role of each of the determinants of gait.
3. The muscle activity that occurs in the upper extremities and trunk during walking gait.

Compare

1. Motion of the upper extremities and trunk with motion of the pelvis and lower extremities during walking gait.
2. The traditional gait terminology with the newer terminology.
3. Normal walking gait with a gait in which there is a weakness of the hip extensor and hip abductor muscles.
4. Normal gait with a gait in which there is unequal leg length.
5. Normal walking gait with stair gait in relation to range of motion and muscle activity.
6. Normal walking gait with running gait.

· ·

Introduction

Preceding chapters in this text introduced the reader to the basic elements of human structure and function. In Chapter 13 the reader learned how individual joints and muscles function cooperatively to maintain the body in the erect posture. Knowledge of body structure and function in the static posture forms the basis for study of the human structure in a dynamic situation. In human locomotion (ambulation, gait) the reader is given the opportunity to discover how individual joints and muscles function in an integrated fashion both to maintain upright posture and to produce motion of the body as a whole. Knowledge of the kinematics and kinetics of normal ambulation provides the reader with a foundation for analyzing, identifying, and correcting abnormalities in gait.

One of the most distinctive features of human gait is the fact that it is individualistic. Each person has a characteristic gait pattern. Novelists and dramatists often use gait patterns to help portray the characters in their writings. Gait patterns may reflect a person's occupation, body structure, health status, and personality, as well as many other physical and psychological attributes. For example, the rolling gait that is used to describe a sailor's movement reflects the wide base of support (BOS) needed to maintain balance at sea. The term "waddling" used to describe an obese person's gait reflects his or her unique body structure. Staggering gaits usually are associated with either drunkenness or weakness, and

bouncy gaits are associated with vitality and strength. Swaggering gaits imply an aggressive personality, whereas mincing gaits may imply timidity. Investigations of gait indicate that potential assault victims display unique patterns of movement during walking. These particular patterns presumably communicate vulnerability and, as a result, predispose the person to attack.[1]

General Features

The descriptive terms used by nonscientific writers to describe gait are successful in conveying images of a unique gait but do not provide the information necessary for evaluators of human function. Scientists from many different disciplines have contributed to our present knowledge of gait and have provided us with detailed methods for analyzing gait. Human locomotion, or gait, may be described as a translatory progression of the body as a whole, produced by coordinated, rotatory movements of body segments.[2] Normal gait is rhythmic and characterized by alternating propulsive and retropulsive motions of the lower extremities. The alternating movements of the lower extremities essentially support and carry along the head, arms, and trunk (HAT).[3] HAT constitutes about 75% of total body weight. The head and arms combined constitute about 25% of total body weight, and the trunk accounts for the remaining 50%.[4]

In standing posture, HAT is supported by both lower extremities; in gait, HAT not only must be balanced over one extremity, but also must be transferred from one extremity to the other. The weight of HAT (75% of total body weight) plus the weight of the swinging lower extremity (about 10% of total body weight) must be supported by one extremity during single-limb support. Although single-limb support alternates with periods in which both lower extremities are in contact with the ground, gait places many more demands on the lower extremities than does the static erect posture. Before individuals can walk they must be able to balance HAT in the erect standing posture, transfer HAT from one lower extremity to another, and lift one lower extremity off the ground and place it in front of the other extremity in an alternating pattern. These activities require coordination, balance, intact kinesthetic and proprioceptive senses, and integrity of the joints and muscles.[5]

To simplify the understanding of gait, several authors have defined gait in terms of certain tasks that must be accomplished.[5,6] According to the professional staff at Rancho Los Amigos Medical Center in California, the following three main tasks are involved in walking: (1) weight acceptance, (2) single-limb support, and (3) swing limb advancement.[5] In other words, a person must be able to accept and support the weight of the body on one lower extremity and to swing one extremity forward to progress. Winter[6] also has proposed three main tasks for walking gait that include (1) maintenance of support of HAT against gravity, (2) maintenance of upright posture and balance, and (3) control of the foot trajectory to achieve safe ground clearance and a gentle heel contact. The tasks described by these authors are similar except that Winter[6] has included gentle heel contact and foot clearance as essential tasks. In addition to studying the events occurring during gait and the prerequisite skills, researchers have become interested in determining how gait is initiated.

Gait Initiation

Gait initiation may be defined as the series or sequence of events that occur from the initiation of movement to the beginning of the gait cycle. Gait initiation has been described as a stereotyped activity in both young and old healthy people. The initiation of movement is well defined, but the end of this activity is less

well defined. Gait initiation begins in the erect standing posture with an activation of the tibialis anterior and vastus lateralis, in conjunction with an inhibition of the gastrocnemius. Bilateral concentric contractions of the tibialis anterior (pulling on the tibias) results in a sagittal torque that inclines the body anteriorly from the ankles. Initially, the center of pressure (COP) is described as shifting either posteriorly and laterally toward the swing foot (foot that is preparing to take the first step)[7] or posteriorly and medially toward the supporting limb.[8] Abduction of the swing hip occurs almost simultaneously with contractions of the tibialis anterior and vastus lateralis and produces a coronal torque that propels the body toward the support limb. According to Elbe and colleagues[7] the support limb hip and knee flex a few degrees (3–10°) and now the COP moves anteriorly and medially toward the support limb. This anterior and medial shift of the COP frees the swing limb so that it can leave the ground. The end of the gait initiation activity ends when either the stepping or swing extremity lifts off the ground[7] or when the heel strikes the ground.[8] The total duration of the gait initiation phase is about 0.64 seconds.[8] A healthy individual may initiate gait with either the right or left lower extremity and no changes will be seen in the pattern of events. However, for patients with hemiplegia (one-sided paralysis) a considerable difference exists between gait initiation that begins with a step by the affected leg compared with gait initiation that begins with a step by the nonaffected leg. When the affected leg initiates gait the pattern of events is practically the same as in a nonaffected person, but when the person with paralysis attempts gait initiation with the nonaffected leg the pattern of events is erratic and stability is seriously threatened.[8]

Kinematics

Gait is an extremely complex activity to analyze. Therefore, gait has been divided into a number of segments that make it possible to identify the events that are occurring. It is also worth noting that gait analysis is merely a special case of movement analysis as a whole. Knowledge of the terminology used to describe the events is necessary to be able to understand and analyze gait. Generally, gait is described by using the activities of one lower extremity (referred to as the reference extremity) from the beginning to the end of one gait cycle.

Phases of the Gait Cycle

The **gait cycle** includes the activities that occur from the point of initial contact of one lower extremity to the point at which the same extremity contacts the ground again (Fig. 14–1). During one gait cycle each extremity passes through two phases, a single **stance phase** and a single **swing phase.**

The stance phase begins at the instant that one extremity contacts the ground (heel strike) and continues only as long as some portion of the foot is in contact with the ground (toe off) (Fig. 14–2). During the stance phase of gait some portion of the foot is in contact with the supporting surface at all times. The stance

phase makes up approximately 60% of the gait cycle during normal walking.[9]

The swing phase begins as soon as the toe of one extremity leaves the ground and ceases just before heel strike or contact of the same extremity (Fig. 14–3). When the reference extremity is in the swing phase, it does not contact the ground at any time. The swing phase makes up 40% of the gait cycle.[9,10]

A period of double-limb support occurs in walking, when the lower extremity of one side of the body is beginning its stance phase and the lower extremity on the opposite side is ending its stance phase. Therefore, there are *two* periods of double support in a single gait cycle (Fig. 14–4). During double support *both* lower extremities are in contact with the ground at the same time. At a normal walking speed, stance of one leg and stance of the op-

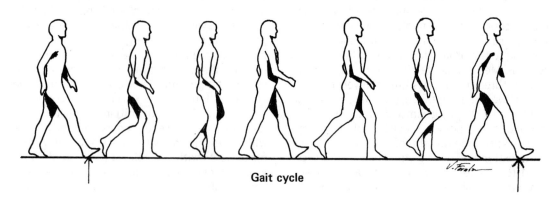

Gait cycle

FIGURE 14–1. A gait cycle consists of the events that occur between initial contact of the reference extremity (right) and the successive contact of the same extremity.

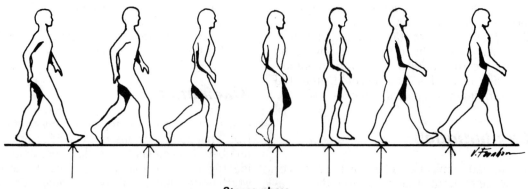

Stance phase

FIGURE 14–2. The stance phase of a gait cycle is defined as the period in which some portion of the foot of the reference extremity is in contact with the supporting surface. The period extends from the point of initial foot contact of the reference extremity (right lower extremity in the diagram) to the point at which only the toes of the same (right) extremity are in contact with this supporting surface.

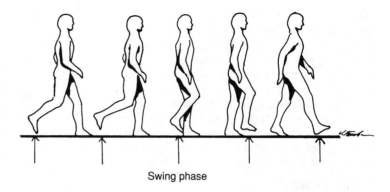

FIGURE 14–3. The swing phase of gait is defined as the period in which the foot of the reference extremity is not in contact with the supporting surface. The swing phase extends from the instant that the toe of the reference extremity (right lower extremity) leaves the ground to just before initial contact of the reference extremity.

Swing phase

posite leg overlap for about 22% of the gait cycle (Fig. 14–5).

Subdivisions

Traditionally, the stance and swing phases of gait have been divided into the following subunits: (1) stance, which consists of heel strike, foot flat, midstance, heel off, and toe off, and (2) swing, which consists of acceleration, midswing, and deceleration. Another set of terms has been introduced to describe the subunits of gait by the Gait Laboratory at Rancho Los Amigos (RLA) Medical Center.[5] The RLA terminology may eventually replace the older descriptive terms. The reader should become

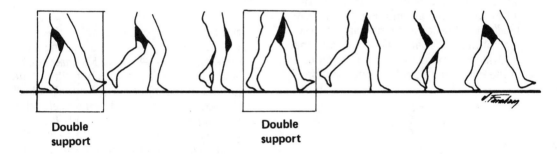

Double support

Double support

FIGURE 14–4. Double support is defined as the period in which some portions of the feet of both extremities are in contact with the supporting surface at the same time. Two periods of double support occur within a single gait cycle. One period occurs early in the stance phase of the reference extremity and the other occurs late in the stance phase of the reference extremity.

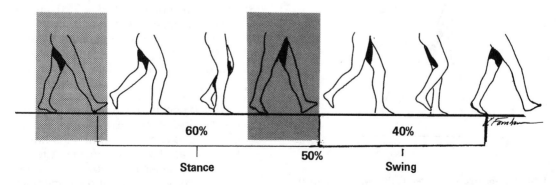

60%

40%

50%

Stance

Swing

FIGURE 14–5. Two periods of double support overlap the stance phases of the two lower extremities for about 22% of the gait cycle at a normal walking speed. The stance phase constitutes 60% of the gait cycle and the swing phase constitutes 40% of the cycle at normal walking speeds. Increases or decreases in walking speeds will alter the percentages of time spent in each phase.

familiar with both the traditional and newer terms because both methods of describing gait may be encountered in the literature. In the following section definitions will be given for the traditional terminology first and for the RLA terminology second. It should be noted, however, that the two terminologies are not exactly equivalent but are placed in the following order to make comparison easier. The traditional terminology refers to points in time, whereas the RLA terminology refers to lengths of time.

STANCE PHASE

1. *Heel strike* refers to the instant at which the heel of the leading extremity strikes the ground (Fig. 14–6). RLA: *Initial contact* refers to the instant the foot of the leading extremity strikes the ground.[5] In normal gait the heel is the point of contact. In abnormal gait it is possible for either the whole foot or the toes rather than the heel to make initial contact with the ground.

2. *Foot flat* occurs immediately after heel strike and is the point at which the foot fully contacts the ground (Fig. 14–7). RLA: *Loading response* occurs immediately following initial contact and continues until the contralateral extremity lifts off the ground at the end of the double-support phase.[5]

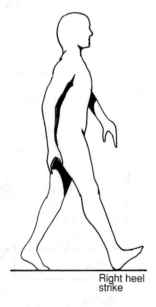

FIGURE 14–6. Heel strike refers to the instant at which the heel of the reference extremity contacts the supporting surface. Right heel strike in the diagram constitutes the beginning of the stance phase of gait for the right lower extremity. Heel strike is analogous to initial contact.

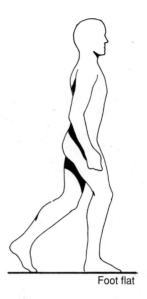

Foot flat

FIGURE 14–7. Foot flat occurs immediately after heel strike and is defined as the point at which the foot is flat on the ground. The period of loading response (RLA) extends from initial contact until the contralateral extremity leaves the ground at the end of the double support period.

3. *Midstance* is the point at which the body weight is directly over the supporting lower extremity (Fig. 14–8). RLA: *Midstance* begins when the contralateral extremity lifts off the ground and continues to a position in which the body has progressed over and ahead of the supporting extremity (Fig. 14–9).

4. *Heel off* is the point at which the heel of the reference extremity leaves the ground (Fig. 14–10). RLA: *Terminal stance* is the period from the end of midstance to a point just prior to initial contact of the contralateral extremity or following heel off of the reference extremity (Fig. 14–11).

5. *Toe off* is the point at which only the toe of the ipsilateral extremity is in contact with the ground (Fig. 14–12). RLA: *Preswing* encompasses the period from just following heel off to toe off (Fig. 14–13).

SWING PHASE

1. *Acceleration* begins once the toe of the reference (ipsilateral) extremity leaves the ground and continues until midswing or the point at which the swinging extremity is directly under the body (Fig. 14–14). RLA: *Initial swing* begins at the same point as acceleration and continues until maximum knee flexion of the reference (ipsilateral) extremity occurs.

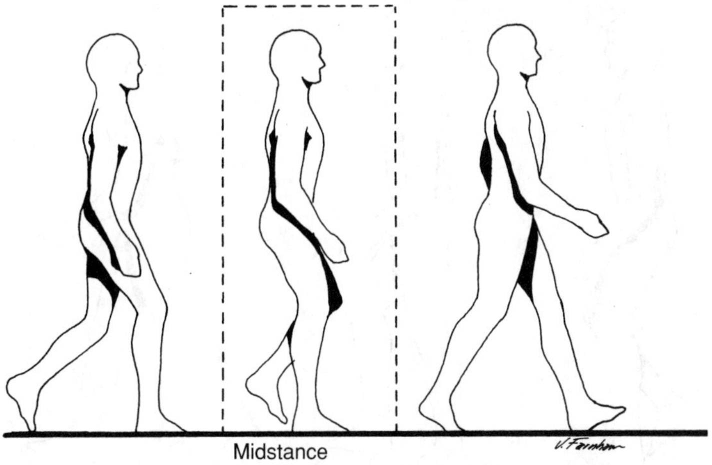

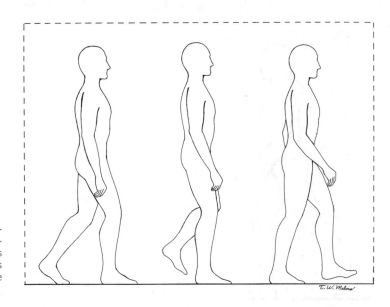

FIGURE 14–8. Midstance is the point at which the body weight passes directly over the supporting lower extremity. The dotted line in the diagram outlines the point of midstance for the right lower extremity. Midstance encompasses the period from the end of foot flat to the beginning of heel off.

Midstance

FIGURE 14–9. Midstance (RLA) begins when the contralateral extremity lifts off the ground and continues to a position in which the body has progressed over and ahead of the supporting extremity.

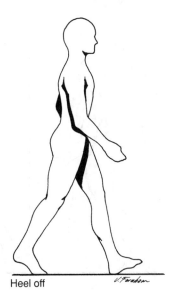

FIGURE 14–10. Heel off is the point at which the heel of the reference extremity (right extremity in the diagram) leaves the supporting surface.

Heel off

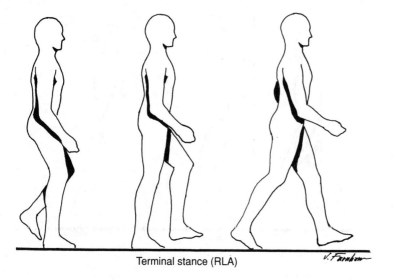

Terminal stance (RLA)

FIGURE 14–11. The period of terminal stance (RLA) includes the interval of the stance phase from the end of midstance (RLA) to just after the heel of the reference extremity (right extremity in the diagram) leaves the ground. Therefore, heel off is included in terminal stance.

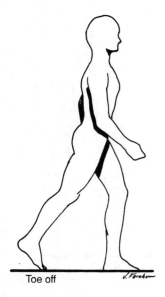

Toe off

FIGURE 14–12. Toe off is defined as the point in which only the toe of the reference extremity (right extremity) is touching the ground. The period from heel off to toe off often is referred to as the push off period of the stance phase.

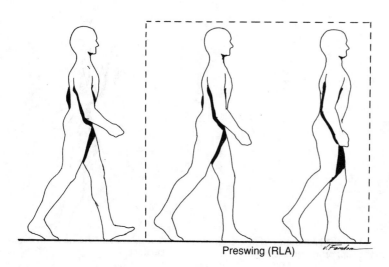

Preswing (RLA)

FIGURE 14–13. Preswing (RLA) includes the interval of stance from the end of terminal stance (just after the right heel leaves the ground and the left heel contacts the ground) until the toe leaves the ground. Preswing is not exactly comparable to push off because preswing does not include heel off. Heel off occurs during terminal stance when using RLA terminology.

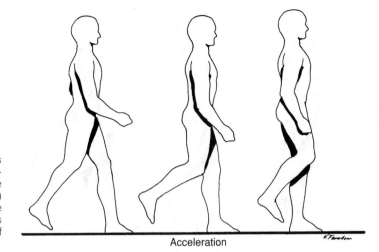

Acceleration

FIGURE 14–14. Acceleration begins once the toe of the reference (right extremity in the diagram) has left the supporting surface. Initial swing (RLA) begins at approximately the same point as acceleration and continues until maximum flexion of the knee of the reference extremity.

2. *Midswing* occurs when the ipsilateral extremity passes directly beneath the body (Fig. 14–15). RLA: *Midswing* encompasses the period immediately following maximum knee flexion and continues until the tibia is in a vertical position (Fig. 14–16).
3. *Deceleration* occurs after midswing when the tibia passes beyond the perpendicular and the knee is extending in preparation for heel strike. RLA: *Terminal swing* includes the period from the point at which the tibia is in the vertical position to a point just prior to initial contact (Fig. 14–17).

A comparison of the traditional and RLA terminology reveals some differences between the two. However, these differences appear to be based primarily on the fact that the RLA terminology better defines a particular interval than the traditional. Sometimes the traditional terminology does not adequately define the end and the beginning of an interval, for example, where foot flat ends and midstance begins. In the RLA terminology each segment has a fairly well-defined beginning and observable end point and reference is made to an interval of gait rather than to a point. The following summary compares the traditional and RLA terminologies. A detailed description of the joint and muscle activity during each subdivision of gait will be present later in the chapter.

Comparison of Gait Terminology

Traditional	RLA
Heel strike	Initial contact
Heel strike to foot flat	Loading response
Foot flat to midstance	Midstance
Midstance to heel off	Terminal stance
Toe off	Preswing
Toe off to acceleration	Initial swing
Acceleration to midswing	Midswing
Midswing to deceleration	Terminal swing

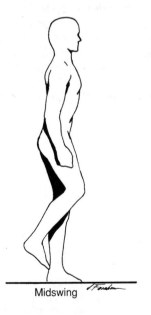

Midswing

FIGURE 14–15. Midswing occurs when the reference extremity passes directly below the body. In the diagram, the right lower extremity has just passed directly beneath the trunk. The midswing period extends from the end of acceleration to the beginning of deceleration.

Distance and Time Variables

Time and distance are two of the basic parameters of motion, and measurements of these

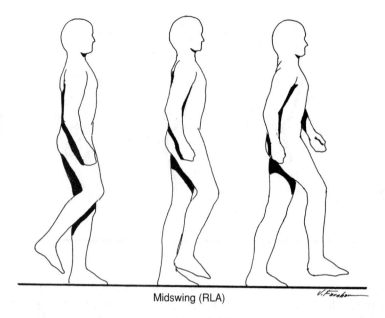

Midswing (RLA)

FIGURE 14–16. Midswing (RLA) is the period from maximal knee flexion to a point at which the tibia attains a vertical position.

variables provide a basic description of gait. **Temporal variables** include stance time, single-limb and double-support time, swing time, stride and step time, cadence, and speed. The **distance variables** include stride length, step length, width of walking base, and degree of toe out. These variables provide essential quantitative information about a person's gait and should be included in any gait description. Each variable may be affected by such factors as age, sex, height, size and shape of bony components, distribution of mass in body segments, joint mobility, muscle strength, type of clothing and footgear, habit, and psychological status. However, a discussion of all the factors affecting gait is beyond the scope of this text.

Stance time is the amount of time that elapses during the stance phase of one extremity in a gait cycle.

Single-support time is the amount of time that elapses during the period when only one extremity is on the supporting surface in a gait cycle.

Double-support time is the amount of time that a person spends with both feet on the ground during one gait cycle. The percentage of time spent in double support may be increased in the elderly and in those with balance disorders. The percentage of time spent in double support decreases as the speed of walking increases.

Stride length is the linear distance between

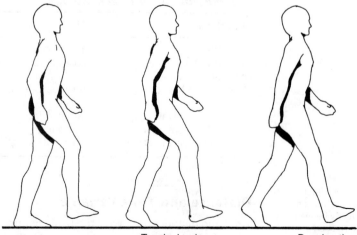

Terminal swing   Deceleration

FIGURE 14–17. Deceleration is the point at which the knee is extending in preparation for heel strike. Terminal swing (RLA) includes the period in which the tibia moves from its vertical position to the point at which the knee is in full extension just before initial contact.

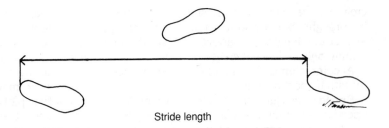

FIGURE 14–18. Stride length is determined by measuring the distance from the point of heel strike of the reference extremity to the next heel strike of the same extremity. Two successive heel strikes of a right lower extremity are shown in the drawing, and a left step.

Stride length

two successive events that are accomplished by the *same* lower extremity during gait.[9] Generally, stride length is determined by measuring the linear distance from the point of heel strike of one lower extremity to the next heel strike of the same extremity (Fig. 14–18). The length of one stride is traveled during one gait cycle and includes all of the events of one gait cycle. Stride length also may be measured by using other events, such as two successive toe offs of the same extremity, but in normal gait two successive heel strikes are used as the reference points. A stride includes two steps, a right step and a left step. However, stride length is not always twice the length of a single step because right and left steps may be unequal. Stride length varies greatly among individuals, because it is affected by leg length, height, age, sex, and other variables. Stride length can be normalized by dividing stride length by leg length or by total body height. Stride length usually decreases in the elderly[10–12] and increases as the speed of gait increases.[13] *The length of one stride is traveled during one gait cycle.*

Stride duration refers to the amount of time it takes to accomplish one stride. Stride duration and gait cycle duration are synonymous. One stride lasts approximately 1 second.[14] Complex fluctuations in stride duration during slow, normal, and fast walking have been identified as being statistically correlated with variations in stride duration thousands of strides earlier. These fluctuations appear to be a characteristic of normal gait.[15]

Step length is the linear distance between two successive points of contact of *opposite* extremities. It is usually measured from heel strike of one extremity to heel strike of the opposite extremity (Fig. 14–19). A comparison of right and left step lengths will provide an indication of gait symmetry. The more equal the step lengths, the more symmetrical is the gait. Variability in step length is at a minimum when the ratio of step length to step rate is about 0.006 m/step or at a person's preferred walking speed.[16]

Step duration refers to the amount of time spent during a single step. Measurement usually is taken in seconds per step. When there is weakness of an extremity or pain, step duration may be decreased on the affected side and increased on the unaffected (stronger or less painful) side.

Cadence is the *number* of steps taken by a person per unit of time. Cadence may be measured as the number of steps per second or per minute.

Cadence = number of steps/time

A shorter step length will result in an increased cadence at any given velocity.[13] Lamoreaux found that when a person walks with a cadence between 80 and 120 steps per minute, cadence and stride length had a linear relationship.[9,13] As one walks with increased cadence, the duration of the double support period decreases. When the cadence of walking approaches 180 steps per minute, the period of double support disappears and running commences. A step frequency or cadence of about 110 steps per minute can be considered as "typical" for adult men; a typical cadence for women is about 116 steps per minute.[4]

Walking velocity is the rate of linear forward motion of the body, which can be measured in centimeters per second, meters per minute, or in miles per hour.

Walking velocity = distance walked/time

Women tend to walk with shorter and faster steps than men at the same velocity.[13] In-

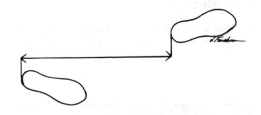

FIGURE 14–19. Step length is the linear distance between two successive points of contact of opposite extremities. Two successive points of contact of a right and left lower extremity are shown in the drawing.

creases in velocity up to 120 steps per minute are brought about by both increases in cadence and stride length but above 120 steps per minute only cadence increases.

Acceleration is the rate of change of velocity with respect to time.

Speed is measured in centimeters per minute. Speed of gait usually is referred to as slow, free, and fast. **Free speed** of gait refers to a person's normal walking speed; **slow** and **fast** speeds of gait refer to speeds slower or faster than the person's normal comfortable walking speed. A fast speed of gait is generally accompanied by increased cadence and stride length and decreased angle of toe out. However, there is a certain amount of variability in the way an individual elects to increase walking speed. Some individuals increase stride length and decrease cadence to achieve a fast walking speed. Other individuals decrease stride length and increase cadence to increase the speed of gait. Walking speed is determined by multiplying step length by step rate.

The **width of the BOS** is found by measuring the linear distance between the midpoint of the heel of one foot and the same point on the other foot (Fig. 14–20). The width of the walking base has been found to increase when there is an increased demand for side-to-side stability such as occurs in the elderly and in small children. In toddlers and young children the center of gravity (COG) is higher than in the adult and a wide BOS is necessary for stability. In the normal population the mean width of the BOS is about 3.5 inches and varies within a range of 1 to 5 inches.

Degree of toe out represents the angle of foot placement and may be found by measuring the angle formed by each foot's line of progression and a line intersecting the center of the heel and the second toe. The angle for men normally is about 7° from the line of progression of each foot at free speed walking (Fig. 14–21).[10] The degree of toe out decreases as the speed of walking increases in normal men.[10]

Joint Motion

Another way in which gait may be described is through measuring the trajectories of the lower

extremities and the joint angles. Sophisticated equipment, such as stroboscopic flash photography, cinematography, electrogoniometers, and computers have been used to provide the information about joint angles and limb trajectories in normal and abnormal gait.[17–20] Diagrams that plot the joint angles of the lower limbs against each other, called **angle-angle diagrams,** may be used to analyze and display data obtained from photography.[19,20] The angle-angle diagrams can provide an objective measure of a patient's progress because various gaits produce characteristic angle-angle diagram displays.[19,20]

Less sophisticated and less objective methods are used in observational gait analysis, whereby an observer makes a judgment as to whether or not a particular joint angle or motion adheres to a norm. For example, an observer may estimate that the walking subject has more knee flexion at the end of midstance than the 5° that represents the norm. The observer then must determine why the subject has increased knee flexion.

One disadvantage of the observational method of analysis is that it requires a great deal of training and practice to be able to identify the particular segment of gait in which a particular joint angle deviates from a norm while a person is walking. Another disadvantage of observational gait analysis methods is that they have low reliability. Observational gait analysis is used in the clinical setting because it has the advantage of being less cumbersome to walking subjects and less expensive than other more sophisticated methods of analysis. In addition, well-trained observers can derive a great deal of information from simple observation.

The gait laboratory at the RLA medical center has developed observational gait analysis recording forms that help the observer to focus attention systematically on different portions of the body during gait.[5] In our experience these forms have been useful for educational purposes. The joint ranges of motion (ROM) that are presented in Table 14–1 have been adapted from the RLA gait analysis forms.[5] The

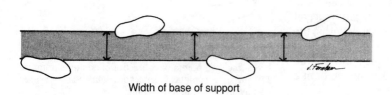

Width of base of support

FIGURE 14–20. Width of the base of support. The midpoint of the heel is used as a point of reference for measuring the width of the base of support.

FIGURE 14–21. Degree of toe out. The angle formed by each foot's line of progression and a line intersecting the center of the heel and the second toe represents the angle of foot placement. The normal angle is 7° for men at free speed walking.

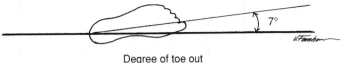

Degree of toe out

degrees of motion presented in the table are the values achieved at the end of each phase. However, neither the population that was used to determine the ranges of joint motion nor the speed of gait used are defined by RLA.[5] Therefore, the reader should expect to find that the degrees of angulation will vary among investigators because the speed of gait may vary and populations used to establish norms may differ in such characteristics as age and sex. The approximate total ROM needed for normal gait may be determined by looking at the value of the joint angle at each joint throughout the gait cycle. For example, in Table 14–1 it can be seen that the knee joint is in extension (0°) at initial contact in the stance phase and in 60° of knee flexion in the swing phase. Therefore, one may conclude that a person needs full extension and up to 60° of knee flexion for normal knee motion to occur during gait. If an individual's knee motion were limited to 10° or 15° of knee flexion, one would expect his or her gait pattern to show considerable deviations from the norm.

Kinematic data on the norms of joint angles at each segment of gait also enable one to describe the changes in joint motion that occur during each phase. For example, a study of Table 14–1 shows that the knee is in extension at initial contact and in 15° of flexion at the end of loading response. Therefore, the knee must be flexing during the loading response period of gait. In the period of midstance the knee is extending because it moves from 15° of flexion at the end of loading response to 5° of flexion at the end of midstance. Again, by referring to Table 14–1, it is possible to determine that the knee continues to extend through terminal stance and flexes again in preswing. The hip begins the stance phase in flexion and extends throughout the phase until it reaches 10° of extension (hyperextension) by the end of terminal stance. Flexion of the hip begins and proceeds through preswing. Similar descriptions of joint motion may be derived for the ankle in stance and for the hip, knee, and ankle during the swing phase by studying the average values given for joint angles at each gait segment at each period of gait in Table 14–1.

Determinants of Gait

Although the reader has been introduced to a number of the variables that are used to describe and define gait, another group of gait components has not yet been mentioned. These components are called the **determinants of gait.** They were first described by Saunders and coworkers in 1953[21] and elaborated on by Inman and colleagues[4] in 1981. The determinants are supposed to represent adjustments made by the pelvis, hips, knees, and ankles that help to keep movement of the body's COG to a minimum. The determinants are credited with decreasing the vertical and lateral excursions of the body's COG and therefore decreasing energy expenditure and making gait more efficient (Fig. 14–22). The six determinants are lateral pelvic tilt in the frontal plane, knee flexion during stance, knee interactions, ankle interactions, pelvic rotation in the transverse plane, and physiologic valgus of the knee. The order of presentation of the determinants that follows is based on their function and is not necessarily related to the order in which they appear in gait. The first four determinants are supposed to help to keep the vertical rise of the body's COG to a minimum. The fifth determinant prevents a drop in the body's COG, and the sixth determinant reduces the side-to-side movement of the COG.

Lateral Pelvic Tilt (Pelvic Drop in the Frontal Plane)

In single-limb support (unilateral weight-bearing) the combined weight of HAT and the swinging leg must be balanced over one lower extremity. During this period the COG reaches its highest point in the sinusoidal curve. Lateral tilting of the pelvis (pelvic drop) on the side of the unsupported extremity (swing leg) keeps the peak of the rise lower than if the pelvis did not drop, because the drop produces a relative adduction of the stance hip in the stance phase and relative abduction of the swinging extremity (Fig. 14–23). The tilting of the pelvis is controlled by the hip abductor muscles of the stance extremity. For example,

Table 14–1. Range of Motion (RLA)

Stance Phase

Joints	Initial Contact	End of Loading Response	End of Midstance	End of Terminal Stance	End of Preswing
Hip	30° of flexion	25° of flexion	0°	10–20° of hyperextension	0°
Knee	0°	15° of flexion	5° of flexion	0°	35–40° of flexion
Ankle	0° (neutral position)	15° of plantarflexion	5–10° of dorsiflexion	0° of dorsiflexion	20° of plantarflexion
Toes (MTP joints)	0°	0°	0°	30° of hyperextension	50–60° of hyperextension

Swing Phase

	End of Initial Swing	End of Midswing	End of Terminal Swing
Hip	20° of flexion	30° of flexion	30° of flexion
Knee	60° of flexion	30° of flexion	0°
Ankle	10° of plantarflexion	0°	0°

Total Range of Motion

	Stance Phase	Swing Phase
Hip	0–30° of flexion, 0–10 or 20° of hyperextension	20–30° of flexion
Knee	0–40° of flexion	0–60° of flexion
Ankle	0–10° of dorsiflexion, 0–20° of plantarflexion	0–10° of plantarflexion

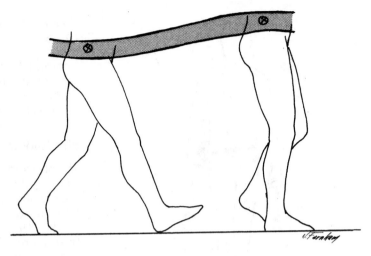

FIGURE 14–22. The vertical displacement of the body's center of gravity (COG) produces a smooth sinusoidal curve in normal walking. The lowest point in the curve is during the period of double support. The highest point in the curve coincides with midstance when the trunk is directly over the stance extremity. The drawing shows the lowest and highest points in the curve.

pelvic drop on the side of the right swing extremity is controlled by isometric and eccentric contractions of the left hip abductor muscles.

Knee Flexion

Knee flexion at midstance when the COG is at its highest point represents another adjust-

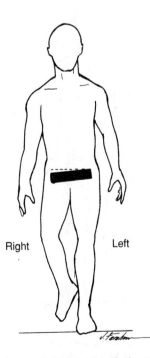

FIGURE 14–23. Lateral pelvic tilt in the frontal plane keeps the peak of the sinusoidal curve lower than it would have been if the pelvis did not drop, because it produces adduction at the stance hip. Lateral pelvic tilt (drop) to the right is controlled by the left hip abductors.

ment that helps to keep the COG from rising as much as it would have to if the body had to pass over a completely extended knee.

Knee, Ankle, and Foot Interactions

Movements at the knee occur in conjunction with movements at the ankle and foot and are responsible for smoothing the pathway of the body's COG so that it forms a sinusoidal curve. Combined knee, ankle, and foot movements prevent abrupt changes in the vertical displacement of the body's COG from a downward to an upward direction. The change from a downward motion of the COG at heel strike to an upward motion at foot flat (loading response) is accomplished by knee flexion, ankle plantarflexion, and foot pronation. These combined motions serve to relatively shorten the extremity and thus prevent an abrupt rise in the body's COG after heel strike. If these motions did not occur in conjunction with each other, the COG would rise abruptly after heel strike as the tibia rides over the talus.

Another instance in which knee, ankle, and foot interactions play an important role is when the body's COG falls after midstance. A combination of ankle plantarflexion, foot supination, and knee extension at heel off slow the descent of the body's COG by a relative lengthening of the stance extremity.

Forward and Backward Rotation of the Pelvis

Forward and backward rotations of the pelvis in the transverse plane accompany forward and

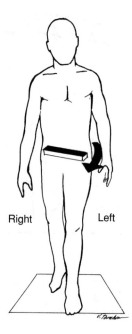

FIGURE 14–24. Pelvic rotation in the transverse plane. The drawing shows left forward rotation of the pelvis on the side of the swinging extremity. The right hip joint serves as the axis for motion. The bar, which represents the pelvis, shows the apparent backward rotation that is occurring simultaneously on the right side of the pelvis. The pelvic rotation relatively lengthens the extremities and therefore minimizes the drop of the body's COG that occurs at double support.

backward movements of the lower extremities during gait (Fig. 14–24). Forward rotation occurs on the side of the swinging extremity with the hip joint of the weight-bearing extremity serving as the axis for pelvic rotation. The pelvis begins to move forward at preswing and continues as the swinging extremity moves forward during initial swing. At the point of maximal elevation of the body's COG in midstance, the forward pelvic rotation has brought the pelvis to a neutral position with respect to rotation. Forward rotation of the pelvis continues beyond neutral on the swing side through terminal swing to initial contact.

The total amount of rotation of the pelvis is small and averages about 4° on the swing and stance sides for a total of 8°. The result of pelvic rotation is an apparent lengthening of the lower extremities. The swinging lower extremity is lengthened in terminal swing by the forwardly rotating pelvis, and the weight-bearing extremity is lengthened in preswing by the posterior position of the pelvis. Therefore both the stance and swing extremities are lengthened as the COG descends to its lowest level in the period of

double support. The relative lengthening helps to prevent an excessive drop of the COG and maintains the COG at a higher level than would be possible if no pelvic rotation occurred. Pelvic rotation functions to minimize the depression of the COG, whereas the first two determinants function to minimize the elevation of the COG.

Physiologic Valgus at the Knee

The physiologic valgus at the knee reduces the width of the BOS from what it would be if the femoral and tibial shafts formed a vertical line from the greater tuberosity of the femur (Fig. 14–25). Therefore, because the BOS is relatively narrow, little lateral motion of the pelvis is necessary to shift the COG from one lower extremity to another over the BOS.

Although the six determinants and their role in decreasing vertical and lateral excursions of the COG generally have been accepted without question for many years, recently a number of researchers have begun to question the validity of the role of the determinants in gait. Gard and

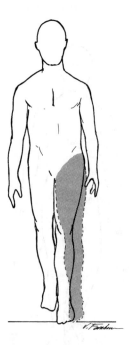

FIGURE 14–25. Physiologic valgus at the knee. The normal physiologic valgus at the knee reduces the width of the base of support from what it would be if the lower extremity were aligned vertically. The darkened left lower extremity in the drawing is supposed to represent a hypothetical vertical alignment of the tibia and femur. It is evident from the drawing that the base of support is considerably wider when the leg is aligned vertically than when the leg is normally aligned.

Childress[22] studied the effect of stance phase knee flexion on the vertical displacement of the trunk in normal walking. These authors compared vertical displacement of the trunk with knee flexion to vertical displacement of the trunk without knee flexion. Although knee flexion reduced the peak values of the trunk's vertical displacement by a few millimeters, the valleys were reduced by the same amount so peak to peak amplitude remained unchanged. Furthermore they found that knee flexion occurred before the peak in the trunk's vertical rise which demonstrated that knee flexion could not play a dominant role in reducing the peak rise of the body's COG. These authors suggest that the function of knee flexion in stance is to absorb and reduce peak impact forces as weight is transferred onto the stance limb at the time of contralateral toe off and not to reduce the vertical excursion of the body's COG.

In a critical examination of the lateral pelvic tilt determinant, Gard and Childress[23] concluded that pelvic tilt had much less influence on the vertical displacement of the body's COG than was previously assumed. The authors based their conclusions on their findings that the vertical excursion of the trunk remained essentially unchanged by pelvic tilt over walking speeds ranging from 1.0 to 2.0 m/s. Childress and Gard[24] found that pelvic tilt peaked early in the swing phase and contributed little to the vertical position of the trunk after 25% of the gait cycle. Peak to peak amplitude of the body's COG was not affected by pelvic motion. Pandy and Berme[25] also concluded that pelvic tilt was not as dominant a factor as previously indicated and these authors suggested that the major role of the hip abductor muscles was to stabilize the pelvis. Additional research undoubtedly will need to be undertaken before the suggested new roles for knee flexion and pelvic tilt are universally accepted. However, the research of these investigators indicates the need for ongoing critical examinations of the theories we operate under and the assumptions we use to explain complex human behavior.

Energy Requirements

The kinematic aspects of human gait have been introduced in the preceding sections. In the following sections the reader will be introduced to some of the forces involved in producing gait. Force must be used to produce accelerations and decelerations of the body and its segments. Muscles use metabolic energy to perform mechanical work by converting metabolic energy into mechanical energy. The overall metabolic cost incurred during locomotion may be measured by assessing the body's oxygen consumption per unit of distance traveled.

Duff-Raffaele and coworkers[26] investigated the proportion of energy consumption used to effect a vertical raise (lift work) in the body's COG during walking. Because kinetic energy is proportional to the square of the velocity, the metabolic energy cost of raising the body's COG during walking is relatively small at slower speeds of gait. These investigators found that at comfortable walking speeds of 1.34 m/s and 1.79 m/s, more than half (5.3.2% and 62.8%, respectively) of the total energy consumption was explained by lift work. At slow speeds of 0.45 m/s and 0.90 m/s only 21.6% and 37.65% of the total energy consumption was accounted for by lift work. Davies[27] found that the total caloric cost to walk 1 mile per unit mass was significantly different between young and older adults. Both older men and women (65–78 years) had increased energy cost and walked at a slower gait speed compared to younger adults. The relatively slow speed of gait adopted by the elderly appears to be the cause of increases in the metabolic energy cost per unit distance in older individuals or in any group of individuals who use a slow gait speed. This finding was rather unexpected because the energy cost of lifting the body's COG is considerably less at a slow gait speed than it is at a normal or average gait speed. Kinetic energy is proportional to the square of the velocity and the metabolic energy cost of changing this energy is relatively small at slower gait speeds. Duff-Raffele and colleagues[26] suggest that increase in energy cost for slow speed of gait compared to normal speed is due primarily to internal muscular work.

The main objective of locomotion is to move the body through space with the least expenditure of energy. If a long distance is traveled, but only a small amount of oxygen is consumed, the metabolic cost of that particular gait is low. Oxygen consumption for a person walking at 4 to 5 km/h averages 100 mL/kg body weight per minute. The highest efficiency is attained when the least amount of energy is required to travel a unit of distance. If the speed of walking increases above an individual's preferred free walking speed, the energy cost per unit of distance walked increases.[28] Also as described above, as the speed of walking decreases below free walking speed the energy cost increases.

Mechanical Energy

The mechanical energy cost of gait involves assessments of mechanical energy exchanges between various segments of the body. The two types of mechanical energy are kinetic energy and potential energy. **Kinetic energy** has translational and rotational components. **Translational energy** refers to energy related to the linear velocity of a segment in space. **Rotational energy** is due to the rotational velocity of a segment in space. **Potential energy** is the quantity of mass raised, multiplied by the height to which it is raised. In other words, whenever a mass is raised, gravity tends to act on it and make it fall, and therefore the mass has potential energy. The amount of potential energy that an elevated mass possesses is equal to the amount of kinetic energy that was required to lift the mass against gravity. When the mass has stopped elevating or is at its peak, kinetic energy is transformed into potential energy. When the mass falls, the potential energy is transformed back into kinetic energy as the mass accelerates. In human gait, kinetic energy must be expended in order to raise the body's mass, which is concentrated at the body's COG. The higher the COG is raised, the greater the amount of kinetic energy that must be expended. When the COG reaches its highest point at midstance, the body has the greatest potential energy. The downward fall of the body is brought about by potential energy, but kinetic energy is required to control the fall. Because potential energy is transformed into kinetic energy during the fall, kinetic energy is available.

Exchanges between kinetic and potential energy occur throughout the gait cycle. If gait is mechanically efficient, energy is conserved and little more energy than the energy required to initiate movement is needed. If changes in the body's COG are large and abrupt, more energy must be expended; therefore, energy expenditure in human gait is often equated with movements of the body's COG. However, because energy exchanges also occur between the segments of the body during gait, a more accurate assessment of energy exchange involves a segment-by-segment calculation to measure the mechanical efficiency of an individual's gait.[28]

Positive and Negative Work

The muscles of the body supply kinetic energy. When muscles do positive work such as in a concentric contraction, they increase the total energy of the body and transfer energy to the bony components. At a cadence of 105 to 112 steps per minute, a brief burst of positive work (energy generation) occurs as the hip extensors contract concentrically between heel strike and foot flat while the knee extensors perform negative work (energy absorption) by acting eccentrically to control knee flexion during the same period.[28,29] Negative work is also performed by the plantarflexors as the leg rotates over the foot during the period of stance from foot flat through midstance. However, positive work of the knee extensors occurs during this period to extend the knee following foot flat.[28,29] Positive work of the plantarflexors and hip flexors in late stance and in early swing increases the energy level of the body. By midswing (which is midstance on the stance side) the potential energy of the body is at a maximum. On the other hand, in late swing negative work is performed by the hip extensors as they work eccentrically to decelerate the leg in preparation for initial contact. At this point there is a decrease in the total energy level of the body.

The positive energy generated by the hip muscles during concentric muscle action for normal men walking at a cadence of 109 steps per minute is approximately double the amount of energy absorbed by the hip muscles during eccentric muscle action.[4] At the ankle the positive energy generated by concentric muscle action during a single gait cycle is almost triple that of the energy absorbed by eccentric muscle action.[4] According to a model developed by Kepple,[30] the eccentric activity of the plantarflexors generates a forward acceleration of the HAT COG because a moment acting across a joint produces a reaction force at that joint, which is transmitted throughout the kinematic chain and accelerates all segments in the linkage. Accelerations produced by a joint are independent of velocity and thus of type of contraction.[30] The knee, in contrast to the hip and ankle, absorbs more energy through eccentric muscle action during a gait cycle than it generates.[4] At slow and normal speeds of walking in healthy subjects, the hip flexors and extensors contribute about 25% of the total concentric work. The ankle plantarflexors contribute about 66% and the knee extensors contribute about 8%.[31] The sum of all of the energy increases over a given period of time results in the net positive work that has been done. Likewise, the sum of all of the energy decreases that have occurred during the same given time period yields the net negative work that has been done. The work required to move the body during gait is the absolute sum of the positive and negative energy changes of the whole body.[29] The total body energy curve gives a measure of the mechanical energy cost per distance traveled.

Eng and Winter[32] found that although 74% of the total hip work was done in the sagittal plane, 23% of the total hip work was in the form of eccentric contraction of the hip abductors to control the pelvic drop in the frontal plane. Kepple[30] found that hip abductor moments did not make a significant contribution to the vertical acceleration of HAT during single-limb support because the hip abduction moment that acts to keep the COG level also produces a knee flexor acceleration that tends to collapse the leg. The knee extensors have to contract to keep the leg from collapsing.

Kinetics

External and Internal Forces

To gain a better understanding of energy requirements and the role of the determinants during gait, it is necessary to acquire knowledge of the forces involved. In gait, the external forces acting on the body are inertia, gravity, and the ground reaction force (GRF).[4] The magnitude and direction of external forces such as the GRFs may be determined through the use of instruments such as force platforms.[33] The inertial force arises from the inertial properties of the body segments and is proportional to the acceleration of the segment. However, the inertial force acts in the opposite direction to the acceleration. The force of gravity acts directly downward through the center of mass of each segment. The GRF represents the force of the ground on the foot and it is equal in magnitude and opposite in direction to the force that the body applies to the floor through the foot[34] (Fig. 14–26). The GRF is probably the most important force during locomotor activities such as walking, skipping, hopping, jumping, and running. The GRFs may actually act on many points on the foot but the center of pressure (COP) is the point at which the forces are considered to act just as the COG of the body is designated as the point where the force of gravity is considered to act.

The COP moves along a path during gait and produces a characteristic pattern. The pattern for normal individuals during barefoot walking differs from the patterns using various types of footgear.[35] In barefoot walking the COP starts

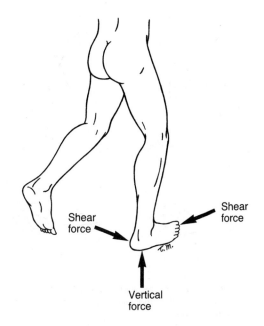

FIGURE 14–26. The ground reaction force (GRF) represents the force of the ground on the foot. GRFs are transmitted through the foot to the leg and rest of the body.

at the posterolateral edge of the heel at the beginning of the stance phase and moves in a nearly linear fashion through the midfoot area, remaining lateral to the midline, and then moves medially across the ball of the foot with a large concentration along the metatarsal break. The COP then moves to second and first toes during terminal stance (Fig. 14–27).

Internal forces are created primarily by the muscles. **Muscle power** is a measure of the rate of doing work, which is equal to the joint moment of force multiplied by the joint angular velocity.[36] The formula $P = Fv$ is used to determine power where F equals force (applied in a certain direction) and v equals the velocity of movement in that direction. P is measured in either Watts or Newton meters per second (Nm/s).[36] The ligaments, tendons, joint capsules, and bony components assist the muscles by resisting, transmitting, and absorbing forces. Muscle activity can be identified by electromyography (EMG), a technique in which the electrical activity generated by an active muscle is recorded. This technique has been used extensively to determine patterns of muscle activity during gait. EMG is often used in conjunction with force plates, cinematography, and electrogoniometry to pinpoint the point in time when muscle activity occurs during the gait cycle. However, the EMG record only pro-

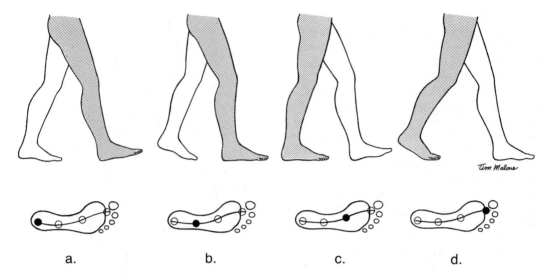

<table>
<tr><td>a.</td><td>b.</td><td>c.</td><td>d.</td></tr>
</table>

FIGURE 14–27. A center of pressure (COP) pathway is shown by the position of the black dot at heel strike (a), at foot flat (b), at the end of midstance (c), and at toe off (d). The COP path may vary among subjects and may be altered by different footwear.

vides information about if and when particular muscles are acting. It does not tell why the muscles are acting or how much force the muscles are generating. EMG studies of gait are used to validate theoretical models that attempt to explain why muscles are needed to counteract the forces acting in gait, and theoretical models are developed to explain the muscle activity found by EMG.[37]

Sagittal Plane Analysis

The analyses that are presented in the following section include the location of the GRF relative to the joints of the lower extremities and kinematic data. The relationship of the ground reaction force vector (GRFV) (anterior-posterior and medial-lateral) to the joint axes of the ankle, knee, and hip is used to show the type of moment (flexion/extension, abduction/adduction) that is acting around a joint. The magnitudes of the moments that are determined by measuring the length of the moment arm (MA) (perpendicular distance of a GRFV from a joint axis) are not represented in the illustrations; that is, no attempt was made to make the distance of the GRFV from the joint axis equivalent to the actual length of the MAs. The location of the GRFV, joint positions, and muscle activity that were used to create the illustrations were derived from published studies on normal human walking.[4,5,34]

In Chapter 13, the concept of flexion and ex-

tension moments was reviewed. In the erect standing posture when the LOG is located at a distance from the joint axis a gravitational moment is created around the joint that threatens to disturb the equilibrium of the forces acting around that joint. To prevent motion at the joint a specific muscle or group of muscles is called into action to oppose the moment, thereby maintaining equilibrium. In a dynamic situation, such as gait, joint movement is necessary and desirable.

> EXAMPLE 1: If flexion of the knee is necessary during a certain phase of gait and a flexion moment is acting at the knee, the flexion moment is desirable. Muscular activity may be required to control knee flexion. If control is necessary, then an eccentric muscle contraction of the knee extensors is required to control flexion (Fig. 14–28a). If, on the other hand, there is a flexion moment at the knee and knee extension is the desired motion, a concentric contraction of the knee extensors is necessary to oppose the flexion moment and to produce knee extension (Fig. 14–28b).

Stance Phase

The type of muscle activity (eccentric, concentric, or isometric) necessary during gait depends on the nature of the moments acting around the joints of the stance extremity and the direction of

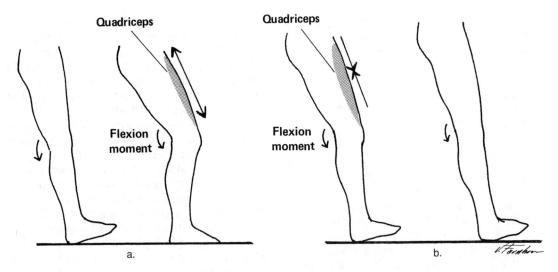

FIGURE 14–28. (a) There is a flexion moment at the knee produced by the GRF and knee flexion is the desired motion; therefore, an eccentric contraction of the quadriceps is necessary to control the amount of knee flexion. (b) There is a flexion moment acting around the knee produced by the GRF and extension is the desired action; therefore, the quadriceps must work concentrically to counteract the flexion moment and to produce knee extension.

the desired motion. If a GRFV moment tends to cause movement of a bony component in a desired direction, muscle function is generally one of control or restraint (eccentric contraction).

EXAMPLE 2: In the period of gait from initial contact through loading response (heel strike to foot flat), a plantarflexion moment is acting around the ankle because the resultant GRFV is posterior to the axis of the ankle joint. Plantarflexion is a desired motion in that plantarflexion is necessary to put the foot on the floor in a position to receive the body weight. However, the foot will slap the floor in an uncontrolled fashion unless muscle activity (eccentric) is used to control the plantarflexion (Fig. 14–29).

A different situation exists at the knee joint during midstance. During this period, the knee is extending as it moves from about 15° of flexion at the end of loading response to 5° of flexion at the end of midstance. A flexion moment exists at the knee, and flexion is an undesired motion. A concentric contraction of the knee extensors is necessary to oppose the flexion moment and to produce extension.

Each segment of the stance phase of gait may be examined in a similar manner by using the location of the resultant GRFV relative to a joint axis to determine the moments acting around a joint in the sagittal, frontal, and transverse planes. Knowledge of the desired joint motion derived from the kinematic analysis is used in conjunction with the location of

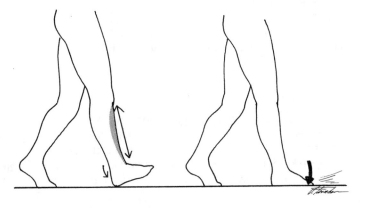

FIGURE 14–29. In the period of gait from heel strike to foot flat there is a plantarflexion moment acting around the ankle. Plantarflexion is the desired motion that is necessary to position the foot on the supporting surface. The dorsiflexors act eccentrically to control plantarflexion and to prevent the foot from slapping to the ground in an uncontrolled motion.

the resultant GRFV to determine the type of muscle activity required to produce or control a desired motion. Sometimes the resultant GRFV changes location *within* as well as *between* periods, and as a consequence, muscle activity changes from eccentric to concentric or vice versa. These changes in the type of muscle activity account for the energy changes that occur during gait.

EXAMPLE 3: In the period of gait from initial contact to the end of midstance, the ankle moves from the neutral position at initial contact to 15° of plantarflexion by the end of loading response and to 10° of dorsiflexion by the end of midstance. The GRFV changes from a location posterior to the ankle joint at initial contact to an anterior position in midstance.

Therefore, at initial contact and during loading response (heel strike to foot flat) there is a plantarflexion moment and the ankle is moving in a direction of plantarflexion. An eccentric contraction of the dorsiflexors controls the motion and negative work is done. The moment acting around the ankle changes at the end of loading response from plantarflexion to dorsiflexion. The dorsiflexion moment continues through midstance while the ankle is dorsiflexing. An eccentric contraction of the plantarflexors is necessary to control the dorsiflexion and prevent the forward progression of the tibia from moving too rapidly. The dorsiflexion moment continues until the end of the stance phase. Mueller[38] found that the peak torque of the plantarflexors and the dorsiflexion ROM are interrelated and are important contributions to plantarflexor moments and power. At the end of the stance phase in preswing, plantarflexion is the desired motion. Therefore, activity of the plantarflexors changes from eccentric to concentric. The energy changes for the lower leg during this phase are the sum of the positive and negative energy changes that occurred as a result of the eccentric and concentric muscle activity.

Swing Phase

During the swing phase of gait there are no GRFs because the foot is not in contact with the ground. The swing extremity is moving in an open kinematic chain. Muscle activity is required to accelerate and decelerate the swing-

ing extremity and to lift and hold the extremity up against the force of gravity so that the foot clears the ground and is placed in an optimum position for heel contact. Acceleration is brought about by early concentric activity of the hip flexor and knee extensor muscles. The hip flexors act concentrically to initiate the forward swing of the lower extremity during initial swing. They are inactive through midswing and terminal swing. Deceleration of the swing leg during terminal swing is accomplished primarily by eccentric muscle activity of the hip extensor and knee flexor muscles. At the ankle the tibialis anterior, extensor digitorum longus, and extensor hallicus longus contract isometrically to keep the ankle in a neutral position and to prevent the foot and toes from dragging on the ground.

Frontal Plane Analysis

During the early part of the stance phase, HAT is moving forward rapidly and shifting laterally over the stance extremity. The rapid lateral shift of HAT onto the stance extremity creates demands for lateral stability at the hip, knee, and ankle (Fig. 14–30). Muscular support is essential when the body weight is being accepted by the stance extremity, partly because the hip,

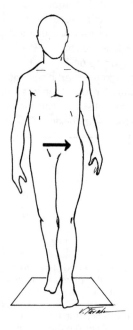

FIGURE 14–30. The rapid lateral weight shift in early stance creates demands for stability at the hip, knee, and ankle.

knee, and ankle are in loose-packed positions. Stabilization of the pelvis at the hip is provided for by activity of the gluteus medius, gluteus minimus, and the tensor fascia latae.[39] The gluteus medius on the stance side controls the lateral drop of the pelvis on the side of the swinging leg. The rapid transfer of weight and demands of single-limb balance create a valgus thrust at the knee and ankle as the body weight is accepted on the extremity.[39] The medial aspect of the knee is given dynamic support by the vastus medialis, semitendinosus, and the gracilis. These muscles counteract the valgus thrust at the knee and thereby prevent an increase in the normal physiologic valgus.[40]

At the ankle and foot, the body weight is transferred from the heel at initial contact along the lateral border of the foot during loading response. At the end of loading response all five metatarsals are weight-bearing. Subsequently, the weight is transferred across the heads of the metatarsals in terminal stance and to the great toe in preswing. The hindfoot bears weight for about 43% of the stance phase.[41] Pronation of the foot at the subtalar joint is initiated at heel strike mostly as a result of the heel being loaded lateral to the axis of motion.[42] Subtalar pronation continues during the first 25% of the stance phase in response to the acceptance of weight.[43] Pronation of the subtalar joint leaves the transverse joint mobile, and therefore permits the foot to adapt to the supporting surface. The tibialis anterior is the only invertor active at the time of heel strike that can restrain eversion. During loading response the valgus thrust at the ankle tends to increase the pronation of the foot, and activity of the tibialis posterior muscle is required to control the thrust toward pronation. At approximately 25% of the stance phase (midstance), the foot begins supinating again and returns to neutral by the end of midstance.[44]

Pronation of the foot in a weight-bearing posture (closed kinematic chain) produces a medial rotatory force on the tibia while supination produces a lateral rotatory force on the tibia.[42] Just as the position of the foot can cause tibial rotation, tibial rotation can cause a change in the position of the foot. Medial rotation of the tibia in a closed kinematic chain with the foot in a weight-bearing posture produces pronation and lateral tibial rotation causes supination.[44] The tibialis posterior, soleus, and gastrocnemius contract eccentri-

cally to control the pronation that occurs after heelstrike and to control internal rotation of the tibia.[45] At the end of loading response and continuing through the remainder of the stance phase (midstance, terminal stance, preswing) the foot is supinating. By heel off the foot has formed a rigid lever and enhances the pulley action for extrinsic muscles.[46] In preswing the toes are weight-bearing.[44] During the middle of the stance phase the demands for medial-lateral stability are somewhat diminished as the valgus thrust decreases. The tensor fascia latae muscle that began activity at loading response continues to provide stabilization of the pelvis during midstance through terminal stance. Activity of the gluteus medius muscle diminishes during midstance and no activity of these muscles is found in preswing once the opposite limb has contacted the ground.[10] The hip adductors (magnus and longus) begin acting in terminal stance and are active eccentrically in preswing to restrain the lateral weight shift onto the opposite extremity. At the knee, the activity of the dynamic stabilizers (semitendinosus, gracilis, and vastus medialis) ceases at midstance as the valgus thrust diminishes. During the last part of stance the weight is being shifted back onto the contralateral extremity, and the hip adductors and the ankle plantarflexors help to control the weight shift. Table 14–2 provides a summary of transverse rotations in the frontal plane for the pelvis, femur, and tibia.

Summary: Lower-Extremity Joint and Muscle Activity

Stance Phase

Tables 14–3 through 14–6 and Figures 14–31 to 14–34 present a summary of joint and muscle activity for one lower extremity during the stance phase of gait. The tables include the joint position in degrees, resultant GRFV, the moment, type of muscle action, and muscle activity (as determined by EMG). The reader should realize that although joint positions and muscle actions are supposed to represent the average of a normal population, these averages are affected by the speed of gait and may vary among different investigators. Dujardin[47] found considerable variation among individuals in hip flexion-extension, which ranged from a minimum of 20° to a maximum of 42°. Oberg[48] found that hip joint ROM for

Table 14–2. Summary of Transverse Rotations at Pelvis, Femur, and Tibia (Right Lower Extremity)*

	Initial Contact	Loading Response	Midstance	Terminal Stance	Preswing
Percent of stance gait cycle	0%	12%	31%	50%	62%
Pelvis	Left side begins to move forward	Left side moving forward	Neutral	Left side moving forward	Left side moving forward
Femur	Medial rotation	Medial rotation	Lateral rotation	Lateral rotation	Lateral rotation
Tibia	Medial rotation	Medial rotation	Lateral rotation	Lateral rotation	Lateral rotation

	Initial Swing	Midswing	Terminal Swing
Percent of swing gait cycle	75%	82%	100%
Pelvis	Right side moving forward	Neutral	Right side moving forward
Femur	Medial rotation	Medial rotation	Medial rotation
Tibia	Medial rotation	Medial rotation	Medial rotation

*The femur and tibia medially rotate to about 10–20% of stance and then begin laterally rotating to the end of preswing. At initial swing the femur and tibia begin medially rotating again. The degree of transverse rotation that occurs during gait as well as the point in the gait where the rotation occurs varies according to the gait speed. Individual variations also are common.

Table 14–3. Sagittal Plane Analysis (Fig. 14–31)

Heel Strike (Initial Contact) to Foot Flat (End of the Loading Response)

Joint	Motion	Ground Reaction Force	Moment	Muscle	Contraction
Hip	Flexion: 30–25°	Anterior	Flexion	Gluteus maximus Hamstrings Adductor magnus	Isometric to eccentric
Knee	Flexion: 0–15°	Anterior to posterior	Extension to flexion	Quadriceps	Concentric to eccentric
Ankle	Plantarflexion: 0–15°	Posterior	Plantarflexion	Tibialis anterior Extensor digitorum longus Extensor hallucis longus	Eccentric to lower foot to the supporting surface and to control ankle plantarflexion

Frontal Plane Analysis*

Joint	Motion	Muscle Activity
Pelvis	Forwardly rotated position on right side of pelvis at initial contact Left side of pelvis begins to move forward	
Hip	Medial rotation of the femur on the pelvis	
Knee	Valgus thrust with increasing valgus Medial rotation of the tibia	Gracilis, vastus medialis, semitendinosus Long head of biceps femoris to control medial rotation of tibia
Ankle	Valgus thrust with increasing pronation Subtalar joint pronation reaches a maximum at the end of loading response Transverse tarsal pronation	Eccentric contraction of tibialis posterior to control valgus thrust on foot.
Thorax	Right side of thorax is in posterior position at initial contact and begins moving forward	
Shoulder	Right shoulder is slightly behind right hip and moving forward	

*Reference limb is the right lower extremity.

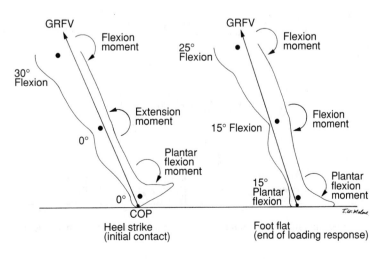

FIGURE 14–31. The period of gait from heel strike (initial contact) to foot flat (end of loading response). The ground reaction force vectors (GRFV) are indicated by the straight arrows. The curved clockwise arrows indicate flexion moments, and the curved counterclockwise arrows indicate extension moments. Notice that the GRFV changes from a position anterior to the axis of the knee at heel strike to posterior to the axis of the knee at foot flat.

Table 14–4. *Sagittal Plane Analysis (Fig. 14–32)**

Foot Flat (End of Loading Response) to Midstance (End of Midstance)

Joint	Motion	Ground Reaction Force	Moment	Muscle	Contraction
Hip	Extension: 25–0° 20° flexion-0°	Anterior to posterior	Flexion to extension	Gluteus maximus	Concentric to no activity
Knee	Extension: 15–5° 15–5° flexion	Posterior to anterior	Flexion to extension	Quadriceps	Concentric to no activity
Ankle	15° of plantar-flexion to 5–10° of dorsiflexion	Posterior to anterior	Plantarflexion to dorsiflexion	Soleus Gastrocnemius Plantarflexors	Eccentric

Frontal Plane Analysis

Joint	Motion	Muscle Activity
Pelvis	Right side rotating backward to reach neutral at midstance. Lateral tilting toward the swinging extremity	Hip abductors are active to prevent excessive lateral tilting (gluteus medius tensor fascia lata)
Hip	Medial rotation of the femur on the pelvis continues to a neutral position at midstance. Adduction moment continues throughout single support	Minimal or no activity
Knee	There is a reduction in valgus thrust and the tibia begins to rotate laterally	Minimal or no activity
Ankle-foot	The foot begins to move in the direction of supination from its pronated position at the end of loading response. The foot reaches a neutral position at midstance	The tibialis posterior helps to produce supination
Thorax	Right side moving forward to neutral	
Thorax	Translating right to neutral	
Shoulder	Moving forward	

*In the period described above, the hip is extending from about 30° of flexion to about 5° of flexion. The GRFV shifts from anterior to posterior and the moment acting around the hip changes from a flexion to an extension moment. The hip extensors cease their activity at or around midstance because the moment is in the desired direction and momentum appears to be sufficient to carry the body forward. Muscle activity at the hip at midstance is mostly abductor activity to stabilize the pelvis. The quadriceps also ceases its activity as the femur advances over the tibia.

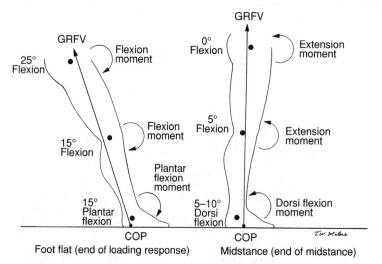

FIGURE 14–32. The period of gait from foot flat (end of loading response) to midstance (end of midstance).

Table 14–5. *Sagittal Plane Analysis (Fig. 14–33)**

Midstance (Middle of Midstance) to Heel Off (Prior to End of Terminal Stance)

Joint	Motion	Ground Reaction Force	Moment	Muscle	Contraction
Hip	Extension: 0° of flexion to 10–20° of hyperextension	Posterior	Extension	Hip flexors	Eccentric
Knee	Extension: 5° of flexion to 0°	Posterior to anterior	Flexion to extension	No activity	
Ankle	Plantarflexion: 5° dorsiflexion to 0°	Anterior	Dorsiflexion	Soleus plantarflexors	Eccentric to concentric
Toes (MTP)	Extension: 0–30° of hyperextension			Flexor hallicus longus and brevis Abductor hallicus Abductor digiti quinti Interossei Lumbricals	

Frontal Plant Analysis

Joint	Motion	Muscle Activity
Pelvis	Right side moving posteriorly from neutral position	Minimal or no muscle activity
Hip	Lateral rotation of femur and adduction	Inconsistent hip adductor activity
Knee	Lateral rotation of tibia	No activity
Ankle-foot	Supination of subtalar joint increases	Concentric plantarflexor activity
Thorax	Right side moving forward	
Shoulder	Right shoulder moving forward	

*A small extension moment exists at the hip and knee and no muscle activity is required at the knee to maintain the knee in extension. The momentum of HAT appears to assist in keeping the knee extended. The dorsiflexion moment at the ankle reaches a peak toward the end of this period and the plantar flexors are active to control the tibia and to raise the heel. Toe extension occurs as a result of a closed-chain response to heel rise.

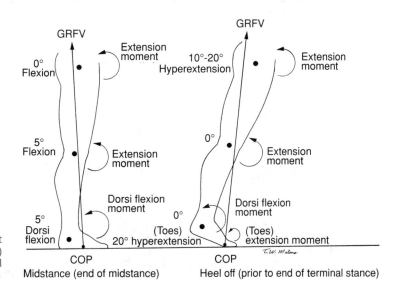

FIGURE 14–33. The period of gait from midstance (end of midstance) to heel off (before end of terminal stance).

Table 14–6. Sagittal Plane Analysis (Fig. 14–34)*

Heel Off (End of Terminal Stance) to Toe Off (End of Preswing)

Joint	Motion	Gravity Line	Moment	Muscle	Contraction
Hip	Flexion: 20° of hypertension to 0°	Posterior	Extension to neutral	Iliopsoas Adductor magnus Adductor longus	Concentric
Knee	Flexion: 0–30° of flexion	Posterior	Flexion	Quadriceps	Eccentric to no activity
Ankle	Plantarflexion: 0–20° of plantarflexion	Anterior	Dorsiflexion	Gastrocnemius Soleus Peroneus brevis Peroneus longus Flexor hallucis longus	Concentric to no activity
Toes (MTP)	Extension: 50–60° of hyperextension			Abductor hallicus Abductor digit quinti Flexor digitorum brevis Flexor hallicus brevis Interossei Lumbricals	Closed-chain response to increasing plantarflexion at the ankle.

Frontal Plane Analysis

Joint	Motion	Muscle Activity
Pelvis	Left side moving forward until left heel contact (right toe off). Lateral tilting to the swing side ceases as the contralateral extremity enters its stance phase and the period of double support begins.	The hip adductors control eccentrically
Hip	Abduction occurs as the weight is shifted onto the opposite extremity. Lateral rotation of femur	
Knee	Inconsistent Lateral rotation tibia	
Foot/Ankle	The weight is shifted to the toes and at toe off only the first toe is in contact with the supporting surface. Supination of subtalar joint	Plantarflexors
Thorax	Translation to the left	
Shoulder	Moving forward	

*Activity in the gastrocnemius and the soleus ceases after the heel leaves the ground. The other plantarflexors cease activity in the order in which they are listed in the sagittal analysis above.

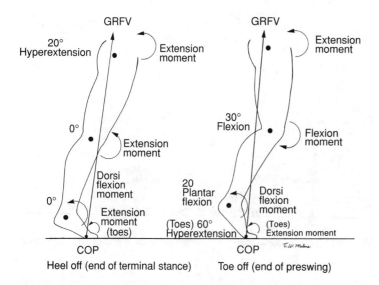

FIGURE 14–34. The period of gait from heel off (end of terminal stance) to toe off (end of preswing).

women varied from 41° at slow walking speed to 52.5°. The hip joint ROM for men varied from 44° at slow walking speed to 53.6° for men at a fast gait speed. Borghese and colleagues[49] determined that the pattern of changes (time course) in angles of flexion, and extension at the hip, knee, and ankle were variable being idiosyncratic to the individual and that they changed with speed of walking.

An examination of the moments acting at the lower extremity during the stance phase show that for the majority of the phase the algebraic sum of all extensor (positive) moments and flexor (negative) moments acting at the hip, knee, and ankle is a positive or extensor moment. Winter[6] calls this quantification of the total limb synergy a **support moment** and he found the extensor support moment to be consistent for all walking speeds for both normal individuals and persons with disabilities. Hip and knee moments may vary considerably among individuals but the net moment remains an extensor moment. The extensor moment keeps the leg from collapsing during the stance phase. If the knee, hip, or ankle is excessively flexed, a larger than normal extensor moment will be generated at another joint so that the net moment remains an extensor moment and the limb is kept from collapsing. The support moment changes from a net extensor to a net flexor moment at late stance (55–60% of the gait cycle), which continues into early swing. The flexor pattern achieves liftoff, weight shifting, and toe clearance. In late swing a net extensor moment appears again, presumably to assist in the final positioning of the limb for heel contact.[6,50]

Swing Phase

Tables 14–7 and 14–8 and Figures 14–35 and 14–36 present a summary of joint and muscle activity during the swing phase. In the swing phase of gait the primary functions of the swing extremity muscles are to maintain a certain joint position, to accelerate or decelerate the swinging extremity, to ensure toe/foot clearance, and to ensure that the foot is positioned for heel strike.

At the ankle, the tibialis anterior, extensor digitorum longus, and extensor hallucis longus contract concentrically to move the foot from the plantarflexed position at toe off to a position of neutral in midswing. These muscles then act isometrically to maintain the ankle in a neutral position throughout the swing phase.[42]

The knee continues to flex after toe off and reaches a maximum flexion angle of 60° at the end of initial swing. At midswing the knee is in about 30° of flexion and by terminal swing the knee is fully extended. Quadriceps femoris activity, which began as an eccentric contraction in preswing to control flexion at the knee, changes after maximum flexion is attained to a brief concentric contraction that initiates forward acceleration of the tibia. Momentum then appears to carry the tibia forward. In the terminal swing period the hamstrings contract eccentrically to control the forward motion of the lower extremity. At the very end of the phase (terminal swing), the knee extensors contract to stabilize the knee in extension, in preparation for heel strike.

The hip is moving from neutral at toe off to about 20° of flexion in early swing. The hip flexes to about 30° of flexion by the end of midswing and is maintained in this position until the end of the swing phase. The hip flexors, which were active to control hip extension at toe off, contract concentrically to initiate swing. The flexors show no activity through midswing and terminal swing. However, the adductor magnus and adductor longus may act to maintain hip flexion, in addition to their function of keeping the extremity near the midline. During terminal swing the hamstrings contract eccentrically to control the forward progression of the lower extremity.

The motor strategies used by healthy individuals to oppose the moments show a considerable amount of variability among individuals and even in the same individual from one bout of walking to another. This variability occurs even though the kinematics of gait and total limb synergies (support moments) appear to be similar.[37] The variety of motor patterns used suggest that peripheral feedback from joint receptors has a strong influence on gait. Input from the visual system that provides information about obstacles in the walking path also appears to affect muscle activity during gait. The fact that muscle activity in the hip flexors and ankle dorsiflexors appears in advance of the appropriate movement may indicate the existence of a feed-forward or preparatory system of control that is based on input from the visual system.[6]

Table 14–7. **Sagittal Plane Analysis (Fig. 14–35)***

Acceleration (Initial Swing Through Midswing)			
Joint	**Motion**	**Muscle**	**Contraction**
Hip	Flexion: 0–20° of flexion to 30° of flexion	Iliopsoas Gracilis Sartorius	Concentric
Knee	Flexion: 30° of flexion to 60° of flexion Extension: 60° of flexion to 30° flexlon	Biceps femoris Sartorius Gracilis	Concentric
Ankle	Dorsiflexion: 20° plantarflexion to neutral	Tibialis anterior Extensor digitorum longus Extensor hallicus longus	Concentric

Frontal Plane Analysis			
Joint	**Motion**	**Muscle**	**Contraction**
Pelvis	Lateral pelvic tilt to the right (right side drops). Right side moving forward	Left gluteus medius	
Hip	Rotation from lateral to medial rotation		
Knee	From lateral to medial rotation		
Foot-ankle	Unweighted subtalar joint returns to slight supination		
Thorax	Right side moving posteriorly		
Shoulder	Right side moving posteriorly		

*Concentric contractions of the hip flexors occur to ensure adequate hip flexion to bring the extremity forward and accomplish foot clearance. The femur and tibia attain the greatest amount of lateral rotation at the beginning of initial swing and then begin to rotate medially.

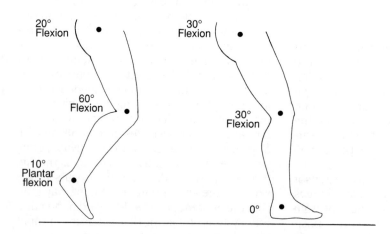

20° Flexion

30° Flexion

60° Flexion

30° Flexion

10° Plantar flexion

0°

FIGURE 14–35. The period of gait from acceleration (initial swing) to midswing (midswing).

Table 14–8. **Sagittal Plant Analysis (Fig. 14–36)***

Midswing Through Deceleration (Terminal Swing)			
Joint	**Motion**	**Muscle**	**Contraction**
Hip	Hip remains at 30° flexion	Gluteus maximus	Eccentric
Knee	Extension: 30° flexion to 0°	Quadriceps	Concentric
		Hamstrings	Eccentric
Ankle	Ankle remains in neutral	Tibialis anterior	Isometric
		Extensor digitorum longus	Isometric
		Extensor hallicus longus	isometric

Frontal Plane Analysis		
Joint	**Motion**	**Muscle Activity**
Pelvis	Right side moving anteriorly	
Hip	Lateral tilting to the left medial rotation	Right gluteus medius
Knee	Medial rotation	
Ankle		
Thorax	Right side moving posteriorly	
Shoulder	Right shoulder moving posteriorly	

*The hip remains in a position of 30° flexion while the pelvis rotates forward to increase step length. The momentum of the swinging extremity is restrained by eccentric contraction of the hamstrings while full knee extension is ensured by a brief concentric contraction of the quadriceps. The ankle is maintained in a neutral position to ensure ground clearance and readiness for initial contact. The medial rotation of the thigh and tibia continue through terminal swing into the first part of the stance phase.

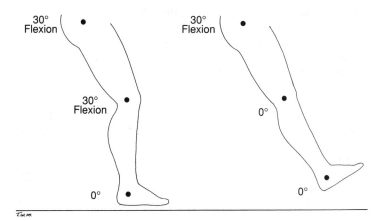

FIGURE 14–36. The period of gait from midswing (midswing) through terminal deceleration (terminal swing).

Kinematics and Kinetics of the Trunk and Upper Extremities

Trunk

The trunk remains essentially in the erect position during normal free speed walking on level ground. However, Krebs and coworkers[51] found that a flexion peak of low amplitude occurred near each heel strike and an extension peak of low amplitude occurred during single limb support. The amount of transverse rotation of the trunk during gait is slight and occurs primarily in a direction opposite to the direction of pelvic rotation (Fig. 14–37). As the pelvis rotates forward with the swinging lower extremity, the thorax on the opposite side rotates forward as well. Actually, the thorax undergoes a biphasic rotation pattern with a reversal directly following lift off of the stance leg. The thorax is rotated backward during double support and then slowly rotates forward during single support. This trunk motion helps to prevent excess body motion and to counterbalance rotation of the

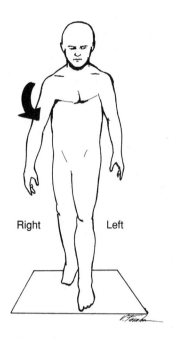

FIGURE 14–37. Trunk rotation in normal gait is slight and occurs in the opposite direction of pelvic rotation. The right side of the pelvis is rotating in a posterior direction; the right side of the trunk is rotating in an anterior direction.

has been shown that the erector spinae exhibit two periods of activity.[54] The first burst of activity occurs at heel strike, and the second occurs at toe off. Supposedly the erector spinae are active to prevent the trunk from falling forward owing to the flexion moment at the hip that is present at each of the bursts of activity. Other muscles that have been found to be active are the quadratus lumborum and the rectus abdominis, although there appear to be conflicting opinions among investigators regarding the activity of these muscles.

Upper Extremities

While the lower extremities are moving alternately forward and backward, the arms are swinging rhythmically. However, the arm swinging is opposite to that of the legs and pelvis but similar to that of the trunk (Fig. 14–38). The right arm swings forward with the forward swing of the left lower extremity while the left arm swings backward. This swinging of the arms provides a counterbalancing action to the forward swinging of the leg and helps to de-

pelvis. Krebs and associates found that at a free speed of gait transverse rotation reached a maximal of 9° at 10% of the cycle after each heel strike.[51] In a study of treadmill walking, Stokes[52] found that the movements and interactions of the trunk and pelvis were extremely complex when translatory and rotatory movements of the trunk were considered along with anterior and posterior pelvic tilting, lateral pelvic tilting, and rotation. Medial-lateral translations of the trunk occur as side to side motions (leans) relative to the pelvis. For example, the trunk is leaning or moving to the right from right heel strike to left foot off at which point the trunk begins a lean to the left until right toe off. The average total ROM that occurs during the medial-lateral trunk leans is about 5.4 cm.[52] Hirasaki and coworkers[53] used a treadmill and a video-based motion analysis system to study trunk and head movements at different walking speeds. These authors found that the relationship between walking speed and head and trunk movements was the most linear in the range of walking speeds from 1.2 to 1.8 m/s. At velocities above and below this range, head and trunk movements were less well coordinated.

Although relatively few EMG studies have been done on the trunk muscles during gait, it

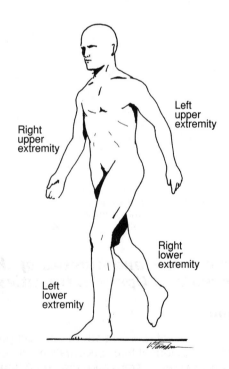

FIGURE 14–38. Arm swinging in gait is opposite to lower extremity motion. The right upper extremity swings forward at the same time that the right lower extremity is moving posteriorly. The right upper extremity and left lower extremity are both moving forward at the same time.

celerate rotation of the body, which is imparted to it by the rotating pelvis. The total ROM at the shoulder is not very large. At normal free velocities the ROM is only approximately 30° (24° extension and 6° of flexion).

The normal shoulder motion is the result of the combined effects of gravity and muscle activity. During the *forward* portion of arm swinging, the following medial rotators are active: subscapularis, teres major, and latissimus dorsi. In *backward* swing the middle and posterior deltoid are active throughout, and the latissimus dorsi and teres major are active only during the first portion of backward swing.[54] The supraspinatus, trapezius,[54] and posterior and middle deltoid[55] are active in both backward and forward swing. It is interesting to note that little or no activity was reported in the shoulder flexors in these studies.[54,55] It would appear that during forward swing the medial rotators are acting eccentrically to control external rotation of the arm at the shoulder as the posterior deltoid acts eccentrically to restrain the forward swing. The latissimus dorsi and teres major as well as the posterior deltoid may then act concentrically to produce the backward swing. The role of the middle deltoid is unclear, although it has been suggested that it functions to keep the arm abducted so that it may clear the side of the body.[50] Activity in all muscles increases as the speed of gait increases.[54]

Stair and Running Gaits

Stair Gait

Ascending and descending stairs are common forms of locomotion that are required for performing normal activities of daily living such as shopping, using public transportation, or simply getting around in a multistory home or building. Although many similarities exist between level-ground locomotion and stair locomotion, the difference between the two modes of locomotion may be significant for a patient population. The fact that a patient has adequate muscle strength and joint ROM for level walking does not ensure that the patient will be able to walk up and down stairs. For example Krebs and coworkers[51] found that trunk ROM during level gait was similar to trunk ROM during descending stairs but differed from trunk ROM during ascending stairs in all planes. The maximum ROM of trunk flexion relative to the room during ascending stairs was at least dou-

ble the amount of trunk flexion found in either descending stairs or in level walking.[51]

Locomotion on stairs is similar to level-ground walking in that stair gait involves both swing and stance phases in which forward progression of the body is brought about by alternating movements of the lower extremities. Also in both stair and level gait the lower extremities must balance and carry along HAT. McFayden and Winter (using step dimensions of 22 cm for the stair riser and 28 cm for the tread) performed a sagittal plane analysis of stair gait.[56] These investigators collected kinetic and kinematic data for one subject during eight trials. The stair gait cycle for stair ascent presented in Figure 14–39 is based on data from McFayden and Winter's study.[56]

The investigators divided the stance phase of the stair gait cycle into the three subphases and the swing phase into two subphases. The subdivisions of the stance phase are weight acceptance (WA), pull up (PU), and forward continuance (FCN). The subdivisions of the swing phase are foot clearance (FCO) and foot placement (FP). As can be seen in Figure 14–39, WA comprises approximately the first 14% of the gait cycle and is somewhat comparable to the heel strike through loading phase of walking gait. However, in contrast to walking gait, the point of initial contact of the foot on the stairs usually is located on the anterior portion of the foot and travels posteriorly to the middle of the foot as the weight of the body is accepted. The PU portion, which extends from approximately 14% to 32% of the gait cycle, is a period of single-limb support. The initial portion of PU is a time of instability, as all of the body weight is shifted onto the stance extremity when it is flexed at the hip, knee, and ankle. During this period the task is to pull the weight of the body up to the next stair level. The knee extensors are responsible for most of the energy generation required to accomplish pull up. The FCN period is from approximately 32% to 64% of the gait cycle and corresponds roughly to the midstance through toe-off subdivisions of walking gait. In the FCN period the ankle plantarflexors exhibit the greatest amount of energy generation.

Some of the data regarding joint ROM and muscle activity for ascending stairs that was collected by McFayden and Winter[56] is presented in Tables 14–9, 14–10, and 14–11. A review of the tables demonstrates differences between level gait and stair gait in regard to joint ROM as well as some differences in the muscle activity required.

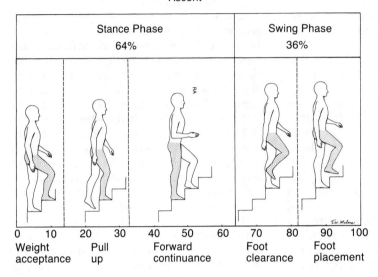

Stair Gait Cycle
Ascent

Stance Phase 64%			Swing Phase 36%	
0 10	20 30	40 50 60	70 80	90 100
Weight acceptance	Pull up	Forward continuance	Foot clearance	Foot placement

FIGURE 14–39. Stair gait.

Table 14–9. *Sagittal Plane Analysis of Stair Ascent (Fig. 14–39)*

Stance Phase—Weight Acceptance (0–14% of Stance Phase) Through Pull-Up (14–32% of Stance Phase)

Joint	Motion	Muscle	Contraction
Hip	Extension: 60–30° of flexion	Gluteus maximus Semitendinosus Gluteus medius	Concentric
Knee	Extension: 80–35° of flexion	Vastus lateralis Rectus femoris	Concentric
Ankle	Dorsiflexion: 20–25° of dorsiflexion Plantarflexion: 25–15° of dorsiflexion	Tibialis anterior Soleus Gastrocnemius	Concentric Concentric

Table 14–10. *Sagittal Plane Analysis of Stair Ascent (Fig. 14–39)*

Stance Phase—Pull Up (End of Pull-Up) Through Forward Continuance (32–64% of the Stance Phase of Gait Cycle)

Joint	Motion	Muscle	Contraction
Hip	Extension: 30–5° flexion	Gluteus maximus Gluteus medius Semitendinosus	Concentric and isometric
	Flexion: 5 to 10–20° of flexion	Gluteus maximus Gluteus medius	Eccentric
Knee	Extension: 35–10° of flexion	Vastus lateralis Rectus femoris	Concentric
	Flexion: 5 to 10–20° of flexion	Rectus femoris Vastus lateralis	Eccentric
Ankle	Plantarflexion: 15° of dorsiflexion to 15–10° of plantarflexion	Soleus Gastrocnemius	Concentric
		Tibialis anterior	Eccentric

Table 14–11. **Sagittal Plane Analysis of Stair Ascent (Fig. 14–39)**

Joint	Motion	Muscle	Contraction
Swing Phase (64–100% of Gait Cycle)—Foot Clearance Through Foot Placement			
Hip	Flexion: 10–20° to 40–60° of flexion Extension: 40–60° of flexion to 50° of flexion	Gluteus medius	Concentric
Knee	Flexion: 10° of flexion to 90–100° of flexion Extension: 90–100° of flexion to 85° of flexion	Semitendinosus Vastus lateralis Rectus femoris	Concentric Concentric
Ankle	Dorsiflexion: 10° of plantarflexion to 20° of dorsiflexion	Tibialis anterior	Concentric and isometric

EXAMPLE 4: In Table 14–10 one can observe that considerably more hip and knee flexion are required in the initial portion of stair gait than are required in normal level-ground walking. Therefore, a patient would require a greater ROM for stair climbing (the same stair dimensions and slope) than they would for normal level-ground walking. Naturally muscle activity and joint ROMs will change if stairs of other dimensions than the ones investigated by McFayden and Winter are used.

Ascending stairs involves a large amount of positive work that is accomplished mainly through concentric action of the rectus femoris, vastus lateralis, soleus, and medial gastrocnemius. Descending stairs is achieved mostly through eccentric activity of the same muscles and involves energy absorption. The support moments during stair ascent, descent, and level walking exhibit similar patterns; however, the magnitude of the moments is greater in stair gait and consequently more muscle strength is required. Kirkwood[57] found that the maximum peak internal abductor moment at the hip occurred during descending stairs and reached 0.96 Nm/kg compared to 0.91 Nm/kg for level walking. The peak hip medial rotation moment during descending stairs also was greater than in level walking. However, these investigators found that internal extensor, lateral rotation, and adductor hip moments were the same as in level walking.

Running Gait

Running is another locomotor activity that is similar to walking, but certain differences need to be examined. As in the case of stair gait, a patient who is able to walk on level ground may not have the ability to run. Running requires greater balance, muscle strength, and ROM than normal walking. Greater balance is required because running is characterized not only by a considerably reduced BOS, but also by an absence of the double-support periods observed in normal walking and the presence of float periods in which both feet are out of contact with the supporting surface (Fig. 14–40). The walking gait cycle presented in Figure 14–41 can be used to compare the gait cycle in walking and running gait. The percentage of the gait cycle spent in float periods will increase as the speed of running increases. Muscles must generate greater energy both to raise HAT higher than in normal walking and to balance and support HAT during the gait cycle. Muscles and joint structures also must be able to absorb more energy to accept and control the weight of HAT.

For example, in normal level walking the magnitudes of the GRFs at the COP in heel strike are approximately 70% to 80% of body weight and rarely exceed 120% of body weight during the gait cycle.[42,58] However, during running, the GRFs at the COP have been shown to reach 200% of body weight and increase to 250% of body weight during the running cycle. Furthermore, the knee is flexed at about 20° degrees when the foot strikes the ground. This degree of flexion helps to attenuate impact forces but also increases the forces acting at the patellofemoral joint. The BOS in running is considerably less than in walking. A typical BOS in walking is about 2 to 4 inches, whereas in running both feet fall in the same line of progression so the entire COG of the body must be placed over a single support foot. To compensate for the reduced BOS the functional limb varus increases. Functional limb varus is the angle between the bisection of the lower leg and the floor.[59] According to Mcpoil and col-

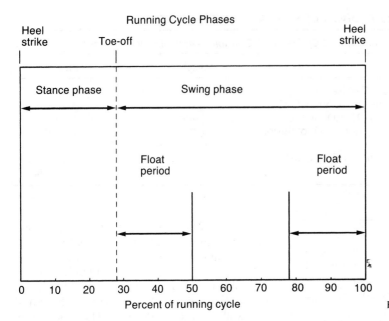

FIGURE 14–40. Running gait cycle.

leagues,[59] the functional limb varus increases about 5° during running compared to walking and causes a greater degree of pronation in running compared to walking.

Joint Motion and Muscle Activity

JOINT MOTION

The ROM varies according to the speed of running and among different researchers. At the be-

ginning of the stance phase of running the hip is in about 45° of flexion at heel strike and extends during the remainder of the stance phase until it reaches about 20° of hyperextension just after toe off.[59] The hip then flexes to reach about 55° to 60° of flexion in late swing. Just prior to the end of the swing phase the hip extends slightly to 45° to 50° in preparation for heel strike.[58] The knee is flexed to about 20° to 40° at heel strike and continues to flex to 60° during the loading

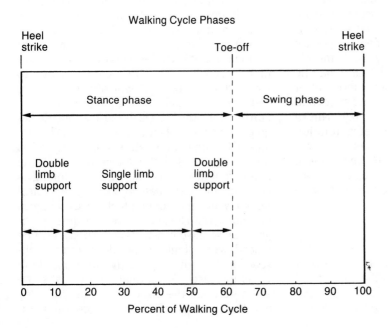

FIGURE 14–41. Walking gait cycle.

response. Thereafter, the knee begins to extend, reaching 40° of flexion just prior to toe off. During the swing phase and initial float period the knee flexes to reach a maximum of approximately 125° to 130° in the middle of the swing phase. In late swing the knee extends to 40° in preparation for heel strike.[58]

The ankle is in about 10° of dorsiflexion at heel strike and rapidly dorsiflexes to reach about 25° to 30° dorsiflexion. The rapid dorsiflexion is followed immediately by plantarflexion, which continues throughout the remainder of the stance phase and into the initial part of the swing phase. Plantarflexion reaches a maximum of 25° in the first few seconds of the swing phase. Throughout the rest of the swing phase the ankle dorsiflexes to reach about 10° in late swing in preparation for heel strike.[58]

The reference extremity begins to medially rotate during the swing phase. At heel strike the extremity continues to medially rotate and the foot pronates. Lateral rotation of the stance extremity and supination of the foot begins as the swing leg passes the stance limb in midstance. The ROM in the lower extremities needed for running compared to the ROM required for norrmal walking is presented in Table 14–12. The largest differences in the total ROM requirements between the two activities appear to be at the knee and hip joints. At the knee joint an additional 90° of flexion is required for running versus walking. At the hip joint running requires about twice the amount of motion that was needed for normal walking.

MUSCLE ACTIVITY

The gluteus maximus and gluteus medius are active both at the beginning of the stance phase and at the end of the swing phase. The tensor fascia lata is also active at the beginning of stance and at the end of swing but also is active between early and midswing. The adductor magnus shows activity for about 25% of the gait cycle from late stance through the early part of the swing phase. Activity in the iliopsoas occurs for about the same percentage of the gait cycle as the adductor longus, but iliopsoas activity also occurs during the swing phase from about 35% to 60% of the gait cycle.

The quadriceps muscle acts eccentrically during the first 10% of the stance phase to control knee flexion when the knee is flexing rapidly. The quadriceps ceases activity after the first part of stance and no activity occurs until the last 20% of the swing phase when concentric activity begins to extend the knee (to 40° of flexion) in preparation for heel strike. The medial hamstrings are active at the beginning of stance and through a large part of swing. For example, the medial hamstrings are active from 18% to 28% of the stance phase, from about 40% to 58% of initial swing and for the last 20% of swing. During part of this time the knee is flexing and the hip is extending and the hamstrings may be acting to extend the hip and to control the knee. During initial swing the hamstrings are probably acting concentrically at the knee to produce knee flexion, which reaches a maximum at midswing. In late swing the hamstrings may be contracting eccentrically to control knee extension and to re-extend the hip.

A comparison of walking and running muscle activity at the ankle shows that in walking, gastrocnemius muscle activity begins just after the loading response at about 15% of the gait cycle

Table 14–12. **Average Peak ROM at the Hip, Knee, and Ankle: Comparison Between Running[58,59] and Walking[5]**

Running			Walking		
Hip Joint			**Hip Joint**		
Flexion	65°		Flexion	30°	
Hyperextension	20°		Hyperextension	20°	
Knee Joint			**Knee Joint**		
Flexion	130°		Flexion	40°	
Extension	5°		Extension	0°	
Ankle Joint			**Ankle Joint**		
Dorsiflexion	10–25°		Dorsiflexion	10°	
Plantarflexion	30°		Plantarflexion	20°	

and is active to about 50% of the gait cycle (just prior to toe off). In running, gastrocnemius muscle activity begins at heel strike and continues through the first 15% of the gait cycle ending at the point where activity begins in walking. The gastrocnemius becomes active again during the last 15% of swing.

The tibialis anterior muscle activity occurs in both stance and swing phases in walking and running. However, the total period of activity of this muscle in walking (54% of the gait cycle) is less than it is in running where it shows activity for about 73% of the gait cycle. The difference in activity of the tibialis anterior between walking and running is due partly to the differences in the length of the swing phases in the two types of gait. The swing period in walking gait is approximately 40% of the total gait cycle, whereas in running gait the swing phase constitutes about 62% of the total gait cycle. Most of the activity in the tibialis anterior during both walking and running gait is concentric or isometric action that is necessary to clear the foot in the swing phase of gait. The longer swing phase in running accounts for at least part of the difference in tibialis anterior activity between walking and running gaits. Tibialis anterior activity in the first half of the stance phase in running gait accounts for the remainder of the difference in activity in this muscle.

Summary

As a result of the efforts of many investigators, our present body of knowledge regarding human locomotion is extensive. However, gait is a complex subject and further research is necessary to standardize methods of measuring and defining kinematic and kinetic variables, to develop inexpensive and reliable methods of analyzing gait in the clinical setting, and to augment the limited amount of knowledge available regarding kinematic and kinetic variables in the gaits of children and the elderly.

Standardization of equipment and methods used to quantify gait variables, as well as standardization of the terms used to describe these variables, would help to eliminate some of the present confusion in the literature and make it possible to compare the findings of various researchers with some degree of accuracy. At the present time inexpensive, quantitative, and reliable clinical methods of evaluating gait are limited to time and distance variables of step length, step duration, stride length, cadence,

and velocity.[59–62] These measures provide a simple means for objective assessment of a patient's status. Increases in step length and decreases in step duration may be used to document a patient's progression toward a more normal gait pattern; however, a normal gait pattern may not be appropriate for many patients. Instead a pattern that is appropriate for a patient's particular disability may be a more appropriate goal of treatment. Advances in gait analysis technology have considerably increased our knowledge of gait. Automated gait analysis programs can provide the clinician with information about all of the kinematic and kinetic gait parameters related to a particular subject or patient. However, the researcher or clinician must have sufficient knowledge of the kinematics and kinetics of normal gait be able to interpret and use the data from automated gait analysis systems for the benefit of the patient.

Effects of Age, Gender, Assistive Devices, Disease States, Muscle Weakness and Paralysis, Asymmetries of the Lower Extremities, Injuries and Malalignments

Age

Adult gait has been the focus of numerous studies, but the gait of young children has not received the same amount of attention. The relatively few studies of children's gait that have been conducted have shown that the age at which independent ambulation begins is extremely variable among individuals and that this variability continues throughout the developmental stages of walking. Cioni and coworkers[63] found that for 25 full-term infants the age at which independent walking (ability to move 10 successive steps without support) was attained, varied between 12.6 and 16.6 months. In the first stage of independent walking none of the 25 toddlers had heel strike, reciprocal arm swinging, or trunk rotation. However, 4 months after attainment of independent walking 11 of 25 children had heel strike and 16 of 25 had reciprocal arm swinging and trunk rotation.

The toddler has a higher COG than the adult and walks with a wider BOS, a decreased single-leg support time, a shorter step length, a slower velocity, and a higher cadence in comparison to normal adult gait. A study of 3- and 5-year-old children showed that some relationships between these variables were similar to the relationships found in adult gaits.[64] For example, as a group, the 3- and 5-year-old children showed significant increases in stride length adjusted for leg length, step length, and cadence from a slow to a free and from a free to a fast speed of gait. However, 5-year-olds differed from 3-year-olds in that they had less variability in step length adjusted for height at slow and free speeds.[64] In a study, which included children from 6 to 13 years of age, Foley and associates[65] reported that the ROM for flexion and extension of the joints of the lower extremities were almost identical to the values obtained for adults. However, linear displacements, velocities, and accelerations were found to be consistently larger for these children than they were for adults.[65] Cadence, stride length, stride time, and other distance and temporal variables have been found to show variability until the child reaches 7 or 8 years of age. A gait pattern that is similar to normal adult gait is demonstrated by children from 8 to 10 years of age.

Sutherland,[66] who studied 186 children from 1 to 7 years of age, suggested that the following five gait parameters could be used as indicators of gait maturity: duration of single-limb support, walking velocity, cadence, step length, and the ratio of pelvic span to ankle spread (indicative of BOS). Increases in all of these parameters except for cadence are indicative of increasing gait maturity. In Sutherland's study the duration of single-limb stance increased from about 32% in 1-year-olds to 38% in 7-year-olds (normal mean adult value is 39%). Walking velocity also increased steadily, whereas cadence decreased with age.[66] Beck[67] found that time and distance measures and GRF measurements depended on speed of gait and age of the child. Increases in height and age were the major factors in determining changes in time and distance measures with age. Average stride length was 76% of the child's height at a walking speed of 104 m/s regardless of a child's age. According to Beck, after 5years of age an adult pattern in the GRF emerged.[67]

Studies involving young children are difficult to perform and often complicated by the fact that the child's musculoskeletal and nervous systems are in various stages of development. However, Sutherland has attempted to provide evaluators with guidelines for assessing children's gait by developing a group of prediction regions for the kinematic motion curves in normal gait. A test of the prediction regions indicated that they were capable of detecting a high percentage of abnormal motion and therefore could be used as an initial screen to identify deficits in lower extremity function in children.[68]

In contrast to the dearth of gait studies of young children, the effects of aging on gait have been and continue to be the object of many studies.[50,69–71] Some of this interest in elderly gait has been prompted by the large number of hip fractures and falls experienced by the elderly. Fifty percent of the elderly who were able to walk prior to a hip fracture are not able to either walk or live independently following the fracture. Furthermore it is estimated that the elderly experience at least two falls per year.[72] Therefore, many studies are directed toward determining what constitutes normal elderly gait and whether or not falls are caused by deficits in motor functioning or control or other deficits that may accompany normal aging.

Lee and Kerrigan[73] found significant differences in kinetic parameters between a group of elderly fallers and an elderly control group. Torque parameters including hip flexion and adduction, knee extension, ankle dorsiflexion, and inversion were higher in the group of fallers than in the control group, but no significant difference in power generation was found between the two groups. The lack of difference in power generation between the two groups led researchers to the conclusion that the fallers might be using co-contraction in an attempt to increase stability. The authors proposed that intervention and prevention strategies should concentrate on activities that promote motor and balance control such as modified Tai Chi. Kaya and coworkers[74] found that healthy elders, aged 67 to 90, tended to limit momentum generation by decreasing gait velocity. The authors suggest that the elderly might lack sufficient strength or balance control to safely dissipate the momentum that accompanies a faster gait speed. Elders with balance impairments had excessive lateral, linear, and angular momentum and walked at a slower pace than healthy elders.

The use of different age groups and levels of activity (sedentary versus active groups) among investigators has made it difficult to draw definitive conclusions about the effects of normal aging. Some investigators have found that the elderly in comparison to younger groups demonstrate a decrease in natural walking speed, shorter stride and step lengths, longer duration of double-support periods, and smaller swing to support phase ratios.[69,70] Hinmann and associates[69] found that between 19 and 62 years of age there was a 2.5% to 4.5% decline in the normal speed of walking per decade for men and women, respectively. After age 62 there was an accelerated decline in normal walking speed; that is, a 16% and 12% decline in walking speed for men and women, respectively.[69] Winter and associates[50] compared the fit and healthy elderly with young adults and found that the natural cadence in the elderly was no different from that in young adults but that the stride length of the elderly was significantly shorter than in young adults and that the period of double support was longer in the elderly than in young adults. Blanke and Hageman[71] compared 12 young men, aged 20 to 32 years, with 12 elderly men, aged 60 to 74 years, and found no effects of aging in regard to step length, stride length, velocity, and vertical and horizontal excursions of the body's COG. However, the ability to generalize Blanke and Hageman's findings is low because of the small size of their sample.

Kerrrigan and associates[75] found that comfortable walking speed and stride length were significantly slower compared to young adults. These authors also found that older persons compared to younger persons had reduced plantarflexion power generation, reduced plantarflexion ROM, peak hip extension ROM, and increased anterior pelvic tilt. The authors suggested that subtle hip flexion contractures and concentric plantarflexor weakness might be causes of the joint changes in the elderly. Judge and colleagues[76] also found that plantarflexor power and ROM in late stance were lower in the elderly (average age 79 years) than in the young (average age 26 years). The elderly appeared to compensate for low plantarflexor power by increasing hip flexor power. Ankle strength was associated with plantarflexor power generation developed in late stance and ankle power was the strongest predictor of step length as it explained 52% of the variance in step length. Mueller and coworkers found that plantarflexor peak torque and ankle dorsiflexion were interrelated. These authors suggested that walking speed and step length might be improved by increasing ankle flexor peak torque and dorsi-

flexion ROM.[38] Bohannon and colleagues[77] found that hip flexor strength was one of the variables that predicted gait speed. These authors did not test plantarflexor strength. Lord and associates[78] conducted an exercise program for women 60 years of age and older. Following the program the authors found significant increases in cadence and stride length as well as reductions in stance time, swing time, and stance duration. Connolly and Vanderwoort[79] measured the effects of detraining (which involved a decline in quadriceps muscle strength) on walking in a group of elderly with a mean age of 82.8 years. Strength values measured 1 year following the training program had declined 68.3% and the speed of self-selected gait declined by 19.5%.

Walking is considered to be a measure of independence and faster walking speed is associated with increased levels of independence. A speed that is faster than comfortable walking is needed in many instances to cross a street. Walking in conjunction with exercise is also considered important to help prevent bone loss in the proximal femur.[57] Although differences of opinion have been found regarding gait speed in the elderly, the consensus of opinion appears to be that in general the elderly select a free speed that is slower than the free speed gait of young people; however, as was shown previously a slow gait requires a greater consumption of energy.

Several investigators have described changes in stride length and speed of gait in the elderly. These changes may represent an attempt to make gait more stable. Falls in the elderly population are common and many of the elderly lead relatively sedentary lifestyles. The inactive elderly may have some muscle atrophy due to disuse and thus be more unsure of themselves while walking. Also, the possibility exists that some of the changes in gait that have been attributed to the aging process may actually be related more to the health and physical fitness status of the individual than to his or her age.

Gender

The research regarding gender differences in gait is fraught with the same difficulties as found in gait research regarding age. Variations among methodologies, technologies, and subjects used in various studies make it difficult to come to many conclusions regarding the effects of gender. When differences in height, weight, and leg length between the genders are considered, gender differences are not very great. Oberg and associates[48] found significant differences between men and women for knee flexion/extension at slow, normal, and fast speeds at midstance and swing. They found a significant increase in joint angles as gait speed increased. For example, the knee angle at midstance increased from 15° to 24° in men and from 12° to 20° in women. However, Oberg and coworkers only looked at the knee and hip. In another study the authors looked at velocity, step length, and step frequency.[80] Gait speed was found to be slower in women compared to men (118–134 cm/s for men and 110–129 cm/sfor women) and step length was smaller in women as compared to men. Kerrigan and colleagues[81] found that women had significantly greater hip flexion and less knee extension during gait initiation, a greater knee flexion moment in preswing and greater peak mechanical joint power absorption at the knee in preswing. Kinetic data were normalized for both height and weight. These authors also found that women had a greater stride length in proportion to their height and that they walked with a greater cadence than their male counterparts.[81]

Assistive Devices

Walking without the use of assistive devices (crutches, canes, and walkers) is the ideal situation. However, such devices often are necessary either after a lower-extremity fracture when the healing bone is unable to bear full body weight or as a more permanent adjunct for a balance or muscle paralysis problem. Canes have typically been used on the contralateral side to an affected lower extremity to reduce forces acting at the affected hip. However, little or no direct evidence of pressure reduction has been available to confirm the validity of this claim. Krebs and associates[82] have been able to test the effect of cane use on reduction of pressure through the use of an instrumented femoral head prosthesis that quantifies contact pressures at the acetabular cartilage. The prosthetic head contains 13 pressure sensing transducers, which are deflected by 0.00028 mm/Mpa pressure from opposing acetabular cartilage. The magnitude of acetabular contact pressure was reduced by 28% on one transducer and by 40% on another transducer in cane-assisted gait compared to

unaided gait. The reduction in pressure at the hip coincided with reductions in EMG amplitude compared to the same pace in unaided gait trials. The authors concluded that the use of a cane on the contralateral side apparently allows the person to increase the BOS and to decrease muscle and GRF forces acting at the affected hip. The hip muscle abductor force was reduced and gluteus maximus activity was reduced approximately 45%. The maximum GRF during cane-assisted gait occurs between heel strike and midstance.

Crosbie compared two types of walking gaits using a walker.[83] In the first gait the person lifted the walker before bringing the affected leg forward. In this type of gait the hip on the affected side was maintained in flexion throughout the gait cycle thus predisposing the hip to degenerative changes and increasing chances of hip flexion contracture. In the second gait the person lifted the walker and brought the walker and the affected leg forward at the same time. Less of a hip flexion posture was assumed in the second gait and therefore the chance of adverse affects at the hip was reduced.

Disease States

Although quantitative evaluation of gait using time and distance measures is being promoted for use by evaluators of human function, qualitative evaluations are useful and should be used in conjunction with the quantitative assessments. An individual's gait pattern may reflect not only physical or psychologic status but also any defects or injuries in the joints or muscles of the lower extremities. Certain disease conditions such as **Parkinson's disease** produce characteristic gaits that are easily recognized by a trained observer. The parkinsonian gait is characterized by an increased cadence, shortened stride, lack of heel strike and toe off, and diminished arm swinging. The muscle rigidity that characterizes this disease interferes with normal reciprocal patterns of movement.

Another gait pattern that results from disturbed neurologic functioning is the **ataxic gait.** In this gait abnormal function of the cerebellum results in a disturbance of the normal mechanisms controlling balance, and therefore, the individual walks with an unusually large BOS. The wider than normal BOS creates a larger than normal side-to-side deviation of the COG and subsequent changes in other gait parameters.

Muscle Weakness or Paralysis

Sometimes an isolated weakness or paralysis of a single muscle will produce a characteristic gait. For example, a unilateral paralysis of the gluteus medius results in a typical gait pattern called a **gluteus medius gait.** The characteristics of this gait pattern can be deduced by reviewing the function of the gluteus medius during normal gait. Normally the gluteus medius stabilizes the hip and pelvis by controlling the drop of the pelvis during single-limb support, especially during the first part of the stance phase. If gluteus medius activity on the side of the stance leg is absent, the pelvis accompanied by the trunk will fall excessively on the swing side resulting in a loss of balance. To prevent the trunk and pelvis from falling to the unsupported side and to maintain HAT over the stance leg, the individual compensates by laterally bending the trunk over the stance leg. The trunk motion enables the person to maintain balance by keeping the COG over the BOS and allows the swing leg to be lifted high enough to clear the ground. The trunk motion reduces the MA of gravity, thus reducing the need for hip abductor contraction and the concomitant compression caused by the hip abductors. The lateral trunk lean characterizes the gluteus medius gait. The use of an assistive device such as a cane on the side opposite to the paralyzed muscle reduces the need for the lateral trunk lean. The use of a cane decreases the energy required in a gluteus medius gait, but increases the energy requirements of ambulation above that of normal gait.

The gluteus maximus in normal gait provides for stability in the sagittal plane and for restraint of forward progression. This muscle helps to counteract the flexion moment at the hip in the early part of stance and restrains the forward movement of the femur in late swing in normal gait. When the gluteus maximus is paralyzed, the trunk must be thrown posteriorly at heel strike, to prevent the trunk from falling forward when there is a flexion moment at the hip. The backward lean is typical of a **gluteus maximus gait** (Fig. 14–42).

The quadriceps is needed during gait at initial contact and loading response when there is a flexion moment acting at the knee. Quadri-

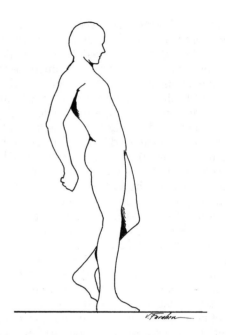

FIGURE 14–42. A backward lean of the trunk is used to compensate for paralysis of the gluteus maximus.

ceps paralysis is easily compensated for if a person has normal hip extensors and plantarflexors. The gluteus maximus and soleus muscles pull the femur and tibia, respectively, posteriorly, which results in knee extension. Additional compensation usually is accomplished by forward trunk bending and a rapid plantarflexion after initial contact. The forward shifting of the weight creates an extension moment at the knee (at initial contact and during the loading response period). It also places the knee in hyperextension and eliminates the need for quadriceps activity. If both the quadriceps and the gluteus maximus are paralyzed, a person may compensate for the loss by pushing the femur posteriorly with his or her hand at initial contact. The arm supports the trunk; it prevents hip flexion and also thrusts the knee into extension.

A paralysis of the plantarflexors (gastrocnemius, soleus, flexor digitorum longus, tibialis posterior, plantaris, and flexor hallucis longus) results in a **calcaneal gait** pattern.[40] This pattern is characterized by greater than normal amounts of ankle dorsiflexion and knee flexion during stance and a less than normal step length on the affected side. The abnormal amount of knee flexion and the fact that the soleus is not pulling the knee into extension require an abnormal amount of quadriceps activity to stabilize the knee during the stance phase. The period of single-limb support is shortened because of the difficulty of stabilizing the tibia and the knee. Step length is shorter than normal because the normal push-off segment of gait is eliminated. The normal heel off and progression to toe off are changed into a rather abrupt lift-off of the entire foot. The asymmetry of this type of gait pattern is obvious through observation and a comparison of right and left step lengths.

Asymmetries of the Lower Extremities

Asymmetries of the lower extremities may be caused by muscle paralysis, contractures of soft tissues around the joints, bony ankylosis, developmental abnormalities, and many other conditions. Any one or a combination of these conditions may cause either a relative or actual shortening of one extremity in comparison with the other. For example, a knee flexion contracture will cause a shortening of the affected extremity. When the affected extremity is weight-bearing, the normal extremity will be proportionately too long to swing through in a normal fashion. A method of equalizing leg lengths is necessary for the swing leg to swing through without hitting the floor. Apparent shortening of the too long normal extremity may be accomplished by a variety of methods. One method of shortening the normal extremity is by increasing the amount of flexion at the hip, knee, and ankle beyond what would normally be required. Other methods that produce relative shortening of the swinging leg are hip hiking (Fig. 14–43) or circumducting the leg (Fig. 14–44). Each of these compensations makes it possible to walk, but they increase the energy requirements above normal levels.

In contrast to shortening of the normal extremity to equalize leg lengths, the person may compensate by using other parts of the body to lengthen the affected extremity. Plantarflexing the foot during stance serves to lengthen the stance extremity as does increasing the amount of pelvic rotation or pelvic tilt during swing. The consequences of either muscle loss

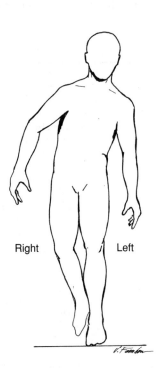

Right   Left

FIGURE 14–43. Hiking of the right hip during the swing phase of the right lower extremity effectively shortens the right lower extremity.

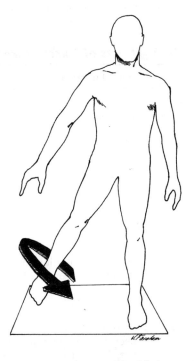

FIGURE 14–44. Circumduction of the right lower extremity during the right swing phase serves as a method of shortening the swing extremity, especially if knee flexion is impossible.

or a loss of ROM may be determined by using the model presented in Chapter 13 on posture.

EXAMPLE 5: Paralysis of dorsiflexors. The normal function of the dorsiflexors in gait is (1) to maintain the ankle in neutral so that the heel strikes the floor at initial contact; (2) to control the plantarflexion moment at heel strike; (3) to dorsiflex the foot in initial swing; and (4) to maintain the ankle in dorsiflexion during midswing and terminal swing. If these functions are absent one would expect that the following would occur: (1) the entire foot or the toes would strike the floor at initial contact; (2) entry into the loading response phase would be abrupt; (3) the amount of flexion at the hip and knee would have to increase to clear the foot in initial swing; and (4) a method of either shortening the swing leg or lengthening the stance would have to be found to clear the plantarflexed joint (Table 14–13).

The human body is remarkable in its ability to compensate for losses or disturbances in function. Most of the compensations that are made are performed unconsciously, and if the disturbance is slight, such as occurs in excessive pronation, the individual may not be aware that the gait pattern is in any way unusual. However, every compensation usually results in an increase in energy expenditure over the optimal and may result in excessive stress on other structures of the body.

Kaufman and coworkers[84] undertook a study to determine the magnitude of limb length inequality that would result in gait abnormalities. Many minor limb inequalities are found in the general population but many of these do not require any particular treatment or intervention because they do not have any significant effects on normal gait. The authors concluded that a limb length discrepancy of 2.0 cm (3.7%) resulted in an asymmetrical gait and had the potential for causing changes in articular cartilage. Song and colleagues[85] evaluated neurologically normal children who had limb discrepancies of 0.8% to 15.8% of the length of the long extremity (0.6–11.1 cm). The compensatory strategies observed were equinus position of the ankle and foot of the short limb (toe walking), vaulting over the long limb, increased flexion of the long limb, and circumduction of the long limb. Children who used toe walking

Table 14–13. **Effects of Muscle Paralysis**

Muscle	Normal Function	Effects on Gait	Possible Compensations
Dorsiflexors	1. Maintain ankle in dorsiflexion in mid-swing, terminal swing, and at heel strike.	1. Functional lengthening of affected extremity. Toe drag during swing and lack of normal heel strike.	1. During the swing phase a functional shortening of the affected extremity can be produced by increased knee and hip flexion to prevent toe drag. 2. During midstance a functional lengthening of the unaffected extremity can be produced by plantarflexion of the unaffected extremity.
	2. Controls plantarflexion from heel strike to foot flat.	2. Lack of control of plantarflexion from heel strike to foot flat.	2. From heel strike to foot flat a toes first position of foot at heel strike eliminates the need for dorsiflexor control.
Quadriceps	1. Helps to position leg at heel strike by maintaining knee in extension.	1. Instability at heel strike.	1. Foot flat at initial contact.
	2. Shock absorption and stability during loading response.	2. Decrease in shock absorption and stability during loading response.	2. From heel strike to foot flat an increase in trunk flexion can help to keep an extension moment at the knee.

had a greater vertical translation of the body's COG during gait compared to normal controls.

Injuries and Malalignments

In running, stresses are greater than in walking, so there is an accompanying increase in the likelihood of injury. In a survey of the records of 1650 running patients between the years 1978 and 1980, 1819 injuries were identified.[86] The knee was the most commonly injured site, and patellofemoral pain was the most common complaint. Increases in the Q angle, tibial torsion, and pronation of the foot are contributing causes to patellofemoral syndromes. Other injuries experienced by runners are iliotibial band syndrome and popliteal tendonitis.[87] Plantar fasciitis caused by repetitive stretching of the planter fascia between its origin at the plantar rim of the calcaneus and its insertion into the metatarsal heads is a common overuse syndrome seen in young athletes.

Structural variations at the hip, knee, and ankle and foot may alter normal gait patterns. At the hip, coxa valga, coxa vara, retroversion, or anteversion all affect gait. At the knee, genu varum, genu valgum or genu recurvatum, and patella alta cause abnormal stresses in walking that may be magnified in running.

Coxa valga may cause alternations at the knee such as genu varum and problems at the ankle such as excessive inversion. In coxa valga abnormal weight-bearing stresses are incurred on the superior medial aspect of the femoral head. Abnormal compressive stress occurs on the medial aspect of the knee joint in genu varum. Abnormal weight-bearing stress occurs on the lateral borders of the feet in excessive inversion. These changes throughout the kinematic chain cause abnormalities in gait.

Coxa vara may lead to changes at the knee and ankle; that is, genu valgum and excessive eversion at the feet. Abnormal weight-bearing in this instance would occur on the superior lateral aspect of the femoral head and excessive shearing forces would be present on the head and neck. In addition, abnormal tensile stresses would occur on the medial knee structures in genu valgum and excessive weight-bearing stresses on the medial aspects of the feet in eversion of the feet. In genu valgum the width of the BOS is considerably wider than in normal gait.

An anteverted hip may cause excessive "toeing in" during gait because of the abnormal amount of medial femoral rotation present in this condition. Conversely, a retroverted hip may cause excessive "out-toeing" during walking because of the abnormal amount of lateral femoral rotation associated with this abnormality.

At the ankle joint, a surgical arthrodesis that fuses the trochlea of the talus in the mortise results in the imposition of greater-than-normal forces on the foot. When the plantarflexors, which are the major source of mechanical energy generation in gait, are affected, muscles at other joints must provide more energy than in normal gait.[4] For example, Winter[88] found that individuals with below-knee amputations used the gluteus maximus, semitendinosus, and knee extensors as energy generators to compensate for loss of the plantarflexors. Olney and associates[31] found that in children who had unilateral plantarflexor paralysis, the involved plantarflexors produced only 33% of the energy generation compared to the 66% produced in normal gait. Greater than normal hip flexor activity in these children compensated for the loss of the plantarflexors.

At the foot, pes cavus and pes planus cause alterations in weight and may cause abnormal stresses at the hip or knee. In pes cavus, the weight is borne primarily on the hindfoot and metatarsal regions and the midfoot provides only minimal support.[41] In running, the metatarsals bear a disproportionate share of the weight. In pes planus, the weight is borne primarily by the midfoot rather than being distributed among the hindfoot, lateral midfoot, metatarsals, and toes, as it is in the normal walking foot. The propulsive phase of gait is severely compromised.

Disturbances in the normal gait pattern cause increases in the energy cost of walking because the normal patterns of transformation from potential to kinetic energy are disturbed. Increases in muscle activity used to compensate for these disturbances lead to increases in the amount of oxygen that is consumed. In a comparison of patients who had an ankle fusion with patients who had a hip fusion, oxygen consumption for patients with the hip fusion was 32% greater than normal and greater than in patients with the ankle fusion.[89] Pain also appears to be a factor that leads to an increase in oxygen consumption. As pain increases, oxygen consumption has been found to increase.[90] In patients with bilateral lower-extremity paralysis, walking usually involves the use of long leg braces and crutches. In this form of gait the trunk and upper extremity muscles must perform all of the work of walking and the energy cost of walking is much greater than normal. A form of electrical stimulation called functional neuromuscular stimulation (FNS) is currently being used to activate the paralyzed lower extremity muscles so that these muscles can generate energy for walking. However, the energy cost of FNS walking is still well above that of normal gait.[91]

Summary

The objectives of gait analysis are to identify deviations from normal and their causes. Once the cause has been determined, it is possible to take corrective action aimed at eliminating or diminishing abnormal stresses and decreasing energy expenditure. Sometimes the corrective action may be as simple as using a lift in the shoe to equalize leg lengths or developing an exercise program to increase flexibility at the hip, knee, or ankle. In other instances, corrective action may require the use of assistive devices such as braces, canes, or crutches. However, an understanding of the complexities of abnormal gait and the ability to detect abnormal gait patterns and to determine the causes of these deviations must be based on an understanding of normal structure and function. The study of human gait, like the study of human posture, illustrates the interdependence of structure and function and the large variety of postures and gaits available to the human species.

REFERENCES

1. Foreman, J: How to tell if you are muggable. *Boston Globe*, January 20, 1981.
2. Steindler, A: Kinesiology. Charles C Thomas, Springfield, Ill., 1955.
3. Winter, DA: Energy assessments in pathological gait. Physiother (Canada) 30; 1978.
4. Inman, VT, et al: Human Walking. William & Wilkins, Baltimore, 1981.
5. Professional Staff Association, Rancho Los Amigos Medical Center: Observational Gait Analysis Handbook. Downey, Calif., 1989.
6. Winter, DA: Biomechanics of normal and pathological gait: Implications for understanding human locomotor control. J Motor Behav 21:337–355, 1989.
7. Elbe, RJ, et al: Gait initiation by patients with lower-half parkinsonism. Brain 119:1705, 1996.
8. Hesse, S, et al: Asymmetry of gait initiation in hemiparetic stroke subjects. Arch Phys Med Rehabil 78:719, 1997.
9. Lamoreaux, LW: Kinematic measurements in the study of human walking. Bull Prosth Res, Spring 1971.
10. Murray, MP: Gait as a total pattern of movement. Am J Phys Med 46:1, 1967.
11. Murray, MP, et al: Walking patterns of normal men. J Bone Joint Surg. 46A:335, 1964.
12. Crowinshield, RD, et al: Effects of walking velocity and age on hip kinematics and kinetics. Bull Hosp Joint Dis 38:1977.
13. Larsson, LE, et al: The phases of stride and their interaction in human gait. Scand J Rehabil Med 12:107, 1980.
14. Wernick, J, and Volpe, RG: Lower extremity function. In Valmassy, RI (ed): Clinical Biomechanics of the Lower Extremities. CV Mosby, St. Louis, 1996.
15. Hausdorf, JM, et al: Fractal dynamics of human gait: Stability of long-range correlations in stride interval fluctuations. J Appl Physiol 80:1448, 1996.
16. Sekiya, N, et al: Optimal walking in terms of variability in step length. Phys Ther 26:266, 1997.
17. Soderberg, GL, and Gavel, RH: A light emitting diode system for the analysis of gait. Phys Ther 58:4, 1978.
18. Grieve, DW: Gait patterns and speed of walking. Biomedicine (Eng) 3:119, 1968.
19. Milner, M, et al: Angle diagrams in the assessment of locomotor function. South Am Med J 47:951, 1973.
20. Hersihler, C, and Milner, M: Angle-angle diagrams in the assessment of locomotion. Am J Phys Med 59:3, 1980.
21. Saunders, JB, et al: The major determinants in normal and pathological gait. J Bone Joint Surg (Am) 35A:543, 1953.
22. Gard, SA, and Childress, DS: The influence of stance-phase knee flexion on the vertical displacement of the trunk during normal walking. Arch Phys Med Rehabil 80:26, 1999.
23. Childress, DS, and Gard, SA: Investigation of vertical motion of the human body during normal walking [abstract]. Gait Posture 5:161, 1997.
24. Gard, SA, and Childress, DS: The effect of pelvic list on the displacement of the trunk during normal walking. Gait Posture 5:233, 1997.
25. Pandy, MG, and Berme, N: Quantitative assessment of gait determinants during single stance via a three-dimensional model. Part 1: Normal gait. J Biomech 22:717, 1989.
26. Duff-Raffaele, M, et al: The proportional work of lifting the center of mass during walking. Am J Phys Med Rehabil 75:375, 1996.
27. Davies, MJ, and Dalsky, GP: Economy of mobility in older adults. J Orthop Sports Phys Ther 26: 69, 1997.
28. Winter, DA: Analysis of instantaneous energy of normal gait. J Biomech 9:253, 1976.
29. Wells, RP: The kinematics and energy variations of swing-through crutch gait. J Biomech 12:579, 1979.
30. Kepple, TM, et al: Relative contributions of lower extremity joint moments to forward progression and support during gait. Gait Posture 6:1–8, 1997.
31. Olney, SJ, et al: Work and power in hemiplegic cerebral palsy gait. Phys Ther 70:431–438, 1990.
32. Eng, JJ, and Winter, DA: Kinetic analysis of the lower limbs during walking: What information can be gained from a three dimensional model? J Biomech 28:753, 1995.
33. Smidt, G: Methods of studying gait. Phys Ther 54:1, 1974.
34. Cerny, K: Pathomechanics of stance: Clinical concepts for analysis. Phys Ther 64:1851–1858, 1984.

35. Kotoh, Y, et al: Biomechanical analysis of foot function during gait and clinical applications. Clin Orthop Rel Res 177:23–33, 1983.
36. Winter, DA, Eng, JJ, and Isshac, MG. A review of kinetic parameters in human walking. In Craik, RL, and Otis, CA (eds): Gait Analysis: Theory and Application. Mosby–Year Book, St. Louis, 1994.
37. Winter, DA, and Yack, HJ: EMG profiles during normal walking: Stride to stride and inter-subject variability. Electroenceph Clin Neurophys (Ireland) 67:402–411, 1987.
38. Mueller, MJ, et al: Relationship of plantar flexor peak torque and dorsiflexion range of motion to kinetic variables during walking. Phys Ther 75:684, 1995.
39. Perry, J, Hislop, H: Principles of Lower Extremity Bracing. American Physical Therapy Association, Washington, DC, 1967.
40. Perry, J: Kinesiology of lower extremity bracing. Clin Orthop 102:18, 1974.
41. Scranton, PE, and McMaster, JH: Momentary distribution of forces under the foot. J Biomech 9:45, 1976.
42. Nuber, GW: Biomechanics of the foot and ankle during gait. Clin Sports Med 7:1–13, 1988.
43. Ramig, D, et al: The foot and sports medicine: Biomechanical foot faults as related to chondromalacia patellae. J Orthop Sports Phys Ther 2:2, 1980.
44. Root, ML, et al: Normal and Abnormal Function of the Foot. Clinical Biomechanics Corp., Los Angeles, 1977.
45. Sutherland, DH, et al: The role of the plantarflexors in normal walking. J Bone Joint Surg 62:3–336, 1980.
46. Donatelli, R: Biomechanics of the Foot and Ankle. FA Davis, Philadelphia, 1990.
47. Dujardin, FH, et al: Interindividual variations of the hip joint motion in normal gait. Gait Posture 5:246, 1997.
48. Oberg, TA, et al: Joint angle parameters in gait: Reference data for normal subjects 10–79 years of age. J Rehabil Res Dev 31:199, 1994.
49. Borghese, NA, et al: Kinematic determinants of human locomotion. J Physiol 494:863, 1996.
50. Winter, DA, et al: Biomechanical walking pattern changes in the fit and healthy elderly. Phys Ther 70:340–347, 1990.
51. Krebs, DE, et al: Trunk kinematics during locomotor activities. Phys Ther 72:505, 1992.
52. Stokes, VP, et al: Rotational and translational movement features of the pelvis and thorax during adult human locomotion. J Biomech 22:43–50, 1989.
53. Hirasaki, E, et al: Effects of walking velocity on vertical head and body movements during locomotion. Exp Brain Res 127:117, 1999.
54. Basmajian, JV: Muscles Alive, ed 4. Williams & Wilkins, Baltimore, 1979.
55. Hogue, RE: Upper extremity muscle activity at different cadences and inclines during normal gait. Phys Ther 49:9, 1969.
56. McFayden, BJ, and Winter, DA: An integrated biomechanical analysis of normal stair ascent and descent. J Biomech 21:733–744, 1988.
57. Kirkwood, RN, et al: Hip moments during level walking, stair climbing and exercise in individuals aged 55 years and older. Phys Ther 79:360, 1999.
58. Mann, RA: Biomechanics of running. In D'Ambrosia, RD, and Drez, D (eds): Prevention and Treatment of Running Injuries, ed 2. Slack, Thorofare, NJ, 1989.
59. Mcpoil, TG, and Cornwall, MW: Applied sports biomechanics in running. In Zachezeweski, JE, et al (eds): Athletic Injuries and Rehabilitation. WB Saunders, Philadelphia, 1996.
60. Craik, RL, and Otis, CA: Gait assessment in the clinic. In Rothstein, JM (ed): Measurement in Physical Therapy. Churchill-Livingstone, London, 1985.
61. Norkin, C: Gait analysis. In O'Sullivan, S, and Schmitz, TJ (eds): Physical Rehabilitation Assessment and Treatment, ed 4. FA Davis, Philadelphia, 2000.
62. Robinson, JL, and Smidt, GL: Quantitative gait evaluation in the clinic. Phys Ther 61:3, 1981.
63. Cioni, G, et al: Differences and variations in the patterns of early independent walking. Early Hum Dev 35:193, 1993.
64. Rose-Jacobs, R: Development of gait at slow, free, and fast speeds in 3 and 5 year old children. Phys Ther 63:1251–1259, 1983.
65. Foley, CD, et al: Kinematics of normal child locomotion: A statistical study based upon TV data. J Biomech 12:1, 1979.
66. Sutherland, DH, et al: The development of mature gait. J Bone Joint Surg 62A:336, 1980.
67. Beck, RJ, et al: Changes in the gait patterns of growing children. J Bone Joint Surg 63A:1452, 1981.
68. Sutherland, DH, et al: Clinical use of prediction regions for motion analysis. Develop Med Child Neurol 38:773, 1996.
69. Hinmann, JE, et al: Age-related changes in speed of walking. Med Sci Sports Exerc 20:161–166, 1988.
70. Finley, FR, et al: Locomotor patterns in elderly women. Arch Phys Med Rehabil 50:140–146, 1969.
71. Blanke, DJ, and Hageman, PA: Comparison of gait of young men and elderly men. Phys Ther 69:144–148, 1989.
72. Rothstein, JM, et al: The Rehabilitation Specialists Handbook, ed 2. FA Davis, Philadelphia, 1998.
73. Lee, LW, and Kerrigan, C: Identification of kinetic differences between fallers and non-fallers in the elderly. Am J Phys Med Rehabil 78:243, 1999.
74. Kaya, BK, et al: Dynamic stability in elders: Momentum control in locomotor ADL. J Gerontol 53A:M126, 1998.
75. Kerrigan, DC, et al: Biomechanical gait alterations independent of speed in the healthy elderly: Evidence of specific limiting impairments. Arch Phys Med Rehabil 79:317, 1998.
76. Judge, JO, et al: Step length reductions in advanced age: The role of ankle and hip kinetics. J Gerontol 51A:M303, 1996.
77. Bohannon, RW, et al: Walking speed: Reference values and correlates for older adults. J Orthop Sports Phys Ther 24:86, 1996.
78. Lord, SR, et al: The effect of exercise on gait patterns in older women: A randomized controlled trial. J Gerontol 51A:M64, 1996.
79. Connelly, DM, and Vandervoort, AA: Effects of detraining on knee extensor strength and functional mobility in a group of elderly women. J Orthop Sports Phys Ther 26:340, 1997.
80. Oberg, T, et al: Basic gait parameters: Reference data for normal subjects 10–79 years of age. J Rehabil Res Dev 30:210, 1993.
81. Kerrigan, DC, et al: Gender differences in joint biomechanics during walking. Am J Phys Med Rehabil 77:2, 1998.
82. Krebs, DE, et al: Hip biomechanics during gait. J Orthop Sports Phys Ther 28: 51, 1998.
83. Crosbie, J: Comparative kinematics of two walking frame gaits. J Orthop Sports Phys Ther 20: 186, 1994.
84. Kaufman, KR, et al: Gait asymmetry in patients with limb-length inequality. J Pediatr Orthop 16:144, 1996.
85. Song, KM, et al: The effect of limb-length discrepancies on gait. J Bone Joint Surg 79A:1690, 1997.

86. Clement, DB, et al: A survey of overuse running injuries. Phys Sports Med 9:5, 1981.

87. Taunton, JE, et al: Non-surgical management of overuse knee injuries in runners. Can J Sports Sci 12:11–18, 1987.

88. Winter, DA: Biomechanics of below knee amputee gait. J Biomech 21:361–367, 1988.

89. Waters, RWL, et al: Comparable energy expenditure after arthrodesis of the hip and ankle. J Bone Joint Surg 70A:1032–1037, 1988.

90. Gussoni, M, et al: Energy cost of walking with hip impairment. Phys Ther 70:295–301, 1990.

91. Marsolais, EB, and Edwards, BG: Energy costs of walking and standing with functional neuromuscular stimulation and long leg braces. Arch Phys Med Rehabil 69:243–249, 1988.

Study Questions

1. The stance phase constitutes what percentage of the gait cycle in normal walking? How does an increase in walking speed affect the percentage of time spent in stance?

2. What percentage of the gait cycle is spent in double support? How is double support affected by increases and decreases in the walking speed?

3. Maximum knee flexion occurs during which period of the gait cycle?

4. What is the total ROM required for normal gait at the knee, hip, and ankle?

5. How does the total ROM required for normal gait at the knee, hip, and ankle compare with the ROMs required for running and stair gait?

6. Which of the determinants of gait help to keep the vertical rise of the body's COG to a minimum?

7. Which determinant helps to minimize a drop in the body's COG?

8. Which determinant helps to keep the lateral shift of the body's COG to a minimum?

9. What is the role of the tibialis posterior during walking gait?

10. How is the swinging motion of the upper extremities related to movements of the trunk, pelvis, and lower extremities during walking gait?

11. How do the traditional terms used to describe walking gait compare with the RLA terms? Describe the similarities and differences between the terms.

12. Describe the subdivisions of the stance and swing phases of the walking gait cycle using the traditional terminology.

13. Describe the subdivisions of the stance and swing phase of the walking gait cycle using the RLA terminology.

14. What is the function of the plantarflexors during walking gait?

15. Describe the transverse rotations in the frontal plane at the pelvis, femur, and tibia during walking gait.

16. When does the foot begin supinating in normal walking gait?

17. What are the functions of the dorsiflexors in normal walking gait?

18. Compare muscle action in walking gait with muscle action in running gait.

19. Where does the GRFV fall in relation to the ankle, knee, and hip at initial contact? What type of moments are acting at the ankle, knee, and hip at initial contact? Answer the same question using different subdivisions, that is, loading response, midstance, terminal stance, and preswing.

20. Explain valgus thrust. Identify where it occurs in the gait cycle and the muscles that help to control it.

21. Explain what would happen in walking and running if a person's plantarflexors were paralyzed. What compensations might you expect?

INDEX

An "f" following a page number indicates a figure, and a "t" following a page number indicates a table.